The Behavioral and Cognitive Neurology of Stroke

The care of stroke patients has changed dramatically in recent years. As well as improvements in the emergency care of the condition, there have been marked advances in our understanding, management and rehabilitation of residual deficits. This book is about the care of stroke patients, focusing on behavioral and cognitive problems. It provides a comprehensive review of the field covering the diagnostic value of these conditions, in the acute and later phases, their requirements in terms of treatment and management, and the likelihood and significance of long-term disability. This book will appeal to all clinicians involved in the care of stroke patients, as well as to neuropsychologists, other rehabilitation therapists and research scientists investigating the underlying neuroscience.

Olivier Godefroy is Professor of Neurology and Chief of the Neurology Department, University Hospital of Amiens, France.

Julien Bogousslavsky is Head of Neurology, Swiss Medical Network, Valmont-Genolier, Montreux, Switzerland.

The Behavioral and Cognitive Neurology of Stroke

Edited by

Olivier Godefroy
Professor of Neurology and Chief of Neurology Department
University Hospital of Amiens, France

Julien Bogousslavsky
Head of Neurology
Swiss Medical Network
Valmont-Genolier, Switzerland

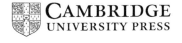

CAMBRIDGE
UNIVERSITY PRESS

CAMBRIDGE UNIVERSITY PRESS
Cambridge, New York, Melbourne, Madrid, Cape Town, Singapore, São Paulo, Delhi

Cambridge University Press
The Edinburgh Building, Cambridge CB2 8RU, UK

Published in the United States of America by Cambridge University Press, New York

www.cambridge.org
Information on this title: www.cambridge.org/9780521106955

First published 2007
This digitally printed version (with corrections) 2009

A catalogue record for this publication is available from the British Library

ISBN 978-0-521-84261-7 hardback
ISBN 978-0-521-10695-5 paperback

Additional resources for this publication at www.cambridge.org/9780521106955

A colour version of Figs. 7.1, 8.3, 9.3, 9.4, 9.6, 15.1B and 16.1 are available for download

Contents

v

Behavioral and mood disorders

Dementia and anatomical left/right syndromes

Contributors

Michael P. Alexander
Behavioral Neurology Unit
Department of Neurology
Beth Israel Deaconess Medical Center
330 Brookline Avenue, Boston, MA 02215
USA

Jean-Marie Annoni
Neuropsychology Unit
Department of Neurology
Lausanne University Hospital
Rue de Bugnon 46
1011 Lausanne
Switzerland

Pascal Auzou
Service d'Explorations
Fonctionnelles Neurologique
47, rue du Dr Calot
62600 Berck sur Mer
France

Selma Aybek
Department of Neurology
University Hospital
Lausanne
Rue du Bugnon 46
CH-1011 Lausanne
Switzerland

Philippe Azouvi
Department of Physical Medicine
and Rehabilitation
Univ de Versailles-Saint-Quentin
INSERM
UPMC 731
Raymond Poincaré Hospital
92380 Garches
France

Francoise Bernasconi
Neuropsychology Unit
Department of Neurology
Geneva University Hospitals
24 rue Micheli-du-Crest
1211 Geneva 14
Switzerland

Julien Bogousslavsky
Department of Neurology
Swiss Medical Network
Valmont-Genolier
1823 Glion-Sue-Montreux
Switzerland

Lara Caeiro
Servico de Neurologia (piso 6)
Hospital de Santa Maria
Av. Prof. Egas Moniz
1649-035 Lisboa
Portugal

Antonio Carota
Service de Neurologie
CHUV
CH-1011 Lausanne
Switzerland

Mathieu Ceccaldi
Department of Neurology and
Neuropsychology
INSERM U751
University Hospital
La Timone
Marseille
France

Hugues Chabriat
Department of Neurology
University Hospital Lariboisière and IFR 49
Paris
France

Laurent Cohen
Service de Neurologie 1
Hôpital de la Salpêtrière
Paris
France

Alexandre Croquelois
Neurorehabilitation Unit
University Hospital
CH-1011 Lausanne
Switzerland

Luc Defebvre
Department of Neurology &
Movement Disorders
Hopital Salengro
CHRU, 59037 Lille Cedex
University Hospital, Lille
France

Stanislas Dehaene
Cognitive Neuroimaging Unit
INSERM U562
CEA/DSV
Orsay
France

Sebastian Dieguez
Laboratory of Cognitive Neuroscience
Brain Mind Institute
Swiss Federal Institute of Technology (EPFL)
Station 15
1015 Lausanne
Switzerland

Diane Dupuy
Department of Neurology
Laboratoire de Neurosciences
Fontionnelles et Pathologies
(CNRS FRE 2726)
University Hospital F-80054, Amiens
France

Frédérique Etcharry-Bouyx
Department of Neuropsychology
UPRES EA 2646
University Hospital
Angers
France

José Ferro
Servico de Neurologia (piso 6)
Hospital de Santa Maria
Av. Prof. Egas Moniz
1649-035 Lisboa
Portugal

Olivier Godefroy
Department of Neurology & Laboratoire
de Neurosciences
Fonctionnelles et Pathologies
(CNRE FRE 2726)
University Hospital, F-80054, Amiens
France

Georg Goldenberg
Neuropsychological Department
Krankenhaus Munchen
Bogenhausen
Englschalkingerstrasse 77
D 81925 Munchen
Germany

Hilde Henon
E.A. 2691
Department of Neurology
Stroke Unit
University Hospital of Lille
59037 Lille
France

Argye Hillis
Department of Neurology
Johns Hopkins University School
of Medicine
Johns Hopkins Hospital
Phipps 126, 600 N Wolfe Street
Baltimore, MD 21287
USA

Veronique Izard
Cognitive Neuroimaging Unit
INSERM U562
CEA/DSV
Orsay
France

Andrew Kertesz
St Joseph's Health Care
University of Western Ontario
268 Grosvenor Street
London
Ontario, N6A 4V2
Canada

Asaid Khateb
Lab of Experimental Neuropsychology and
Neuropsychology Unit
Department of Neurology
Geneva University Hospitals
24 rue Micheli-du-Crest
CH 1211 Geneva 14
Switzerland

Pierre Krolak-Salmon
Hôpital Neurologique Pierre
Wertheimer
Service de Neurologie D
59 Boulevard Pinel
69677 Bron Cedex
France

Pierre Krystkowiak
Department of Neurology &
Movement Disorders
Hopital Salengro
CHRU, 59037 Lille Cedex
University Hospital, Lille
France

Jany Lambert
INSERM E.0218
Service de Neurologie
CHU de Caen
F - 14000
France

Laurent Lavanchy
Neuropsychology Unit
Department of Neurology
Geneva University Hospitals
24 rue Micheli-du-Crest
1211 Geneva 14
Switzerland

Bernard Lechevalier
Service de Neurologie
CHU de Caen
F - 14000
France

Didier Leys
E.A. 2691
Department of Neurology
Stroke Unit
University Hospital of Lille
59037 Lille
France

Chun Lim
Behavioral Neurology Unit
Department of Neurology
Beth Israel Deaconess Medical Center
330 Brookline Avenue, Boston,
MA 02215
USA

Ursula Lopez
Neuropsychology Unit
Department of Neurology
Geneva University Hospitals
24 rue Micheli-du-Crest
1211 Geneva 14
Switzerland

Steve Majerus
Cognitive Psychopathology Unit
Department of Cognitive Sciences
Boulevard du Rectorat B33
400 Liège
University of Liège
Belgium

Isabel P. Martins
Servico de Neurologia (piso 6)
Hospital de Santa Maria
Av. Prof. Egas Moniz
1649-035 Lisboa
Portugal

Eugene Mayer
Neuropsychology Unit
Neurology Clinic
Geneva University Hospitals
24, Micheli du Crest
1211 Geneva 14
Switzerland

Sylvain Moreau
Service d'ORL
CHU de Caen
F − 14000
France

Stefano Paolucci
I.R.C.C.S.
Fondazione Santa Lucia
Roma
Italy

Bertille Perin
Service de Neurologie
CHU d'Amiens
Hôpital Nord
Place Victor Pauchet
80054 Amiens Cedex 1
France

Anne Peskine
Department of Physical Medicine
and Rehabilitation
Univ de Versailles-Saint-Quentin
Raymond Poincaré Hospital
92380 Garches
France

Hervé Platel
INSERM E.0218
Université de Caen
CHU de Caen
F − 14000
France

Martine Poncelet
Neuropsychology of Language Unit
Department of Cognitive Sciences
Boulevard du Rectorat, B33
4000 Liège
University of Liège
Belgium

Marc D. Reichhart
XIGEN SA, and CHUV
17, rue des terreaux
1003 Lausanne
Switzerland

Bruno Rossion
Unite Cognition & Developpement
Université Catholique de Louvain
10 Place du Cardinal Mercier
1348 Louvain-la-Neuve
Belgium

Fabienne Staub
Service de Neurologie
CHUV
CH-1011 Lausanne
Switzerland

Donald Stuss
The Rotman Research Institute
Baycrest Centre for Geriatric Care
University of Toronto
Toronto, Ontario M6A 2E1
Canada

Pierre Thomas
Department of Psychiatry &
UMR-CNRS 8160
Höpital Fontan CHRU
University Hospital
59037 Lille
France

Fausto Viader
Service de Neurologie
CHU de Caen
F-14000
France

Martial Van der Linden
Cognitive Psychopathology &
Neuropsychology Unit
Psychology Department
University of Geneva
Uni-Mail, 40 Bd Pont d'Arve
CH-1205 Geneva
Switzerland

Alain Vighetto
Service de Neurologie D et
Consultation de Neuro-Opthalmologie,
Hôpital Neurologique Pierre Wertheimer
Lyon Université Claude Bernard
Lyon 1
France

Patrik Vuilleumier
LABNIC
Département de Neuroscience &
Service de Neurologie
Centre Médical Universitaire
Bldg A, Rm 7008
1 rue Michel-Servet
1211 Geneva
Switzerland

Anna Wilson
Cognitive Neuroimaging Unit
INSERM U562
CEA/DSV
Orsay
France

Preface

During the last years, the care of stroke patients has dramatically changed with the advent of new treatments such as thrombolysis, and the development of specialized units such as stroke units. Following the acute phase, the management of residual signs is also evolving with the development of specialized rehabilitation units, the treatment of dementia and new hopes for the future such as cell transplantation, Transcranial Magnetic Stimulation or cortical stimulation. Theses advances stress the need for an accurate determination of stroke signs and complications both at the acute and late phases. This is a vast domain considering the extraordinary complexity of the brain and the multiple mechanisms of stroke. This domain is also rapidly evolving owing to the major advances in neurosciences and neuropsychology.

For the clinician, the development of cognitive and clinical neurosciences has shed light on the interpretation, assessment, diagnosis and prognosis value of stroke signs and their treatments. The objectives of cognitive examination differ according to the phase. At the hyperacute phase, the recognition of stroke signs is essential for diagnosis and prognosis purposes. Unusual and misleading clinical presentations (e.g. delirium-like state due to cortical blindness or to acute dysexecutive syndrome), the high frequency of some deficits in the first hours (e.g. right hemineglect in left hemisphere stroke), the fast course of deficits in the first hours (e.g. global aphasia evolving to Broca aphasia of lower severity; severe right hemisphere syndrome evolving to left hemineglect of mild severity) which parallels the course of ischemia territory, and the characteristics of behavioral changes and reactions to acute distress are now better documented. Following the hyperacute phase, the identification of complications and their significance (e.g. the presence of delirium state and its relation with pre-existing dementia), the recognition of persisting signs and the determination of appropriate care are essential and this covers a very wide range of cognitive and behavioral changes. Such purpose is also present after the acute phase where the functional assessment of stroke forms the basis of the rehabilitation strategy at home or in a specialized center. At the late phase, it is essential to identify residual signs and sequels, (including post-stroke dementia which is underdiagnosed and due to multiple mechanisms) and complications which appear in the long term (e.g. dystonia and other movement disorders).

Following the initial report of aphasia, stroke has long been a unique window on brain functions and functional organization. The examination of functional deficits in stroke patients has provided a major contribution to our knowledge on cognitive functions of the human brain. Research in this still active area now requires precise information on lesion location and brain pathology in order to analyze more deeply the relations between brain structures and functions.

In order to fill the gap between clinical and cognitive neurosciences in the domain of stroke, our objective was to provide basis on the main brain functions (perception, motor, behavior and cognition) and their disorders according to recent developments from basic neurosciences, to provide a comprehensive review of the specificity of disorders observed in stroke patients (including the hyperacute phase), their relations with stroke mechanisms, their assessments (including validated tests) and management.

We hope this book will provide valuable information for all clinicians involved in care of stroke patients from the acute to the late phase, in stroke unit, neurology and rehabilitation departments. We also hope that it will be useful for neuroscientists and neuropsychologists and that it will contribute to further research in the domain of cognitive neurosciences and neuropsychology.

Olivier Godefroy and Julien Bogousslavsky

1

Evaluation of cognitive and behavioral disorders in the stroke unit

Asaid Khateb,[1] Jean-Marie Annoni,[1] Ursula Lopez,[1] Françoise Bernasconi,[1] Laurent Lavanchy,[1] and Julien Bogousslavsky[2]

[1]Geneva University Hospitals, Geneva, Switzerland
[2]Swiss Medical Network, Montreux, Switzerland

Introduction

The general aim of a clinical neuropsychological examination is to assess language, memory, attention, adaptive behavior, motivation, and emotion impairments that result from a brain dysfunction. This behavioral and cognitive evaluation can be performed during the first hours following cerebral damage either in a classical bedside approach or by means of standardized tests and may thus help establish a precise diagnostic. In the hyperacute or acute phase of stroke, neuropsychological intervention may also be necessary to establish communication with the patient (e.g. in the case of aphasia) or to set up adequate strategies to be used by healthcare providers (e.g. in the case of spatial neglect). In this context, the patient is most often tested while lying in bed and in the presence of other patients in the same room. Due to this context, as well as other disturbing factors, the evaluation of cognitive–behavioral deficits in the stroke unit is generally difficult, of relatively short duration, and must thus be repeated in order to correctly track the clinical evolution and to advise when the symptoms become more stable. Moreover, effective rehabilitation of cognitive deficits often relies on modular neuropsychological models (e.g. Pilgrim and Humphreys, 1994), which are often incompatible with clinical fluctuations and global dysfunction such as confusional states, frequently found in the acute phase. So, actual neuropsychological rehabilitation does not rely on acute evaluation.

In this chapter, we will first emphasize the difficulties in undertaking systematic neurocognitive evaluations in the stroke unit. We will also highlight the necessity of tracking the evolution of cognitive and behavioral disorders, since they constitute important predictors of stroke outcome. We will then briefly recall some common neuropsychological disorders that occur after focal cortical damage and will describe the clinical approach in the stroke unit to the disorders most frequently found following left hemisphere, right hemisphere, or posterior strokes.

Difficulty in evaluating cognitive functions in the stroke unit

Neuropsychological literature very often concentrates on post-acute or chronic cognitive impairments which persist after three months following stroke onset. Studies investigating cognitive deficits during the hyperacute or the acute phase of stroke (i.e. the first week, 1–4 days, or 1–7 days) generally refer to small cohort descriptive studies or to case reports that illustrate representative or unusual symptoms. Despite the fact that such clinical observations are of outstanding interest, detailed neuropsychological and/or behavioral evaluations remain less systematic than studies on chronic patients. At three months post-stroke, about 60% of patients are estimated to suffer from major or residual deficits in at least one cognitive domain (Pohjasvaara *et al.*, 1998). In the stroke unit, the difficulty in obtaining systematic and reproducible evaluations during the acute phase is in part due to the concurrent intensive medical care, which does not always allow for easy and careful analysis. Due to this, but also to other reasons, cognitive disorders are often either overlooked or underestimated in acute stroke (Merino and Heilman, 2003). Of these other reasons, the following two appear as the most important to consider:

1. The attitude of the patients towards their stroke and the resulting cognitive deficits is distorted by false beliefs (Croquelois and Bogousslavsky, 2004). More than half of the patients do not initially recognize their symptoms as a stroke (Meijer *et al.*, 2003). Acute stroke is an active injury to the "self" that makes the patient underestimate the ongoing changes in the sensory-motor interactions with both the internal and external world, and thus leads the patient to a certain degree of anosognosia (Vuilleumier, 2004), and consequently to an underestimation of cognitive impairments by the emergency care-givers. With respect to the importance of mental alterations that can occur during the hyperacute phase of the stroke, it has been observed that at least one-third of the patients have no, or have only a poor, memory of the events of the first 24 hours (Grotta and Bratina, 1995), and this independently of the affected hemisphere. Whenever therapeutical decisions must be applied, this point has to be carefully examined in order to determine whether or not the patient's judgment and decision-making capacities are altered (Bogousslavsky, 2003; Hacke *et al.*, 2000).

2. The second major reason making it difficult to conduct systematic evaluations in the stroke unit is the fact that the hyperacute and the acute phases represent unstable conditions during which symptoms can change very rapidly (Croquelois and Bogousslavsky, 2004). In this context, the major causes of fluctuations are the evolution of the ischemic penumbra in the surrounding

territories and the regression of the cerebral diaschisis that may involve areas distant from the infarct (e.g. Cappa *et al.*, 1997). These unstable conditions do not allow for the adequate testing of anatomo-functional hypotheses as can be undertaken in stabilized patients, and reduce the efficiency of possible neurorehabilitation interventions.

The necessity of steadily evaluating cognitive functions in acute stroke

Despite the fact that systematic cognitive evaluations may encounter considerable difficulties in the stroke unit, there are at least two main reasons that strongly motivate such evaluation during the first days.

1. First, the effect of therapeutic intervention on cognitive deficits can be underscored when assessed by the global stroke scales. For example, Hillis *et al.* (2003) have shown that the National Institute of Health Stroke Scale (NIHSS) is not reliable in assessing stroke severity and outcome because of the lack of items assessing the neuropsychological aspects of the deficits. The authors showed that while perfusion indices did not correlate with NIHSS scores, these measures correlated in acute right hemisphere stroke with spatial neglect scores and with aphasia scores in left hemisphere strokes. In line with this observation, previous studies have suggested that aphasia (Wade *et al.*, 1986) and neglect (Kalra *et al.*, 1997) might have a direct impact on stroke outcome.

2. Second, increasing evidence in animal studies and clinical settings suggests that early therapy is associated with a better long-term outcome in both sensory-motor and cognitive functions. For instance, animal models have recently shown that motor recovery could be maximally enhanced by training, and negatively affected by limiting beam-walking experience during early recovery periods (Brown *et al.*, 2004). These findings raise questions about the role of early neuropsychological intervention in enhancing cognitive recovery after stroke, like, for instance, motor impairment (Crisostomo *et al.*, 1988). However, since cognitive functioning is an important predictor for the successful treatment and rehabilitation of stroke patients, it is therefore mandatory to assess cognitive status during the acute period with a clinical bedside examination (Paolucci *et al.*, 1996). Under the practical constraints of an acute stroke unit ward, such a screening should be repeatedly performed with little technical equipment in a reasonable time, and only at a subsequent juncture can a formal assessment be undertaken to specify the persistent cognitive−behavioral deficits.

Cognitive–behavioral disorders in the stroke unit

Neuropsychological syndromes or cognitive–behavioral disorders in the stroke unit constitute the clinical manifestations of the acute dysfunction of complex and largely distributed neural systems that subserve cognition and adaptive behavior. In the acute phase, these clinical manifestations depend not only on the infarct area, but also on other transient factors such as the diaschisis, the ischemic penumbra, and intracerebral pressure that can be induced by hemorrhagic strokes. The most common cortical neuropsychological syndromes in the stroke unit are aphasia and spatial neglect that result respectively from left and right hemisphere damage (Croquelois *et al.*, 2003; Pedersen *et al.*, 1995). To a lesser extent amnesia, the different forms of visual agnosia (apperceptive, associative, prosopagnosia, color agnosia, and pure alexia), and Bálint's syndrome are encountered following damage to the posterior areas (Ferro, 2001). Less localized disorders include disorientation, abulia, and delirium (or confusional syndrome) (Ferro, 2001). Delirium is particularly frequent in older patients with medical complications but also in hemorrhagic strokes where it can be associated with neglect (Caeiro *et al.*, 2004). With respect to behavioral disorders, these most frequently include overt sadness, disinhibition, lack of adaptation, crying, anosognosia, anosodiaphoria (or lack of concern), passivity, and aggressiveness (Ghika-Schmid *et al.*, 1999). Overt sadness and crying are more frequently associated with left hemisphere lesions. In right brain-damaged patients, anosognosia and ansodiaphoria are frequently associated with neglect. Paradoxically, anosognosia may also co-exist with severe sadness. Finally, although of a very low incidence, catastrophic reaction constitutes a particular emotional modification in the acute phase (Carota *et al.*, 2001). Its high association with aphasia and left insular lesions suggests that this emotional disturbance is induced by damage to a specific neural module.

Clinical approach of right hemispheric strokes at different steps of evolution: The example of spatial neglect

The most frequent deficit following right hemispheric strokes is the so-called "syndrome of contralesional neglect" or hemi-spatial neglect. This syndrome denotes the impaired or lost ability to react to, or to process, sensory stimuli (visual, auditory, somato-sensory, or olfactory) presented in the hemi-space opposite to the lesion side (e.g. Kerkhoff, 2001). Most frequently, spatial neglect occurs following right hemisphere (RH) damage that involves parietal, temporo-parietal, frontal, limbic, and subcortical areas (Husain and Rorden, 2003; Mesulam, 1999). At the cortical level, these lesions include the angular and supramarginal gyri of the inferior parietal lobe, the temporo-parietal junction, the superior temporal gyrus, and the inferior and middle frontal gyri (Parton *et al.*, 2004).

Although neglect is classically related to RH lesions, the occurrence of this phenomenon is more diffuse in the hyperacute phase. Actually, it has been suggested that, within the first three days following a stroke, neglect could be found with quasi-equal frequency in patients with right and left lesions (72% vs. 62%) (Stone *et al.*, 1991). Nevertheless, it is more severe following right strokes and resolves more frequently in patients with left strokes. At two months post-stroke, visuo-spatial neglect could still be observed in 40% of right-brain-damaged patients (Robertson and Halligan, 1998).

Behavioral assessment in daily life is often the most sensitive initial evaluation of spatial neglect (Azouvi *et al.*, 2002). In the hyper and acute phases, inability to cross the midline with the eyes or to explore left space is the typical feature. With right parietal damage, the patients may have head and eyes turned to the extreme right and never orient to the left spontaneously and thus pay attention only to items situated to their right (such as dinner or newspaper). When approached from their left, they may orient themselves to the right and respond with gaze directed away from the speaking person (Parton *et al.*, 2004). This particular behavior can even be increased on repetitive stimulation, so that the patient tries to turn over by more than 180 degrees to the right (Ghika *et al.*, 1995). Assessing the severity of the trouble and associated symptoms allows for tracking of the clinical evolution of the patient in the stroke unit. Clinical evaluation must thus initially rely on questions and simple tests. Psychometric testing, although not easy to undertake in acute stroke, can be conducted using "paper and pencil" tests (e.g. line bisection). Letter cancellation (Halligan *et al.*, 1990) and star cancellation tests (Halligan *et al.*, 1991) are some of the most sensitive tests and allow for the identification of up to 74% of neglect patients. Drawing (e.g. the sun, or a clock), copying pictures situated in near space, or describing a picture situated in far space will give other information about different modalities of neglect. Starting the description of a picture on the extreme right, as well as omitting the contralesional part of a drawing, represent positive signs of neglect. Reading sentences and composite words (i.e. rainbow, water lily, seat belt) may reveal spatial dyslexia when the left parts of words or text are omitted. In the same way, spatial dysgraphia is revealed when written words are far away from the contralesional paper's margin. Clinical evaluation may also concern motor impairments (motor neglect) and imagined spatial scenes (representational neglect). Questions based on the patient's or the examiner's body parts ("whose hand is it?") will give information on hemiasomatognosia or even on alien hand, often associated with neglect (Motomura *et al.*, 1988). Visual extinction as well as auditory and tactile extinction must also be clinically tested (De Renzi *et al.*, 1989).

After a few days, further assessment of neglect implies evaluation of the various aspects of spatial cognition. Hemineglect can affect the allocentric space (that refers to the spatial relationship between two stimuli separated in the space) and the egocentric space (which is related to the patient's own body or specific body parts, see Hillis *et al.*, 2005) differently. Neglect can also affect the diverse subdivisions of the subjective near and far space, commonly referred to as body space (personal), reaching space (peripersonal), and extrapersonal space (far space or walking space) differently. With respect to far space, representational neglect may be tested, relying on a memory description of a public place (Bisiach and Luzzatti, 1978). A memory description of the inside of a car while the patient is successively seated in the conductor's and the passenger's seat also allows for testing of representational neglect in the near space (Ortigue *et al.*, 2003).

Rehabilitation of spatial neglect can be undertaken in the acute phase (Bowen *et al.*, 2002; Pierce and Buxbaum, 2002). However, patients are usually not receptive or unable to collaborate enough for the neuropsychologist to start a full rehabilitation. Usually, clinicians have to work with the patient in order to go beyond anosognosia. Depending on the patient's complaints, spatial representation can be slightly improved in the hyperacute or acute phase. Trying to attract the patient's gaze from his ipsilesional to his contralesional visual space (i.e. asking the patient to describe left-cued pictures can help him to pay attention to neglected space), asking the patient to move his contralesional body parts (in the left or right mid-sagittal plan), or attracting the patient's attention by loudly speaking in his ipsilesional and then contralesional space (by moving around the bed) can be done without use of particular materials.

Clinical approach to left hemispheric strokes: The example of aphasia

Aphasia, which refers to an acquired deficit of receptive/expressive language abilities in oral and/or written codes, is considered the most important cognitive impairment that occurs following left hemisphere strokes. This is observed in nearly 40% of all strokes, (Pedersen *et al.*, 1995) and constitutes an important predictor of persistent disability, particularly if the initial form is global and associated with hemiplegia, hemisensory loss, hemianopia, and reduced consciousness (Heinsius *et al.*, 1998). During the acute phase, the most important factors for aphasia recovery are the initial severity of the symptoms and the size and location of the infarct (Basso, 1992; Kertesz, 1988; Pedersen *et al.*, 1995), but also the presence of other associated cognitive deficits (Pashek and Holland, 1988). Stationary language functions are reached after 2–10 weeks, depending on the severity of aphasia (Pedersen *et al.*, 1995). The frequency of aphasic symptoms decreases to about 20–30% after two weeks, of which one half is considered moderate to severe (Engelter *et al.*, 2004).

When a patient shows communication difficulties, the objective of the first clinical evaluation within the stroke unit is to help in establishing a differential diagnostic. Actually, it is important to determine if these difficulties are due to aphasia, dysarthria, confusional syndrome, locked-in syndrome, akinetic mutism, or other speech-associated disorders. This differential diagnosis is particularly important, since acute aphasia is often severe, either global or unclassified in 50% of cases (Godefroy *et al.*, 2002). On the basis of the neurological clinical examination only, a portion of these disorders cannot be adequately diagnosed during the first days (Trapl *et al.*, 2004). Therefore, clinical examination in the stroke unit should be rapidly accompanied by standardized simple aphasiological tests, so that every patient can be correctly treated as a function of the posited diagnostic and its severity.

Depending on the context facilities (i.e. patient in the room with others, in bed, in an armchair) and the general state of the patient, the clinical evaluation can be divided into several sessions. In severe cases, the sessions may last less than 10 minutes. The oral production will be limited to very automated spontaneous productions (answers to questions, use of "yes/no" series, singing), to the repetition of simple words or isolated phonemes and to the naming of objects belonging to different lexical fields (window, key, bottle, clock . . .). Word fluency tasks and propositional language are usually impossible at this level. The oral comprehension can be investigated using closed questions (i.e. that can be answered by *yes* or *no*), designation in the room, and execution of increasingly complex orders. Instead of reading, the patient can be asked to associate written words to an object on a forced-choice basis. Spelling should be tested with particular attention, since patients who have not already noticed a deficit at this level can show catastrophic reactions or refuse to take a pencil with their left hand in case of right hemiplegia.

At this level and up to the stabilization of the symptoms, the decision to set up systematic speech therapy cannot be taken. However, it is inconceivable to leave the patient without any linguistic stimulation, given the importance of early training (Aichner *et al.*, 2002). The therapist thus proposes a follow-up that aims to maximally engage the patient's residual abilities. Informing the patient about improvement, even if very modest, leads to a better awareness and subsequently to a better adaptation to the handicap. An important part of the intervention will also be centered on the awareness of the deficits, mainly when considering that the persistence of language difficulties will constitute a major problem for professional reintegration. The therapist's intervention with the family and the nursing personnel is also important in the acute phase, with special attention to the attitudes that care-givers and family members have to avoid. With regard to the patient's family, the nature of the disorder has to be clearly explicated in order to facilitate exchanges and prevent misinterpretations. Furthermore, the patient's relatives must be informed that the difficulties are not necessarily short-lasting and that they are not related simply to tiredness or to lack of motivation.

Clinical approach to posterior strokes: The example of visual agnosia

Strokes involving the posterior cerebral artery can induce brainstem, cerebellar, thalamic, and occipital dysfunctions. Cognitive deficits may prevent resuming occupational activities, even in infratentorial strokes (Aichner *et al.*, 2002), and thus necessitate an attentive screening. Moreover, vascular damage involving the thalamus or intrahemispheric white matter pathways can lead to severe cognitive deficits that meet the criteria of a particular form of vascular dementia (Auchus *et al.*, 2002). However, in cortical posterior infarcts, cognitive deficits related to visual integration processes are the most frequent. Clinical bedside examination of patients with posterior strokes aims first to uncover specific disorders of visuo-cognitive functions that can be dissociated from other sensorial and cognitive disturbances, such as language or memory. Of these, visual disorders such as agnosias or dyschromatopsia appear as a difficulty to recognize respectively visual stimuli and colors in the absence of any elementary disturbance of perception or intellect. However, agnosic deficits are not always easy to demonstrate in the acute phase due to the importance of visual field defects (such as hemianopia, quadranopia, hemiachromatopsia, cortical blindness, etc.), and to the presence of other perceptive—cognitive symptoms such as visual hallucinations, neglect, dysphasia, or memory disorders (Cals *et al.*, 2002). Acute clinical evaluation, using simple tests (asking the patient about their visual acuity, naming objects presented in the visual, tactile, and auditory modalities, copying objects, drawings, etc), should be conducted to specify the nature of the agnosia. An example of the importance of acute repeated evaluations is suggested by the difficulty in obtaining a consistent picture of Anton's syndrome. That syndrome, the denial of blindness by patients who are clinically unable to see (Argenta and Morgan, 1998), has often been found in the very acute phase of cortical blindness after eclampsia and is accompanied by confabulations or excuses for their symptoms ("there is not enough light to see"). This syndrome is less frequent in systematic sub-acute evaluations (Argenta and Morgan, 1998), suggesting that cortical blindness and related symptoms evolve rapidly during the first days. Moreover, follow-up evaluations suggest that cortically blind patients later develop visual agnosia, or may partially recover blind sight, perception of color, movement, or selective perception of emotional stimuli (Aldrich *et al.*, 1987; Pegna *et al.*, 2005) but the pattern of such recovery is not clear.

Patients with apperceptive visual agnosia are generally aware of their impairment: they spontaneously complain about it and try to use hands in an attempt to recognize what they see (Landis *et al.*, 1982). Despite the relative preservation of elementary visual functions, such patients have difficulties in recognizing visually presented objects, whereas the same objects can be correctly identified through the other sensorial channels (e.g. touch or hearing) (Grossman *et al.*, 1997). In contrast, patients with associative agnosia, who are generally unaware of their difficulty, will not complain about it, and will adopt a normal visual behavior without attempting to explore objects using the tactile modality. Clinically, they are able to correctly describe (or copy) a visually presented item despite their failure to recognize it.

The evolution of these visual deficits can take the form of more specific agnosic impairment. Prosopagnosia refers to the failure to recognize previously known faces and occurs more frequently after right hemisphere posterior stroke. Since some patients are aware of the deficit and can spontaneously describe their troubles, the easiest way to identify the problem consists in asking them whether or not they have difficulties in recognizing familiar people. The crucial test consists of confronting the patient with several people (which should be very similar for various criterions, such as stature, dressing . . . .), one of who ought to be known by them (Rentschler *et al.*, 1994).

The counterpart of prosopagnosia but following left posterior lesions is pure alexia or agnosic alexia that concerns the visual and not the language system *per se* (Grüsser and Landis, 1991). This reading impairment, which occurs without agraphia or other language impairments, is due to a lesion in the inferior occipito-temporal cortex (Déjerine, 1892). Pure alexia has been thought to result from damage that affects the visual word-form (Cohen *et al.*, 2000; Warrington and Shallice, 1980). Clinically, in the most severe forms the patients are not able to recognize isolated letters and indicate whether the letters "a" and "A" represent the same grapheme (Miozzo and Caramazza, 1998). In moderate cases, recognition errors may depend on the configuration complexity of the letters (e.g. I and O vs. G and H), on the difficulty in discriminating between the graphic features of the letters (O vs. Q), and of the phonemic similarity between the letters (M vs. N, or P vs. B).

Cognitive evaluation of color vision following posterior strokes aims at specifying whether a given deficit is related to achromatopsia, color agnosia, or color anomia. Since these different deficits can result from impairment at different levels of color processing, clinical screening should be undertaken according to three successive steps (Gil, 1996). The first step consists of exploring the perceptive stage with, for example, a matching color tokens test. The second step should evaluate the associative level using tests such as coloring objects, matching color/objects (i.e. red/cherry). In the third step, visuo-verbal tests, like naming the color of objects, can simply be used. According to this schema, it is possible to decide if color impairment is due to achromatopsia (impairment of the first stage), color agnosia (deficit at the second and third stage), or color anomia (impairment of the third stage only). Finally, akinetopsia or motion blindness is an often-misdiagnosed symptom in the acute phase (Blanke *et al.*, 2003). All these specific syndromes are difficult, but important to detect in a stroke unit, to improve assessment, follow-up, rehabilitation, and information to the family.

There are few data about acute intervention in visual impairment. A cognitive–behavioral assessment in the acute phase is, however, mandatory as cognitive impairment is a predictor of poor functional outcome in stroke survivors. Patients with deficits should then have neuropsychological support in order, for example, to reduce their anosognosia, and later on to fully specify their residual deficits (for example, it is important in the case of visual agnosia to determine which visual processes are impaired). Later, after an extensive neuropsychological investigation, therapy targeting the impaired processes will be designed (Burns, 2004).

Conclusion

This short introduction has emphasized the importance of cognitive assessment in acute stroke, despite ongoing modifications to the clinical picture and the difficulty in obtaining reliable and clear responses. Patients with cognitive deficits should first benefit from neuropsychological support (if no contraindications are detected such as acute confusional state), and later from a more extensive assessment with a neuropsychological rehabilitation program oriented to their specific deficits. The evaluation, clinical and bedside in a first attempt, and inspired by cognitive models in a second step, is important in determining severity, evolution, and prognosis in the stroke unit. Ultimately, the questions that have to be answered by a cognitive evaluation in the acute phase are:

1. Is the clinical picture due to a single or multiple infarcts?
2. Is there a specific or a global cognitive impairment or a confusional state?
3. What is the pattern of stabilization or recovery during the first week?
4. Which therapy programs should be conducted at a given time, specific or more global?

REFERENCES

Aichner, F., Adelwohrer, C. and Haring, H. P. (2002). Rehabilitation approaches to stroke. *J. Neural Transm. Suppl.*, 59–73.

Aldrich, M. S., Alessi, A. G., Beck, R. W. and Gilman, S. (1987). Cortical blindness: etiology, diagnosis, and prognosis. *Ann. Neurol.*, **21**, 149–58.

Argenta, P. A. and Morgan, M. A. (1998). Cortical blindness and Anton syndrome in a patient with obstetric hemorrhage. *Obstet. Gynecol.*, **91**, 810−12.

Auchus, A. P., Chen, C. P., Sodagar, S. N., Thong, M. and Sng, E. C. (2002). Single stroke dementia: insights from 12 cases in Singapore. *J. Neurol. Sci.*, **203/204**, 85−9.

Azouvi, P., Samuel, C., Louis-Dreyfus, A., *et al.* (2002). Sensitivity of clinical and behavioural tests of spatial neglect after right hemisphere stroke. *J. Neurol. Neurosurg. Psychiatry*, **73**, 160−6.

Basso, A. (1992). Prognostic factors in aphasia. *Aphasiology*, **6**, 337−48.

Bisiach, E. and Luzzatti, C. (1978). Unilateral neglect of representational space. *Cortex*, **14**, 129−33.

Blanke, O., Landis, T., Mermoud, C., Spinelli, L. and Safran, A. B. (2003). Direction-selective motion blindness after unilateral posterior brain damage. *Eur. J. Neurosci.*, **18**, 709−22.

Bogousslavsky, J. (2003). William Feinberg lecture 2002: emotions, mood, and behavior after stroke. *Stroke*, **34**, 1046−50.

Bowen, A., Lincoln, N. B. and Dewey, M. E. (2002). Spatial neglect: is rehabilitation effective? *Stroke*, **33**, 2728−9.

Brown, A. W., Bjelke, B. and Fuxe, K. (2004). Motor response to amphetamine treatment, task-specific training, and limited motor experience in a postacute animal stroke model. *Exp. Neurol.*, **190**, 102−8.

Burns, M. S. (2004). Clinical management of agnosia. *Top Stroke Rehabil.*, **11**, 1−9.

Caeiro, L., Ferro, J. M., Albuquerque, R. and Figueira, M. L. (2004). Delirium in the first days of acute stroke. *J. Neurol.*, **251**, 171−8.

Cals, N., Devuyst, G., Afsar, N., Karapanayiotides, T. and Bogousslavsky, J. (2002). Pure superficial posterior cerebral artery territory infarction in the Lausanne Stroke Registry. *J. Neurol.*, **249**, 855−61.

Cappa, S. F., Perani, D., Grassi, F., *et al.* (1997). A PET follow-up study of recovery after stroke in acute aphasics. *Brain Lang.*, **56**, 55−67.

Carota, A., Rossetti, A. O., Karapanayiotides, T. and Bogousslavsky, J. (2001). Catastrophic reaction in acute stroke: a reflex behavior in aphasic patients. *Neurology*, **57**, 1902−5.

Cohen, L., Dehaene, S., Naccache, L., *et al.* (2000). The visual word form area: spatial and temporal characterization of an initial stage of reading in normal subjects and posterior split-brain patients. *Brain*, **123**, 291−307.

Crisostomo, E. A., Duncan, P. W., Propst, M., Dawson, D. V. and Davis, J. N. (1988). Evidence that amphetamine with physical therapy promotes recovery of motor function in stroke patients. *Ann. Neurol.*, **23**, 94−7.

Croquelois, A. and Bogousslavsky, J. (2004). Cognitive deficits in hyperacute stroke. *Stroke*, **35**, 25.

Croquelois, A., Wintermark, M., Reichhart, M., Meuli, R. and Bogousslavsky, J. (2003). Aphasia in hyperacute stroke: language follows brain penumbra dynamics. *Ann. Neurol.*, **54**, 321−9.

De Renzi, E., Gentilini, M. and Barbieri, C. (1989). Auditory neglect. *J. Neurol. Neurosurg. Psychiatry*, **52**, 613−17.

Déjerine, J. (1892). Contribution à l'étude anatomo-pathologique et clinique des différentes variétés de cécité verbale. *Mémoires de la Société de Biologie*, **4**, 61−90.

Engelter, S., Gostynski, M., Papa, S., *et al.* (2004). Prevalence and severity of aphasia due to first ischemic stroke: a prospective population based study. European Stroke Conference. Mannheim-Heidelberg.

Ferro, J. M. (2001). Hyperacute cognitive stroke syndromes. *J. Neurol.*, **248**, 841–9.

Ghika, J., Bogousslavsky, J. and Regli, F. (1995). "Hyperneglect," a sequential hemispheric stroke syndrome. *J. Neurol. Sci.*, **132**, 233–8.

Ghika-Schmid, F., van Melle, G., Guex, P. and Bogousslavsky, J. (1999). Subjective experience and behavior in acute stroke: the Lausanne Emotion in Acute Stroke Study. *Neurology*, **52**, 22–8.

Gil, R. (1996). *Abrégé de Neuropsychologie*, Paris: Masson.

Godefroy, O., Dubois, C., Debachy, B., Leclerc, M. and Kreisler, A. (2002). Vascular aphasias: main characteristics of patients hospitalized in acute stroke units. *Stroke*, **33**, 702–5.

Grossman, M., Galetta, S. and D'Esposito, M. (1997). Object recognition difficulty in visual apperceptive agnosia. *Brain Cogn.*, **33**, 306–42.

Grotta, J. and Bratina, P. (1995). Subjective experiences of 24 patients dramatically recovering from stroke. *Stroke*, **26**, 1285–8.

Grüsser, O.-J. and Landis, T. (1991). Lost letters: pure alexia. In J. R. Cronly-Dillon, ed., *Visual Agnosias and Other Disturbances of Visual Perception and Cognition.* Vol 12. London: Macmillan Press, pp. 333–56.

Hacke, W., Kaste, M., Skyhoj Olsen, T., Orgogozo, J. M. and Bogousslavsky, J. (2000). European Stroke Initiative (EUSI) recommendations for stroke management. The European Stroke Initiative Writing Committee. *Eur. J. Neurol.*, **7**, 607–23.

Halligan, P., Wilson, B. and Cockburn, J. (1990). A short screening test for visual neglect in stroke patients. *Int. Disabil. Stud.*, **12**, 95–9.

Halligan, P. W., Cockburn, J. and Wilson, B. A. (1991). The behavioural assessment of visual neglect. *Neuropsychol. Rehab.*, **1**, 5–32.

Heinsius, T., Bogousslavsky, J. and Van Melle, G. (1998). Large infarcts in the middle cerebral artery territory: etiology and outcome patterns. *Neurology*, **50**, 341–50.

Hillis, A. E., Wityk, R. J., Barker, P. B., Ulatowski, J. A. and Jacobs, M. A. (2003). Change in perfusion in acute nondominant hemisphere stroke may be better estimated by tests of hemispatial neglect than by the National Institutes of Health Stroke Scale. *Stroke*, **34**, 2392–6.

Hillis, A. E., Newhart, M., Heidler, J., *et al.* (2005). Anatomy of spatial attention: insights from perfusion imaging and hemispatial neglect in acute stroke. *J. Neurosci.*, **25**, 3161–7.

Husain, M. and Rorden, C. (2003). Non-spatially lateralized mechanisms in hemispatial neglect. *Nat. Rev. Neurosci.*, **4**, 26–36.

Kalra, L., Perez, I., Gupta, S. and Wittink, M. (1997). The influence of visual neglect on stroke rehabilitation. *Stroke*, **28**, 1386–91.

Kerkhoff, G. (2001). Spatial hemineglect in humans. *Prog. Neurobiol.*, **63**, 1–27.

Kertesz, A. (1988). What do we learn from recovery from aphasia? *Adv. Neurol.*, **47**, 277–92.

Landis, T., Graves, R., Benson, D. F. and Hebben, N. (1982). Visual recognition through kinaesthetic mediation. *Psychol. Med.*, **12**, 515–31.

Meijer, R., Ihnenfeldt, D. S., van Limbeek, J., Vermeulen, M. and de Haan, R. J. (2003). Prognostic factors in the subacute phase after stroke for the future residence after six months to one year, a systematic review of the literature. *Clin. Rehabil.*, **17**, 512–20.

Merino, J. G. and Heilman, K. M. (2003). Editorial comment: Measurement of cognitive deficits in acute stroke. *Stroke*, **34**, 2396–8.

Mesulam, M. M. (1999). Spatial attention and neglect: parietal, frontal and cingulate contributions to the mental representation and attentional targeting of salient extrapersonal events. *Philos. Trans. R. Soc. Lond. B. Biol. Sci.*, **354**, 1325–46.

Miozzo, M. and Caramazza, A. (1998). Varieties of pure alexia: the case of failure to access graphemic representations. *Cogn. Neuropsych.*, **15**.

Motomura, N., Sawada, T., Inoue, N., Asaba, H. and Sakai, T. (1988). Neuropsychological and neuropsychiatric findings in right hemisphere damaged patients. *Jpn. J. Psychiatry Neurol.*, **42**, 747–52.

Ortigue, S., Viaud-Delmon, I., Michel, C. M., *et al.* (2003). Pure imagery hemineglect of far space. *Neurology*, **60**, 2000–2.

Paolucci, S., Antonucci, G., Gialloreti, L. E., *et al.* (1996). Predicting stroke inpatient rehabilitation outcome: the prominent role of neuropsychological disorders. *Eur. Neurol.*, **36**, 385–90.

Parton, A., Malhotra, P. and Husain, M. (2004). Hemispatial neglect. *J. Neurol. Neurosurg. Psychiatry*, **75**, 13–21.

Pashek, G. V. and Holland, A. L. (1988). Evolution of aphasia in the first year post-onset. *Cortex*, **24**, 411–23.

Pedersen, P. M., Jorgensen, H. S., Nakayama, H., Raaschou, H. O. and Olsen, T. S. (1995). Aphasia in acute stroke: incidence, determinants, and recovery. *Ann. Neurol.*, **38**, 659–66.

Pegna, A. J., Khateb, A., Lazeyras, F. and Seghier, M. L. (2005). Discriminating emotional faces without primary visual cortices involves the right amygdala. *Nat. Neurosci.*, **8**, 24–5.

Pierce, S. R. and Buxbaum, L. J. (2002). Treatments of unilateral neglect: a review. *Arch. Phys. Med. Rehabil.*, **83**, 256–68.

Pilgrim, E. and Humphreys, G. W. (1994). Rehabilitation of a case of ideomotor apraxia. In M. J. Riddoch and G. W. Humphreys, eds., *Cognitive Neuropsychology and Cognitive Rehabilitation*. Hove, Hillsdale: Lawrence Erlbaum Associates, pp. 271–85.

Pohjasvaara, T., Erkinjuntti, T., Ylikoski, R., *et al.* (1998). Clinical determinants of poststroke dementia. *Stroke*, **29**, 75–81.

Rentschler, I., Treutwein, B. and Landis, T. (1994). Dissociation of local and global processing in visual agnosia. *Vision Res.*, **34**, 963–71.

Robertson, I. H. and Halligan, P. W. (1998). *Spatial Neglect: A Clinical Handbook for Diagnosis and Treatment*, East Sussex, UK: Psychology Press.

Stone, S. P., Wilson, B., Wroot, A., *et al.* (1991). The assessment of visuo-spatial neglect after acute stroke. *J. Neurol. Neurosurg. Psychiatry*, **54**, 345–50.

Trapl, M., Eckhardt, R., Bosak, P. and Brainin, M. (2004). Early recognition of speech and speech-associated disorders after acute stroke. *Wien. Med. Wochenschr.*, **154**, 571–6.

Vuilleumier, P. (2004). Anosognosia: the neurology of beliefs and uncertainties. *Cortex,* **40,** 9—17.

Wade, D. T., Hewer, R. L., David, R. M. and Enderby, P. M. (1986). Aphasia after stroke: natural history and associated deficits. *J. Neurol. Neurosurg. Psychiatry,* **49,** 11—16.

Warrington, E. K. and Shallice, T. (1980). Word-form dyslexia. *Brain,* **103,** 99—11.

2

Motor and gestural disorders: Abnormal movement and motor behavior

Luc Defebvre and Pierre Krystkowiak

Hôpital Salengro, CHRU, France and University Hospital, Lille, France

Introduction

Focal brain lesions can induce several types of abnormal involuntary movement (AIM): dystonia, chorea, hemiballism, tremor, myoclonus, parkinsonism, and asterixis for example (Bhatia and Marsden, 1994; Lee and Marsden, 1994). The most frequent cause is stroke, followed by tumor, trauma, anoxia, vascular malformation, or multiple sclerosis. For some causes (and for stroke in particular), AIM can occur immediately after the brain lesion (for example, hemiballism during the acute phase of the stroke (Destée *et al.*, 1990) whereas initial motor deficit may improve or be recovered rapidly. However, in other situations, AIMs (e.g. dystonia) emerge following a long period (a few months or years) of stable motor impairment (Marsden *et al.*, 1985; Scott and Jankovic, 1996). AIMs can also be subdivided into transient (hemiballism, often in the acute phase) and persistent (dystonia, tremor, etc.). Whatever their timescales of appearance or disappearance, AIM may be the main symptom of stroke. This induces a delay in diagnosis or even a lack of knowledge of the specific diagnosis, since for the same underlying cause, the type of AIM can be quite different. This problem is sometimes clinically evident when the AIM is intense (hemiballism) or, in contrast, very moderate and focalized (asterixis). It is clear that a delay in diagnosis may have unhelpful consequences in terms of the patient's clinical and therapeutic management.

In stroke, AIM is attributed to lesions of various structures, including the striato-pallidal complex, mesencephalon, thalamus, and (more rarely) the cortex. Stroke can usually induce unique localized lesions with well-defined boundaries that facilitate anatomoclinical correlations but unfortunately only a few neuropathological studies have been published (Dooling and Adams, 1975; Garcin, 1955; Oppenheimer, 1967). CT scan and MRI studies have produced many reports of clinicopathological correlations based upon single cases or small series of patients with lesions in the above-mentioned structures. This enables

Table 2.1. Clinical classification of post-stroke abnormal involuntary movements

Transient movements	Permanent movements
Hemiballism−Hemichorea	Dystonia
Asterixis	Tremor
Paroxysmal dyskinesia	Vascular parkinsonism
	Vascular chorea

researchers to establish the pathophysiological mechanisms of the various types of AIM (Bhatia and Marsden, 1994; Krystkowiak *et al.*, 1998; Lehéricy *et al.*, 2001; Lehéricy *et al.*, 1996). In this chapter, we review the abnormal involuntary movements and motor behaviors observed in stroke. We also draw up a clinical classification based on the progression of the condition and whether the movement is transient or persistent (Table 2.1).

Transient movement disorders

For some patients, AIM occurs immediately after the stroke and may regress spontaneously and progressively. This kind of hyperkinetic movement disorder is uncommon in acute stroke, with a prevalence of 1% (Ghika-Smith *et al.*, 1997), and may sometimes be the only clearly observed clinical symptoms. Indeed, they are often masked by the motor deficit (hemiplegia). The most common types are hemiballism−hemichorea and (more rarely) transient asterixis, myoclonic and dystonic hand syndrome, and paroxysmal dyskinesia.

Hemiballism−hemichorea

Classically, hemiballism−hemichorea is considered as one of the most frequent post-stroke involuntary movements (Chung *et al.*, 2004; Ghika-Smith *et al.*, 1997). These two terms are often used interchangeably and designate continuous, non-patterned, and involuntary movements involving one side of the body. Ballism is characterized by irregular, violent, flinging movements of the limbs due to a contraction of the proximal muscles, whereas chorea consists of continuous, random, jerking movement involving both distal and proximal muscles. Some clinicians prefer to differentiate between these two hyperkinetic disorders on the basis of etiology, pathology, and severity. However, in clinical practice many patients with hemiballism perform choreiform movements and vice versa. This is especially true after a stroke where hemiballism often evolves into hemichorea. Consequently, it appears more sensible to use the term hemiballism−hemichorea to describe this clinical entity: in fact, these should be considered as two different signs (or two points on a spectrum) of the same underlying disease process.

Hemiballism—hemichorea is induced by stroke in 50—60% of cases, generally by a hemorrhagic rather than an ischemic lesion (Dewey and Jankovic, 1989). A few previous studies (often including just a small number of patients) have reported clinical outcomes and have tried to precisely localize the lesion responsible for post-stroke hemichorea (Chung *et al.*, 2004; Dewey and Jankovic, 1989; Ghika-Smith *et al.*, 1997; Vidakovic *et al.*, 1994; Zagnoli *et al.*, 1996). Other principal causes of hemiballism—hemichorea include the presence of abscesses (cerebral toxoplasmosis), metastatic lesions, acquired immunodeficiency syndrome, L-Dopa (levodopa) therapy, Sydenham's chorea, neonatal anoxic brain injury, multiple sclerosis, and central nervous system lupus. In this latter group of patients, the mean age of onset is lower (35 years) than in the stroke subgroup (61 years) (Dewey and Jankovic, 1989).

In one study, AIM onset occurred suddenly on the day of the stroke in 85% of cases (Chung *et al.*, 2004). However, the movements sometimes worsen gradually over a period of a few weeks or begin after a latency period of several months (Dewey and Jankovic, 1989). Pure hemiballism, pure hemichorea, or a combination of hemiballism and hemichorea are observed on the contralateral side of the stroke (Defebvre *et al.*, 1990). Bilateral symptoms appear only if bilateral basal ganglia damage is observed on CT scans or brain MRI. The arm and the leg are typically involved (sometimes along with face), although in some cases only a single part of the body may be affected (neck, arm, or leg). Some patients have also other combinations of abnormal movement — mainly dystonia and segmental myoclonus (depending on the location of the ischemic lesions) but also athetosis (a slow form of choreic movement), orofacial movements, and parkinsonian tremor. As the patient's condition progresses, the AIM is intermittent, typically with spontaneous disappearance in more than half of the patients (AIM can often be voluntarily but temporarily suppressed and then decreases progressively, in terms of intensity). However, some patients may experience moderate or severe persistent symptoms (including induced pain), with a level of disability which depends on both the intensity and duration of the involuntary movement. The functional prognosis may sometimes be permanently impaired. Neurological examination mainly reveals decreased muscle tone in the affected limbs, a possible sensory deficit, and mild motor weakness (Chung *et al.*, 2004). Neurobehavioral changes were also described in a case of post-hematoma hemiballism syndrome in the left subthalamic nucleus: this disinhibition syndrome was characterized by logorrhea and euphoria (Trillet *et al.*, 1995).

Classically, hemichorea and hemiballism are associated with caudate nucleus or subthalamic nucleus lesions (Bhatia and Marsden, 1994; Lee and

Marsden, 1994). However, this clinicopathological correlation is not so simple, since we know that lesions of the caudate nucleus rarely cause movement disorders (such as dystonia). In fact, hemichorea–hemiballism syndrome has been described in association with lesions of the lentiform nucleus (putamen and/or globus pallidus) (Figure 2.1), striatum (caudate nucleus and putamen), subthalamic nucleus, and thalamus (Bhatia and Marsden, 1994; Chung et al., 2004; Lee and Marsden, 1994). Certain authors report that the striatum is the most commonly involved region (Chung et al., 2004; Defebvre et al., 1990; Destée et al., 1990; Zagnoli et al., 1996). In some cases, the infarct lesion involved the cortex in the superficial territory of the middle cerebral artery (parietal, insular, and temporal areas) (Mizushima et al., 1997). This was observed in 6 patients out of 27 in a study by Chung et al. (2004). Ischemic lesions appeared to be more frequent (80%) than hemorrhagic ones: however, patients with an isolated lesion of the subthalamic nucleus tended to have suffered from hemorrhagic stroke (Chung et al., 2004).

The pathogenesis of the hemichorea caused by contralateral lesion of the striatal neurons of the indirect striato-thalamo-cortical pathways may be explained by the interruption of GABA transmission from the striatum to the external globus pallidus (GPE), which may thus increase GPE neuronal activity

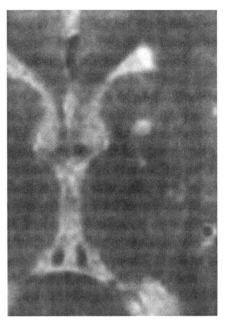

Figure 2.1   T2 weighted MRI. Left lentiform nucleus infarct inducing transient hemiballism–hemichorea syndrome.

and inhibit the subthalamic nucleus. Consequently, this inhibition would induce a loss of control of the internal globus pallidus (GPI) neurons, which may finally lead to disinhibition of the motor thalamus. In the same way, lesion of the subthalamic nucleus may induce the same dysfunction, with disinhibition of the motor thalamus creating AIM. When hemichorea—hemiballism is caused by a cortical lesion, one can assume that an excitatory neuronal circuit from some part of the frontal or parietal cortex (somatosensory cortex projecting to the caudate nucleus and the putamen) must be interrupted and thus produces AIM. The functional prognosis is significantly better in patients with cortical strokes compared to those with subthalamic lesions (Chung *et al.*, 2004): in the former group, AIMs are probably induced by transient hypoperfusion or functional "disconnection" rather than destruction of the basal ganglia circuitry.

It is surprising to note that hemichorea—hemiballism after stroke is uncommon, whereas stroke in the above-mentioned arterial territory is rather frequent. Several explanations for this scarcity may be proposed (Zagnoli *et al.*, 1996):

1. A selective impairment of the indirect pathway is necessary to induce AIM, whereas the indirect pathway represents only one-third of the total motor striatal neuronal population.
2. The striatal infarct is too large and also involves the pyramidal tract with a motor deficit.
3. The transient character of these AIMs may be due to the regulation of accessory striato-nigro-striatal, cortico-striato-nigro-thalamo-cortical, and cortico-subthalamic pathways.

Certain drugs can be proposed in the event of permanent and disabling hemichorea—hemiballism. These are mainly neuroleptics, which are effective in the control of this type of AIM (Dewey and Jankovic, 1989; Johnson and Fahn, 1977). Clonazepam and tetrabenazine are also sometimes administered with success (Chung *et al.*, 2004). Patients with mild and non-disabling AIM are not given medication, in order to avoid the potential side-effects (both acute and chronic) of neuroleptic therapy.

Key points Ballism and chorea

Ballism: irregular, violent, flinging movements of the limbs due to a contraction of the proximal muscles

Chorea: continuous, random, jerking movement involving both distal and proximal muscles

Hemiballism—hemichorea: contralateral lesion of the caudate nucleus or subthalamic nucleus; rarely perisylvian cortex lesion

Generalized chorea: bilateral lacunar infarctions of the basal ganglia

Treatment in severe cases: neuroleptics; clonazepam; tetrabenazine

---

Asterixis

Asterixis (negative myoclonus) is an involuntary movement with spontaneous and intermittent interruptions of muscle tone occurring during posture maintenance. It is usually bilateral and in such a case is accompanied by metabolic encephalopathy. Unilateral asterixis is less common, and occurs in patients with focal brain lesions. Some authors have reported that asterixis is the most common post-stroke hyperkinetic movement disorder, with a prevalence of 1.9% (Kim, 2001a). Transient asterixis (lasting from 2 to 12 days) is associated with contralateral lesions mainly involving the thalamus (accounting for more than half of the cases, and notably the ventrolateral and ventroposterior nucleus), although other structures (such as the frontal lobe, lenticular nucleus, internal capsule, precentral cortex, midbrain, and cerebellum) are sometimes affected (Kim, 2001a; Tatu *et al.*, 1996). The prevalence of asterixis after thalamic infarction ranges between 2 and 7.5%. Ipsilateral asterixis is more rarely observed after a lesion in the pons, medulla, or cerebellum (Peterson and Peterson, 1987; Pullicino *et al.*, 1990). This post-stroke AIM is often discrete and associated with other symptoms such as motor or sensory deficits and cerebellar syndrome (limb and/or gait ataxia); in this case, AIM is observed after the disappearance of these symptoms and has to be differentiated from a proprioceptive deficit ("unstable ataxic hand"). Both myoclonic (positive myoclonus) and dystonic hand syndrome is also possible and is generally observed with small thalamic lesions. Electromyographic recording can detect an asterixis which is in fact a negative myoclonus caused by intermittent failure in maintaining sustained muscle contraction. The asterixis may be caused by abnormal control of arm posture maintenance due to functional dysregulation of the brainstem-spinal tracts from the cerebello-brainstem-thalamo-frontal lobe system (Kim, 2001a). An antiepileptic drug may be proposed in case of persistent asterixis which induces a functional impairment.

Key points Asterixis

Asterixis (negative myoclonus): involuntary movement with spontaneous and intermittent interruptions of muscle tone occurring during posture maintenance
Contralateral lesion of the thalamus (more rarely frontal lobe, lenticular nucleus, internal capsule, midbrain and cerebellum or ipsilateral lesion of the pons, medulla or cerebellum)
Treatment: Antiepileptic drug may be proposed in case of persistent asterixis which induces a functional impairment

Paroxysmal dyskinesia

Other uncommon, transient post-stroke AIMs have been reported, such as paroxysmal kinesigenic dystonia or stimulus-induced paroxysmal dyskinesia related to lesions in the basal ganglia (Bhatia and Marsden, 1994), the postero-lateral thalamus (Nijssen and Tijssen, 1992), or the medulla (Riley, 1996). Unusual movements (such as undulating tongue) have been observed in such cases.

Permanent movement disorders

Movement disorders induced by stroke may occur after several months or years of stable motor impairment. The most common movement disorder caused by basal ganglia lesion is dystonia, which accounts for more than 60% of all the cases of movement disorder (Marsden *et al.*, 1985). Tremor is also reported, especially after thalamic stroke. This latter symptom may also be included in vascular parkinsonism which appears often to be heterogeneous both in terms of lesions (type and localization), clinical presentation, progression, and sensitivity to therapy (mainly levodopa). Finally, generalized and permanent chorea has only rarely been related to bilateral, vascular lesions of the basal ganglia.

Dystonia

Various post-stroke clinical subtypes of dystonia have been described according to the anatomical sites (mainly the striato-pallidal complex (Dooling and Adams, 1975; Marsden *et al.*, 1985; Pettigrew and Jankovic, 1985) and the thalamus (Garcin, 1955; Lehéricy *et al.*, 1996; Marsden *et al.*, 1985). Dystonia may also occasionally be caused by midbrain lesions affecting the dopaminergic nigro-striatal system, the red nucleus, and the superior cerebellar peduncle (Lee and Marsden, 1994). The clinical expression of dystonia may differ according to lesion location. They are presented separately in this chapter. Classically, the topography and delineation of the ischemic lesions are determined precisely using three-dimensional (3D) reconstruction and then compared to the anatomical boundaries of the nuclei as described in human atlases and Hassler's stereotaxic atlas. Moreover, the determination of precise clinicoradiological correlations in cases of single, localized, vascular lesion allows one to establish pathophysiological mechanisms of striato-pallidal and thalamic dystonia (Krystkowiak *et al.*, 1998; Lehéricy *et al.*, 1996).

Dystonia and striato-pallidal Lesions

Clinically, dystonia is focal or segmental: it is first observed distally and then progressively spreads to the proximal limb segment or to the ipsilateral lower limb extremity (hemidystonia). Dystonia consists of spasms and abnormal posture, induced and increased by voluntary movements: hyperextension of the fingers with flexion of the metacarpo-phalangeal joints, "claw-like" posture with flexion of the interphalangeal joints, hyperextension of the big toe, or flexion of the toes (especially when walking) and, more rarely, contraction of the face spontaneously and when talking (Bhatia and Marsden, 1994).

Vascular lesions are always contralateral to the dystonic movements. The sensorimotor part of the striato-pallidal complex plays an important role in the induction of dystonia (Lehéricy *et al.*, 1996; Narbona *et al.*, 1984) (Figure 2.2), as opposed to the associative (more rostral) and limbic (ventral) parts of the striatum. The infarction area corresponds to the deep zone around the middle cerebral artery. Lesions are mostly located posterior to the anterior commissure and centered on the putamen, which is always involved. Taking into account the somatotopic organization of this structure, there is a trend towards somatotopic distribution with a correspondence between the localization of the lesion within the putamen and the dystonic part of the body: the lesions of the face were more posterior and inferior, and the lesions associated with foot dystonia extended more dorsally and rostrally (Krystkowiak *et al.*, 1998; Lehéricy *et al.*, 1996). The lateral segment of the globus pallidus is involved occasionally but often less than the putamen. In a previous study, we were unable to determine whether the sensorimotor part of the pallidum was also predominantly affected (with or without a somatotopic distribution), since the sensorimotor and associative

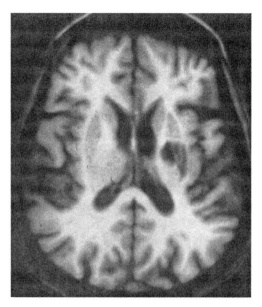

Figure 2.2   T1 weighted MRI. Left lentiform nucleus infarct inducing post-stroke dystonia.

areas in the pallidum are usually less well defined than in the putamen (Krystkowiak *et al.*, 1998; Percheron *et al.*, 1994). The medial segment of the globus pallidus was not damaged. Finally, lesions of the caudate nucleus mainly involve the structure's body and the dorsolateral part of the head.

From a physiopathological point of view, putaminal lesions might interrupt both direct and indirect pathways of the basal ganglia. The underactivity of the indirect pathway might predominate, and this disruption could increase the thalamocortical drive and induce dystonia. This hypothesis is backed up by a recent PET study of hemidystonia induced by striatopallidal lesions: there was an increased activity in cortical motor areas receiving inputs from the pallidonigral thalamic region (Ceballos-Baumann *et al.*, 1995).

Anticholinergic therapy may be considered for controlling this type of post-stroke dystonia: however, high doses are necessary and the effect is often limited. Subjective improvement may occur after injection of botulinum toxin but objective evaluation failed to demonstrate significant improvement (Yoshimura *et al.*, 1992).

Dystonia and thalamic lesions

In the case of thalamic lesions, dystonia is associated with an irregular myoclonus described as "myoclonic dystonia". Dystonia is localized to the hand, with flexion of the metacarpo-phalangeal joints and extension of the interphalangeal joints. Marked actions and postural, myoclonic jerks of variable amplitude and duration occurred irregularly and were sometimes more severe than the dystonic posture. In some patients, pure myoclonus and irregular postural and kinetic tremor were observed (Ghika *et al.*, 1994; Kim, 1992). Hemianesthesia, impairment of proprioceptive discrimination, proximal tremor, and a mild cerebellar syndrome may also be present.

Thalamic infarctions are localized within the area around the inferolateral thalamic artery territory (Lehéricy *et al.*, 1996). The lesion mainly involved the ventral intermediate (Vim) and the ventral caudate (Vc) nucleus according to Hassler's terminology, which correspond to the ventral parts of the ventral lateral posterior and the ventral posterior nuclei in the terminology of Hirai and Jones. The Vim receives cerebellar, kinesthetic, and vestibular afferents: in this case, dystonia may be induced by lesions of the cerebellar pathways which pass through the Vim (Ohye *et al.*, 1989).

Lesions may also be localized in the centromedian nucleus (CM), which is a regulator of the cortico-striato-pallido-thalamo-cortical loop (Flaherty and Graybiel, 1994). Lesion of the CM could play an important role in the induction of dystonia. This hypothesis is supported by experiments which suggest an inhibition by the mesial thalamus (including the CM) of the ventrolateral nucleus, which receives pallidal inputs (Milhorat, 1967). A PET study — in which hyperactivity was observed in motor areas after thalamic lesions (Ceballos-Baumann *et al.*, 1995) — is in agreement with the increased thalamocortical drive hypothesis. Moreover, Mitchell *et al.* (1990) have suggested that the CM could also induce dystonia via lesion of the inputs from the pedunculo-pontine complex. Hence, the pathophysiology of myoclonic dystonia may result from a combined dysfunction of the cerebello-thalamic and cortico-striato-pallido-thalamo-cortical circuits.

The ventral oral anterior and posterior nuclei of Hassler (corresponding to the ventral lateral nucleus of Hirai and Jones and constituting a relay of the efferent projections from the GPI) are undamaged, suggesting that the region involved is distinct from the striato-pallidal circuits.

Dystonia and midbrain lesions

Dystonia affects the distal part of the upper limb without involvement of the lower limb. The severity of the dystonia (often characterized by abnormal posture of the hand, with permanent hyperextension of one or more fingers) depends upon its intensity at the onset of the condition: mild dystonia disappears within a few weeks; but when it is more severe, progression is variable and ranges from modest improvement to spreading. The structures most frequently involved are the ventromedial mesencephalon (including the ventral tegmental area and the medial part of the substantia nigra), the nigrostriatal pathways, the superior cerebellar peduncle, and the red nucleus area (Leenders *et al.*, 1986; Remy *et al.*, 1995). Concurrent cerebellar syndrome may also be observed. Vascular mesencephalic lesions may also induce a levodopa-sensitive rest and postural tremor with a slow frequency of 3–4 Hz. A PET study has suggested that dystonia is severe and persistent when the dopaminergic nuclei and the nigrostriatal pathway are involved (Vidhailhet *et al.*, 1999). However, the lack of improvement in dystonia after prolonged, high-dose levodopa treatment may be explained by the fact that lesions of non-dopaminergic structures (such as the cerebello-thalamic fibers, the serotoninergic system, and the cholinergic efferent projections of the pedunculopontine nucleus) also play a role in midbrain dystonia. In contrast, in a case of dystonia associated with tremor markedly improved by levodopa, the lesion was located more laterally and dorsally in the substantia nigra and affected also the peri- and retro-rubral areas. The occurrence of rest and postural tremor due to stroke has been observed solely in patients with mesencephalic lesion including the substantia nigra.

Antiparkinsonian therapy may be proposed for controlling this type of post-stroke dystonia with tremor, but the effect is often limited.

Key points Dystonia

Dystonia: spasms and abnormal posture induced and increased by voluntary movements
Lesions: contralateral putaminal stroke
Treatment: anticholinergic therapy, botulinum toxin
Myoclonic dystonia due to thalamic lesions (inferolateral thalamic artery territory) dystonia
(hand) associated with an irregular actions and postural myoclonus
Dystonia (distal part of the upper limb) due to ventromedial mesencephalic lesion often with
rest and postural tremor
Treatment: antiparkinsonian therapy may be proposed

Thalamic tremor

The thalamus plays an important role in the pathophysiological mechanisms that underlie several types of tremor:

1. Tremor-synchronous neurons were evidenced within the thalamus, especially in the ventral intermediate nucleus (the Vim, according to Hassler).
2. The thalamus (and particularly the Vim) is known to be a target for stereotaxic surgery for alleviation of parkinsonian tremor.
3. Interruption of the cerebellar outflow tract to the thalamus (within the brainstem) may induce severe action tremor which is usually called "midbrain tremor". As with other AIMs like dystonia and myoclonus, tremor may be observed after thalamic infarction. However, cases of tremor associated with a precise limitation of single focal vascular thalamic lesions have rarely been reported (Bastian and Thach, 1995; Krystkowiak *et al.*, 2000; Lehéricy *et al.*, 2001; Miwa *et al.*, 1996; Qureshi *et al.*, 1996).

Clinically, the condition is characterized by a low-frequency (2–4 Hz) tremor of the upper limb with a postural and kinetic component affecting the proximal and distal parts contralateral to the side of the thalamic lesion. Sometimes, there is a mild rest component. Occasionally, tremor also appears in the lower limbs and the trunk. The index stroke (infarction or hemorrhage) usually results in mild or transient hemiparesis: occasionally, mild or severe sensory disturbances are present.

The lesions are mainly located in the contralateral ventral lateral posterior nucleus (according to the classification of Hirai and Jones), this latter including the Vim (according to Hassler's classification) (Figure 2.3). However, other authors have noted that the Vim is not damaged (Krystkowiak *et al.*, 2000). These data suggest a possible role of the thalamic cerebellar region represented by the ventral lateral posterior nucleus. Furthermore, it is well known that lesion or high-frequency stimulation of the ventrolateral nucleus (and especially the Vim, which contains neurons discharging synchronously with the tremor) provides

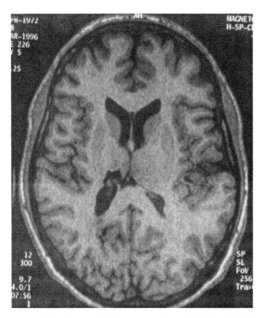

Figure 2.3   T1 weighted MRI. Right posterolateral thalamic infarct inducing tremor.

alleviation of different types of tremor (Benabid *et al.*, 1991), including midbrain tremors (Andrew *et al.*, 1982). If the Vim is not damaged, thalamic tremor might thus be induced by a lesion of the cerebellar outflow pathway to the thalamus (within the thalamus) prior to entry into the Vim. Experimental data in animals bear out this hypothesis: cerebello-thalamic inputs exert a tonic depolarization on recipient neurons located in the Vim (Steriade *et al.*, 1991), and removal of this input could produce a profound hyperpolarization of the Vim's thalamic neurons so that they could generate low-frequency oscillations (0.5–4 Hz), similar to those of thalamic tremor. These oscillations might be synchronized by thalamo-reticular and thalamo-cortico-reticular pathways (Llinàs and Paré, 1995).

One can observe that thalamic tremor and midbrain tremor frequently share similar clinical features – namely a low-frequency, high-amplitude postural and kinetic tremor present in the proximal and/or distal part of the limb and sometimes associated with a rest component. Nevertheless, these two kinds of tremor are related to lesions whose respective topographies are completely different. Midbrain tremor is known to be caused by lesions affecting the cerebello-thalamic pathway, the dento-rubro-olivary loop, and the nigro-striatal pathway (Hopfensperger *et al.*, 1995). The involvement of the nigro-striatal pathway might be responsible for the rest component. Thus, the only link between the two types of tremor might be the cerebellar outflow pathway to the thalamus.

This is borne out by animal experiments: lesion of the dento-thalamic tract in the monkey induces a kinetic tremor similar to that observed in cases with thalamic or midbrain tremors (Growdon *et al.*, 1967).

Various treatments may be proposed in the case of thalamic tremor. Levodopa may be systematically used when a resting component is present. A beneficial effect of lisuride has been observed, possibly due to the dopaminergic effect of this drug (Krystkowiak *et al.*, 2000). Since cerebellar tremor can be improved by 5-hydroxytryptophan (a serotonin precursor) in combination with benzeraside (Trouillas, 1984), this drug should be considered because of the involvement of cerebellar pathways in thalamic tremor. Finally, botulinum toxin may sometimes temporarily limit the tremor intensity (Cordivari *et al.*, 2004).

Key points Thalamic tremor

Thalamic tremor: low frequency (2–4 Hz) tremor of the upper limb with a postural and kinetic component and sometimes, a mild rest component
Contralateral to lesion of ventral lateral posterior nucleus
Treatment: Levodopa, systematically used when a resting component is present; beneficial effect of lisuride in some cases; 5-hydroxytryptophan (with benzeraside) or botulinum toxin could be considered

---

Vascular parkinsonism

The concept of vascular parkinsonism, initially controversial, is now clearly accepted, although confusion does sometimes arise because the incidence of vascular lesions in true idiopathic Parkinson's disease is up to 10 times higher than that in parkinsonism due to cerebrovascular disease (Fénélon and Houéto, 1998). Observations of vascular parkinsonism have demonstrated a heterogeneous collection of lesions with different localizations (which do not just concerned the basal ganglia), clinical expressions, and clinical courses. In light of this clinical heterogeneity, it is difficult to determine the epidemiology of vascular parkinsonism: about 8–12% of cases of parkinsonism may be due to cerebrovascular disease, whereas patients diagnosed during their lifetime as having idiopathic Parkinson's disease and then reclassified post-mortem as having vascular parkinsonism represented between 1% and 3% of the UK Parkinson's Disease Brain Bank series (Hughes *et al.*, 2001; Sibon *et al.*, 2004).

The lesions responsible for vascular parkinsonism are mostly basal ganglia lacunae and/or Biswanger-type subcortical white matter vasculopathies (Yamanouchi and Nagura, 1995). Single striatal infarction (of the lenticulostriate arteries), striatal cribiform cavities ("état criblé"), and ischemic or hemorrhagic lesions in the substantia nigra have been more rarely described. Finally, stroke in the cerebral anterior artery region with lesions of the supplementary motor area may also induce parkinsonism. Consequently, lesions that induce vascular parkinsonism can be situated anywhere in the cortico-subcortical basal ganglia motor loops (Kim, 2001b).

Clinically, two rare circumstances can be identified: vascular parkinsonism similar to Parkinson's disease and unilateral vascular parkinsonism due to contralateral basal ganglia lesions. In contrast, many more atypical parkinsonism syndromes are frequently reported (Demirkiran *et al.*, 2001). These syndromes differ from Parkinson's disease by their parkinsonism symptomatology: no typical resting tremor of the upper limbs, the absence of true akinesia (lower limb bradykinesia predominates over upper limb bradykinesia), a predominance of gait disorders and postural instability, the presence of associated neurological signs (transient deficits, pyramidal tracts signs, pseudobulbar palsy, dementia), and finally lower sensibility to levodopa. Later age at onset, acute onset, rapid or stepwise progression of the disease, and multiple vascular risk factors have all been reported as counter-indicating idiopathic Parkinson's disease. Vascular parkinsonism with isolated gait disorders is also called "lower-body parkinsonism," "frontal-type gait disorders," or "gait ignition failure." Gait abnormalities are marked by start and turn hesitation, slow and short steps, wide base, freezing, and postural instability, whereas festination is absent and arm swing is unaffected. Exceptionally, vascular parkinsonism may mimic other degenerative diseases, such as progressive supranuclear palsy (resembling a primary form with more asymmetric limb and lower body involvement), multiple system atrophy (patients with cerebellum and pyramidal signs due to stroke with hypotension induced by antihypertensive drugs), or corticobasal degeneration (combined basal and parietal infarctions).

There is still a need for accurate criteria of clinical diagnosis of vascular parkinsonism. A vascular parkinsonism rating scale (derived from the Hachinski ischemia scale) has been proposed (Winikates and Jankovic, 1999) and takes into account the following points: pathologically or angiography proven diffuse vascular disease (2 points), onset of parkinsonism within one month of stroke (1 point), history of two or more strokes (1 point), history of two or more vascular risk factors for stroke (1 point), neuroimaging evidence of vascular disease in two or more vascular territories (1 point). The diagnosis of vascular parkinsonism is established if there is a Parkinson syndrome plus vascular score of 2 or more.

The attribution of the parkinsonism disorders to vascular lesions identified during imaging is often unreliable; however, certain anatomoclinical observations have confirmed that vascular parkinsonism does exist. Basal ganglia lacunae (Figure 2.4) and subcortical white matter MRI lesions are more frequent in vascular parkinsonism than in Parkinson's disease (Zijlmans *et al.*, 1995); on rare occasions, one merely observes striatal cribiform cavities ("état criblé") (Figure 2.5) or an isolated ischemic or hemorrhagic (Figure 2.6) lesion of the substantia nigra (Hunter *et al.*, 1978; Leduc *et al.*, 1997).

Vascular parkinsonism usually does not improve with dopaminergic drugs. The effect of the L-threo-DOPS norepinephrine precursor appears to be limited and unconfirmed. Recently Ondo *et al.* (2002) reported a beneficial effect of lumbar puncture on gait in 37.5% of patients with a clinical diagnosis of vascular parkinsonism.

The pathophysiology of vascular parkinsonism is poorly understood. Hypoxic and ischemic mechanisms may lead to both presynaptic (substantia nigra), postsynaptic (striatal outflow pathways), and pallido-thalamo-cortical loop dysfunction (Sibon *et al.*, 2004). Focal lesions of the basal ganglia rarely cause parkinsonism. Indeed, vascular parkinsonism would require a lesion in the territory of both the medial and lateral lenticulostriate arteries – this would affect the putamen and external globus pallidus but not the internal globus pallidus, motor cortex, and motor pathways (Fénélon and Houéto, 1997).

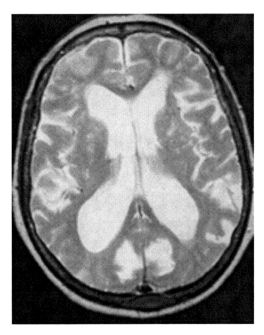

Figure 2.4   T2 weighted MRI. Basal ganglia lacunae inducing vascular parkinsonism.

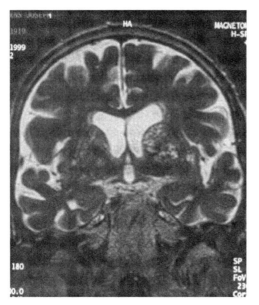

Figure 2.5   T2 weighted MRI. Striatal cribiform cavities ("état criblé") inducing vascular parkinsonism.

Key points Vascular parkinsonism

To be considered when: late age at onset, acute onset, rapid or stepwise progression of the disease and multiple vascular risk factors

Characteristics:
– no typical resting tremor of the upper limbs,
– absence of true akinesia
– predominance of lower limb bradykinesia, gait disorders and postural instability ("frontal-type gait disorders")
– presence of associated neurological signs
– lower sensibility to levodopa.

Lesions basal ganglia lacunae and/or Biswanger-type subcortical white matter vasculopathies; single striatal infarction, striatal cribiform cavities ("état criblé") and lesions in the substantia nigra; rarely, stroke of the supplementary motor area (cerebral anterior artery territory)

Treatment: dopaminergic drugs tried systematically but have usually poor effect, L-threo-Dops norepinephrine?; beneficial effect of lumbar puncture?

Vascular generalized chorea

Although hemichorea is often described attributed to a vascular lesion, generalized adult-onset chorea is often induced by a degenerative disease such as Huntington's disease. However, in very rare cases, generalized chorea has been related to bilateral

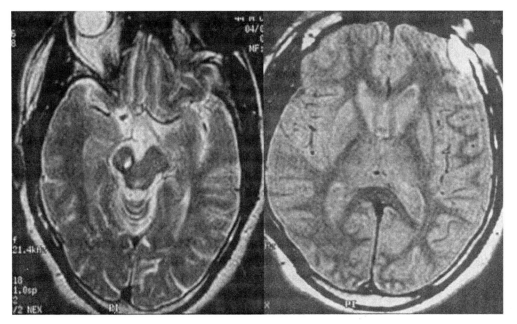

Figure 2.6   T2 weighted MRI. Hemorrhagic lesion of the right substantia nigra without other lesions in the basal ganglia inducing a left parkinsonian syndrome.

vascular lesions of the basal ganglia with multiple lacunar infarctions in patients with a history of vascular disease (Bhatia *et al.*, 1994; Sethi *et al.*, 1987; Tabaton *et al.*, 1985). Generalized chorea with dementia may mimic Huntington's disease: consequently, this diagnosis must be systematically excluded by molecular genetic analysis, even in the absence of a family history of chorea. Acute-onset, generalized chorea with spontaneous disappearance argues in favor of a vascular mechanism, as for hemichorea–hemiballism syndrome (Sethi *et al.*, 1987; Tabaton *et al.*, 1985). However, progressive-onset, generalized chorea followed by chronic worsening is also possible (Bhatia *et al.*, 1994; Krystkowiak *et al.*, 1996). The diagnosis of generalized vascular chorea is classically established by cerebral MRI showing bilateral hypersignal in the basal ganglia (suggesting vascular lesions) and is proved definitively by autopsy (revealing multiple lacunar infarctions of the basal ganglia). As in disabling hemichorea–hemiballism, neuroleptics may be considered for treatment of generalized, vascular chorea.

REFERENCES

Andrew, J., Fowler, C. J. and Harrison, M. J. (1982). Tremor after head injury and its treatment by stereotaxic surgery. *J. Neur. Neurosurg. Psychiatry*, **45**, 815–19.

Bastian, A. J. and Thach, W. T. (1995). Cerebellar outflow lesions: a comparison of movement deficits resulting from lesions at the levels of the cerebellum and thalamus. *Ann. Neurol.*, **38**, 881–92.

Benabid, A. L., Pollak, B., Gervason, C., *et al.* (1991). Long-term suppression of tremor by chronic stimulation of the ventral intermediate thalamic nucleus. *Lancet*, **337**, 403–6.

Bhatia, K. P., Lera, G., Luthert, P. J. and Marsden, C. D. (1994). Vascular chorea: case report with pathology. *Mov. Disorders*, **9**, 447–50.

Bhatia, K. P. and Marsden, C. D. (1994). The behavioral and motor consequences of focal lesions of the basal ganglia in man. *Brain*, **117**, 859–76.

Ceballos-Baumann, A. O., Passingham, R. E., Marsden, C. D. and Brooks, D. J. (1995). Motor reorganization in acquired hemidystonia. *Ann. Neurol.*, **37**, 746–57.

Chung, S. J., Im, J. H., Lee, M. C. and Kim, J. S. (2004). Hemichorea after stroke: clinical-radiological correlation. *J. Neurol.*, **251**, 725–29.

Cordivari, C., Misra, V. P., Catania, S. and Lee, A. J. (2004). New therapeutic indications for botulinum toxins. *Mov. Disorders*, **19**(Suppl. 8), S157–S161.

Defebvre, L., Destée, A., Cassim, F., Muller, J. P. and Vermersch, E. (1990). Transient hemiballism and striatal infarct. *Stroke*, **21**, 967–8.

Demirkiran, M., Bozdemir, H. and Sarica, Y. (2001). Vascular parkinsonism: a distinct, heterogeneous clinical entity. *Acta. Neurol. Scand.*, **104**, 63–7.

Destée, A., Muller, J. P., Vermersch, P., Pruvo, J. P. and Warot, P. (1990). Hémiballisme. Hémichorée. Infarctus striatal. *Rev. Neurol.*, **146**, 150–2.

Dewey, R. B. and Jankovic, J. (1989). Hemiballism-Hemichorea: Clinical and pharmacologic findings in 21. *Arch. Neurol.*, **46**, 862–7.

Dooling, E. C. and Adams, R. D. (1975). The pathological anatomy of posthemiplegic athetosis. *Brain*, **98**, 29–48.

Fénélon, G. and Houéto, J. L. (1997). Unilateral parkinsonism following a large infarct in the territory of the lenticulostriate arteries. *Mov. Disorders*, **12**, 1086–90.

Fénélon, G. and Houéto, J. L. (1998). Les syndromes parkinsoniens vasculaires: un concept controversé. *Rev. Neurol.*, **154**, 291–302.

Flaherty, A. W. and Graybiel, A. M. (1994). Anatomy of the basal ganglia. In *Movement Disorders 3*, ed. C. D. Marsden and S. Fahn. Butterworth Heinemann Ltd., pp. 3–27.

Garcin, R. (1955). Syndrome cérébello-thalamique par lésion localisée du thalamus avec une digression sur le "signe de la main creuse" et son intérêt séméiologique. *Rev. Neurol.*, **93**, 143–9.

Ghika, J., Bogousslavski, J., Henerson, J., Maeder, P. and Regli, F. (1994). The "jerky dystonic unsteady hand": a delayed motor syndrome in posterior thalamic infarctions. *J. Neurol.*, **241**, 537–42.

Ghika-Smith, F., Ghika, J., Regli, F. and Bogousslavsky, J. (1997). Hyperkinetic movement disorders during and after acute stroke: the Lausanne Stroke Registry. *J. Neurol. Sci.*, **146**, 109–16.

Growdon, H., Chambers, W. W. and Liu, C. N. (1967). An experimental dyskinesia in the rhesus monkey. *Brain*, **90**, 603–32.

Hopfensperger, K. J., Busenbark, K. and Koller, W. C. (1995). Midbrain tremor. In *Handbook of Tremor Disorders*, ed. L. J. Findley and W. C. Koller. New York, pp. 1455−9.

Hughes, A. J., Daniel, S. E. and Lees, A. J. (2001). Improved accuracy of clinical diagnosis of Lewy body parkinson's disease. *Neurology*, **57**, 1497−9.

Hunter, R., Smith, J., Thomson, T. and Dayan, A. D. (1978). Hemiparkinsonism with infarction of the ipsilateral substantia nigra. *Neuropathol. Appl. Neurobiol.*, **4**, 297−301.

Johnson, W. G. and Fahn, S. (1977). Treatment of vascular hemiballism and hemichorea. *Neurology*, **27**, 634−6.

Kim, J. S. (1992). Delayed onset hand tremor caused by cerebral infarction. *Stroke*, **23**, 292−4.

Kim, J. S. (2001a). Asterixis after unilateral stroke: lesion location of 30 patients. *Neurology*, **56**, 533−6.

Kim, J. S. (2001b). Involuntary movements after anterior cerebral artery territory infarction. *Stroke*, **32**, 258−61.

Krystkowiak, P., Defebvre, L. and Destée, A. (1996). Vascular chorea causing a phenocopy of Huntington's disesase. *4th International Congress of Movement Disorders*, June 17−21, 1996, Vienne. *Movement Disorders*, **11**, 56.

Krystkowiak, P., Martinat, P., Cassim, F., *et al.* (2000). Thalamic tremor: correlations with 3D MRI data and pathophysiological mechanisms. *Mov. Disorders*, **15**, 911−18.

Krystkowiak, P., Martinat, P., Defebvre, L., *et al.* (1998). Dystonia following thalamic and striatopallidal stroke: radioclinic correlations and pathophysiological mechanisms. *J. Neurol. Neurosurg. Psychiatry*, **65**, 703−8.

Leduc, V., Montagne, B. and Destée, A. (1997). Parkinsonism consecutive to an hemorrhagic lesion of the substantia nigra. *Mov. Disorders*, **12**(Suppl. 1), 2.

Lee, M. S. and Marsden, C. D. (1994). Movement disorders following lesions of the thalamus or subthalamic region. *Mov. Disorders*, **9**, 493−507.

Leenders, K. L., Frackowiak, R. S., Quinn, N., *et al.* (1986). Ipsilateral blepharospasm and contralateral hemidystonia and parkinsonism in a patient with unilateral rostral brainstem-thalamic lesion: structural and functional abnormalities studied with CT, MRI and PET scanning. *Mov. Disorders*, **1**, 51−8.

Lehéricy, S., Grand, S., Pollak, P., *et al.* (2001). Clinical characteristics and topography of lesions in movement disorders due to thalamic lesions. *Neurology*, **57**, 1055−66.

Lehéricy, S., Vidailhet, M., Dormont, D., *et al.* (1996). Striatopallidal and thalamic dystonia: a magnetic resonance imaging anatomoclinical study. *Arch. Neurol.*, **53**, 241−50.

Llinàs, R. and Paré, D. (1995). Role of intrinsic neuronal oscillations and network ensembles in the genesis of normal and pathological tremors. In *Handbook of Tremor Disorders*, ed. L. J. Findley and W. C. Koller. New York, pp. 7−36.

Marsden, C. D., Obeso, J. A., Zarranz, J. J. and Lang, A. E. (1985). The anatomical basis of symptomatic hemidystonia. *Brain*, **108**, 463−83.

Milhorat, T. H. (1967). Experimental myoclonus of thalamic origin. *Arch. Neurol.*, **17**, 365−78.

Mitchell, I. J., Luquin, R., Boyce, S., *et al.* (1990). Neural mechanisms of dystonia: evidence from a 2-deoxyglucose uptake study in a primate model of dopamine agonist-induced dystonia. *Mov. Disorders*, **5**, 49−54.

Miwa, H., Hatori, K., Kondo, T., Imai, H. and Mizuno, Y. (1996). Thalamic tremor: case reports and implications of the tremor-generating mechanism. *Neurology*, **46**, 75−9.

Mizushima, N., Park-Matsumoto, Y. C., Amakawa, T. and Hayashi, H. (1997). A case of Hemichorea-Hemiballism associated with parietal lobe infarction. *Eur. Neurol.*, **37**, 65−6.

Narbona, J., Obeso, J., Tunon, T., Martinez-Lage, J. M. and Marsden, C. D. (1984). Hemidystonia secondary to localised basal ganglia tumour. *J. Neurol. Neurosurg. Psychiatry*, **47**, 704−9.

Nijssen, P. C. and Tijssen, C. C. (1992). Stimulus-sensitive paroxysmal dyskinesias associated with a thalamic infarct. *Mov. Disorders*, **7**, 364−6.

Ohye, C., Shibazaki, T., Hirai, T., *et al.* (1989). Further physiological observations on the ventralis intermedius neurons in the human thalamus. *J. Neurophysiol.*, **61**, 488−500.

Ondo, W. G., Chan, L. L. and Levy, J. K. (2002). Vascular parkinsonism: clinical correlates predicting motor improvement after lumbar puncture. *Mov. Disorders*, **17**, 91−7.

Oppenheimer, D. R. (1967). A case of striatal hemiplegia. *J. Neurol. Neurosurg. Psychiatry*, **30**, 134−9.

Percheron, G., Yelnik, J., Francois, C., Fenelon, G. and Talbi, B. (1994). Analyse informationnelle du système lié aux ganglions de la base. *Rev. Neurol.*, **150**, 614−26.

Peterson, D. I. and Peterson, G. W. (1987). Unilateral asterixis due to ispilateral lesions in the pons and medulla. *Ann. Neurol.*, **22**, 661−3.

Pettigrew, L. C. and Jankovic, J. (1985). Hemidystonia: a report of 22 patients and a review of the literature. *J. Neurol. Neurosurg. Psychiatry*, **48**, 650−7.

Pullicino, P., Xuereb, M. and Farrugia, B. (1990). Hémorragie cérébelleuse et asterixis unilateral. *Rev. Neurol.*, **146**, 687−98.

Qureshi, F., Morales, A. and Elble, R. J. (1996). Tremor due to infarction in the ventrolateral thalamus. *Mov. Disorders*, **11**, 440−59.

Remy, P., De Recondo, A., Defer, G., *et al.* (1995). Peduncular « rubral » tremor and dopaminergic denervation: a PET study. *Neurology*, **45**, 472−7.

Riley, D. E. (1996). Paroxysmal kinesigenic associated with a medullary lesion. *Mov. Disorders*, **11**, 738−40.

Scott, B. L. and Jankovic, J. (1996). Delayed-onset progressive movement disorders after static brain lesions. *Neurology*, **46**, 68−74.

Sethi, K. D., Nichols, F.T. and Yaghmai, F. (1987). Generalized chorea due to basal ganglia lacunar infarcts. *Mov. Disorders*, **2**, 61−6.

Sibon, I., Fénelon, G., Quinn, N. P. and Tison, F. (2004). Vascular parkinsonism. *J. Neurol.*, **251**, 513−24.

Steriade, M., Currò-Dossi, R. and Nunez, A. (1991). Network modulation of a slow intrinsic oscillation of cat thalamocortical neurons implicated in sleep delta waves: cortically induced synchronization and brainstem cholinergic suppression. *J. Neurosci.*, **11**, 3200−17.

Tabaton, M., Mancardi, G. and Loeb, C. (1985). Generalized chorea due to bilateral small, deep cerebral infarcts. *Neurology*, **35**, 588−9.

Tatu, L., Moulin, T., Martin, V., *et al.* (1996). Asterixis unilatéral et lésions cérébrales focales: douze cas. *Rev. Neurol.*, **152**, 121−7.

Trillet, M., Vighetto, A., Croisile, B., Charles, N. and Aimard, G. (1995). Hémiballisme avec libération thymo-affective et logorrhée par hématome du noyau sous-thalamique gauche. *Rev. Neurol.*, **151**, 416–19.

Trouillas, P. (1984). Regression of cerebellar syndrome with long term administration of 5-HTP or the combination 5-HTP-benzeraside. *Ital. J. Neurol. Sci.*, **5**, 253–66.

Vidakovic, A., Dragasevic, N. and Kostic, V. S. (1994). Hemiballism: report of 25 cases. *J. Neurol. Neurosurg. Psychiatry*, **57**, 945–9.

Vidhailhet, M., Dupel, C., Lehericy, S., *et al.* (1999). Dopaminergic dysfunction in midbrain dystonia: anatomoclinical study using 3-dimensional magnetic resonance imaging and fluorodopa F 18 positron emission tomography. *Arch. Neurol.*, **56**, 982–9.

Winikates, J. and Jankovic, J. (1999). Clinical correlates of vascular parkinsonism. *Arch. Neurol.*, **56**, 98–102.

Yamanouchi, H. and Nagura, H. (1995). Cerebrovascular parkinsonism-clinicopathologic study. *Rinsho Shinkeigaku*, **35**, 1457–8.

Yoshimura, D. M., Aminoff, M. J. and Olney, R. K. (1992). Botulinum toxin therapy for limb dystonias. *Neurology*, **42**, 627–30.

Zagnoli, F., Rouhart, F., Perotte, P., Bellard, S. and Goas, J. Y. (1996). Hémichorée et infarctus striatal. *Rev. Neurol.*, **152**, 615–22.

Zijlmans, J. M. C., Thijssen, H. O. M., Vogels, O. J. M., *et al.* (1995). MRI in patients with suspected vascular parkinsonism. *Neurology*, **45**, 2183–8.

3

Gestural apraxia

Frédérique Etcharry-Bouyx[1] and Mathieu Ceccaldi[2]

[1]University Hospital, Angers, France
[2]University Hospital, La Timone, Marseille, France

Introduction

The term apraxia was introduced by Liepmann in 1908 (Liepmann, 1908) in order to describe an inability to properly execute a learned skilled movement which cannot be accounted for by weakness, incoordination or sensory deafferentation, or by language comprehension deficits or a global intellectual impairment. All patients described by Liepmann had suffered strokes in parietal or frontal regions. Although described in the early twentieth century, the clinical features of apraxia remain relatively unknown. Two old ideas contribute to underestimation of the critical role of apraxia after a stroke: the first is related to the concept that apraxia spontaneously and rapidly improves after a stroke, and the second is that, in view of the dissociation between automatic and voluntary motor skills, repercussion of apraxia in everyday life is mild.

Nevertheless, systematic studies of apraxia lead to different conclusions. For example, Basso *et al.* (1987) re-examined after several months 26 patients with focal left hemisphere vascular lesions who presented with ideomotor apraxia (IMA) in the acute period. They had to imitate 24 meaningful or meaningless movements with the hand ipsilateral to the lesion. The first examination was performed at between 15 and 30 days post-stroke, the second assessment at between 5 and 23 months. On the second examination the improvement was significant but half of the patients were still apraxic. Eleven of the 13 subjects were examined a third time. Five patients (1/4) presented with long-lasting apraxia (from 13.5 to 60 months after the stroke).

Activities of daily living (ADL) are not expected to be affected by apraxia because they concern overlearned routine actions that are automatically performed when the appropriate context is provided (De Renzi, 1990). However, in practice, it is not rare to observe difficulties of routine occupations such as dressing, eating, or lighting a cigarette (Pradat-Diehl *et al.*, 1999) and recent studies have shown that apraxia may interfere with many naturalistic situations (Goldenberg and Hagmann, 1998; Donkervoort *et al.*, 2002; Hanna-Pladdy *et al.*, 2003).

The aim of this chapter is first to recall the clinical features of subtypes of apraxia and the basis for the clinical examination of gestures; second, to consider relationships between strokes and apraxia, especially in terms of laterality and intra-hemispheric topography of lesions; third, to describe the technical basis of rehabilitation of gestural impairments; and finally to point out some issues concerning neural substrates of action.

Approach to gestural apraxia in clinical practice

Qualifying apraxia remains difficult because of confused terminology, still unknown issues concerning physiopathology and poorly defined protocols of examination (Le Gall and Etcharry-Bouyx, 2003; Le Gall and Peigneux, 2003). It refers to a variety of sensorimotor transformations that concern either multimodal sensory inputs (which correspond to the classical gestural apraxias as defined by Liepmann) or modality-selective movements (which has been called "unimodal apraxias" (Freund, 2001)).

Bilateral limb apraxias: Ideomotor apraxia and ideational apraxia

In most cases, gestural apraxia affects both upper limbs (or, in case of paresis, the non-paretic limb, ipsilateral to the cerebral lesion), resulting from an inability to mentally evoke actions from stored motor representations (Jeannerod and Decety, 1995). According to the classical nomenclature of Liepmann, ideomotor apraxia (IMA) corresponds to disorders of realization of symbolic gestures, of pantomimes and of imitation of actions, while the term ideational apraxia (IA) is retained when the disorder concerns the use of actual objects. In fact, the same clinical disorder may be caused by different mechanisms. Cognitive neuropsychological models that have been developed over the past twenty years allow a discriminating analysis of the mechanisms of the apraxias, distinguishing distinct tasks in clinical testing corresponding to distinct components of generation of gestures. For example, Rothi *et al.* (1991, 1997) have proposed a model with three different accesses to mental representation of gestures: an auditory-verbal entry ("show me the gesture of using a key"), a visual entry with sight of objects ("show me the gesture for using this object . . ."), and a visual entry with gesture imitation tasks ("made the same gesture as me"). Roy and Square (1985) have suggested that two distinct levels may be discriminated when performing gestures. The first level would be a conceptual level composed of abstract knowledge about the object functions ("what that object is used for"), about the actions ("which object can be used to achieve such an action"), and about the seriation of elementary gestures in order to complete a complex action. The second level would be implicated in the actual production of actions and would activate and monitor motor plans ("how to do a gesture" with that object).

In clinical practice, distinction between IMA and IA may be difficult. Clinically, IMA corresponds to deterioration of learned skills, of meaningful (hand actions with a semantic connotation, e.g. signaling "stop"), and of meaningless gestures performed to verbal command and/or imitation. But IMA can be considered from two distinct points of view: motor behavior and comprehension of actions. In clinical practice, the motor component can be evaluated by imitation of meaningless gestures, while the comprehension of actions can be examined by matching a pantomime performed by the examiner and the corresponding object by multiple choices. Other tasks used in clinical practice implicate both levels, production and comprehension – for example, realization of symbolic actions to verbal command, or pantomimes to verbal command and to visual presentation of corresponding object. As we will see later, these two components of praxis – production and comprehension – may be differently affected depending on the site of the lesion. Labeling limb apraxia is based on the type of the patient's errors observed in clinical testing. In IMA four types of errors are observed:

1. temporal errors, either in speed or in occurrence and in sequencing elementary movements;
2. spatial errors, either in amplitude or insertion point of the gesture;
3. errors of content, using a body part as an object (using an index finger instead of putting the hand into the position of holding a key), perseverating on the previous gesture, producing wrong movements with morphological similarities (ironing instead of brushing) or with semantic similarities (playing trombone instead of playing trumpet) to the expected movement;
4. others: absence of gesture, verbalization, non-recognizable productions.

Ideational apraxia would be due to alteration of stored gestural representations, resulting in difficulties in handling actual objects. Patients with IA make content errors during realization of actions, by for example choosing the bad object (this last type of deficit is sometimes referred to as "conceptual apraxia" by some authors), or they are impaired in sequencing a series of actions when using objects. Some tasks are designed to evaluate patients' knowledge about objects: functional and categorical matching of objects, recognition of the correct use of the presented object among multiple choices, knowledge about the goals of action (functional equivalence of different gestures), and knowledge about sequencing distinct actions in order to complete one goal (scripts). In clinical practice, testing is done with objects used in daily life, by varying their number and choosing them according to semantic links or morphological similarities.

In IA, perseverations or pauses are in favor of impaired representations of action sequences. Deficit on the object-choice level is suggested by different kinds of error:

1. no action (sometimes substituted by giving the name of the presented object, often accompanied by a modification of the patient's behavior such as perplexity...);
2. substitution of the target object by another one (either one object closely related to the target or one object from a preceding task);
3. errors of handling;
4. confusions between actions (either performing an action closer to the target one – for example brushing oneself with a toothbrush, or perseverating with a preceding action);
5. errors in sequencing (addition or omissions of actions);
6. spatial errors (for example, stamp stuck on the wrong part of an envelope).

Unilateral limb apraxias: Limb kinetic apraxia and callosal apraxia

Limb-kinetic apraxia (LKA) (also referred to as melokinetic apraxia or motor apraxia) is generally considered as a form of unilateral movement disorder that is intermediate between paresis and apraxia. Patients with LKA present with elementary motor deficits in the absence of weakness, sensory loss, ataxia, or changes in muscular tonus: movements are rare, slow, imprecise, and stiff, especially at the level of the hand where a loss of independent finger movements may be observed; disorders affect all kinds of gestures – transitive and intransitive, meaningful and meaningless – and there is no dissociation between automatic and intentional actions; although imprecise, they are correctly sequenced and orientated in space and conceptual; conceptual knowledge of gestures is spared. LKA has been attributed to an inability to correctly link independent muscle groups that have separate innervations (Kleist, 1912). LKA is restricted to the contralesional limb.

Callosal apraxia (CA) often concerns the left hand. It is characterized by an inability to correctly perform movements to verbal command with the left hand, contrasting with preserved right-hand movements. In most spontaneous cases, CA is caused by infarctions in the territory of the anterior cerebral artery. In these cases, the anterior part of the corpus callosum is damaged. CA has also been described after a left hemisphere watershed infarct following internal carotid artery occlusion (Habib *et al.*, 1990). Left-sided callosal apraxia could be due to the loss of access of left hemisphere visuokinesthesic motor engrams to the right hemisphere motor areas that control movement of the left hand. Sometimes, in right-handed patients, CA is associated with a very unusual behavior, diagonistic dyspraxia. The association of a left CA and a right diagonistic dyspraxia has been reported in a left-handed patient presenting with an association of infarctions in the zones respectively supplied by the left anterior cerebral artery and the left posterior cerebral artery (Poncet *et al.*, 1978).

Unimodal apraxias: The example of optic ataxia

Optic ataxia (OA), which is also called visuomotor ataxia or visuomotor apraxia, consists of the inability to direct the arm adequately toward a visual target (Perenin and Vighetto, 1988; Goodale and Milner, 1992). Freund (2001) considers OA as a form of "unimodal apraxia" because it represents a modality-selective disturbance of arm movements: only movements in relation to one particular sensory modality – vision – are disturbed while other aspects of motor behavior are preserved. Patients with OA have been shown to exhibit defective trajectories and preshaping of the hand in several visuo-motor situations: reaching, aiming, gripping.... Generally, OA affects both arms and is observed as one of the components of Bálint's syndrome with psychic paralysis of gaze and restricted visual attention. Bálint's syndrome is always caused by bilateral lesions of the parietal-occipital regions, affecting the cortex and adjacent subcortical white matter, and causing an occipito-frontal disconnection. Unilateral OA may be seen in the contralesional arm after small lesions of either hemisphere in the superior parietal lobule (SPL) and the underlying white matter. The SPL is thought to be implicated in online control of the spatial configuration of movement during it execution.

Apraxia testing

Diagnosis and evaluation of apraxia cannot be done without a complete neurological examination of the patient – physical and neuropsychological. Especially, language comprehension and knowledge about body schema have to be evaluated (Goldenberg, 1995). The clinical approach is guided by reports of selective deficits. For example, cases in which transitive gestures (i.e. involving the use of a tool) but not intransitive gestures were selectively impaired have been reported (Rapcsak *et al.*, 1993; Dumont *et al.*, 1999). By contrast, some patients presented an impairment restricted to intransitive actions (Heath *et al.*, 2001). This double dissociation supports the view that transitive and intransitive actions might be processed differently. Apraxia examination has to be carried out under various conditions (imitation, actual realization, recognition) and for several types of gesture (overlearned skills, meaningful and meaningless gestures, using actual objects). Both upper limbs might be examined, and it is recommended to use configurations implicating distinct parts of the limb, especially for imitation. Indeed, in apraxia, hand posture may be impaired in contrast to relatively preserved arm posture and trajectory for skilled actions

(Sirigu *et al.*, 1995). Moreover, imitation of hand and finger postures may be differently impaired depending on the side of the lesion: whereas imitation of finger configurations was about equally impaired in patients with left hemisphere damage (LHD) and right hemisphere damage (RHD), defective imitation of hand positions is almost exclusively observed in patients with LHD (Goldenberg, 1996; Goldenberg *et al.*, 2003). Several protocols have been designed to provide a systematic and complete examination of praxis, either in English (Florida Battery) or in French (Le Gall *et al.*, 2000; Peigneux and Van der Linden, 2000). Nevertheless, if a detailed evaluation of apraxia is necessary to establish a precise diagnosis and to provide a program for rehabilitation, systematic administration of these batteries is not always possible in clinical practice. Shortened versions devoted to the detection of gestural difficulties have been developed (Peigneux and Van Der Linden, 2000; Etcharry-Bouyx and Le Gall, 2003). Relative agreement about the methodological basis under which movements should be studied seems to emerge (verbal order, imitation, actual use of object), but there is still a debate on the nature of actions to be considered (transitive, symbolic, meaningless, simple, or complex ones) and on theoretical validity of comparisons between them (Peigneux *et al.*, 2003). However, advances in the comprehension of neural substrates of distinct components of action, especially from microelectrode recordings in animals and from neuroimaging studies in humans, may contribute to improving the clinical approach to apraxia.

Gestural apraxia in strokes

According to De Renzi *et al.* (1986), in comparison with degenerative diseases: "the consequences of an abrupt disease, such as stroke, are much more disruptive and likely to bring out true apraxia deficits" (p. 1036). Nevertheless, the site of stroke is critical for occurrence of apraxia. We will focus on studies devoted to IMA, the most frequent clinical type of apraxia in strokes.

Left and right hemisphere contributions to IMA in strokes

According to Liepmann, approximately half of patients with LHD present with apraxia involving the non-paretic left hand. Several studies have focused on frequency of apraxia in patients suffering from unilateral stroke. Donkervoort *et al.* (2000) found apraxia in 28% of patients in a rehabilitation center for a first left hemisphere stroke. More recently, Zwinkels *et al.* (2004) examined 100 patients with a first stroke. The frequency of apraxia was 25.3% in the total group, 51.3% in LHD patients, and 6% in RHD patients. There is a general agreement on a preferential association of LHD with apraxia, but discrepancies about the exact frequency of IMA in left hemisphere stroke suggest that sensitivity of assessment should be considered.

Pantomime / imitation

Roy *et al.* (2000) have studied frequency and severity of limb apraxia in patients with left or right hemisphere stroke in both pantomime and imitation. They compared the frequency of apraxia in each stroke group across the three patterns of apraxia described in Roy's model. Performance was scored on the basis of five performance dimensions: orientation, action, hand posture, plane of hand movement, and hand spatial location in from body's referential. LHD patients were significantly less accurate on location and posture dimensions than RHD patients who were more impaired than controls. Further, the LHD group was impaired on action and plane dimensions in comparison to the control group, while the RHD did not differ from controls. In the pantomime condition there was a higher proportion of apraxic patients with LHD. In the imitation condition the distribution of apraxic patients in the two stroke groups did not differ significantly. The performance of the apraxic patients with LHD was not significantly less accurate than the RHD group, suggesting a comparable severity of apraxia. However, a greater percentage of LHD patients (43%) than RHD patients (23%) were impaired on both pantomime and imitation.

Transitive / intransitive movements

There is evidence that transitive gesture imitation is more impaired in patients with IMA than is symbolic gesture imitation such as waving goodbye or beckoning "come here" (Mozaz *et al.*, 2002). Heath *et al.* (2001) examined the frequency and severity of praxis errors related to the production of intransitive gestures according to lesion side in 119 stroke patients (57 LHD, 62 RHD). They had to perform eight intransitive gestures to pantomime and imitation. The patients were separated in three groups: apraxic, "borderline," and non-apraxic patients. Among apraxic patients, for both pantomime and imitation conditions, the proportions of LHD (68% for gestural pantomime, 38% for imitation) and RHD (64% and 27% respectively) were similar. These authors noted a relationship between imitation and neglect for RHD and between language function and praxis pantomime errors for LHD. These findings suggest that the ability to generate intransitive limb gestures can be impaired whichever the stroke side. However, the proportion of patients with an alteration of pantomimes was higher in this last study, compared to that of Roy's (38% vs. 5% in LHD, 42% vs. 6% in RHD). This discrepancy could be due to the possibility to see the tool associated with action in Roy *et al.*'s study. This difference appears to be critical: Goldenberg and Hagmann (1997) have argued that the accurate pantomime of transitive actions can be accomplished via selection/evocation of a response from memory or the ability to infer function from the tool's structure. Furthermore, Roy *et al.* demonstrated that LHD patients exhibit praxis errors more frequently than RHD patients when transitive actions are elicited in response to verbal command. In addition Heath *et al.* suggested that apraxia was equally common in LHD and RHD groups in the context of pantomiming intransitive gestures. Together these studies underscore the importance of regarding gesture type (transitive versus intransitive) as a separate source of variance when studying the relationship between apraxia and lesion side.

Pantomimes / actual using

Several studies described better performance with actual tools compared to miming in IMA. To test modality specific effects, De Renzi *et al.* (1982) examined aphasic patients in two conditions. Patients were asked to mime the use of tools presented either verbally or visually (without any contact with the object) or to use the tools while blindfolded. Use with only tactile input was generally much better than miming to either verbal or visual input. They concluded that the same motor programs are employed for pantomime and actual use. Recently, Goldenberg *et al.* (2004) investigated whether better performance was due to the tactile feedback provided by holding the tool. Ten patients with left hemisphere lesions were asked to demonstrate the use of tools under three conditions: miming, miming with an implement shaped like the handle of the tool, and using the real tool. Using the real tool was much better than pantomime, but there was no significant improvement with tactile feedback from the isolated handle. Tactile feedback from real tools provides specifications of the appropriate action – probably based on mechanical affordances – which are not evident from tactile exploration limited to the shape of the handle. The higher frequency and severity of apraxia for miming than for using real tools in patients with aphasia and LHD suggest that success of this "virtual" act depends crucially on left hemisphere integrity. There is a close link between disorders of single familiar tools or tool/object pairs use and left hemisphere damage, but how do patients perform everyday actions in a natural environment? Buxbaum *et al.* (1998) found that patients with RHD had more difficulties than those with LHD. Recently, Hartmann *et al.* (2005) studied the role of hemispheres in naturalistic actions – for example preparing coffee with a drip coffee or fixing a cassette recorder – which require multi-step actions and involve technical equipment. Patients with LHD and aphasia scored lower than RHD but both patient groups were impaired. Analysis of experimental tests assessing retrieval of functional knowledge from semantic memory, inference of function from structure, and their correlations to naturalistic actions suggest that the multi-step character of an action is a feature sensitive to RHD patients whereas the LHD patients difficulties may be related to inability to retrieve script-like instructions for use from semantic memory. This study suggests that several abilities and strategies, based on different cerebral substrates, are needed to complete actions in daily life. Each hemisphere brings its own contribution to praxis functions. Whereas the left hemisphere appears to be more important for the spatial aspects of the praxis program, the right hemisphere appears to be more important for temporal aspects (timing and extrapersonal representations).

Cortical and subcortical contributions to IMA in stroke

Apraxia in association with subcortical lesions has been repeatedly reported (Della Sala *et al.*, 1992; De Renzi *et al.*, 1986). However, in a review of "deep apraxia", Pramstaller and Marsden (1996) found that, in most cases, the lesion was not confined to the basal ganglia, but extended into peristriatal white matter, damaging corticocortical fiber pathways, and sometimes into the cortex. Moreover, in vascular lesions, decreased blood flow can be observed in cortical areas situated at distance from the subcortical site of infarction. To ascertain the role of subcortical structures lesions in apraxia, Hanna-Pladdy *et al.* (2001) have compared gestural performance on several tasks in patients with left hemisphere cortical and subcortical strokes. Distinct profiles were described. Patients with cortical damage presented with deficits in the production of transitive and intransitive gestures to verbal command and imitation as well as impaired gesture discrimination. In contrast, patients with subcortical lesions demonstrated mild production−execution deficits for transitive pantomimes, but normal imitation and discrimination. Qualitative analysis of errors revealed that the subcortical group made more postural errors whereas the cortical group produced sequencing, unrecognizable and no-response errors. In a study devoted to the influence of intrahemispheric location of lesion on apraxia in 40 patients with LHD, Goldenberg *et al.* (2003) found that patients with lesions of the basal ganglia scored lower than those without such lesions on pantomime of object use. Further, pure thalamic infarction may be associated with apraxia and that could be explained by rich connections from the pulvinar nucleus to the inferior parietal cortex and the lateral prefrontal cortex, which are both implicated in motor representations (Nadeau *et al.*, 1994).

Parietal cortex and other cortical contributions to IMA in stroke

The observation that IMA is often observed after large strokes involving the left middle artery territory strongly supports the assumption that lesions of areas situated in suprasylvian and perirolandic region of the left dominant hemisphere lead to apraxia. Patients with isolated left pre-frontal or premotor convexity lesions frequently show buccofacial apraxia *and* limb apraxia associated with Broca aphasia (Mohr *et al.*, 1978). In addition, patients with left supplementary motor area (SMA) lesions, due to infarct in the territory of the anterior cerebral artery, presenting with bilateral IMA for transitive movements have been reported (Watson *et al.*, 1986). These observations emphasize the putative role of frontal cortex lesions in IMA. Nevertheless, systematic studies of praxis in LHD patients tend to confirm the prominent role of parietal areas, and suggest that praxis is mediated by a distributed modular network which also implicates other cortical areas. For example, Goldenberg *et al.* (2003) found that patients with occipital lesions had lower scores than those without such lesions on imitation of hand positions. Temporal lesions were associated with lower scores on pantomime and imitation of hand postures, and both temporoparietal and parietal lesions led to a marked deterioration of imitation of hand postures. Moreover, results obtained in studies comparing effects of parietal and frontal lesions show that left parietal lesions are associated with both production and recognition deficits of gestures while frontal lesions only impair production (Heilman *et al.*, 1982; Halsband *et al.*, 2001). There is evidence that patients with left inferior parietal lobe lesion associated to IMA have a particular deficit in recognizing the hand postures appropriate for skilled object-related actions, especially for familiar objects, contrasting with preserved ability to reach and grasp geometric three-dimensional shapes (Buxbaum *et al.*, 2003; Buxbaum *et al.*, 2005a). Recently Buxbaum *et al.* (2005b) showed that in stroke patients, the lesion associated with deficits in the recognition of transitive gesture and the hand posture component of transitive gesture, are located in the inferior parietal lobe and intraparietal sulcus. These data converge to growing evidence from very recent fMRI studies that the left inferior parietal lobe and intraparietal sulcus are especially implicated in both imitation of gestures and movement execution on verbal command (Makuuchi *et al.*, 2005; Mühlau *et al.*, 2005). Several neuroimaging studies have also emphasized the relations between IMA and the role of the left inferior parietal lobe in body schema (Goldenberg *et al.*, 2001; Chaminade *et al.*, 2005).

Recovery and rehabilitation of gestural apraxia after stroke

Long-lasting apraxia: a critical factor for recovering autonomy in everyday life

Follow-up of patients with left hemisphere stroke shows that improvement from IMA requires a long period of time, and that this is not related to age, education, sex, type of aphasia, initial severity, and lesion size (Basso *et al.*, 1987). On the basis of a CT scan study, these authors suggested that sparing of posterior temporoparietal and occipital regions was important for recovery from IMA, although recovery might be observed whatever the lesion location. Long-lasting

IMA leads to disability in daily life. Goldenberg and Hagmann (1998) administered a test of three activities of daily living (spreading margarine on a slice of bread, putting on a pullover or a T-shirt, brushing teeth) to 35 patients with left hemisphere stroke. The number of errors correlated strongly with clinical measures of limb apraxia. Donkervoort *et al.* (2002) demonstrated that ADL can measure apraxia with more sensitivity than a conventional functional scale based on motor impairments and that their dysfunction was correlated with severity of apraxia. Hanna-Pladdy *et al.* (2003) examined pantomime to verbal command in 10 patients with a left unilateral stroke. They determined independence in physical self maintenance skills for six categories (toileting, dressing, feeding, grooming, ambulation, bathing). There was a close relationship between severity of apraxia and the subject's independence in physical ADL. The analyses revealed that the apraxic group was more dependent in bathing, toileting, and grooming. Recently Wetter *et al.* (2005) demonstrated that severity of apraxia was the best predictor of a test which simulates activities of daily living for a group with LHD. Moreover, limb apraxia has been reported to predict poorer outcome after rehabilitation than other deficits such as aphasia (Sundet *et al.*, 1988). In a long-term follow-up study, the absence of apraxia was a significant predictor of return to work after stroke (Saeki *et al.*, 1995). These studies suggest that IMA may be a major source of disability.

Apraxia therapy: Usefulness of selective programs

Studies on apraxia rehabilitation generally suggest that apraxic deficits (in particular, the spatial and temporal errors associated with IMA) are amenable to treatment but that there is poor generalization toward gestures not included in the training programs (Maher and Ochipa, 1997; Ochipa *et al.*, 1995). Goldenberg and Hagmann (1998) examined the effects of ADL training in 15 patients with the objective of finding out whether training improvement can be reliably distinguished from spontaneous recovery. The influence of therapy on the reduction of severe errors was highly significant, suggesting that specific training can restore independence for trained activities. However the improvement did not generalize and it persisted only if the activities were practiced in daily routines after leaving the institution. Using a greater number and a wider variety of gestures for training, Smania *et al.* (2000) showed that patients who received therapy achieved a significant improvement of performance in both IA and IMA, while control patients – who received conventional treatment for aphasia – did not show any significant change in performance. These results are in favor of the effectiveness of a specific training program for the treatment of limb apraxia. Rehabilitation programs can be designed in reference to cognitive models. Based on Roy's model, two main directions for training programs can be distinguished, depending on whether the deficit concerns production or conception of gestures (Etcharry-Bouyx *et al.*, 2000).

A production deficit can be observed in IMA or IA (errors in gripping or misorientation of the object contrasting with preserved recognition of the gesture). In this case, the relearning program is based on a spatio-temporal analysis of the movement. Guidance with sensorimotor support or verbal indications (taking into account presence and severity of aphasia) is proposed to the patient. For spatial aspects, preference is given to the verbal modality for emphasizing spatial coordinates of the gesture or of the target (in terms of direction, distance, lateralization, and concerned joints) and to passive positioning of all the joints involved in the action. For temporal aspects, movement monitoring, kinesthetic support, and verbal indications about the chronological development of action are given. Technical assistances are gradually blurred. The action is carried out repeatedly by the patient from a stage of total guidance with passive positioning and verbal monitoring by the therapist, through a stage of exclusively verbal guidance to a final stage of total independence without any aid. Two single case studies have illustrated the possible success of rehabilitation programs. Bergego *et al.* (1994) have reported a six months training program, with daily sessions, which enabled the patient to use more objects (from 7 to 19 out of 20), and to regain autonomy for daily life. Using a method based on verbalization of sequential order of actions, Pilgrim and Humphreys (1991) obtained positive results in a 29-year-old patient presenting with a left unilateral apraxia.

In the case of conceptual disorders, two main types of error are observed: errors in sequencing and planning actions and errors of object-choices sometimes associated with difficulties in gripping or orientating the object. In these cases, rehabilitation programs try to re-establish knowledge about actions with different tasks:

1. categorization and matching of objects;
2. retrieval of the missing object considering a given device;
3. identification of the correct gesture.

Unusual objects or materials which are not compatible with a given task may be included in trials. Actual use of objects may be carried out by visual imitation of gesture and with support of contextual cues. Such a program may contribute to recover autonomy for elementary daily acts as was the case for the patient reported by Bergego *et al.* (1994). Direct global training in situations supported by specific verbal instructions seem to be more effective than exploration of functionally critical details of objects to be used, in recovering routine actions, with the limit that there is no generalization to non trained gestures (Goldenberg *et al.*, 2001). In order to treat disorders in sequencing actions, patients are invited to conform to scripts, i.e. to organize and plan a goal directed action by segregating it in distinct stages from verbal or visual material. Achievement of this type of task requires adaptive behavior. It depends on the environment and ability to segment action with therapist's aids varying from cuing action using verbal or gestural encouraging to total assistance.

Neural substrates of action: a distributed network where the parietal lobe may be an interface

A great number of studies conducted in animals and in humans suggest a division of functions between a ventral stream of cortical areas (visual and inferotemporal cortex) which are implicated in object recognition and a dorsal stream (posterior parietal cortex and premotor cortex) which plays a crucial role in sensorimotor integration and action. This view has been extended by the "mirror neuron" framework (Rizzolatti et al., 1996) and distinct functions have been respectively attributed to the premotor cortex (thought to mediate the sensory cueing of movement – "what to do") and to the posterior parietal lobe (whose pragmatic role in actions has been emphasized – "how to do"). Moreover, a functional subdivision of the posterior parietal lobe has been advanced. The superior parietal lobe is thought to be crucial for monitoring spatial components of contralateral hand movements during execution. The inferior parietal lobe/intraparietal sulcus system may convey information about object/action structure from the ventral pathway to the dorsal pathway, integrate sensory information for the purpose of planning action and select adaptive motor commands in order to plan actions.

REFERENCES

Basso, A., Capitani, E., Della Sala, S., Laiacona, M. and Spinnler, H. (1987). Recovery from ideomotor apraxia a study on acute stroke patients. *Brain*, **110**, 747–60.

Bergego, C., Pradat-Diehl, P., Taillefer, C. and Migeot, H. (1994). Evaluation et rééducation de l'apraxie d'utilisation des objets. In *l'Apraxie*, ed. D. Le Gall and G. Aubin. Marseille: Solal, pp. 214–23.

Buxbaum, L. J., Schwartz, M. F. and Montgomery, M. W. (1998). The role of semantic memory in object use. *Cogn. Neuropsych.*, **75**, 617–44.

Buxbaum, L. J., Sirigu, A., Schwartz, M. F. and Klatzky, R. (2003). Cognitive representations of hand posture in ideomotor apraxia. *Neuropsychologia*, **41**, 1091–1113.

Buxbaum, L. J., Johnson-Frey, S. H. and Barlett-Williams, M. (2005a). *Neuropsychologia*, **43**, 917–29.

Buxbaum, L. J., Kyle, K. M. and Menon, R. (2005b). On beyond mirror neurons: internal representations subserving imitation and recognition of skilled object-related actions in humans. Cognitive Brain Res., **25**, 226–39.

Chaminade, T., Meltzoff, A. N. and Decety, J. (2005). An fMRI study of imitation: action representation and body schema. *Neuropsychologia*, **43**, 115–27.

Della Sala, S., Basso, A., Laiacona, M. and Papagno, C. (1992). Subcortical localization of ideomotor apraxia: a review and an experimental study. In G. Vallar, S. F. Cappa, and C.-W. Wallesch, eds., *Neuropsychological Disorders Associated with Subcortical Lesions.* Oxford: Oxford University Press, pp. 357–80.

De Renzi, E. (1990). Apraxia. In *Handbook of Clinical Neuropsychology*, Vol **2**, ed. F. Boller and J. Grafman. Amsterdam, New York, Oxford: Elsevier, pp. 245–63.

De Renzi, E., Faglioni, P. and Sorgato, P. (1982). Modality-specific and supramodal mechanisms of apraxia. *Brain*, **105**, 301–12.

De Renzi, E., Faglioni, P., Scarpa, M. and Crisi, G. (1986). Limb apraxia in patients with damage confined to the left basal ganglia and thalamus. *J. Neurol. Neurosurg. Psychiatry*, **49**, 1030–8.

Donkervoort, M., Dekker, J. and Deelman, B. J. (2002). Sensitivity of different ADL measures to apraxia and motor impairments. *Clin. Rehab.*, **16**(3), 299–305.

Donkervoort, M., Dekker, J., Van Den Ende, E., Stehmann-Saris, J. C. and Deelman, B. J. (2000). Prevalence of apraxia among patients with a first left hemisphere stroke in rehabilitation centres and nursing homes. *Clin. Rehab.*, **14**(2), 130–6.

Dumont, C., Ska, B. and Schiavetto, A. (1999). Selective impairment of transitive gestures: An unusual case of apraxia. *Neurocase*, **5**, 447–58.

Etcharry-Bouyx, F. and Le Gall, D. (2003). Comment j'examine l'apraxie gestuelle. *Rev. Neurol.*, **159**(2), 231–4.

Etcharry-Bouyx, F., Le Gall, D. and Pradat-Diehl, P. (2000). La prise en charge rééducative de l'apraxie. In *Traité de Neuropsychologie Tome II*, ed. X. Seron and M. Van der Linden. Marseille: Solal, pp. 245–52.

Freund, H.-J. (2001). The parietal lobe as a sensorimotor interface: a perspective from clinical and neuroimaging data. *Neuroimage*, **14**, 142–6.

Goldenberg, G. (1995). Imitating gestures and manipulating a manikin. The representation of the human body in ideomotor apraxia. *Neuropsychologia*, **33**, 63–72.

(1996). Defective imitation of gestures in patients with damage in the left or right hemispheres. *J. Neurol. Neurosurg. Psychiatry*, **61**, 176–80.

Goldenberg, G. and Hagmann, S. (1997). The meaning of meaningless gestures: a study of visuo-imitative apraxia. *Neuropsychologia*, **35**, 333–41.

(1998). Therapy of activities of daily living in patients with apraxia. *Neuropsych. Rehab.*, **8**(2), 123–41.

Goldenberg, G., Daumüller, M. and Hagmann, S. (2001). Assessment and therapy of complex ADL in apraxia. *Neuropsych. Rehab.*, **11**, 147–68.

Goldenberg, G., Hartmann, K. and Schloot, I. (2003). Defective pantomime of object use in left brain damage: apraxia or asymbolia? *Neuropsychologia*, **41**, 1565–73.

Goldenberg, G., Hentze, S. and Hermsdörfer, J. (2004). The effect of tactile feedback on pantomime of tool use in apraxia. *Neurology*, **63**, 1863–7.

Goodale, M. A. and Milner, A. D. (1992). Separate visual pathways for perception and action. *Trends Neurosci.*, **15**, 20–5.

Habib, M., Ceccaldi, M. and Poncet, M. (1990). Syndrome de déconnexion calleuse par infarctus jonctionnel hémisphérique gauche. *Rev. Neurol. (Paris)*, **146**, 19–24.

Halsband, U., Schmitt, J., Weyers, M., *et al.* (2001). Recognition and imitation of pantomimed motor acts after unilateral parietal and premotor lesions: a perspective on apraxia. *Neuropsychologia*, **39**, 200–16.

Hanna-Pladdy, B., Heilman, K. M. and Foundas, A. L. (2001). Cortical and subcortical contributions to ideomotor apraxia analysis of task demands and error types. *Brain*, **124**, 2513–27.

(2003). Ecological implications of ideomotor apraxia evidence from physical activities of daily living. *Neurology*, **60**, 487–90.

Hartmann, K., Goldenberg, G., Daumüller, M. and Hermsdörfer, J. (2005). It takes the whole brain to make a cup of coffee: the neuropsychology of naturalistic actions involving technical devices. *Neuropsychologia*, **43**, 625–37.

Heath, M., Roy, E. A., Black, S. E. and Westwood, D. A. (2001). Intransitive limb gestures and apraxia following unilateral stroke. *J. Clin. Exp. Neuropsychol.*, **23**(5), 628–42.

Heilman, K. M., Rothi, L. J. and Valenstein, F. (1982). Two forms of ideomotor apraxia. *Neurology*, **32**, 342–6.

Jeannerod, M. and Decety, J. (1995). Mental motor imagery: a window into the representational stages of action. *Curr. Opin. Neurobio.*, **5**, 727–32.

Kleist, K. (1912). Der gang und der gegenwurtige stand der apraxie-forschung. *Ergebnisse der Neurologie und Psychiatrie*, **1**, 342–452.

Le Gall, D. and Etcharry-Bouyx, F. (2003). Sémiologie des troubles apraxiques. *La Revue du Praticien*, **53**, 382–7.

Le Gall, D. and Peigneux, P. (2003). Les apraxies: formes cliniques et modèles théoriques. In *L'apraxie*, ed. D. Le Gall and G. Aubin. Marseille: Solal, pp. 91–132.

Le Gall, D., Morineau, T. and Etcharry-Bouyx, F. (2000). Les apraxies: formes cliniques modèles théoriques et méthodes d'évaluation. In *Traité de Neuropsychologie Tome I*, ed. X. Seron and M. Van der Linden. Marseille: Solal, pp. 225–49.

Liepmann, H. (1908). *Drei Aufsatze aus dem Apraxie Gebiet*, Berlin: Karger.

Maher, L. M. and Ochipa, C. (1997). Management and treatment of limb apraxia. In *Apraxia. The Neuropsychology of Action*, ed. L. J. G. Rothi and K. M. Heilman. Hove: Psychology Press. pp. 75–91.

Makuuchi, M., Kaminaga, T. and Sugishita, M. (2005). Brain activation during ideomotor apraxia: imitation and movements executed by verbal command. *J. Neurol. Neurosurg. Psychiatry*, **76**(1), 25–33.

Mohr, J. P., Pessin, M. S., Finkelstein, S., *et al.* (1978). Broca aphasia: pathologic and clinical. *Neurology*, **28**, 311–24.

Mozaz, M., Rothi, L., Anderson, J., Crucian, G. P. and Heilman, K. (2002). Postural knowledge of transitive pantomimes and intransitive gestures. *J. Int. Neuropsychol. Soc.*, **8**, 958–62.

Mühlau, M., Hermsdörfer, J., Goldenberg, G., *et al.* (2005). Left inferior parietal dominance in gesture imitation: an fMRI study. *Neuropsychologia*, **43**, 1086−98.

Nadeau, S. E., Roeltgen, D. P., Sevush, S., Ballinger, W. E. and Watson, R. T. (1994). Apraxia due to a pathologically documented thalamic infarction. *Neurology*, **44**, 2133−7.

Ochipa, C., Maher, L. M. and Rothi, L. J. G. (1995). Treatment of ideomotor limb apraxia. *Twenty Third Annual International Neuropsychology Society Meeting Abstracts*, **149**.

Peigneux, P. and Van der Linden, M. (2000). Présentation d'une batterie neuropsychologique et cognitive pour l'évaluation de l'apraxie gestuelle. *Revue de Neuropsychologie*, **10**(2), 311−62.

Peigneux, P., Van der Linden, M. and Le Gall, D. (2003). Evaluation des apraxies gestuelles. In *L'apraxie*, ed. D. Le Gall and G. Aubin. Marseille: Solal, pp. 133−66.

Perenin, M. T. and Vighetto, A. (1988). Optic ataxia: a specific disruption in visuomotor mechanisms. *Brain*, **111**, 643−4.

Pilgrim, E. and Humphreys, G. W. (1991). Impairment of action to visual objects in a case of ideomotor apraxia. *Cogn. Neuropsychol.*, **8**, 459−73.

Poncet, M., Ali Cherif, A., Choux, M., Boudouresques, J. and Lhermitte, F. (1978). Etude neuropsychologique d'un syndrome de déconnexion calleuse totale avec hémianopsie latérale homonyme droite. *Rev. Neurol. (Paris)*, **134**, 633−53.

Pradat-Diehl, P., Taillefer, C. and Migeot, H. (1999). Rééducation de l'apraxie gestuelle pour l'utilisation des objets. In *La Rééducation en Neuropsychologie: Études de Cas*, ed. P. Azouvi, D. Perrier and M. Van der Linden. Marseille: Solal, pp. 265−73.

Pramstaller, P. P. and Marsden, C. D. (1996). The basal ganglia and apraxia. *Brain*, **119**, 319−40.

Rapcsak, S. Z., Ochipa, C., Beeson, P. M. and Rubens, A. B. (1993). Praxis and the right hemisphere. *Brain Cogn.*, **23**, 181−202.

Rizzolatti, G., Fadiga, L., Gallese, V. and Fogassi, L. (1996). Premotor cortex and the recognition of motor actions. *Cogn. Brain Res.*, **3**, 131−41.

Rothi, L. J. G., Ochipa, C. and Heilman, K. M. (1991). A cognitive neuropsychological model of limb praxis. *Cogn. Neuropsychol.*, **8**, 443−58.

(1997). A cognitive neuropsychological model of limb praxis. In *Apraxia. The Neuropsychology of Action*, ed. L. J. G. Rothi and K. M. Heilman. Hove: Psychology Press. pp. 29−50.

Roy, E. A. and Square, P. A. (1985). Common considerations in the study of limb, verbal and oral apraxia. In *Neuropsychological Studies of Apraxia and Related Disorders*, ed. E. A. Roy. Amsterdam: North-Holland, pp. 111−62.

Roy, E. A., Heath, M., Westwood, D., *et al.* (2000). Task demands and limb apraxia in stroke. *Brain Cogn.*, **44**, 253−79.

Saeki, S., Ogata, H., Okubo, T., Takahashi, K. and Hoshuyama, T. (1995). Return to work after stroke. *Stroke*, **26**, 399−401.

Sirigu, A., Cohen, L., Duhamel, J. R., *et al.* (1995). A selective impairment of hand posture for object utilization in apraxia. *Cortex*, **31**, 41−55.

Smania, N., Girardi, F., Domenicali, C., Lora, E. and Aglioti, S. (2000). The rehabilitation of limb apraxia: a study in left brain damaged patients. *Arch. Phys. Med. Rehabil.*, **81**, 379−88.

Sundet, K., Finset, A. and Reinvang, I. (1988). Neuropsychological predictors in stroke rehabilitation. *J. Clin. Exp. Neuropsychol.*, **10**(4), 363–79.

Watson, R. T., Fleet, S., Gonzalez-Rothi, L. and Heilman, K. (1986). Apraxia and the supplementary motor area. *Arch. Neurol.*, **43**, 787–92.

Wetter, S., Poole, J. L. and Haaland, K. Y. (2005). Functional implications of ipsilesional motor deficits after unilateral stroke. *Arch. Phys. Med. Rehabil.*, **86**, 776–81.

Zwinkels, A., Geusgens, C., Van de Sande, P. and Van Heugten, C. (2004). Assessment of apraxia: inter-rater reliability of a new apraxia test, association between apraxia and other cognitive deficits and prevalence of apraxia in a rehabilitation setting. *Clin. Rehabil.*, **18**(7), 819–27.

4

Aphasia in stroke

Andrew Kertesz
University of Western Ontario

Introduction

Stroke related aphasia occurs in certain patterns, forming predictable aphasic syndromes, creating a basis for cortical localizationist models and providing reliable diagnosis and prognosis. Approximately 25% of stroke patients have significant aphasia (Leske, 1981), making this a common neurological and rehabilitation issue. Broca (1861) established the importance of the left hemisphere in language and Wernicke (1874) extended the description of aphasic syndromes including comprehension deficit, recognizing the sensorimotor organization of language accompanying anteroposterior anatomical distinction. Upon these foundations, a number of aphasic syndromes have been described subsequently. The taxonomy of these syndromes has been much debated, but in Table 4.1 the most commonly accepted classification and terminology are defined.

The cerebral cortex, specialized for language, functionally unique and anatomically localizable, similar to the primary motor or visual cortex, has become an important topic for research. There is anatomical and physiological evidence for overlapping networks specialized for language, output and comprehension. The characteristics of such networks can be summarized as follows:

1. A function is usually represented at multiple sites, so that lesions from multiple sites can produce a similar deficit.
2. Each area may belong to several overlapping networks, so a lesion in a single area often produces multiple deficits.
3. Severe and lasting deficit of function occurs when all or most structural components of a network are involved.

Language deficits can be described at several levels. Linguists have compartmentalized language processing as follows:

1. *Phonology*, or the knowledge of the rules of pronunciation and perception of the sounds of language. Native speakers of any language acquire the processes of phonology in the first two or three years of their lives, but the rules of phonology can be learned later for other languages as well, even though

Table 4.1. Major aphasic stroke symptoms

	Output	Comprehension	Repetition	Naming	Other feature
Broca's aphasia — expressive aphasia	−	+	−	−	Agrammatic
Pure motor aphasia — aphemia	−	+	−	±	Better writing
Transcortical motor aphasia	−	+	+	±	Not paraphasic
Global aphasia	−	−	−	−	Mute or stereotypy
Wernicke's aphasia — sensory aphasia	+	−	−	−	Paraphasic
Pure word deafness — cortical deafness	+	−	−	−	Better reading
Transcortical sensory aphasia	+	−	+	±	Semantic jargon
Anomic aphasia	+	+	+	−	Only naming deficit
Conduction aphasia	+	+	−	+	Mainly repetition deficit
Isolation or mixed transcortical aphasia	−	−	+	−	Only repetition spared

it becomes more difficult beyond a critical period after puberty. Most of us cannot acquire a foreign language without an accent beyond this critical period.

2. *Semantics* or the systematic knowledge of the meaning of words.

3. *Syntax or grammar* incorporating the rules of the relationship and shape of words, phrases, and sentences, essential to convey accurate meaning.

4. *Pragmatics*, or the rules of maintaining the give and take of conversation, including responsiveness, coherence, relevance, topic maintenance etc.

All these linguistic processes seamlessly intertwine to produce the most complex and unique of human skills, *communication*. Although here we talk about the far-reaching effects of impaired verbal communication, it should be remembered that sign language for instance has similar elements, including syntax, semantics, and pragmatics (but not phonology of course, which is replaced by sign morphology), and stroke produces aphasic syndromes in the deaf, which involve these components of sign language analogously to spoken speech.

Broca's aphasia, expressive aphasia, motor aphasias

Articulated language is an example of complex cognitive function subserved by a neural network. Speech output is an easily available, clinically and scientifically much studied function. It is elaborated differently whether it is in response to questions (responsive speech), spontaneous (internally generated) expression of ideas, descriptive speech, or repetition.

Spoken language incorporates many subfunctions, which have been categorized by linguists as articulation, fluency, prosody, phonological processing, lexical retrieval, syntax, pragmatics, etc. Nevertheless, all or most of the functional components tend to be involved to some extent in the clinical syndrome of Broca's aphasia, which can be reliably defined by standardized test scores (Kertesz, 1979) or by careful clinical description. Many identifiable, even dissociable, central processes such as agrammatism or dysprosody contribute to the syndrome, but these do not have nearly as reliable localization as the syndrome as a whole. Articulation and language output are affected in other syndromes as well and these will be discussed further.

Broca's aphasia

Broca's aphasia is defined as effortful speech output with hesitations, pauses, word-finding difficulty, phonemic errors (verbal apraxia) consisting of substitutions, deletions, transpositions and anticipations, occasional semantic errors, and agrammatism, but relatively preserved comprehension (Goodglass and Kaplan, 1972).

Agrammatism, which is the hallmark of Broca's aphasia, in many western languages is characterized by short utterances, omission of small grammatical words such as articles, prepositions, auxiliary verbs, and inflexions. Nouns or single-word substantive utterances predominate and the verb is often deleted. Speech becomes telegraphic suggesting to some that it represents an "economy of effort" (Pick, 1913). Agrammatism has different manifestations in other languages (Goodglass, 1997). Although in English for example it is manifested by the loss of closed class grammatical words, mentioned above, in highly inflected languages the loss of inflectional morphology, in others the loss of word order and in tonal languages the loss of grammatical prosody are characteristic. The other characteristic feature of Broca's aphasia is verbal apraxia, a disorder of motor programming, defined as stumbling, repetition, distortion of words, phonemes, especially the first syllable, or the initial consonants, phonetic groping ("conduite d'approach"), alteration of prosody, emphasis, slowing, and segmentation. More about this aspect of articulated language is discussed below under "Pure motor aphasia".

Lesions producing Broca's aphasia have been described from Broca's area which is the "foot" of the inferior frontal convolution or F3, although they often extend beyond this to involve the rolandic operculum, anterior insula, subcortical (capsulostriatal) area, and periventricular or centrum semiovale lesion (Moutier, 1908; Henschen, 1922; Mohr, 1976, Kertesz *et al.*, 1979; Levine and

Sweet, 1983). Involvement of only Broca's area is usually followed by good recovery (Mohr, 1976). The variation in lesion size and location is related to the extent of middle cerebral artery occlusion. The overlap of acute aphasic lesions, based on our study, is summarized in Figure 4.1 (Kertesz *et al.*, 1979).

Persisting Broca's aphasia is associated with large lesions including not only Broca's area (posterior third of F3 and the frontal operculum), but also the inferior parietal and often the subcortical regions (Kertesz, 1988; Kertesz *et al.*, 1979; Mohr, 1976). Persistent nonfluency has been associated with lesions extending to the rolandic cortical region and underlying white matter in previous studies (Mayendorf, 1930; Lecours and Lhermitte, 1976; Levine and Sweet, 1983). The involvement of the central white matter was also important for the fluency deficit in the head injured population of Russell and Espir (1961) and Ludlow *et al.* (1986), and in stroke (Naeser *et al.*, 1989). The centrum semiovale or periventricular white matter, which is involved in persistent cases of global Broca's aphasia, often includes the pyramidal tract, thalamocortical somatosensory projections, striatocortical connections, callosal radiations, the subcallosal fasciculus (Muratoff, 1893), thalamocortical projections from the dorsomedial and ventrolateral nuclei (Yakovlev and Locke, 1961), and the occipitofrontal fasciculus (Dejerine and Dejerine-Klumpke, 1895). The overlap of lesions with persisting aphasic syndromes is summarized in Figure 4.2.

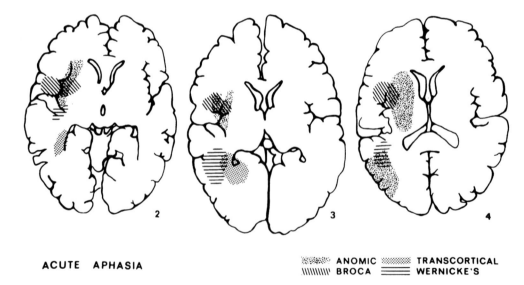

ACUTE APHASIA

ANOMIC   TRANSCORTICAL
BROCA   WERNICKE'S

Figure 4.1   The overlap of lesions in acute aphasic syndromes. Reprinted with permission (Kertesz *et al.*,1979).

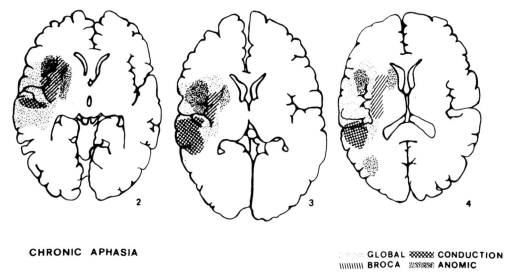

Figure 4.2   The overlap of persisting aphasic lesions. Reprinted with permission (Kertesz *et al.*, 1979).

Lesion location was evaluated in Broca's aphasics, who were divided at the median for poor and good recovery. The structures with significant involvement (more than 50%) were the inferior frontal gyrus, especially the pars opercularis and triangularis, and the insula in both groups. The difference between the persisting cases of Broca's aphasics and those who showed good recovery was most prominent in the involvement of the precentral, postcentral, and supramarginal gyri in cases of poor recovery. The subcortical regions showed significant differences in the involvement of the putamen and the caudate, which was twice as frequent in the persistent cases (Kertesz, 1988). Outcome measures had a high negative correlation with lesion size throughout. Naming was an interesting exception, indicating possibly a ceiling-effect combined with the relative persistence of even moderate naming deficit. All of these patients were treated with a variable amount of language therapy; many of them for the duration of the study. Some of them participated in a formal study of language therapy (Shewan and Kertesz, 1984).

There are several patterns by which a vascular lesion could produce Broca's aphasia. The most common pattern involves the frontal opercular and central cortex, and the anterior insula, with or without significant subcortical involvement. These patients often recover quite well, with the exception of those who had cortical, central, insular, and subcortical involvement together. There is, however, a certain amount of variability in how the components of the network are affected producing different varieties of the syndrome and various degrees of recovery.

This region was considered crucial in aphasia by Pierre Marie (who called it "the Quadrilateral", and the anterior insula was singled out more recently as a "novel" center of articulation (Dronkers, 1996). This and other overlap studies have been criticized because the overlap represents ischemic lesions, not necessarily functional localization. A more recent study using MRI diffusion and perfusion weighted images in acute stroke reclaimed Broca's area as the crucial localization of articulated speech (Hillis *et al.*, 2004). The debate has come around a full circle since Broca (1861).

Another form of nonfluent aphasia named Primary Progressive Aphasia (Mesulam, 1987) recognized increasingly as part of clinical Pick's disease (Kertesz *et al.*, 1994), but the temporal characteristic of this syndrome is the opposite from stroke-induced aphasia. The onset is insidious and deterioration instead of improvement takes place with time. Language impairment in Alzheimer's disease is also common, but it is always fluent initially and logoclonia (syllabic repetition) and mutism are late features (Appel *et al.*, 1982).

Global aphasia

Global aphasia is defined by the loss of speech output, as well as comprehension, usually associated with destruction of both the anterior and posterior language areas (Kertesz *et al.*, 1979). Large middle cerebral artery stroke, occasionally hemorrhage, is the usual etiology. However, in patients who are initially globally aphasic, Wernicke's area may be spared. These patients tend to recover towards Broca's aphasia. Even "Broca's area" cortex may not be destroyed, although it is usually disconnected from the rest of the language cortex by white matter involvement (von Mayendorf, 1930; Naeser *et al.*, 1989). Occasionally, mostly white matter lesions can produce persistent global aphasia. There are also case reports of patients with initial global aphasia without hemiplegia, who recover dramatically when they have posterior-frontal and posterior temporal lesions but sparing of the central structures (Van Horn and Hawes, 1982; Ferro, 1983).

The classification of severely non-fluent aphasics influences the results of localization and recovery studies. For instance, in the Boston Diagnostic Aphasia Examination (BDAE; Goodglass and Kaplan, 1972), a large group of what others would classify as severe Broca's aphasics may be labeled, at times, as "mixed anterior aphasics." In the classification system of the Aachen Aphasia Test (AAT; Huber *et al.*, 1983), many global aphasics would be reclassified as Broca's aphasics in other clinics. Some of these problems in taxonomy have been systematically studied in the comparison of aphasia batteries (Ferro and Kertesz, 1987). Global and Broca's aphasics, as defined by our taxonomy and methods of measurements, have similar spontaneous language characteristics. In our previous taxonomic studies (Kertesz and Phipps, 1977), these were the two closest groups in the nearest-neighbor-network analysis. The major difference between the two groups is in the extent of comprehension deficit. Since comprehension often recovers well, there are a great number of patients who change from global to Broca's aphasia during recovery, producing a change in syndrome label (*Syndromenwandeln*) (Leischner, 1976).

Pure motor aphasia

Pure motor aphasia, also called cortical motor aphasia, aphemia, or verbal apraxia, has been associated with Broca's area anterior subcortical, inferior rolandic, and insular cortical lesions. Verbal apraxia is frequently used by speech pathologists to denote hesitation, stuttering, dysprosody, initial consonant substitution, deletions, repetition, transposition, and anticipation (Darley *et al.*, 1975) that can occur as part of non-fluent or Broca's aphasia, or occasionally alone, as a "pure motor aphasia" also known as aphemia, or cortical dysarthria. All forms of speech output are affected, including repetition, in contrast to transcortical motor aphasia, but writing is usually spared (unlike in Broca's aphasia). However the patient is not agrammatic and anomia or naming difficulty is not severe. Localization is generally considered to involve Broca's area and surrounding motor cortex and insula, but recovery is usually complete as other areas of the articulatory network usually take over the function.

Transcortical motor aphasia

Transcortical motor aphasia is characterized by poor spontaneous speech but good repetition and comprehension. There is a variable naming deficit and the written output is also poor. The localization of lesions is characteristically in the superior mesial frontal region or the supplementary speech area in the dominant hemisphere (Goldstein, 1948; Kornyey, 1975; Rubens, 1975; Arseni and Botez, 1961). These are often caused by an anterior cerebral artery stroke. The importance of the *supplementary motor area* on the left was recognized by Penfield and Roberts (1959), who renamed it the "supplementary speech area" because of the frequent speech arrest that was found during stimulation of this region. Cytoarchitecturally, the supplementary motor cortex appears to represent a paralimbic extension of the limbic cortex (Sanides, 1970). This suggests a link between the limbic system and initiation of the motor mechanisms of speech. The lack of speech initiation is often considered a part of a general hypokinetic syndrome associated with frontal lobe lesions. The term "adynamic aphasia" has also been used to describe this behavior since Arnold Pick and Kleist. Recovery is usually excellent and these patients are generally only seen in acute units.

Wernicke's aphasia, sensory aphasia

Language comprehension is a complex process involving analysis of acoustic and phonological properties of input, as well as a recognition of syntactic and lexical elements (Liebermann *et al.*, 1967). This rapid parallel processing of input and matching it to linguistic precepts is a highly specialized, left hemisphere, analytical function. The most likely candidate to perform this is the auditory association cortex, localized to the superior temporal gyrus region and the planum temporale located behind Heschl's gyrus and well connected to the rest of the temporal parietal and frontal lobes. It has special cytoarchitectonics, suited to carry out sophisticated feedback and feed forward procedures.

Wernicke's aphasia

Wernicke's aphasia is characterized by fluent, paraphasic speech with impaired comprehension, repetition, and naming. Syntax and morphology are relatively preserved, but the substantive words are often substituted by semantic or phonological paraphasias. At times a large number of paraphasias, almost all nouns, distort the speech output to the extent it sounds like jargon. At times this is produced under pressure in great quantities and the patients are not aware of their disability (anosognosia for language impairment). Reading and writing are similarly affected. The taxonomic boundaries for Wernicke's aphasia can be defined with language scores, although this may be considered arbitrary (Kertesz, 1982).

Pure word deafness

"Pure word deafness" is used when the patient complains of not understanding speech, but hearing, reading, and speech output remain undisturbed (Kleist, 1962). One type is called "word form deafness" (Kohn and Friedman, 1986). These patients often "mishear" phonologically similar words, and they cannot tell words from non-words (lexical decision). The other type is "word meaning deafness" where patients can perform lexical decision tasks but cannot access semantics (Franklin *et al.*, 1994). *Auditory agnosia* for nonverbal sounds and amusia is often associated, although these symptoms may be seen with right-sided lesions without the verbal component. In *cortical deafness*, which is the result of bilateral temporal lesions, the patient appears clinically deaf with preserved primary hearing, but impaired central auditory processes (Kertesz, 1983).

Neologistic jargon

Neologistic jargon output is distinctive and occurs in severe Wernicke's aphasia, associated with lesions of both the superior temporal and inferior parietal regions

(Kertesz and Benson, 1970). The superior posterior temporal branch of the middle cerebral artery is usually involved. Neologistic jargon is said to occur when most substantive words are substituted with unintelligible phonological paraphasias. Linguistic explanations of jargon are numerous; one postulates anomic gaps that are filled with semantic paraphasias, which are unstable, when they come to the phonological stage, before speech output. The jargon words carry the phonology of the language spoken, and when a bilingual jargon aphasic attempts to communicate in another language the jargon phonology resembles the second language. Only occasionally will all be words substituted (the *phonetic* jargon of Alajouanine). *Semantic jargon* consists of substitutions of words by meaningful words, often related to the target (semantic paraphasias). However, when most words are replaced and the meaning is undecipherable, the use of jargon is descriptive. Less severe versions are called irrelevant or tangential speech. These may have more meaning than jargon.

Wernicke's aphasia with semantic jargon is correlated with lesions that are somewhat smaller, inferior, and more temporal than those with neologisms or phonemic paraphasia (Kertesz, 1983). Other CT studies indicated that patients with semantic substitutions have lesions posterior to those with phonemic paraphasia (Cappa *et al.*, 1981). Wernicke has postulated that the auditory association area plays a monitoring role in language output (presaging modern concepts of feedback and parallel processing), and its damage results in paraphasic, faulty speech.

Conduction aphasia

Conduction aphasia is distinguished by poor repetition with relatively fluent, but phonologically paraphasic speech and good comprehension. The term was originated by Wernicke (1874) on the basis of the theory that conduction of sensory impulses to motor patterns is impaired. However, it was Lichtheim (1885) who specified the disturbance of repetition as a feature of conduction aphasia. Goldstein (1948) considered it "central aphasia," central in the language area and central to input and output processes and many others subsequently accepted it as a separate form. Some conduction aphasics have a great deal of struggle to approximate target phonemes (conduits d'approche or phonemic approximations), and some investigators consider conduction aphasia a form of expressive aphasia – such as Luria, who called these patients "afferent motor aphasics." The patients are aware of their mistakes and their efforts are considered corrective. The repetition deficit in conduction aphasia has been viewed a a disturbance in short-term verbal memory (Warrington and Shallice, 1969) as an ordering deficiency (Tzortis and Albert, 1974). The more fluent varieties can be distinguished on taxonomic studies (Kertesz and Phipps, 1977) and their lesions are also more posterior. More recently, some patients have been renamed "deep dysphasics" as they had difficulty in accessing meaning through phonology, lexicalized non-words, and produced semantic paraphasias (Katz and Goodglass, 1990).

Lesions are characteristically located in the posterior temporoparietal region at the end of the Sylvian fissure, and involve the posterior insula as Wernicke postulated, or the arcuate fasciculus transmitting language information from Wernicke's area forward to the articulatory network, to Broca's area.

Transcortical sensory aphasia

Transcortical sensory aphasia is characterized by fluent, semantic jargon, poor comprehension, and good repetition. These patients usually have far more posterior lesions, usually in the watershed area between the middle cerebral and posterior cerebral circulation (Kertesz *et al.*, 1982), although at times thalamic lesions are described with "transcortical sensory" features. Recovery is usually rapid unless the syndrome evolves from a more severe lesion initially producing Wernicke's aphasia. A progressive variety of this syndrome is seen with frontotemporal dementia, and interest has concentrated on the loss of meaning of words as the primary feature; hence the designation "semantic dementia" (Snowden *et al.*, 1989). Although the clinical pattern can be similar, the course is progressive, the opposite of the stroke syndrome.

Isolation syndrome

Isolation syndrome, or mixed transcortical aphasia, has features of both motor and sensory transcortical aphasia, and tends to have a poor prognosis with nonfluency persisting and not all comprehension returning, depending on the etiology. It is called isolation syndrome because the lesions tend to surround the middle cerebral artery territory, often in watershed areas, isolating the language areas (Goldstein, 1948). It occurs relatively uncommonly and the recovery patterns have not been described extensively. In our experience, persisting cases occur with strokes and with post-traumatic lesions. Both frontal and parietal association areas are disconnected from the central perisylvian language core.

Anomic aphasia

Anomic aphasia is the mildest form of aphasic syndromes characterized by fluent output, good comprehension, and only naming and word finding difficulty. Word finding or word access, the retrieval of lexical items (often tested by naming), is a fundamental process in language, and *anomia* is a feature of most aphasic syndromes. Various types of anomia have been distinguished, and certain differences in brain damage associated with these types have been described

(Benson, 1979). Anterior and central lesions are more likely to produce lexical retrieval deficit without a loss of semantic representation. Posterior temporoparietal lesions often produce naming difficulty, which is associated with some comprehension deficit for the same lexical item or a loss of meaning of words, even though they may be used in a correct grammatical sentence. Head (1926) called these cases "semantic aphasia." The study of lexical access and semantic processing is a major scientific and clinical topic. Recent advances in this field include the study of modality-specific fields (verbal vs. visual) and the category specificity of recognition and retrieval of lexical items. Lexical retrieval is thought to be dependent on a widely distributed cortical network (Berndt and Mitchum, 1997). Lesion studies have suggested the role of left temporoparietal and temporo-occipital cortex, and functional activation has added the frontal lobe as having a role in semantic processing (Petersen *et al.*, 1990). Considering the complex nature of semantic association, narrowly restricted localization of this function is not likely. This is already evidenced from the wide distribution of lesions resulting in anomia or anomic aphasia. Patients who only have anomic aphasia *de novo* usually recover well. Mild word finding and naming difficulty are very common in acute stroke. They can be seen transiently with subcortical, anterior cortical, and posterior cortical lesions. Rapid recovery is the rule even before these patients are transferred to rehabilitation.

Subcortical stroke aphasias

The role of subcortical structures in language is not fully agreed upon. Marie (1906; 1926) proposed a role for subcortical structures in language, and some of these results have been recently duplicated. Motor impairments often dominate the deficit in lesions of the basal ganglia. These range from dysarthria and hypophonia (which has been known to occur commonly after thalamotomies) to severe global aphasia. Anomic aphasia is often observed, presenting as a disturbance of word retrieval and rather hesitant speech (Mazzocchi and Vignolo, 1979; Alexander and Loverme, 1980). The often-preserved repetition is called a "transcortical feature" (Selby, 1967; Cappa and Vignolo, 1979). Bell (1968) considered the deficit to be similar to the aphasias of the frontal regions. Lesions in the putamen and the anterior internal capsule produces slow, anomic, dysarthric speech, and with posterior extension comprehension is also impaired with paraphasic speech and jargon (Barat *et al.*, 1981; Naeser *et al.*, 1982; Damasio *et al.*, 1982).

Isolated lesions of the caudate or putamen are rare, but both have been described as causing transient speech deficits (Hier *et al.*, 1977).

Damasio *et al.* (1982) found infarcts in the anterior limb of the internal capsule and in the striatum caused aphasia, while non-aphasics had more lateral or caudal lesions. Naeser *et al.* (1982) divided nine patients with capsuloputaminal lesions into three syndromes related to lesion site. Patients with lesions extending into anterior-superior periventricular white matter had good comprehension and grammatical, but slow, dysarthric speech. Posterior extension across the temporal isthmus resulted in fluent speech with poor comprehension. Patients with both anterior-superior and posterior extension had global aphasia. Alexander *et al.* (1987) presented a more detailed model. Only minor language disorders were seen with lesions confined to striatum and internal capsule, and it was postulated that subcortical aphasia is due to disruption of intra-hemispheric white matter pathways. Thalamic lesions produce fluctuating jargon aphasia alternating with relatively nonfluent speech (Mohr *et al.*, 1975). Although subcortical lesions are often said to produce atypical syndromes (Damasio *et al.*, 1982) when an attempt is made to compare the scores of patients with subcortical lesions with equivalent sized cortical lesions, the differences are not significant (Kertesz, 1984; Basso *et al.*, 1987; Kirk and Kertesz, 1994). Distant cortical hypometabolism or diaschisis are considered possible reasons for the deficit, in addition to whatever intrinsic coordinating or processing may take place in the basal ganglia (Metter *et al.*, 1981; Perani *et al.*, 1987; Baron *et al.*, 1986).

Alexia and agraphia

Disturbance of reading and writing may occur in isolation with distinct cortical localization, but also in various combinations with aphasia. Written language functions are also subserved by networks and therefore more than one lesion site will account for the same syndrome. Dejerine (1892) made the classical distinction between pure alexia *without* agraphia with left occipital lesions, which usually involve the splenium or its radiation, and alexia *with* agraphia which are associated with parietal, at times specifically angular gyrus lesions on the dominant side. Dejerine's description of the lesion in alexia without agraphia was the prime model for the disconnection theories postulating the existence of white matter lesions disconnecting various cortical language processors (Geschwind, 1965). Pure alexia is at times called *visual alexia*. One variety is called *spelling dyslexia*, because the patients try to spell or sound out each word and guess their meaning from the sound. The recent linguistic distinction between *deep* and *surface* dyslexia (deep and surface refers to linguistic, not anatomical structures), based on error analysis of the reading of non-words and orthographically irregular words, is partially correlated with anatomical differences (Ellis, 1984). Deep dyslexia seems related to large perisylvian infarcts and corresponds to what other authors describe as aphasic alexia (or the third alexia) (Benson, 1979). Surface dyslexia or reading without comprehension is seen mainly with temporal damage (Bub and Kertesz, 1982). Other varieties of lesions disconnecting primary visual input from the angular gyrus were termed "preangular" or "subangular" alexias by Greenblatt (1983).

Agraphia is associated with partial lobe lesions on the dominant side but agraphia is common with any lesion producing aphasia, although dissociations have also been observed (Bub and Kertesz, 1982). Frontal lobe lesions can produce agraphia, although the existence of Exner's center in the second frontal convolution in front of the hand area of the precentral gyrus has not been generally supported. Recent studies showed a considerable amount of agraphia with purely subcortical lesions, which is somewhat different from agraphia due to cortical lesions because it seems mostly the graphomotor aspects rather than grammatical and semantic aspects are involved (Kertesz, 1984). This type of agraphia used to be designated as "apraxic agraphia."

Ideographic (Kanji) and syllabic (Kana) writing in Japanese have been reported to be affected by different lesion localization, suggesting different neuronal network in processing. Kanji processing is semantic and context-dependent. Kana, on the other hand, can be read aloud without semantic processing. Iwata (1984) suggested semantic processing takes place through inferior occipitotemporal connections, because lesions in this area interfered with Kanji selectively (Kawahata *et al.*, 1988; Kawamura *et al.*, 1987). Dorsal connections through the angular gyrus are involved in Kana (or phonological) processing, similar to Indo-European languages. Pure agraphia for Kanji has also been reported with subcortical damage undercutting the left inferior temporal gyrus (Mochizuki and Ohtomo, 1988).

Recovery from aphasic stroke syndromes

Clinicians have recognized that aphasic stroke syndromes are not stable and recovery takes place to a considerable extent. Wernicke (1886) postulated that much of the recovery from aphasic symptoms is affected by right hemisphere compensation. von Monakow (1914) stated: "the temporary nature is one of the most important characteristics of aphasia." He based his diaschisis theory on observations with aphasics and on the analogy of spinal shock, well established by physiologists. Diaschisis means that acute brain damage deprives the surrounding, functionally connected areas from a trophic influence causing a severe deficit initially. As the surrounding areas recover by acquiring reinnervation from somewhere else, or become active after adapting to the state of parietal denervation, recovery takes place. Recovery alters not only the severity but also the pattern of the language disturbance. The same clinical pattern is seen with larger lesions in the chronic stage and results in a different overlap of lesions. These differences are illustrated in Figures 4.1 and 4.2.

There are certain structural limitations of recovery, allowing compensation to take place only in certain areas, such as the adjacent cortex, contralateral homologous cortex or hierarchically connected structure, such as the subcortical ganglia (Lashley, 1938; Bucy, 1934). The principle of contralateral homologous cortical substitution was based on large left hemisphere lesions with relatively good recovery where there was very little left hemisphere remaining to take over. More recently, CAT scan studies made the same point (Cummings *et al.*, 1979; Landis *et al.*, 1980). In addition, in some patients who became aphasic with a single left hemisphere stroke but recovered, a second, right hemisphere, stroke produced a language deficit again (Nielsen, 1946; Levine and Mohr, 1979; Cambier *et al.*, 1983). These cases, however, may have represented bilateral language organization to begin with, rather than a commonly operating mechanism of functional transfer to the contralateral hemispheres.

The idea of compensation through right hemisphere function, even after partial left hemisphere damage, was also supported by studies of sodium amytal given to aphasics who had recovered (Kinsbourne, 1971; Czopf, 1972). These studies indicated that, even though the aphasic disturbance occurred from a left hemisphere lesion, it was the right hemispheric injection that increased the language disturbance, implying the right hemisphere compensated for the previous deficit produced by the left-side lesion.

The variation in recovery, which cannot entirely be explained by the extent and location of lesions, has been postulated to relate to differences in language laterality, handedness, age, and gender. Subirana's (1969), Gloning *et al.*'s (1969), and Geschwind's (1974) suggestion that left handers and right handers, with a family history of left handedness, recover better from aphasia because more bilateral language distribution is based on anecdotal evidence. Recent studies of anatomical asymmetry on CT scans, inspired by the demonstration of commonly larger planum temporale on the left by Geschwind and Levitsky (1968), have correlated better outcome with atypical or less asymmetry (Pieniadz *et al.*, 1983). This is also based on the idea that this pattern may be associated with more right hemisphere language. We have studied the factor of anatomical asymmetry on CT, as measured by occipital width, frontal width, and protuberance (petalia), and could not confirm that atypical asymmetry played a role in recovery in any of the aphasic groups (Kertesz, 1988). It could be that anatomical asymmetries relate more to handedness variables rather than language distribution, as suggested by some of our studies in normals (Kertesz *et al.*, 1992); therefore, we are not seeing an effect on language recovery. It has been suggested that women have more bilaterally distributed language (McGlone, 1980). However, when we looked at sex differences in recovery, we found none and no evidence to support better right hemisphere substitution by women (Kertesz, 1988). We did not find sex differences in the anterior–posterior distribution of language impairment either (Kertesz and Benke, 1989).

Cerebral blood flow (CBF) and positron emission tomography (PET) studies of cerebral metabolism provide methodologies that add functional information to structural or lesion studies of recovery. Recent studies of CBF with xenon-133 have also revealed a right-hemisphere hypometabolism in aphasic strokes, the extent of which has correlated with recovery to a modest degree (Knopman *et al.*, 1984). PET studies of cerebral metabolism have shown a great deal of hypometabolism surrounding, but also remote from, cerebral infarcts, suggesting that not only surrounding areas but also homologous areas in the contralateral hemisphere play a role in compensation (Metter *et al.*, 1981). Recent studies with perfusion and diffusion MRI imaging have shown that recovery in the acute stage is probably dependent on improving circulation in surrounding areas (Hillis *et al.*, 2004). Some CBF studies showed no significant change while clinical recovery occurred in severe aphasics (Demeurisse *et al.*, 1983). Patients who improved more showed more blood flow in the left hemisphere. This appears to be the consequence of the size of the lesion, which correlates with the CBF changes. Another CBF study showed better than 60% hemispheric flow in patients with good recovery (Nagata *et al.*, 1986). More recent studies of PET activation suggested right hemisphere, as well as ipsilateral, compensation (Weiller *et al.*, 1992).

Functional activation of language

More recent functional activation confirms the importance of the posterior temporal area in auditory perception of language, and the central and premotor cortex in articulation, in addition to some newly emphasized components to the language network, such as the mesial frontal and lateral areas in word retrieval and semantic association (Petersen *et al.*, 1990). The anterior cingulate gyrus appeared part of an anterior attentional system indicated by its activation while monitoring lists of words for semantic category (Petersen *et al.*, 1990). Some of the continuing work with PET and O^{15} and recent efforts on magnetic resonance functional activation promises to shed further light on these issues (Weiller *et al.*, 1992; Binder and Rao, 1994; Chertkow and Murtha, 1997). Functional activation is complementary to the clinical study of aphasic stroke syndromes.

Conclusion

The size and location of lesions, time-from-onset, etiology, and initial severity are complex, interdependent factors in clinical symptomatology and the recovery of language loss. Other biological factors, such as age, education, handedness, and sex play a less significant role when an adult stroke population is followed. Lesion size is undoubtedly a significant factor in the extent of recovery and can be easily determined by CT or MRI scanning. An exception to the negative correlation between language recovery and lesion size is comprehension. In some patients, even with large lesions, the amount of comprehension recovery is considerable; while patients with small lesions demonstrate a relatively small degree of recovery. One of the unresolved issues remains whether ipsilateral connected adjacent, or distant, even contralateral, cortex plays a major role in compensation. The answer is probably both, but our studies of lesion location and recovery in Broca's and Wernicke's aphasias suggest ipsilateral connected structures play the major role in restoration of function after damage. These are structures that are likely used normally in the language network, although for somewhat different functions at different times. The functional participation by these structures implies neuro-plasticity rather than built-in redundancy when recovery from damage occurs. The cytoarchitectonic similarity and anatomical contiguity make adjacent structures prime candidates for substitution. The language network of the left hemisphere is capable of a considerable degree of compensation, producing various clinical patterns of deficit, but its complete destruction results in permanent loss in the majority of individuals. Functional activation and cortical stimulation provides convergent evidence of such networks, as well as bilateral activation and integration in language function.

The addition of cognitive neuropsychology and functional neuroimaging to the clinical knowledge of aphasic syndromes has deepened our understanding of language organization in the brain. In clinical practice, the value of clinical symptoms and aphasic syndromes in predicting localization of stroke lesions and prognosis remains undiminished.

REFERENCES

Alexander, M. P. and Loverme, S. R. (1980). Aphasia after left hemispheric intracerebral hemorrhage. *Neurology*, **30**, 1193–202.

Alexander, M. P., Naeser, M. A. and Palumbo, C. L. (1987). Correlations of subcortical CT lesion sites and aphasia profiles. *Brain*, **110**, 961–92.

Appell, J., Kertesz, A., & Fisman, M. (1982). A study of language functioning in Alzheimer patients. *Brain Lang.*, **17**, 73–91.

Arseni, C. and Botez, M. I. (1961). Speech disturbances caused by tumors of the supplementary motor area. *Acta Psychiatr. Scand.*, **36**, 279–99.

Barat, M., Mazaux, J. M., Bioulac, B., *et al.* (1981). Troubles du langage de type aphasique et lesions putamino-caudees: observation anatome-clinique. *Rev. Neurol.*, **137**, 343–56.

Baron, J. C., D'Antona, R., Serdaru, M., *et al.* (1986). Hypometabolisme cortical après lesion thalamizue chez l'homme: etude par la tomography a postions. *Rev. Neurol.*, **142**, 465–74.

Basso, A., Della, S. S. and Farabola, M. (1987). Aphasia arising from purley deep lesions. *Cortex*, **23**, 29–44.

Bell, D. S. (1968). Speech functions of the thalamus inferred from the effects of thalamotomy. *Brain*, **91**, 619–38.

Benson, D. F. (1979). *Aphasia, Alexia, and Agraphia.* Edinburgh and London: Churhill-Livingstone.

Berndt, R. S. and Mitchum, C. C. (1997). Lexical-semantic organization: evidence from aphasia. *Clin. Neurosci.*, **4**, 57–63.

Binder, J. R. and Rao, S. M. (1994). Human brain mapping with functional magnetic resonance imaging. In A. Kertesz, ed., *Localization and Neuroimaging in Neuropsychology.* San Diego: Academic Press, pp. 185–212.

Broca, P. (1861). Remarques sur le siège de la faculté du langage articulé suivies d'une observation d'amphemie (perte de la parole). *Bulletin et Memories de la Societé Anatomique de Paris*, **36**, 330–57.

Bub, D. and Kertesz, A. (1982). Deep agraphia, *Brain Lang.*, **17**, 146–65.

Bucy, P. C. (1934). The relation of the premotor cortex to motor activity. *J. Nerv. Ment. Dis.*, **79**, 621–30.

Cambier, J., Elghozi, D., Signoret, J. L. and Henin, D. (1983). Contribution of the right hemisphere to language in aphasic patients. Disappearance of this language after a right-sided lesion. *Rev. Neurol.*, **139**, 55–63.

Cappa, S. F., Cavallotti, G. and Vignolo, L. A. (1981). Phonemic and lexical errors in fluent aphasia; correlation with lesion site. *Neuropsychologia*, **19**, 171–9.

Cappa, S. F. and Vignolo, L. A. (1979). "Transcortical" features of aphasia following left thalamic hemorrhage. *Cortex*, **15**, 121–30.

Chertkow, H. and Murtha, S. (1997). PET activation and language. *Clin. Neurosci.*, **4**, 78–86.

Cummings, J. L., Benson, D. F., Walsh, M. J. and Levine, J. L. (1979). Left-to-right transfer of language dominance: a case study. *Neurology*, **29**, 1547–50.

Czopf, J. (1972). Role of the non-dominant hemisphere in the restitution of speech in aphasia. *Archiv fur Psychiatrie und Nervenkrankheiten*, **216**, 162–71.

Damasio, A. R., Damais, H., Rizzo, M., Varney, N. and Gersh, F. (1982). Aphasia with nonhemorrhagic lesions in the basal ganglia and internal capsule. *Arch. Neurol.*, **39**, 15–20.

Darley, F. L., Aronson, A. E. and Brown, J. R. (1975). *Motor Speech Disorders.* Toronto: W. B. Saunders.

Dejerine, J. (1892). Contribution a l'étude anatomo-pathologique et clinique des differentes varietés de cecite verbale. *Comptes Randus des Séances de la Société de Biologie et de Ses Fillales*, **4**, 61–90.

Dejerine, J. and Dejerine-Klumpke, A. (1895). *Anatome des centres nerveus*. Paris: Ruef et Cie.

Demeurisse, G., Verhas, M., Capon, A. and Paternot, J. (1983). Lack of evolution of the cerebral blood flow during clinical recovery of stroke. *Stroke*, **14**, 77–81.

Dronkers, N. F. (1996). A new brain region for coordinating speech articulation. *Nature*, **384**, 159–61.

Ellis, A. W. (1984). *Reading, Writing and Dyslexia: A Cognitive Analysis*. Hilldale, NJ : Lawrence Erlbaum Associates, Inc.

Ferro, J. M. (1983). Global aphasia without hemiparesis. *Neurology*, **33**, 1106.

Ferro, J. M. and Kertesz, A. (1987). Comparative classification of aphasic disorders. *J. Clin. Exp. Neuropsychol.*, **9**, 365–75.

Franklin, S., Howard, D. and Patterson, K. (1994). Abstract word meaning deafness. *Cogn. Neuropsychol.*, **11**, 1034.

Geschwind, N. (1965). Disconnexion syndromes in animal and man. *Brain*, **88**, 237–94, 585–644.

(1974). Late changes in nervous system: An overview in plasticity and recovery of function in the central nervous system. In *Plasticity and Recovery of Function in the Central Nervous System*, ed. D. Stein, J. Rosen and N. Butters. New York: Academic Press, pp. 467–508.

Geschwind, N. and Levitsky, W. (1968). Human brain, left-right asymmetries in temporal speech regions. *Science*, **161**, 186–7.

Gloning, I., Gloning, K., Haub, G. and Quartember, R. (1969). Comparison of verbal behavior in right-handed and nonright-handed patients with anatomically verified lesion of one hemisphere. *Cortex*, **5**, 43–52.

Goldstein, K. (1948). *Language and Language Disturbances*. New York: Grune and Stratton.

Goodglass, H. (1997). Agrammatism in aphasiology. *Clin. Neurosci.*, **4**, 51–6.

Goodglass, H. and Kaplan, E. (1972). *Assessment of Aphasia and Related Disorders*. Philadelphia: Lea and Febiger.

Greenblatt, S. H. (1983). Localization of lesions in alexia. In *Localization in Neuropsychology*, ed. A. Kertesz. New York: Academic Press, pp. 324–56.

Head, H. (1926). *Aphasia and Kindred Disorders of Speech*. Cambridge: Cambridge University Press.

Henschen, S. E. (1922). *Klinische und Anatomische Beitrage zur Pathologie des Gehirns*, Vols. **5–7**. Stockholm: Nordisa Bokhandel n.

Hier, D. B., Davis, K. R., Richardson, E. P. and Mohr, J. (1977). Hypertensive putaminal hemorrhage. *Ann. Neurol.*, **1**, 152–9.

Hillis, A. E., Work, M., Barker, P. B., Jacobs, M. A., Breese, E. L. and Maurer, K. (2004). Re-examining the brain regions crucial for orchestrating speech articulation. *Brain*, **127**(7), 1479–87.

Huber, W., Poeck, K., Weniger, D. and Willmes, K. (1983). *Aachener-Aphasie Test*. Toronto Verlag fur Psychologie Gottingen.

Iwata, M. (1984). Kanji versus Kana: Neuropsycholological correlations of the Japanese writing system. *Trends Neurosci.*, **7**, 290–3.

Katz, R. and Goodglass, H. (1990). Deep dysphasia: An analysis of a rare form of repetition disorder. *Brain Lang.*, **39**, 153–85.

Kawahata, N., Nagata, K. and Shishido, F. (1988). Alexia with agraphia due to the left posterior inferior temporal lobe lesions – Neuropsychological analysis and its pathogenic mechanisms. *Brain Lang.*, **33**, 296–310.

Kawamura, M., Hirayama, K., Hasegawa, K., Takashahi, N. and Yamaura, A. (1987). Alexia with agraphia of kanji (Japanese morphograms). *J. Neurol. Neurosurg. Psychiatry*, **5**, 1125–9.

Kertesz, A. (1979). *Aphasia and Associated Disorders: Taxonomy, Localization and Recovery.* New York: Grune and Stratton.

(1982). *The Western Aphasia Battery.* New York: Grune and Stratton.

(1983). Localizaton of lesions in Wernicke's aphasia. In *Localization in Neuropsychology*, ed. A. Kertesz. New York: Academic Press, pp. 209–30.

(1984). Subcortical lesions and verbal apraxia. In *Apraxia of Speech: Physiology. Acoustics. Linguistics. Management*, ed. J. C. Rosenbek, M. R. McNeil and A. E. Aronson. San Diego, CA : College-Hill Press, pp. 73–90.

(1988). What do we learn from recovery from aphasia? In *Advances of neurology, Vol. 47: Functional Recovery in Neurological Disease*, ed. S. G. Waxman. New York: Raven Press, pp. 277–92.

Kertesz, A. and Benke, T. (1989). Sex equality and intrahemispheric language organization. *Brain Lang.*, **37**, 401–8.

Kertesz, A. and Benson, D. F. (1970). Neoloistic jargon – a clinicopathological study. *Cortex*, **6**, 362–86.

Kertesz, A., Harlock, W. and Coates, R. (1979). Computer tomographic localization, lesion size, and prognosis in aphasia and nonverbal impairment. *Brain Lang.*, **8**, 34–50.

Kertesz, A., Hudson, L., Mackenzie, I. R. A. and Munoz, D. G. (1994). The pathology and nosology of primary progressive aphasia. *Neurology*, **44**, 2065–72.

Kertesz, A. and Phipps, J. (1977). Numerical taxonomy of aphasia. *Brain Lang.*, **4**, 1–10.

Kertesz, A., Polk, M., Black, S. E. and Howell, J. (1992). Anatomical asymmetries and functional laterality. *Brain*, **115**, 589–605.

Kertesz, A., Sheppard, A. and MacKenzie, R. A. (1982). Localization in transcortical sensory aphasia. *Arch. Neurol.*, **39**, 475–8.

Kinsbourne, M. (1971). The minor cerebral hemisphere as a source of aphasic speech. *Arch. Neurol.*, **25**, 302–6.

Kirk, A. and Kertesz, A. (1994). Cortical and subcortical aphasias compared. *Aphasiology*, **8**, 65–82.

Kleist, K. (1962). *Sensory Aphasia and Amusia.* Pergamon: Oxford.

Knopman, D. S., Rubens, A. B., Selnes, O. R., *et al.* (1984). Mechanisms of recovery from aphasia: evidence from serial xenon 133 cerebral blood flow studies. *Ann. Neurol.*, **15**, 530–5.

Kohn, S. and Friedman, R. (1986). Word meaning deafness: a phonological–semantic dissociation. *Cogn. Neuropsychol.*, **3**, 291–308.

Kornyey, E. (1975). Aphasie transcorticale et echolalie: Le problème de l'initiative de la parole. *Rev. Neurol.*, **131**, 347–63.

Landis, T., Cummings, J. L. and Benson, D. F. (1980). Passage of language dominance to the right hemisphere: Interpretation of delayed recovery after global aphasia. *Rev. Med. Suisse Romande*, **100**, 171–7.

Lashley, K. S. (1938). Factors limiting recovery after central nervous lesions. *J. Nerv. Ment. Dis.*, **88**, 733–55.

Lecours, A. R. and Lhermitte, F. (1976). The 'pure form' of the phonetic disintegration syndrome (pure anarthria): anatomo-clinical report of a historical case. *Brain Lang.*, **3**, 88–113.

Leischner, A. (1976). Aptitude of aphasics for language treatment. In *Recovery in Aphasics*, ed. Y. Lebrun and R. Hoops. Amsterdam: Swets and Zeitlinger B. V., pp. 112–24.

Leske, M. C. (1981). Prevalence estimates of communicative disorders in the U.S. Language, hearing and vestibular disorders. *ASHA*, **23**, 229–37.

Levine, D. M. and Mohr, J. P. (1979). Language after bilateral cerebral infarctions: role of the minor hemisphere. *Neurology*, **29**, 927–38.

Levine, D. N. and Sweet, E. (1983). Localization of lesion in Broca's motor aphasia. In *Localization in Neuropsychology*, ed. A. Kertesz. New York: Academic Press, pp. 185–208.

Lichtheim, L. (1885). On aphasia. *Brain*, **7**, 443.

Liebermann, A. M., Cooper, F. S., Shankweiler, D. R. and Staddert-Kennedy, M. (1967). Perception of the speech code. *Psychol. Rev.*, **74**, 431–61.

Ludlow, C., Rosenberg, J., Fair, C., *et al.* (1986). Brain lesions associated with nonfluent aphasia fifteen years following penetrating head injury. *Brain*, **109**, 55–80.

Marie, P. (1906). Que faut-il penser des aphasies sous-corticales? *Seminaires Medicales*, **26**, 493.

Marie, P. (1926). *Travaux et mémoires*, Paris: Masson.

Mayendorf, N. von, E. (1930). *Vom Lokalisationsproblem der artikulierten Sprache*. Leipzig: Barth.

Mazzocchi, F. and Vignolo, L. A. (1979). Localisation of lesions in aphasia: Clinical CT scan correlation in stroke patients. *Cortex*, **15**, 627–54.

McGlone, J. (1980). Sex differences in human brain asymmetry: a critical survey. *Behav. Brain Sci.*, **5**, 215–64.

Mesulam, M.-M. (1987). Primary progressive aphasia–differentiation from Alzheimer's disease. *Ann. Neurol.*, **22**, 533–34.

Metter, E. J., Wasterlain, C. G., Kuhl, D. E., Hanson, W. R. and Phelps, M. E. (1981). FDG positron emission tomography computed tomography in a study of aphasia. *Ann. Neurol.*, **10**, 173–83.

Mochizuki, H. and Ohtomo, R. (1988). Pure alexia in Japanese and agraphia without alexia in kanji. *Arch. Neurol.*, **45**, 1157–9.

Mohr, J. P. (1976). Broca's area and Broca's aphasia. In *Studies in Neurolinguistics (Vol. 1)*, ed. H. Whitaker and H. A. Whitaker. New York: Academic Press, pp. 201–35.

Mohr, J. P., Walters, W. C. and Duncan, G. W. (1975). Thalamic hemorrhage and aphasia. *Brain Lang.*, **2**, 3–17.

Monakow, C. von (1914). *Die Lokalisation im Grosshirn und der Abbau der Funktionen durch kortikale Herde*. Wiesbaden, Bergmann.

Moutier, F. (1908). *L'aphasie de Broca*. Paris: Steinheil.

Muratoff, W. (1893). Secundare Degenerationen nach Durchschneidung des Balkens. *Neurologisches Centralblatt*, **12**, 714—29.

Naeser M. A., Alexander, M. P., Helm-Estabroks, N., *et al.* (1982). Aphasia with predominantly subcortical lesion sites. Description of three capsular/putaminal apshasia syndromes. *Arch. Neurol.*, **39**, 2—14.

Naeser, M. A., Palumbo, C. L., Helm-Estabrooks, N., Sitassny-Eder, D. and Albert, M. L. (1989). Severe nonfluency in aphasia: role of the medial subcallosal fasiculus and other white matter pathways in recovery of spontaneous speech. *Brain*, **112**, 1—38.

Nagata, K., Yunoki, K., Kabe, S., Suzuki, A. and Araki, G. (1986). Regional cerebral blood flow correlates of aphasia outcome in cerebral hemorrhage and cerebral infarction. *Stroke*, **17**, 417—23.

Nielsen, J. M. (1946). *Agnosia, Apraxia and Aphasia*. New York: Hoeber.

Penfield, W. and Roberts, L. (1959). *Speech and Brain Mechanisms*. Princeton, NJ: Princeton University Press.

Perani, D., Vallar, G., Cappa, S., Messa, C. and Fazio, F. (1987). Aphasia and neglect after subcortical stroke: a clinical/cerebral perfusion correlation study. *Brain*, **110**, 1211—29.

Petersen, S., Fox, P. T., Snyder, A. Z. and Raichle, M. E. (1990). Activation of extrastriate and frontal cortical areas by visual words and word-like stimuli. *Science*, **249**, 1041—4.

Pick, A. (1913). "*Die agrammatischen Sprachstorungen. Studien zur psychologischen Grundlegung der aphasielehre.*" Berlin: J. Springer.

Pieniadz, J. M., Naeser, M. A., Koff, E. and Levine, H. L. (1983). CT scan cerebral hemispheric asymmetry measurements in stroke cases with global aphasia: atypical asymmetries associated with improved recovery. *Cortex*, **19**, 371—91.

Rubens, A. B. (1975). Aphasia with infarction in the territory of the anterior cerebral artery. *Cortex*, **11**, 239—50.

Russell, W. and Espir, M. (1961). *Traumatic Aphasia: A Study of Aphasia in War Wounds of the Brain*. London: Oxford University Press.

Sanides, F. (1970). Functional architecture of motor and sensory cortices in primates in the light of a new concept of neocortex evolution. In *The Primate Brain*, ed. C. R. Noback and W. Montagna. New York: Appleton.

Selby, G. (1967). Sterotaxic surgery for the relief of Parkinson's disease II. An analysis of the results of a series of 303 patients (413 operations). *J. Neurol. Sci.*, **5**, 343—75.

Shewan, C. M. and Kertesz, A. (1984). Effects of speech and language treatment on recovery aphasia. *Brain Lang.*, **23**, 272—300.

Snowden, J. S., Goulding, P. J., and Neary, D. (1989). Semantic dementia: a form of circumscribed cerebral atrophy. *Behav. Neurol.*, **2**, 167—82.

Subirana, A. (1969). Handedness and cerebral dominance. In *Handbook of Clinical Neurology*, ed. P. Vinken and G. W. Bruyn. Amsterdam: North Holland, pp. 248—72.

Tzortis, C. and Albert, M. L. (1974). Impairment of memory for sequences in conduction aphasia. *Neuropsychologia*, **13**, 355—66.

Van Horn, G. and Hawes, A. (1982). Global aphasia without hemiparesis: a sign of embolic encephalopathy. *Neurology*, **32**, 403—6.

Warrington, E. K. and Shallice, T. (1969). The selective impairment of auditory-verbal short-term memory. *Brain*, **92**, 885–96.

Weiller, C., Chollet, F., Friston, K. J., Wise, R. J. S. and Frackowiak, R. S. J. (1992). Functional reorganization of the brain in recovery from striatocapsular infarction in man. *Ann. Neurol.*, **31**, 463–72.

Wernicke, C. (1874). *Der aphasische symtomenkomplex.* In Boston Studies on the Philosophy of Science, Vol. **IV**. Dordrecht, Reidel, Breslau: Cohn and Weigart.

Wernicke, C. (1886). Einige neueren Arbeiten uber Aphasie. *Fortschritte der Medizin*, **4**, 371–7.

Yakovlev, P. I. and Locke, S. (1961). Limbic nuclei of thalamus and connections of limbic cortex. *Arch. Neurol.*, **5**, 364–400.

5

Acute vascular aphasia

Alexandre Croquelois,[1] Olivier Godefroy,[2] and Julien Bogousslavsky[3]

[1]University Hospital, Lausanne, Switzerland
[2]University Hospital, Amiens, France
[3]Swiss Medical Network, Montreux, Switzerland

Introduction

Aphasia has been studied extensively at the acute and subacute stages of stroke (see Chapter 4). However, these important studies do not adequately cover the initial stage (i.e. the first hours and days post-stroke), a critical period for the diagnosis and treatment of stroke. With the development of hyperacute management of stroke, a few studies have re-examined the characteristics, determinants, and prognosis of acute aphasia.

Aphasia at the acute stage of stroke

Aphasia is observed with a prevalence ranging from 21% to 33% of patients admitted for acute stroke (Brust *et al.*, 1976; Laska *et al.*, 2001; Godefroy *et al.*, 2002). A very high prevalence (from 38% to 45%) has been observed at the hyperacute stage with tests including non-aphasic disturbances such as the language subtest of stroke scale (Pedersen *et al.*, 1995) or a naming subtest (Riepe *et al.*, 2004) and this presumably inflates the prevalence of aphasia (Thommessen *et al.*, 2002).

Aphasic syndromes evolve rapidly during the first days post-stroke. Global aphasia is the most frequent syndrome observed with a frequency of about 25% (Laska *et al.*, 2001; Godefroy *et al.*, 2002); Wernicke's aphasia is also frequent (15–25%) followed by anomic aphasia, usually associated with various degrees of minor disorders of oral expression, transcortical motor aphasia, frequently associated with hypophonia in subcortical lesions (Kreisler *et al.*, 2000), and Broca's aphasia (Brust *et al.*, 1976; Laska *et al.*, 2001; Godefroy *et al.*, 2002). Improvement seems to be more frequent and rapid in the first days and this influences the distribution of aphasic syndromes:

1. Global aphasia may progress to Broca's aphasia (or less frequently to Wernicke type).

2. Broca's aphasia and transcortical motor aphasia may progress to anomic-plus aphasia.

3. Wernicke's aphasia may progress to conduction aphasia.

The main determinants of the type of aphasia are the sites of the lesions and, in infarct only, the patient's age (Kertesz and Shepard, 1981; Ferro and Madureira, 1997; Kreisler *et al.*, 2000; Godefroy *et al.*, 2002). In addition, recent studies at the hyperacute stage have shown that aphasic disturbances have a parallel course to that of cortical hypoperfusion, and that reversal of cortical hypoperfusion (following thrombolysis or intervention) is associated with resolution of aphasia (Hillis *et al.*, 2002; Croquelois *et al.*, 2003).

Characteristics of acute aphasia

Despite the rapid course of aphasia in the first days post-stroke, several studies performed in stroke units have examined its characteristics.

Aphasia characteristics were described in 207 consecutive inpatients (85% infarct, 15% hemorrhage) who underwent a complete language evaluation in the first month after stroke onset (median delay 11 days) (Godefroy *et al.*, 2002). It used a composite battery associating subtests from the Montreal–Toulouse (Nespoulous *et al.*, 1986) and Boston Diagnosis Aphasia Evaluation (Goodglass and Kaplan, 1983) validated in the study. The administration of the battery took less than one hour and could be performed in the patient's room. Global and unclassified aphasias (mainly anomic-plus aphasia of mild severity) accounted for half of aphasic syndromes at the acute stage, whereas classic aphasia syndrome was less frequent with motor transcortical, Wernicke's, and Broca's aphasia representing 40% of aphasias. Other aphasia types (conduction, sensory transcortical, pure anomia) were very rare. Nonfluent types accounted for 54% of aphasia, 25% with mutism or expression restricted to stereotyped utterances. The main determinant of aphasia type was the lesion location (Kreisler *et al.*, 2000) and the presence of previous stroke, more frequent in unclassified aphasia. Conversely the effect of age was marginal and observed only in infarcts (conduction aphasics were younger, and patients with subcortical aphasia were older), suggesting that it was due to its influence on infarct location. Thus the age effect of aphasia type at the acute stage of stroke acts mainly through its effect on infarct type and perhaps on pattern of recovery. Conversely it does not seem to be explained by variation of the cerebral organization of language areas with age (see also Coppens, 1991).

In the Lausanne Stroke Registry (LSR), aphasia was classified as mainly expressive, mainly receptive or expressive–receptive, with a somehow basic bedside evaluation performed at admission, assessing spontaneous verbal fluency, comprehension (simple, semicomplex, and complex commands), naming, and repetition. Among 4802 first-ever stroke patients between 1978 and 2000, 1273 had aphasia (27%), 88% having ischemic and 12% hemorrhagic strokes. The more frequent clinical presentation was expressive–receptive aphasia (38%) and mainly expressive aphasia (37%), whereas mainly receptive aphasia was less frequently observed (25%). Ischemic lesions were found in the MCA territory in 88% of the cases (in 11% the lesion was restricted to the deep MCA territory), in 2% in the ACA territory, in 7% in the PCA territory (2% in thalamus) and in 3% in the junctional territory. On the other hand, hemorrhagic lesions were found more frequently in the striatum (39%) than in parieto-occipital lobe (21%), frontal lobe (19%), temporal lobe (12%), or thalamus (9%). In 70% of striatal hemorrhage cases, patients presented with expressive–receptive aphasia which was often associated with hemiparesis, hypoesthesia, and hemianopia (49%). Ninety percent of patients with aphasia had left hemispheric strokes, whereas in 5% they had a right hemispheric lesion and in 5% bilateral lesions. Nineteen percent of patients with right hemispheric strokes and aphasia were left-handed. Mean age at stroke onset was significantly different between patients with and without aphasia (64.9 vs. 63.1 years respectively), as well as between patients with different types of language disorder (63.5, 66.4, and 65.2 for expressive, receptive, and expressive–receptive aphasia respectively).

Two-third of infarcts with aphasia are due to arterio-arterial or cardiac emboli, with a slight preponderance for arterio-arterial emboli in expressive and expressive–receptive aphasia, whereas in receptive aphasia cardioembolic origin is more frequent. The main clinical association with expressive aphasia was hemiparesis (49%) and hemiparesis + hypoesthesia (25%); with

Key points Main characteristics of hyperacute aphasia

Incidence	Frequent (about one fourth to one third of stroke patients)
Clinical presentation	Rapidly evolving in the first hours/days after symptoms onset
	Expressive-receptive aphasia and expressive aphasia: more frequent than receptive aphasia
	Aphasic syndrome: global, anomic-plus, more frequent
	Wernicke, Broca and motor transcortical types: intermediate
	Rare: conduction, sensory transcortical, pure anomic aphasia

expressive—receptive aphasia it was hemiparesis + hypoesthesia + hemianopsia (44%) and hemiparesis + hypoesthesia (25%); whereas for receptive aphasia no dominant clinical picture was found (hemiparesis + hypoesthesia + hemianopsia 16%, hemiparesis + hypoesthesia 15%, hypoesthesia 12%, hemianopsia 11%, hemiparesis 10%).

Clinical radiological correlation

Clinical radiological correlation in aphasia has been widely discussed. Despite some studies demonstrating exceptions to the standard correlation (Basso *et al.*, 1985; Willmes and Poeck, 1993), other works have shown that, in most patients, language modalities such as spontaneous verbal fluency, repetition, comprehension, and naming are affected by lesions confined to precise brain regions (Kreisler *et al.*, 2000; Hillis *et al.*, 2001; Godefroy *et al.*, 2002; Croquelois *et al.*, 2003). In general, a 10—20% unexpected lesion site according to clinical deficit can be retained. Basso *et al.* (1985) found 17% exceptions to the classical aphasia localization, mainly fluent aphasia with lesion of the anterior middle cerebral artery (MCA) territory and nonfluent aphasia with posterior MCA lesions. Exceptions to the classical aphasia localization were also present in the LSR: in 471 patients with defined CT or MRI lesions and mainly expressive aphasia, 18 (4%) had posterior MCA lesions and 27 (6%) had large anteroposterior MCA lesions, whereas in over 295 patients with mainly receptive aphasia a defined lesion was found in the anterior MCA territory in 14 (5%) and large anteroposterior stroke was found in 13 (4%). Expressive—receptive aphasia was found in 478 patients; among them 47 (10%) had defined anterior MCA lesions and 46 (10%) posterior MCA infarcts. The overall exceptions percentage in the LSR was of about 13%. Studies using MRI, which allows visualization of small lesions outside the scope of CT imaging, could lower this percentage to 6%, especially when analysis is restricted to specific language modalities (Kreisler *et al.*, 2000). Reduction in spontaneous verbal fluency was associated with inferior frontal gyrus, putamen and anterior subcortical lesions, repetition deficits were found in insular, external, and posterior internal capsular lesions, oral comprehension was affected in lesions of the posterior part of the superior and middle temporal gyri, of the external capsule, of the insula as well as of the inferior frontal gyrus, whereas naming deficits were found with lesions in a more extensive territory (insula, external capsule, posterior subcortical, head of caudate nucleus, medial temporal, middle and inferior frontal gyri, and genu of internal capsule).

Deep MCA and thalamic strokes

In a review of the literature, Nadeau and Crosson (1997) stated that the finding of nearly every conceivable pattern of language impairment in different reported cases of striatocapsular infarction and the absence of aphasia in reported cases of dominant hemisphere striatocapsular infarction provide strong evidence against a major direct role of the basal ganglia in language. They formulated two hypotheses for aphasic symptoms related to subcortical infarcts. One is a possible sustained cortical hypoperfusion and infarction not visible on structural imaging studies (Godefroy *et al.*, 1994; Hillis *et al.*, 2004), the other being a possible thalamic disconnection, as may occur with striatocapsular infarcts. Data from the Lausanne Stroke Registry showed aphasia in 24% of left deep MCA infarcts, the more frequent presentation being expressive aphasia (59%) and expressive–receptive aphasia (32%), receptive aphasia being infrequent in this localization (9%). Poor speech volume (hypophonia) has been described in subcortical aphasias (Puel *et al.*, 1984; Alexander *et al.*, 1987), but is not always present.

In aphasia due to thalamic lesion, fluent and nonfluent aphasia have been described. Nevertheless, a clinical picture of thalamic aphasia is sometimes described with a predominance of expression deficit, verbal paraphasias, and no or slight comprehension and repetition deficits (Puel *et al.*, 1984; Verstichel, 2003). Again, in the majority of the cases, the participation of cortical dysfunction cannot be ruled out, except when DWI is performed. In the Lausanne Stroke Registry,

Key points Main types of stroke responsible for hyperacute aphasia

Stroke type	Characteristics
Infarct (≈80–90%)	Anterior MCA: expressive aphasia, hemiparesis
	Posterior MCA: receptive aphasia, hemiparesis ± hypoesthesia ± hemianopia
	Complete MCA: expressive–receptive aphasia, hemiparesis + hypoesthesia + hemianopia
	Deep MCA: expressive aphasia, hypophonia
	Thalamic: expressive aphasia, verbal paraphasias
Hemorrhage (≈10–20%)	Striatal: expressive–receptive aphasia, hemiparesis + hypoesthesia + hemianopia
	Frontal, temporal and parietal
Aneurysm	Infarct/hemorrhage due to MCA aneurysm
Venous thrombosis	Infarct/hemorrhage due to thrombosis of lateral or superior sagittal sinus

aphasia was present in 18% (expressive–receptive 8%, expressive 6%, and receptive 4%) of left thalamic infarcts.

Uncommon localization

Acute aphasia was described in superficial posterior cerebral artery infarction (without thalamic infarction) (Maulaz *et al.*, 2005); it was mainly characterized by receptive aphasic symptoms (83%). It was also described in a lesion restricted to the insular cortex (Cereda *et al.*, 2002), with no evidence for a dominant clinical subtype of aphasia. Although the cerebellum has been described as possibly contributing to language skills by the way of its anatomical connections (Abe *et al.*, 1997), no case study describing aphasia in a single cerebellar lesion has been reported, except with diaschisis (Marien *et al.*, 1996).

Other clinical entities mimicking stroke aphasia

Migraine with aura can be evoked in patients with a past history of migraine. The clinical presentation is generally somehow more progressive than with stroke aphasia. Severe headache is often present but acephalgic auras have been described. In all cases, this represents an exclusion diagnostic as headache is often present with stroke, brain imaging being therefore always necessary. Epileptic seizures can be evoked in cases with repetitive and transient aphasic symptoms. Ictal electroencephalography generally shows epileptic discharges. Aphasia is usually considered to be rare in multiple sclerosis (MS). In a recent multicenter study, Lacour *et al.* (2004) found an incidence of less than 1%. A majority of cases involved nonfluent aphasia. In one-third of MS patients with aphasia, it was the first clinical manifestation of the disease; nevertheless all of them met the criteria for MS. Infections, and particularly herpes simplex encephalitis, have also been described as a cause of acute aphasia (Kennedy, 1988); nevertheless flu-like symptoms, fever or meningism generally orientate the diagnostic workup.

Functional imaging techniques

New hyperacute-period imaging techniques allow confirmation of the standard clinical–radiological correlation. Perfusion CT, measuring cerebral blood flow and volume, can generate maps of *penumbra* (decreased cerebral blood flow and normal or increased cerebral blood volume) and *infarct* (decreased cerebral blood flow and volume) in the very first hours after stroke onset. It has been shown that penumbra dynamics are the major determinant for aphasia changes; rescuing a brain region known to be involved in a specific language modality clinically improved this modality (Hillis *et al.*, 2001; Croquelois *et al.*, 2003).

Following these results, an fMRI study provided evidence that brain tissue at risk of infarction, as shown by the PWI/DWI (perfusion-weighted-imaging–diffusion-weighted-imaging) mismatch, can survive if recanalization occurs and constitutes the major site underlying post-ischemic recovery as demonstrated by language-task-specific activation adjacent to the infarct lesion within the former PWI/DWI mismatch area (Kleiser *et al.*, 2005). A positron emission tomography (PET) study demonstrated that reactivation of the left superior temporal gyrus was related to a favorable outcome, while activation of other eloquent regions or of contralateral areas was accompanied by some improvements but never a complete recovery (Heiss *et al.*, 1999).

Outcome

Aphasia symptoms often evolve quickly over the first 24 hours after stroke onset (Croquelois *et al.*, 2003). As a general rule they become less severe during the first year after stroke, and even patients with severe speech impairment have considerable potential for recovery, particularly in the first three months. Nonfluent aphasia could evolve into fluent aphasia, whereas fluent aphasia never evolved into a nonfluent aphasia (Pedersen *et al.*, 2004). The outcome of aphasia is dependent on initial aphasia severity, but also on general stroke severity. Influence of sex, age, and aphasia type on outcome has been widely studied with conflicting results. In a prospective study, Pedersen *et al.* (2004) found no influence of theses factors on aphasia evolution over the first year. Nevertheless, severe comprehension deficits are often considered as a negative factor for overall stroke recovery, as the patients could not understand the rehabilitation tasks.

Assessment and management at the acute stage

The use of an extensive aphasia battery is rarely feasible during the first days post-stroke. Assessment must be brief, should not require extensive test material, and must be able to be performed at bedside. However, it should provide an overall index of aphasia severity and its validity must be assessed. In addition, its ability to classify aphasia into main syndromes could be useful in clinical practice. Several short aphasia tests have been designed for this purpose (Godefroy *et al.*, 2002; Hillis *et al.*, 2002; Croquelois *et al.*, 2003; Doesborgh *et al.*, 2003), some of which use certain subtests of previously validated batteries, such as the Boston Diagnostic Aphasia Examination (Goodglass and Kaplan, 1983) and the Montreal–Toulouse battery (Nespoulous *et al.*, 1986). Our studies comparing clinical examination

Key points Assessment and management of hyperacute aphasia

Acute management
Emergency: rapid transport and admission
   to a stroke unit
Perfusion-CT or PWI-DWI (penumbra)
Early restoration of cortical hypoperfusion
   if feasible
Speech and language therapy
Short aphasia battery
Assessment
Spontaneous verbal fluency:
BDAE sentence length subtest (number of words consecutively pronounced in a sentence during
   spontaneous speech; normal: >7 words)
Comprehension:
BDAE command subtest (3 simple, 3 semicomplex, and 3 complex commands; normal: at least 2
   complex commands fully executed)
Subtests of the Montreal–Toulouse battery
Repetition:
BDAE repetition subtest (6 trisyllabic words, 3 non-words and 1 sentence; normal: no paraphasias or
   omissions)
Subtests of the Montreal-Toulouse battery
Naming:
BDAE command subtest (8 images; normal: at least 7 images correctly named)
Subtest of the Montreal-Toulouse battery
Others: reading, writing, buccofacial apraxia
Treatment
Language therapy usually offered as soon as permitted by clinical condition
Pharmacotherapy: remains to be evaluated

BDAE: Boston Diagnostic Aphasia Examination

with battery assessment support the use of a short aphasia battery. A large number of clinical misdiagnoses are due to two main types of error:

1. Clinical examination frequently underestimates oral comprehension deficits, leading to erroneous classification of global and of Wernicke's aphasia into Broca's and conduction aphasia, respectively.
2. It frequently confounds verbal stereotypes (e.g. 'tan, tan') that are observed in global and Broca's aphasia with jargon aphasia (characteristic of Wernicke's aphasia).

   Aphasia is a marker of stroke severity and is associated with a higher risk of mortality (Pedersen *et al.*, 1995; Laska *et al.*, 2001) and post-stroke dementia (Tatemichi *et al.*, 1994; Pohjasvaara *et al.*, 1998). Therefore, recovery from aphasia influences the overall neurological outcome and should be an early main goal of management. Currently, treatments designed to restore cortical perfusion during the first hours post-stroke constitute the main management. Efficacy of pharmacological treatments needs to be demonstrated at the hyperacute stage of stroke aphasia. In the chronic phase, preliminary positive results were found using piracetam when started soon after the stroke. The benefit of bromocriptine seems to be restricted to nonfluent aphasias, and cholinergic agents such as donepezil need further randomized controlled trials (Berthier, 2005).

Speech and language therapy

There is an extensive, but often contradictory, literature on aphasia recovery and the impact of therapy. Speech and language therapy (SLT) has raised a number of questions about its efficacy, the time at which it should begin, and the optimal intensity required. In spite of a great number of studies dedicated to SLT efficacy, in a review Greener *et al.* (2000) could not determine whether formal SLT is more effective than informal support. Since then, Bhogal *et al.* (2003) speculated that the conflicting results demonstrated across post-stroke aphasia therapy studies might be related to differences in therapy intensity. They reviewed ten studies and found that intense therapy over a short time (about 9 hours of therapy per week for 12 weeks) can improve outcomes of SLT for stroke patients with aphasia, while less intense SLT (2 hours a week) over a longer period (> 20 weeks) did not significantly improve the outcome as compared with informal support. Community-based aphasia treatment programs that provided therapy of known intensity using a structured and consistent therapeutic model and standardized measurement tools were developed and were responsible for a significant language improvement regardless of starting times after stroke onset (Aftonomos *et al.*, 1999). In spite of this statement and the lack of trials specifically assessing when to start SLT (for Cochrane reviews of aphasia treatments, see Greener *et al.*, 2000; 2001), following general rules of neurorehabilitation, speech therapy should be typically offered as soon as the clinical condition becomes favorable – which nowadays is generally possible in the acute stroke unit.

REFERENCES

Abe, K., Ukita, H., Yorifuji, S. and Yanagihara, T. (1997). Crossed cerebellar diaschisis in chronic Broca's aphasia. *Neuroradiology*, **39**, 624–6.

Aftonomos, L. B., Appelbaum, J. S. and Steele, R. D. (1999). Improving outcomes for persons with aphasia in advanced community-based treatment programs. *Stroke*, **30**, 1370–9.

Alexander, M. P., Naeser, M. A. and Palumbo, C. L. (1987). Correlations of subcortical CT lesion sites and aphasia profiles. *Brain*, **110**, 961–91.

Basso, A., Lecours, A. R., Moraschini, S. and Vanier, M. (1985). Anatomoclinical correlations of the aphasias as defined through computerized tomography: exceptions. *Brain Lang.*, **26**, 201–29.

Berthier, M. L. (2005). Poststroke aphasia: epidemiology, pathophysiology and treatment. *Drugs Aging*, **22**, 163–82.

Bhogal, S. K., Teasell, R. and Speechley, M. (2003). Intensity of aphasia therapy, impact on recovery. *Stroke*, **34**, 987–93.

Brust, J. C., Shafer, S. Q., Richter, R. W. and Bruun, B. (1976). Aphasia in acute stroke. *Stroke*, **7**, 167–74.

Cereda, C., Ghika, J., Maeder, P. and Bogousslavsky, J. (2002). Strokes restricted to the insular cortex. *Neurology*, **59**, 1950–5.

Coppens, P. (1991). Why are Wernicke's aphasia patients older than Broca's? A critical view of the hypotheses. *Aphasiology*, **5**, 279–90.

Croquelois, A., Wintermark, M., Reichhart, M., Meuli, R. and Bogousslavsky, J. (2003). Aphasia in hyperacute stroke: language follows brain penumbra dynamics. *Ann. Neurol.*, **54**, 321–9.

Doesborgh, S. J., van de Sandt-Koenderman, W. M., Dippel, D. W., *et al.* (2003). Linguistic deficits in the acute phase of stroke. *J. Neurol.*, **250**, 977–82.

Ferro, J. M. and Madureira, S. (1997). Aphasia type, age and cerebral infarct localization. *J. Neurol.*, **244**, 505–9.

Godefroy, O., Rousseaux, M., Pruvo, J. P., Cabaret, M. and Leys, D. (1994). Neuropsychological changes related to unilateral lenticulostriate infarcts. *J. Neurol. Neurosurg. Psychiatry*, **57**, 480–5.

Godefroy, O., Dubois, C., Debachy, B., Leclerc, M. and Kreisler, A. (2002). Vascular aphasias: main characteristics of patients hospitalized in acute stroke units. *Stroke*, **33**, 702–5.

Goodglass, H. and Kaplan, E. (1983). *The Assessment of Aphasia and Related Disorders.* Philadelphia: Lea and Febiger.

Greener, J., Enderby, P. and Whurr, R. (2000). *Speech and Language Therapy for Aphasia Following Stroke.* Cochrane Database Syst Rev CD000425.

(2001) *Pharmacological Treatment for Aphasia Following Stroke.* Cochrane Database Syst Rev CD000424.

Heiss, W. D., Kessler, J., Thiel, A., Ghaemi, M. and Karbe, H. (1999). Differential capacity of left and right hemispheric areas for compensation of poststroke aphasia. *Ann. Neurol.*, **45**, 430–8.

Hillis, A. E., Kane, A., Tuffiash, E., *et al.* (2001). Reperfusion of specific brain regions by raising blood pressure restores selective language functions in subacute stroke. *Brain Lang.*, **79**, 495–510.

Hillis, A. E., Wityk, R. J., Barker, P. B., *et al.* (2002). Subcortical aphasia and neglect in acute stroke: the role of cortical hypoperfusion. *Brain*, **125**, 1094–104.

Hillis, A. E., Barker, P. B., Wityk, R. J., *et al.* (2004). Variability in subcortical aphasia is due to variable sites of cortical hypoperfusion. *Brain Lang.*, **89**, 524–30.

Kennedy, P. G. (1988). A retrospective analysis of forty-six cases of herpes simplex encephalitis seen in Glasgow between 1962 and 1985. *Q. J. Med.*, **68**, 533–40.

Kertesz, A. and Sheppard, A. (1981). The epidemiology of aphasic and cognitive impairment in stroke: age, sex, aphasia type and laterality differences. *Brain*, **104**, 117–28.

Kleiser, R., Wittsack, H. J., Butefisch, C. M., Jorgens, S. and Seitz, R. J. (2005). Functional activation within the PI-DWI mismatch region in recovery from ischemic stroke: preliminary observations. *Neuroimage*, **24**, 515–23.

Kreisler, A., Godefroy, O., Delmaire, C., *et al.* (2000). The anatomy of aphasia revisited. *Neurology*, **54**, 1117–23.

Lacour, A., De Seze, J., Revenco, E., *et al.* (2004). Acute aphasia in multiple sclerosis: A multicenter study of 22 patients. *Neurology*, **62**, 974–7.

Laska, A. C., Hellblom, A., Murray, V., Kahan, T. and von Arbin, M. (2001). Aphasia in acute stroke and relation to outcome. *J. Intern. Med.*, **249**, 413–22.

Marien, P., Saerens, J., Nanhoe, R., *et al.* (1996). Cerebellar induced aphasia: case report of cerebellar induced prefrontal aphasic language phenomena supported by SPECT findings. *J. Neurol. Sci.*, **144**, 34–43.

Maulaz, A. B., Bezerra, D. C. and Bogousslavsky, J. (2005). Posterior cerebral artery infarction from middle cerebral artery infarction. *Arch. Neurol.*, **62**, 938–41.

Nadeau, S. E. and Crosson, B. (1997). Subcortical aphasia. *Brain Lang.*, **58**, 355–402.

Nespoulous, J. L., Lecours, A. R. and Lafond, D. (1986). *Protocole Montréal-Toulouse de l'examen de l'aphasie, Module Standard Initial (Version Beta)*. Montréal, Canada: L'Ortho Édition.

Pedersen, P. M., Jorgensen, H. S., Nakayama, H., Raaschou, H. O. and Olsen, T. S. (1995). Aphasia in acute stroke: incidence, determinants, and recovery. *Ann. Neurol.*, **38**, 659–66.

Pedersen, P. M., Vinter, K. and Olsen, T. S. (2004). Aphasia after stroke: type, severity and prognosis. The Copenhagen aphasia study. *Cerebrovasc. Dis.*, **17**, 35–43.

Pohjasvaara, T., Erkinjuntti, T., Ylikoski, R., *et al.* (1998). Clinical determinants of poststroke dementia. *Stroke*, **29**, 75–81.

Puel, M., Demonet, J. F., Cardebat, D., *et al.* (1984). Aphasie souscorticale. Etude neurolinguistique et scangraphique de 25 cas. *Rev. Neurol. (Paris)*, **140**, 695–710.

Riepe, M. W., Riss, S., Bittner, D. and Huber, R. (2004). Screening for cognitive impairment in patients with acute stroke. *Dement. Geriatr. Cogn. Disord.*, **17**, 49–53.

Tatemichi, T. K., Desmond, D. W., Stern, Y., *et al.* (1994). Cognitive impairment after stroke: frequency, patterns, and relationship to functional abilities. *J. Neurol. Neurosurg. Psychiatry*, **57**, 202–7.

Thommessen, B., Thoresen, G. E., Bautz-Holter, E. and Laake, K. (2002). Validity of the aphasia item from the Scandinavian Stroke Scale. *Cerebrovasc. Dis.*, **13**, 184–6.

Verstichel, P. (2003). Thalamic aphasia. *Rev. Neurol. (Paris)*, **159**, 947–57.

Willmes, K. and Poeck, K. (1993). To what extent can aphasic syndromes be localized? *Brain*, **116**, 1527–40.

6

Dysarthria

Pascal Auzou

Service d'Explorations Fonctionnelles Neurologique, France

Introduction

Speech motor disorders are one of the most common forms of movement disorder and are typical symptoms of numerous neurological diseases. They can be broadly categorized as apraxia of speech and dysarthria. Dysarthria has been defined as "a collective name for a group of speech disorders resulting from disturbances in muscular control over the speech mechanism due to damage of the central or peripheral nervous system. It designates problems in oral communication due to paralysis, weakness, or poor coordination of the speech musculature" (Darley et al., 1969a; 1969b; 1975). The disorder is due to abnormal neuromuscular execution and may affect the strength, speed, range, timing, and accuracy of speech movements. It can involve respiration, phonation, articulation, and prosody, either singly or in combination.

Dysarthria is a classical symptom of stroke observed in up to 30% of cases (Kumral et al., 1998; 1999; 2002; Bogousslavsky et al., 1988). It is included as a sign in the National Institutes of Health Stroke Scale (NIHSS) (Lyden et al., 1999). Melo et al. (1992) observed dysarthria in 29% of patients with isolated hemiparesis. It was also estimated to occur in about one-quarter of patients with lacunar infarction (Arboix et al., 1990). In some cases, dysarthria may be the sole sign of stroke (Fisher, 1982; Ichikawa and Kageyama, 1991; Kim, 1994).

Some studies suggest that the presence of dysarthria can have negative influences on the outcome of the stroke (Tilling et al., 2001). However Arboix et al. (2003) observed improvement in 44% of patients with lacunar stroke, such as the "dysarthria / clumsy hand" syndrome.

Speech production

Speech production requires a complicated biological system that may include as many as 100 different muscles, various types of physiological variable, and a neural control that may involve extensive areas of the nervous system. The physiological systems involved in speech production (Figure 6.1) are the

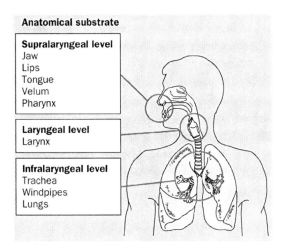

Anatomical substrate

Supralaryngeal level
Jaw
Lips
Tongue
Velum
Pharynx

Laryngeal level
Larynx

Infralaryngeal level
Trachea
Windpipes
Lungs

Figure 6.1   Anatomical substrate of speech components.

respiratory system, the larynx and the supralaryngeal system (pharynx, velum, jaw, tongue, lips). The respiratory system is primarily the energy source of speech, as the larynx enables vibration of the air column. The supralaryngeal system mainly contributes to the production of speech sounds (phonemes). Sound formation is the result of two basic processes: articulation, which is movement of structures to form strictures and shapes, and resonance, which is a matter of adjusting the length and shape of air-filled cavities to reinforce certain frequency regions of sound energy.

The motor neurons controlling speech articulation are located in various nuclei in the pons (trigeminal motor nucleus), medulla (facial nucleus, nucleus ambiguous, hypoglossal nucleus) and ventral horn of the spinal cord (cervical, thoracic and lumbar region). Coordination of the different motor neurons is carried out by an extensive network in the brainstem. Voluntary control over the initiation and suppression of vocal utterances is carried out by the mediofrontal cortex (including anterior cingulate gyrus and supplementary as well as pre-supplementary motor area). Voluntary control over the acoustic structure of vocalizations is carried out by the motor cortex via the pyramidal/corticobulbar as well as extrapyramidal pathways. The most important extrapyramidal pathway seems to be the connections between the motor cortex, putamen, substantia nigra, parvocellular reticular formation, and phonatory motoneurones. The motor cortex receives several inputs: cerebellar input via the ventrolateral thalamus, proprioceptive input from the phonatory organs, input from the ventral premotor and prefrontal cortex, including Broca's area, for motor planning of longer purposeful utterances, and input from the supplementary motor area (Duffy, 1995).

After a stroke or other brain injury, the muscles of the mouth, face, and respiratory system may become weak, move slowly, or not move at all, resulting in dysarthria. The type and severity of dysarthria depends on which area of the nervous system is affected. A person with dysarthria may experience any of the following symptoms, depending on the extent and location of damage to the nervous system: (1) "slurred" speech, (2) speaking softly or barely able to whisper, (3) slow rate of speech, (4) rapid rate of speech with a "mumbling" quality, (5) limited tongue, lip, and jaw movement, (6) abnormal intonation (rhythm) when speaking, (7) changes in vocal quality ("nasal" speech or sounding "stuffy"), (8) hoarseness, and (9) breathiness.

Classification of dysarthria

The current classification of dysarthria was developed by Darley *et al.* (1969a; 1969b; 1975) from physiological abnormalities in clinical non-speech motor performance or other signs. These works continue to serve as a standard for the fundamental understanding of neurogenic disorders of speech production (Duffy, 1995). The seven subtypes of dysarthria considered by Darley *et al.* (1975) were spastic, flaccid, mixed spastic–flaccid in amyotrophic lateral sclerosis, ataxic, hypokinetic, hyperkinetic in chorea, and hyperkinetic in dystonia (Table 6.1). The dysarthria associated with unilateral upper motor neuron lesion

Table 6.1. Major types of dysarthria

Type of dysarthria	Localization	Neuromotor basis
Flaccid	Lower motor neuron (final common pathway, motor unit)	Weakness
Spastic	Bilateral upper motor neuron (direct and indirect activation pathways)	Spasticity
Ataxic	Cerebellum (cerebellar control circuit)	Incoordination
Hypokinetic	Basal ganglia control circuit (extrapyramidal)	Rigidity/reduced range of movement
Hyperkinetic	Basal ganglia control circuit (extrapyramidal)	Involuntary movements
Unilateral upper motor neuron	Unilateral upper motor neuron	Weakness/ Incoordination
Mixed	Variable	

Source: adapted from Darley *et al.*, 1975

constitutes an additional subtype following more recent reports (Duffy, 1995; Kent *et al.*, 2001).

In contrast to other etiologies, dysarthria due to stroke has received little systematic perceptual description. The studies of neural lesions related to dysarthria following stroke are much more informative concerning the size and location of lesions than on the characteristics of dysarthria. Moreover, the dysarthria is frequently neither classified nor described in a way that adequately portrays the speech disturbance. Although all kinds of dysarthria may be observed after stroke, the most prominent are the spastic, unilateral upper motor neuron and ataxic types.

Key points Main characteristics of dysarthria

Dysarthria: disturbances in muscular control over the speech mechanism
impaired language articulation due to paralysis, weakness, or poor coordination of the speech musculature
Characteristics: Reduced intelligibility, loss of naturalness, impaired voiced quality, impaired articulation (consonants and vowels), prosodic troubles
Classification: spastic, flaccid, mixed spastic—flaccid (amyotrophic lateral sclerosis), ataxic, hypokinetic, hyperkinetic (chorea, dystonia) and unilateral upper motor neuron lesion

Evaluation of dysarthria

The speech examination can be divided into different parts (Duffy, 1995; Özsancak and Auzou, 2003): (1) history, (2) auditory—perceptual characteristics, (3) assessment of intelligibility, (4) examination of the oral mechanism during non-speech activities, (5) acoustic and physiological analyses, and (6) self-evaluation.

Vascular dysarthria usually has a sudden onset. The dysarthria is recognized primarily and sometimes exclusively by the speaker's auditory—perceptual characteristics. In clinical practice, only some salient features are usually considered, such as slurred speech or monotony. In their seminal work, Darley *et al.* (1969a; 1969b; 1975) rated speech characteristics on 38 dimensions of deviant speech. Different perceptual scales have been developed from these works and are available (Joanette and Dudley, 1980; Ludlow and Bassich, 1983; 1984; Kluin *et al.*, 1988; 1993; 1996; Chenery *et al.*, 1988; 1990; 1992; Theodoros *et al.*, 1994; Duffy, 1995). They usually take into account several aspects of speech production such as prosody, articulation, resonance, voice quality, respiration, overall intelligibility, and naturalness. Clinical experience suggests that the primary deviant dimensions of vascular dysarthria vary in relation to the topography of lesions.

Dysarthria after stroke can be mild and not affect intelligibility significantly. Nevertheless an evaluation of intelligibility constitutes a major component of a dysarthria assessment as it has great face and ecological validity as an index of severity. Intelligibility testing can range from a judgment during interaction with the patient to formal standardized quantitative testing. For diagnostic purposes and treatment indications, a general rating of intelligibility is usually sufficient. Usually at least one item of the auditory perceptual systematic scale concerns intelligibility. A quantified assessment of speech intelligibility is important for measuring improvement during treatment. A few tools have been developed for assessing intelligibility. The Assessment of Intelligibility in Dysarthric Speakers (AIDS) (Yorkston and Beukelman, 1981) is a widely used standardized test. A computerized version is available (Yorkston *et al.*, 1984). It quantifies intelligibility of single words and sentences and provides an estimate of communication efficiency by examining the rate of intelligible words per minute in sentences. Other tests are available (Enderby, 1983; Kent *et al.*, 1989).

Darley *et al.* (1975) discussed six salient neuromuscular features that influence speech production. They include strength, speed of movement, range of movement, accuracy, steadiness, and tone. They form a useful framework for integrating observations made during examination. Moreover, dysarthrias are necessarily accompanied by impairment of non-speech functions of the musculature involved in speech. An attempt is made to identify significant dysfunctions that may be important in the assessment, treatment, or understanding of the dysarthria. Specific sensorimotor dysfunctions include non-speech oral

Key points Assessment of dysarthria in stroke patients

Clinical examination
Auditory perceptual examination: spontaneous speech, reading, words and phonemes repetition
Maximum repetition rate
Motor examination of orofacial area
Published test for dysarthria
Assessment of Intelligibility in dysarthric speakers (Yorkston and Beukelman, 1981)
Frenchay Dysarthria Assessment (Enderby, 1983)
Evaluation Clinique de la dysarthrie (Auzou *et al.*, 1998)
Optional and developing area
Acoustical analysis
Aerodynamic analysis

alternating motion rate or diadochokinesis, dysphagia, orosensory impairments, altered tonus and resting tremor or postural instability. Dysarthria may also be related to other co-occurring dysfunctions in cognitive, sensory, or motor domains.

Beside clinical evaluation, instrumental evaluations such as acoustical analysis, aerodynamic testing, fiberoptic and cinefluorographic videotaping, and force, movement, and electromyographic recording, are also important in understanding the physiological bases for the perceived speech deviations (why speakers sound as they do) (Netsell and Rosenbek, 1985).

Varieties of vascular dysarthria

Spastic dysarthria

Spastic dysarthria is produced by bilateral damage to the upper motor neuron pathways with involvement of muscles innervated by pontine and medullary cranial nerves nuclei. It may alter respiratory, phonatory, resonatory, and articulatory components of speech and is usually not confined to a single component. Its characteristics reflect the combined effects of weakness and spasticity which result in slow movement with reduced range and force. Stroke is a major cause of spastic dysarthria. As Duffy (1995) wrote: "although no general etiologic category is uniquely associated with spastic dysarthria, vascular disorders are more frequently associated with spastic dysarthria than with most other dysarthria types." Darley *et al.* (1969a) rated the perceptual speech characteristics of 30 subjects with pseudobulbar palsy, resulting from bilateral upper motor neuron damage, on 38 dimensions of deviant speech. Unlike the flaccid dysarthria, the spastic one is not easily described by listing each cranial nerve and the speech characteristics associated with its abnormal function. This is because spastic dysarthria is associated with impaired movement patterns rather than weakness of individual muscles. This reflects the organization of the central nervous system pathway for control of movement patterns rather than isolated muscle movements. Therefore, spastic dysarthria is usually associated with deficits at all of the speech physiological systems (respiration, larynx, etc.). This broad involvement may explain why it frequently affects intelligibility.

The predominant perceptual features of spastic dysarthria are imprecise consonants, monopitch, reduced stress, harsh voice quality, monoloudness, low pitch, slow rate, hypernasality, strained/strangled voice quality, short phrases, distorted vowels, pitch breaks, continuous breathy voice, excess, and equal stress (Darley *et al.*, 1969a; 1969b). These features were confirmed in stroke patients with or without pseudobulbar palsy (Chenery *et al.*, 1992; Thompson and Murdoch, 1995a; 1995b).

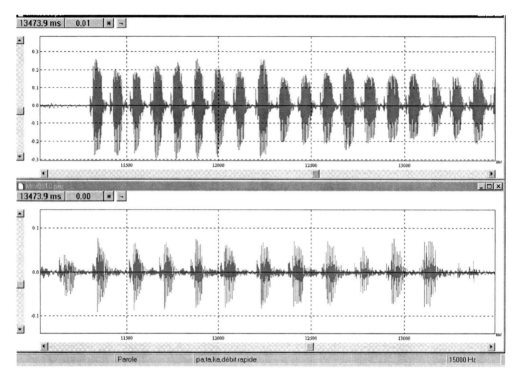

Figure 6.2   Waveform of the repeated syllable /ta/ at maximum rate. Control at 9 Hz (top) and spastic patient at 6 Hz (bottom).

The task of alternating motion rate (AMR) (syllable repetition or diadochokinesis) (Figure 6.2) has been studied with both perceptual and acoustic methods in subjects with spastic dysarthria. AMRs are slower in subjects with spastic dysarthria than in control speakers (Darley *et al.*, 1969a; 1969b; 1975; Enderby, 1986). In their original description, Darley *et al.* (1975) concluded that syllables were repeated at a slower rate but with a normal rhythm. Other authors found an abnormal variability of syllable rhythms. Thompson *et al.* (1995a; 1995b) and Thompson and Murdoch (1995a; 1995b) assessed physiological function in patients with spastic dysarthria. They measured overall articulation, intelligibility, tongue strength, rate of repetition movements, and sustained tongue contraction (endurance). Both tongue strength and rates of tongue movement were reduced compared to a control group. The patients also had a reduced endurance, which may indicate that muscle fatigue adversely affects tongue function.

Unilateral upper motor neuron dysarthria

Unilateral upper motor neuron (UUMN) dysarthria is due to damage to the upper motor neurons that carry impulses to the cranial and spinal nerves supplying speech muscles. The lesion may concern either the direct pathways (corticobulbar or corticospinal) or the indirect pathways. Stroke is by far the most common cause of UUMN damage. It is especially observed in unilateral infarcts in the territory of the middle cerebral artery. Infarcts in the territory of the posterior cerebral, basilar and anterior cerebral arteries are less frequent causes of UUMN deficit. UUMN dysarthria often co-occurs with aphasia, apraxia of speech, or neglect. However, dysarthria can be the patient's most obvious communication disorder and in some cases the only manifestation of stroke. It has been considered a mild and temporary problem (Darley *et al.*, 1975) and has received little systematic perceptual description.

The description of the dysarthria in patients with UUMN lesions is usually limited to vague terms such as "slow dysarthria," "slurred," "unintelligible, or "defective articulation." The most precise description of UUMN dysarthria features has been reported by Duffy (1995). In this study, 91% of the patients had stroke. The dysarthria severity was usually mild. Only half of the patients received therapy and of those 92% improved during therapy. The main characteristic of their speech was an articulatory impairment (98%). Phonation was altered in 57% of cases, with predominantly harsh voice qualities. Articulation rate and prosody were altered in 23% of patients. Studies by Hartman and Abbs (1992), Benke and Kertesz (1989), and Ropper (1987) reported similar features.

UUMN dysarthria is more frequently studied in small infarcts (Kim *et al.*, 2003) and lacunar strokes. It contributes to some classical lacunar syndromes (Fisher, 1982) such as pure motor hemiparesis, ataxic hemiparesis, and dysarthria clumsy-hand syndrome.

The dysarthria clumsy-hand syndrome represents 6% of the lacunar syndromes (Arboix *et al.*, 2004; Chamorro *et al.*, 1991). It includes dysarthria, facial weakness, and dysphagia as prominent signs. It is associated with mild weakness and clumsiness of the hand. The lesion mainly concerns the internal capsule, pons, and corona radiata (Arboix *et al.*, 2004; Schonewille *et al.*, 1999). Outcome is usually good (Arboix *et al.*, 2003; 2004).

Pure dysarthria may be associated with face and tongue weakness. It is observed in 1% of lacunar strokes (Arboix *et al.*, 1991). The lesion mainly concerns the corona radiata and the internal capsule (Ozaki *et al.*, 1986; 1991; Ichikawa and Kageyama, 1991; Bogousslavsky and Regli, 1990; Urban *et al.*, 1999). Okuda *et al.* (1999) found that pure dysarthria is usually due to bilateral lacunes.

These syndromes are probably due to a partial involvement of the motor fibers along the course of the pyramidal tract. Pure dysarthria has been attributed to a lesion of the cortico-lingual tract (and to a lesser extent of the cortico-orofacial tract) with sparing of the cortico-spinal and cortico-ponto-cerebellar tracts (Urban *et al.*, 1999).

Ataxic dysarthria

Ataxic dysarthria is the motor speech disorder due to damage to the cerebellar circuit. It clearly reflects a breakdown in motor organization and control, rather than in neuromuscular execution that characterizes other dysarthria types. When the examiner listens to a patient with ataxic dysarthria, the impression is not one of underlying weakness, resistance to movement, or restriction of movement, but rather one of an activity that is being poorly controlled or coordinated (Duffy, 1995). Patients with ataxic dysarthria often complain of slurred speech like in other dysarthria types, but they also frequently insist on the "drunken quality" of their speech. They may also report dramatic deterioration in their speech with limited alcohol intake.

The first main deviation of ataxic dysarthria is articulatory inaccuracy that comprised imprecise consonants, irregular articulatory breakdowns, and vowel distortions. These features reflect inaccuracy in the direction of articulatory movements and dysrhythmia of repetitive movements. There is also a prosodic impairment. Some speakers exhibit explosive loudness and poorly modulated pitch and loudness variation. This deviance is striking when present. A slow voice tremor of approximately 3 Hz may be observed due to tremor of the laryngeal and respiratory muscles (Ackermann and Ziegler, 1991). Abnormal resonance is considered as infrequent in ataxic dysarthria. However, intermittent hypo or hypernasality may be perceived. They presumably reflect improper timing of the velar and articulatory gestures for nasal consonants (Auzou et al., 2000).

Finally, cerebellar mutism is a possible complication mainly described after posterior fossa surgery. It is usually observed in children after resection of a cerebellar mass lesion. However, rare cases have also been reported after stroke lesions (Nishikawa et al., 1998).

Most of the acoustic and physiological data on ataxic dysarthria were obtained from patients with neurodegenerative diseases. An altered respiratory patterning with poor coordination between chest wall components has been reported. Acoustical studies found abnormal variability in fundamental frequency and intensity during vowel prolongation and speech maximum articulation rate tasks.

Lechtenberg and Gilman (1978) suggested that cerebellar dysarthria due to focal cerebellar damage was most often associated with a lesion of the left superior paravermal region. Amarenco et al. (1991) described a patient with an isolated cerebellar dysarthria due to an infarction located precisely in the left paravermal zone of the rostral cerebellum, demonstrating the major role of this area in the control of speech. Dysarthria is more frequent in infarcts in the territory of the superior cerebellar artery (Onnient et al., 1994; Amarenco and Hauw 1990; Amarenco et al., 1988; 1991).

Many aspects of ataxic dysarthria seem to be explained by assuming that the cerebellum is involved in the temporal processing of sensory and motor information. Analysis of the articulatory pattern of ataxic subjects shows inconsistency in both range and velocity of movement, particularly in sequences of repeated monosyllables, while the maximum velocity is decreased or sometimes almost normal. In EMG analysis of articulators' functions, the pattern of rhythmical activation and suppression is generally distorted and irregular.

Flaccid dysarthria

Flaccid dysarthria is produced by injury or malfunction of one or more of the cranial or spinal nerves. It reflects a dysfunction at the level of the final common pathway (i.e. nuclei, axons, or neuromuscular junctions), and it affects to various degrees the respiratory, phonatory, resonatory, and articulatory components of speech (Duffy, 1995). The perceptual characteristics are due to muscular weakness and reduced muscle tone and their effects on the speed, range, and accuracy of speech movements. Unlike the other dysarthria types, flaccid dysarthria may result from damage confined to isolated muscle groups. The clinical presentation varies according to the damaged neuronal structure. The salient perceptual speech characteristics are a marked hypernasality with nasal emission of air, continuous breathiness during phonation, and audible inspiration (Darley *et al.*, 1975).

Table 6.2 summarizes the innervation of major subsystems of speech production and the consequences of damage to specific cranial nerves. Brainstem stroke affecting cranial nerve nuclei can lead to flaccid dysarthria. Wallenberg's lateral medullary syndrome is the most common vascular syndrome

Table 6.2. Peripheral innervation of major muscles system involved in speech production

Cranial Nerve	Muscle System
V, IX, X, XI	Nasopharyngeal system
IX, X	Pharyngeal muscles
XI, XII	Tongue muscles
VII	Lips and circumoral muscles
V	Mandibular muscles
X	Larynx, intrinsic muscles
V, VII and spinal nerves	Larynx, extrinsic muscles
XI and spinal nerves	Respiratory system

associated with flaccid dysarthria. It leads to ipsilateral nucleus ambiguous involvement with subsequent palatal, pharyngeal, and laryngeal weakness and associated dysarthria and dysphagia.

Key points Main types of stroke associated with dysarthria

Infarct type	Territory/characteristics
Territorial infarct	middle cerebral artery
	anterior cerebral artery
	posterior cerebral artery
	basilar artery
	laterobulbar (Wallenberg syndrome)
	cerebellar infarct: superior cerebellar artery
Lacunar infarct	Corona radiata
	Internal capsule
	Pons

Treatments

It is necessary first to determine the severity and type of involvement in each functional component, defined as a structure (or a set of structures) that works to generate or valve the speech air stream. The approach focuses on neurological signs. In many speech disorders, orofacial muscle strength and mobility is compromised. Management strategies undertaken by speech therapist are summarized in Table 6.3.

Single case studies and small group studies of dysarthric patients have suggested that therapy may improve their intelligibility (Robertson, 2001; Ray, 2002). Current practice in speech therapy often involves different kinds of oromotor exercises using various techniques and devices (e.g. tongue depressors, straws). In stroke patients, the preferred strategy relies on the treatment of all systems (phonatory, articulatory, resonatory, and respiratory) to enhance intelligible utterances (Freed, 2000; Robertson and Thomson, 1986). A recent study by Robertson (2001) suggested that the combination of a standardized clinic-based program and home exercises was beneficial in a group of patients with vascular dysarthria. Using a program based on orofacial myofunctional exercises, Ray (2002) showed a significant improvement of strength and mobility of buccal, facial, labial, and lingual musculature. The intelligibility also improved at the level of single words. However, a Cochrane review shows that available

Table 6.3. Speech therapy: main strategies

---

1. Attempted normalization of muscle tone and/or increasing strength and movement precision and co-ordination (Netsell, 1984).
2. Behavioral compensation, e.g. reducing rate of speech beyond an already slower rate to promote improved intelligibility (Yorkston *et al.*, 1999).
3. Elimination of maladaptive responses such as increasing rate of speech in order to reduce a speaking rate wrongly perceived as being too slow (Tudor and Selley, 1974).
4. Provision of prosthetic devices such as the palatal lift or training appliance to compensate for hypernasality in speech (Tudor and Selley, 1974).
5. Provision of assistive devices. These can range from very low-tech aids such as an alphabet board to a highly sophisticated computerized system. They may be intended to facilitate a single function such as improving rate of speech completely (Crow and Enderby, 1989).
6. Reducing the handicap by altering the environment, listener training, and promoting positive attitudes in those regularly communicating with the dysarthric individual (Berry and Sanders, 1983)

Source: From Sellars *et al.*, 2002

Key points Management and treatment of vascular dysarthria

Speech therapy
Further randomized controlled trial required
Usually performed in selected patients
No selection criteria available so far

---

studies cannot support or refute the effectiveness of speech therapy for vascular dysarthria (Sellars *et al.*, 2002). This highlights the need for future studies in this area.

REFERENCES

Ackermann, H. and Ziegler, W. (1991). Cerebellar voice tremor: an acoustic analysis. *J. Neurol. Neurosurg.* Psychiatry, **54**, 74–6.

Amarenco, P., Chevrie-Muller, C., Roullet, E. and Bousser, M. G. (1991). Paravermal infarct and isolated cerebellar dysarthria. *Ann. Neurol.*, **30**, 211–13.

Amarenco, P., Debroucker, T. and Cambier, J. (1988). Dysarthrie et instabilité révélant un infarctus distal de l'artére cérébelleuse supérieure gauche. *Rev. Neurol. (Paris)*, **144**, 459–61.

Amarenco, P. and Hauw, J. J. (1990). Cerebellar infarction in the territory of the superior cerebellar artery. A clinicopathologic study of 33 cases. *Neurology*, **40**, 1383–90.

Amarenco, P., Roullet, E., Goujon, C., *et al.* (1991). Infarction of the anterior rostral cerebellum. *Neurology*, **41**, 253–8.

Arboix, A., Bell, Y., Garcia-Eroles, L., *et al.* (2004). Clinical study of 35 patients with dysarthria–clumsy hand syndrome. *J. Neurol. Neurosurg. Psychiatry*, **75**, 231–4.

Arboix, A., Garcia-Eroles, L., Comes, E., *et al.* (2003). Predicting spontaneous early neurological recovery after acute ischemic stroke. *Eur. J. Neurol.*, **10**, 429–35.

Arboix, A., Marti-Vilalta, J. L. and Garcia, J. H. (1990). Clinical study of 227 patients with lacunar infarcts. *Stroke*, **21**, 842–7.

Arboix, A., Massons, J., Oliveres, M. and Titus, F. (1991). Isolated dysarthria. *Stroke*, **22**, 531.

Auzou, P., Gaillard, M. J., Özsancak, C., *et al.* (1998). Evaluation clinique de la dysarthrie. *L'Ortho-Editions*, Isbergues.

Auzou, P., Özsancak, C., Jan, M., *et al.* (2000). Intérêt de l'évaluation motrice des organes de la parole dans le diagnostic des dysarthries. *Rev. Neurol. (Paris)*, **156**, 47–52.

Benke, T. and Kertesz, A. (1989). Hemispheric mechanisms of motor speech. *Aphasiology*, **3**, 627–41.

Berry, W. and Sanders, S. B. (1983). Environmental education: the universal management approach for adults with dysarthria. In W. R. Berry, ed., *Clinical Dysarthria*. San Diego: College-Hill Press, pp. 203–16.

Bogousslavsky, J. and Regli, F. (1990). Capsular genu syndrome. *Neurology*, **40**, 1499–502.

Bogousslavsky, J., Van Melle, G. and Regli, F. (1988). The Lausanne Stroke Registry: analysis of 1,000 consecutive patients with first stroke. *Stroke*, **19**, 1083–92.

Chamorro, A., Sacco, R. L., Mohr, J. P., *et al.* (1991). Clinical-computed tomographic correlations of lacunar infarction in the Stroke Data Bank. *Stroke*, **22**, 175–81.

Chenery, H. J., Ingram, J. C. and Murdoch, B. E. (1990). Perceptual analysis of speech in ataxic dysarthria. *Aust. J. Hum. Commun. Dis.*, **18**, 19–28.

Chenery, H. J., Murdoch, B. E. and Ingram, J. C. (1988). Studies in Parkinson's disease: 1. Perceptual speech analyses. *Aust. J. Hum. Commun. Dis.*, **16**, 17–29.

(1992). The perceptual speech characteristics of persons with pseudobulbar palsy. *Aust. J. Hum. Commun. Dis.*, **20**, 21–30.

Crow, E. and Enderby, P. (1989) The effects of an alphabet chart on the speaking rate and intelligibility of speakers with dysarthia. In K. M. Yorkston and D. R. Beukelman, eds., *Recent Advances in Clinical Dysarthria*. Boston: College-Hill, pp. 99–108.

Darley, F. L., Aronson, A. E. and Brown, J. R. (1969a). Differential diagnostic patterns of dysarthria. *J. Speech Hear. Res.*, **12**, 246–69.

(1969b). Clusters of deviant speech dimensions in the dysarthrias. *J. Speech. Hear. Res.*, **12**, 462–96.

(1975). *Motor Speech Disorders*. Philadelphia: W.B. Saunders.

Duffy, J. R. (1995). *Motor Speech Disorders*. St Louis: Mosby-Year book.

Enderby, P. (1983). *Frenchay Dysarthria Assessment*. San Diego: College-Hill Press.

(1986). Relationships between dysarthric groups. *Br. J. Disord. Commun.*, **21**, 189–97.

Fisher, C. M. (1982). Lacunar strokes and infarcts: a review. *Neurology*, **32**, 871–6.

Freed, D. B. (2000). *Motor Speech Disorders*. United States Singular Thompson Learning.

Hartman, D. E. and Abbs, J. H. (1992). Dysarthria associated with focal unilateral upper motor neuron lesion. *Eur. J. Disord. Commun.*, **27**, 187–96.

Ichikawa, K. and Kageyama, Y. (1991). Clinical anatomic study of pure dysarthria. *Stroke*, **22**, 809–12.

Joanette, Y. and Dudley, J. G. (1980). Dysarthric symptomatology of Friedreich's ataxia. *Brain Lang.*, **10**, 39–50.

Kent, R. D., Duffy, J. R., Slama, A., Kent, J. F. and Clift, A. (2001). Clinicoanatomic studies in dysarthria: review, critique, and directions for research. *J. Speech Lang. Hear. Res.*, **44**, 535–51.

Kent, R. D., Weismer, G., Kent, J. F. and Rosenbek, J. C. (1989). Toward phonetic intelligibility testing in dysarthria. *J. Speech Hear. Dis.*, **54**, 482–99.

Kim, J. S. (1994). Pure dysarthria, isolated facial paresis, or dysarthria-facial paresis syndrome. *Stroke*, **25**, 1994–8.

Kim, J. S., Kwon, S. U. and Lee, T. G. (2003). Pure dysarthria due to small cortical stroke. *Neurology*, **60**, 1178–80.

Kluin, K. J., Foster, N. L., Berent, S. and Gilman, S. (1993). Perceptual analysis of speech disorders in progressive supranuclear palsy. *Neurology*, **43**, 563–6.

Kluin, K. J., Gilman, S., Lohman, M. and Junck, L. (1996). Characteristic of the dysarthria of multiple system atrophy. *Arch. Neurol.*, **53**, 545–8.

Kluin, K. J., Gilman, S., Markel, D., *et al.* (1988). Speech disorders in olivopontocerebellar atrophy correlate with Positron Emission Tomography findings. *Ann. Neurol.*, **23**, 547–54.

Kumral, E., Bayulkem, G. and Evyapan, D. (2002). Clinical spectrum of pontine infarction. Clinical-MRI correlations. *J. Neurol.*, **249**, 1659–70.

Kumral, E., Evyapan, D. and Balkir, K. (1999). Acute caudate vascular lesions. *Stroke*, **30**, 100–8.

Kumral, E., Ozkaya, B., Sagduyu, A., *et al.* (1998). The Ege Stroke Registry: a hospital-based study in the Aegean region, Izmir, Turkey. Analysis of 2,000 stroke patients. *Cerebrovasc. Dis.*, **8**, 278–88.

Lechtenberg, R. and Gilman, S. (1978). Speech disorders in cerebellar disease. *Ann. Neurol.*, **3**, 285–90.

Ludlow, C. L. and Bassich, C. J. (1983). The results of acoustical and perceptual assessment of two types of dysarthria. *Clinical Dysarthria*. San Diego: College-Hill Press, pp. 121–53.

(1984). Relationships between perceptual ratings and acoustic measures of hypokinetic speech. *The dysarthrias: Physiology, Acoustics, Perception, Management*. San Diego: College-Hill Press, pp. 163–5.

Lyden, P., Lu, M., Jackson, C., *et al.* (1999). Underlying structure of the National Institutes of Health Stroke Scale: results of a factor analysis. *Stroke*, **30**, 2347–54.

Melo, T. P., Bogousslavsky, J., van Melle, G. and Regli, F. (1992). Pure motor stroke: a reappraisal. *Neurology*, **42**, 789–98.

Netsell, R. (1984). Physiological studies of dysarthria and their relevance to treatment. In J. C. Rosenbek, ed., *Seminars in Language*. New York: Thieme-Stratton, pp. 279–92.

Netsell, R. and Rosenbek, J. (1985). Treating the dysarthrias. In: J. K. Darby, eds., *Speech and Language Evaluation in Neurology: Adult Disorders*. Orlando: Grune and Stratton, pp. 363–92.

Nishikawa, M., Komiyama, M., Sakamoto, H., Yasui, T. and Nakajima, H. (1998). Cerebellar mutism after basilar artery occlusion–case report. *Neurol. Med. Chir. (Tokyo)*, **38**, 569–73.

Okuda, B., Kawabata, K., Tachibana, H. and Sugita, M. (1999). Cerebral blood flow in pure dysarthria: role of frontal cortical hypoperfusion. *Stroke*, **30**, 109–13.

Onnient, Y., Mihout, B., Guegan-Massardier, E. and Samson, M. (1994). Aspects clinique et évolutif des infarctus cérébelleux. *Rev. Neurol. (Paris)*, **150**, 209–15.

Ozaki, I., Baba, M., Matsunaga, M., Takebe, K. and Narita, S. (1991). Capsular genu syndrome. *Neurology*, **41**, 1853–4.

Ozaki, I., Baba, M., Narita, S., Matsunaga, M. and Takebe, K. (1986). Pure dysarthria due to anterior internal capsule and/or corona radiata infarction: a report of five cases. *J. Neurol. Neurosurg. Psychiatry*, **49**, 1435–7.

Özsancak, C. and Auzou, P. (2003). Comment examiner une dysarthrie. *Rev. Neurol. (Paris)*, **159**, 466–9.

Ray, J. (2002). Orofacial myofunctional therapy in dysarthria: a study on speech intelligibility. *Int. J. Orofacial Myology*, **28**, 39–48.

Robertson, S. (2001). The efficacy of oro-facial and articulation exercises in dysarthria following stroke. *Int. J. Lang. Commun. Disord.*, **36** (Suppl), 292–7.

Robertson, S. J. and Thomson, F. (1986). Working with dysarthrics. A practical guide to therapy for dysarthria. Oxon: Winslow Press.

Ropper, A. H. (1987). Severe dysarthria with right hemisphere stroke. *Neurology*, **37**, 1061–3.

Schonewille, W. J., Tuhrim, S., Singer, M. B. and Atlas, S. W. (1999). Diffusion-weighted MRI in acute lacunar syndromes. A clinical-radiological correlation study. *Stroke*, **30**, 2066–9.

Sellars, C., Hughes, T. and Langhorne, P. (2002). Speech and language therapy for dysarthria due to nonprogressive brain damage: a systematic Cochrane review. *Clin. Rehabil.*, **16**, 61–8.

Theodoros, D. G., Murdoch, B. E. and Chenery, H. J. (1994). Perceptual speech characteristics of dysarthric speakers following severe closed head injury. *Brain Injury*, **8**, 101–24.

Thompson, E. C. and Murdoch, B. E. (1995a). Disorders of nasality in subject with upper motor neuron type dysarthria following cerebrovascular accident. *J. Commun. Dis.*, **28**, 261–76.

(1995b). Respiratory function associated with dysarthria following upper motor neuron damage. *Aust. J. Hum. Commun. Dis.*, **23**, 61–87.

Thompson, E. C., Murdoch, B. E. and Stokes, P. D. (1995a). Lip function in subjects with upper motor neuron type dysarthria following cerebrovascular accidents. *European J. Dis. Com.*, **30**, 451–66.

(1995b). Tongue function in subjects with upper motor neuron type dysarthria following cerebrovascular accidents. *J. Med. Speech Lang. Pathol.*, **3**, 27–40.

Tilling, K., Sterne, J. A., Rudd, A. G., *et al.* (2001). A new method for predicting recovery after stroke. *Stroke*, **32**, 2867–73.

Tudor, C. and Selley, W. G. (1974). A palatal training appliance and a visual aid for use in the treatment of hypernasal speech. *Br. J. Disord. Commun.*, **9**, 117–22.

Urban, P. P., Wicht, S., Hopf, H. C., Fleischer, S. and Nickel, O. (1999). Isolated dysarthria due to extracerebellar lacunar stroke: a central monoparesis of the tongue. *J. Neurol. Neurosurg. Psychiatr.*, **66**, 495–501.

Yorkston, K. M. and Beukelman, D. R. (1981). *Assessment of Intelligibility of Dysarthric Speech.* Tigard, OR: C. C. Publications.

Yorkston, K. M., Beukelman, D. R., Strand, E. A. and Bell, K. (1999). *Management of Speech Motor Disorders.* Austin, Texas: Pro-Ed Inc.

Yorkston, K. M., Beukelman, D. R. and Traynor, C. D. (1984). *Computerized Assessment of Intelligibility of Dysarthric Speech.* Austin, TX: Pro-Ed Inc.

7

Alexia and agraphia in acute and chronic stroke

Argye E. Hillis

Johns Hopkins University School of Medicine

Introduction

Reading and writing are increasingly important in society. More transactions and communications take place over the internet each day. Stroke or other focal brain injuries can selectively impair reading and/or writing, causing important deficits in these daily interactions. Although not immediately apparent on the traditional neurological examination, alexia and agraphia can be disabling and dehumanizing. Furthermore, these deficits may be the only functional sequel of certain types of stroke, such as posterior watershed infarct, embolism to the left posterior parietal cortex, or occlusion of the left posterior cerebral artery. Therefore, assessment of reading and writing is an essential component of a complete neurological examination in cases of suspected stroke.

Presentations of disordered reading and writing

Reading and spelling are complex tasks with a number of processing components, each of which can be individually impaired by focal brain lesions. It is possible to determine the component of the task that is disrupted by evaluating performance across a variety of tasks and by considering the types of error made by the patient.

In order to read a printed word, the sequence of letters must first be seen and attended to. This early visual processing involves computation of a sequence of increasingly abstract spatial representations of the visual stimulus. In this process, specific letter shapes must be converted to graphemes (abstract letter identities), so that the word *chair* written in lower-case script in the left-hand corner of the page is recognized as the same word as the stimulus CHAIR written in upper-case block letters at the bottom of the page. Then, the sequence of graphemes must be recognized as a familiar word (on the basis of stored knowledge of how words are spelled; sometimes known as the lexical orthographic representation).

This component of processing allows us to recognize *chair* but not *chare* as a familiar word. An orthographic representation activates the corresponding meaning of the word, or semantic representation (e.g. chair: furniture, for one, for sitting) as well as stored knowledge about its pronunciation. The pronunciation can be derived from orthography—phonology conversion mechanisms (or "phonics") or can rely on stored pronunciations of words – lexical phonological representations. Unfamiliar words can only be pronounced by "sounding them out" (using orthography-to-phonology conversion, OPC, mechanisms), as we do when reading aloud an unfamiliar family name. To read aloud, it is also necessary to access specific motor programs for articulating the word.

Similarly, to spell a familiar word to dictation, the spoken word can be recognized and understood by accessing the corresponding stored phonological representation and semantic representation, and can be spelled by accessing a stored orthographic representation. Alternatively, the spoken word can be spelled using phonology-to-orthography conversion mechanisms (POC mechanisms, essential for spelling unfamiliar words). In either case, the sequence of graphemes that comprise the spelling of the word must be held in a short-term memory system, or buffer, while motor programs for forming the written letters are executed. Finally, motor programs for writing specific letter shapes must be implemented.

Each of these component processes in reading or spelling can be individually impaired by brain damage. Although damage to any one component will affect reading and/or writing, the presentation will differ in terms of types of error and pattern of performance across tasks, as described below.

Impaired spatial attention: Neglect dyslexia

Hemispatial neglect is a common manifestation of nondominant hemisphere stroke. It can disrupt reading in a variety of ways.

Patients who neglect the side of space contralateral to brain damage (the "contralesional" side) as defined by the midplane of the viewer (called "viewer-centered" or "egocentric" neglect) will often fail to read words on the contralesional side of the paper (Hillis *et al.*, 1998).

Other patients, who neglect the contralesional sides of individual stimuli on both sides of the viewer (called "stimulus-centered" or "allocentric" neglect), make errors on the contralesional side in individual words on both sides of the paper (Ellis *et al.*, 1987a; Riddoch *et al.*, 1990; Hillis and Caramazza, 1991 and 1995b; Young *et al.*, 1991; Arguin and Bub, 1993; Nichelli *et al.*, 1993; Subbiah and Caramazza, 2000). For example, such patients might read *chair* as "hair" or "fair." Patients with both egocentric and allocentric neglect dyslexia generally recognize words correctly if the words are spelled aloud to them or written in vertical print (Hillis and Caramazza, 1995a). Their errors in spelling consist of failures to use visual feedback on the contralesional side of what has just been written, so that they fail to dot i's, cross t's, and make perseverative strokes in writing n, m, u, etc. (Ellis *et al.*, 1987b).

Still other patients neglect the contralesional side of the internal spatial representations of the string of graphemes in languages with left to right reading; they make errors on the initial letters of the word after right brain damage (or final letters of the word after left brain damage), whether the word is written in standard print or vertical print for reading, spelled aloud to the patient, or dictated for spelling (Baxter and Warrington, 1983; Barbut and Gazzaniga, 1987; Hillis and Caramazza, 1990; Warrington, 1991; see Haywood and Coltheart, 2000 and Hillis and Caramazza, 1995a for review of these distinct patterns of dyslexia due to neglect).

Impaired access to orthography from vision: Alexia without agraphia

Some lesions prevent spatial representations of the visual stimulus from activating stored orthographic representations or knowledge. Such patients typically have trouble recognizing printed letters (e.g. have trouble naming letters and matching letters to identical letters in a different case or font) and have trouble recognizing printed words, but can recognize words that are spelled aloud to them (Dejerine, 1892; Geschwind, 1965; Damasio and Damasio, 1986; Chialant and Caramazza, 1998; Cohen, *et al.*, 2003). Because orthographic knowledge itself is not affected, spelling is spared. Sometimes such patients can slowly recognize individual letters in the printed stimulus, and painstakingly name each letter, often making errors on visually similar letters (e.g. substituting e for o, or m for n). When their *letter-by-letter reading* is correct, they can identify the word. Longer words take longer to read than shorter words using this strategy. Errors tend to be visually similar words or "completion" errors. For example, a patient might identify the first few letters of the word, and then guess the remainder of the word (e.g. chair becomes "c-h-a . . . change"). Some patients read better if they manually trace the letters, to recognize letters through a different sensory modality (Seki *et al.*, 1995). This pattern of performance has classically been considered a "disconnection syndrome," since visual information about the printed word is disconnected from corresponding language cortex critical for accessing stored orthographic representations (as described in greater detail later).

Impaired access to orthography: Alexia with agraphia

Some patients are unable to recognize words whether the words are written or spelled aloud, because they cannot access previously learned knowledge of how words are spelled. Typically, such patients cannot distinguish real written words from pseudowords, cannot read aloud or understand written words, and cannot spell words reliably. Some patients who cannot access stored orthographic representations of familiar words are able to use orthography-to-phonology correspondence (OPC) mechanisms to read and spell "regular" words and pseudowords correctly. Such patients often make "regularization" errors in reading aloud and understanding irregular words (e.g., read *sweat* as "sweet"). This pattern of performance is sometimes called *surface dyslexia*. They may make similar errors in spelling (e.g. "sweat" spelled swet), called *surface dysgraphia* (Behrmann and Bub, 1992).

Impaired access to sublexical orthography-to-phonology correspondence (OPC) mechanisms

Patients who are particularly impaired in applying OPC mechanisms have relatively spared reading of familiar words, but have difficulty pronouncing (and/or spelling) unfamiliar words and pseudowords. They may substitute visually similar words (e.g. read *suite* as "suit" and fleed as "steep" or "flood"). This pattern is sometimes referred to as *phonological dyslexia* and is often accompanied by *phonological agraphia* (Goodglass and Budin, 1988; see Shallice, 1988, for a review).

Impaired access to semantic representations

Selective impairment in accessing semantic representations of words is manifest by poor comprehension of written and spoken words. Characteristically, patients will make "semantic errors" in comprehension tasks, such as matching the word *chair* to a picture of a table. Oral reading, at least of regular words, may be intact, because the patient can use orthography-to-phonology conversion mechanisms. Therefore, they often show "surface dyslexia," making regularization errors (e.g., *flood* read as "flude") (Behrmann and Bub, 1992). They also often show *surface dysgraphia*, making comparable regularization errors in spelling to dictation (e.g. "soup" spelled as *supe*). However, unlike patients with selectively impaired access to orthographic representations, patients with impaired access to semantic representations often misunderstand even words that they read aloud and spell correctly (Hillis and Caramazza, 1991b). This pattern of performance is often observed in cases of dementia.

Impaired access to semantic representations and orthography-to-phonology correspondence mechanisms

This combination of deficits leads to a pattern of performance known as *deep dyslexia*, characterized by production of "semantic errors" (e.g. *flood* read as "rain"; *chair* read as "table") not only in comprehension, but also in oral reading (Coltheart *et al.*, 1980). Such patients may access incomplete meanings of words (e.g. specifying that a chair is a type of furniture, but not specifying that it is used for sitting), and thus would access phonological representations of "table," "chair," "sofa," "bureau" from the incomplete semantic representation of chair. Normally, orthography-to-phonology correspondence mechanisms would "block" reading the word *chair* as "table," but are impaired in these patients. Patients with the combination of impaired access to semantic representations and phonology-to-orthography correspondence (POC) mechanisms typically have *deep agraphia*, characterized by semantic errors in written naming and spelling to dictation. They are unable to spell unfamiliar words, and have trouble comprehending spoken and written words (Bub and Kertesz, 1982; Hillis, 1991).

However, the reading pattern of "deep dyslexia" can also be observed in cases with impaired access to phonological representations along with impaired orthography-to-phonology correspondence mechanisms, in the face of intact semantic representations. In these cases, reading comprehension is spared, but the patient makes semantic errors in oral reading. For example, patient RGB read *blue* as "orange" but defined it as "another color of the flag and the sky is supposed to be." He read *six* as "seven" but defined it as "half a dozen" (Caramazza and Hillis, 1990). Such patients do not characteristically make semantic errors in spelling, since access to orthographic representations is intact.

Impaired access to phonological representations for output in reading: Alexia with anomia

Many patients are impaired in both oral naming and oral reading, because they have trouble accessing learned phonological representations. Such patients understand written (and spoken) words, but make errors in reading them aloud. They may make semantic errors as noted above, if they also have trouble using orthography-to-phonology correspondence mechanisms. In these cases, oral naming and oral reading of the same items are very similar. For example, RGB read the word *celery* as "lettuce," and named a picture of celery as "lettuce," but he demonstrated access to the semantic representation of celery by his written naming of celery as *celry*. Other patients who fail to access the phonological representation of words rely on orthography-to-phonology conversion to sound out either the entire word, or enough of the word to facilitate access to the phonological representation. In these cases, oral reading is better than oral naming of pictures and objects, because objects do not provide the additional information to facilitate access to the pronunciation of the word. To illustrate, patient JSR correctly named only 54% of pictured objects, but correctly read aloud 82% of the names of the same objects (Hillis and Caramazza, 1995c). His errors in oral reading were those characteristic of deep dyslexia: semantic errors (e.g. *accordion* read as "organ"), visually similar words (e.g. *shall* read as "hall"), and morphological errors (e.g. *speak* read as "speech"). Although JSR could not read unfamiliar words or pseudowords, he was able to use orthography-to-phonology correspondence mechanisms to "sound out" the beginning of the word, which cued his oral reading (see also Nickels, 1992). He showed similar accuracy in naming objects (90%) when he was supplied with the beginning of the word as a cue (e.g. a pictured locker +/la/elicited "locker").

Patients with intact orthography-to-phonology conversion, with impaired access to phonological representations, show the errors characteristic for "surface dyslexia" (regularization errors such as *great* read as "greet"; Patterson *et al.*, 1985). However, in contrast to patients with impaired access to orthographic representations, these patients understand the written words that they pronounce incorrectly (e.g. understand the word *great* as meaning excellent).

Pure agraphia

As noted, damage to many of the components of reading described above also disrupt spelling. However, both alexia and agraphia can occur independently. Some patients are able to access orthography in order to read, but *fail to access orthographic representations of words for spelling*. These patients may rely on phonology-to-orthography correspondence mechanisms, manifested by *surface dysgraphia* (e.g. spelling the word *shoe* as *shew*). Those who are also impaired in using phonology-to-orthography correspondence mechanisms often make semantic errors in written naming and in spelling to dictation, as in *deep dysgraphia*. For example, immediately after her stroke, patient RCM (Hillis *et al.*, 1999) was able to read, speak, and understand normally, but could not write. She was able to correctly read aloud the word *tulip*; in naming a picture of a tulip she correctly said "tulip," but wrote the word *rose*. Her written naming and spelling to dictation were severely impaired, but she could write nouns better than verbs, concrete words better than abstract words, and high-frequency better than low-frequency words. She was unable to spell pseudo-words at all.

Other cases of pure agraphia result from an *impairment in holding the spelling of the word in the short-term memory* system or "buffer," resulting in deletion, substitution, insertion, and transposition of letters in written and oral spelling (and even delayed copying) of familiar and unfamiliar words. One hallmark of damage to this component is that spelling accuracy is only affected by word length; longer words are less accurate because they must be held longer in the buffer

(Caramazza *et al.*, 1987). Furthermore, since all stimuli must be held in the buffer while motor programs for writing or saying aloud individual letters are implemented, the frequency and type of spelling errors are comparable across all spelling tasks (oral and written spelling of familiar and unfamiliar words, written naming, and even delayed copying).

Still other patients show pure agraphia because of *impaired access to letter shape-specific motor plans from the abstract graphemes*. These patients (with so-called *apractic agraphia*) have impaired written spelling, but relatively intact oral spelling. Their errors include letter substitutions that share letter strokes with the intended letter (Black *et al.*, 1989; Kinsbourne and Rosenfield, 1974; Rapp and Caramazza, 1997; Rothi and Heilman, 1981; Zangwill, 1954). Since the problem is not in spelling per se, they even have trouble converting upper-case to lower-case print, and vice versa.

The main characteristics of each of these subtypes of alexia and agraphia are summarized in the Key points table.

Alexia and agraphia in stroke

Frequency of written language deficits and clinical presentation

Acutely after stroke, alexia and agraphia that result from damage to most vascular territories are ordinarily accompanied by other language or cognitive deficits. For example, left posterior frontal strokes often result in Broca's aphasia (see Chapter 4) as well as impaired oral reading due to disrupted access to phonological representations or disturbed motor speech, and impaired writing due to disrupted access to orthographic representations and problems with written sentence production. Similarly, in the case of neglect dyslexia and dysgraphia, there are usually non-linguistic spatial deficits, anosognosia, aprosodia, and other cognitive deficits associated with non-dominant hemisphere damage. Likewise, isolated damage to the left angular gyrus can cause alexia and agraphia without other language deficits, but there is often associated acalculia, left–right confusion, impaired reading and writing of music, and/or constructional deficits. Acute alexia without agraphia ("pure alexia") often co-occurs with right homonymous hemianopia, and these deficits may be the only or primary manifestations of left posterior cerebral artery strokes involving the left occipital lobe and splenium. Thus the frequency of written language deficits remains rarely examined at the acute stage of stroke and a few series suggest that it is rarely isolated.

Chronically, alexia and/or agraphia may be the residual deficits from any type of aphasia, either because less attention is paid to reading and spelling than verbal skills in rehabilitation, or because reading and writing are relatively later developed

Key points Alexia and agraphia due to damage to selective processing components

Presentations	Parameters that affect accuracy	Error types (with examples)
Pure alexia		
Viewer-centered (egocentric) *neglect dyslexia*	Location of words with respect to the viewer; orientation of word (few errors on vertical words; errors on opposite side in reading mirror-reversed words); modality (few errors recognizing orally spelled words)	*Reading*: substitution, deletion, or addition errors on words and letters on the side of the viewer contralateral to brain lesion (chair-> "fair" or "air") *Spelling*: writing only on side of paper ipsilateral to brain damage
Stimulus-centered (allocentric) *neglect dyslexia*	Word frequency relative to frequency of words that share letters on the ipsilesional side; orientation of word (e.g., few errors on vertical words); modality (few errors recognizing orally spelled words)	*Reading*: letter substitution, deletion, or addition on side of stimulus contralateral to brain lesion (chair-> "fair" or "air") *Spelling*: perseverative strokes; failure to dot i's and cross t's. ("chain"-> chalmm)
Impaired access to orthography from vision	Word length and frequency; modality of input (few or no errors in recognizing orally spelled words); stimulus presentation rate (worse for brief/faster presentation)	*Reading*: visually similar words; "regularization" errors (leopard-> "leepard"); letter-by-letter reading (*two*-> "t-w-o") *Spelling*: few or none
Alexia with agraphia		
Object-centered *neglect dyslexia* and dysgraphia	Word frequency relative to frequency of words that share letters on the side ipsilateral to brain damage. No effect of location, orientation, or modality	*Reading and spelling*: letter substitution, deletion, or addition on side of canonical representation of word contralateral to brain damage (chair-> "fair" or "air")
Impaired *access* to *stored orthographic* representations	Word frequency, grammatical word class; orthographic regularity	*Reading*: phonologically plausible errors, including "regularization" errors (*one*-> "own") *Spelling*: phonologically plausible errors (*chair*-> chare; "one"-> *wun*)
Impaired use of *OPC* and *POC*	Lexicality (words better than pseudowords); word length	*Reading and/or spelling*: inability to read or spell pseudowords

Key points (cont.)

Presentations	Parameters that affect accuracy	Error types (with examples)
Impaired *semantics* and impaired use of OPC and POC	Word frequency, concreteness (concrete > abstract), grammatical word class (nouns > verbs)	*Reading and spelling:* semantically related words (chair- > table); +/− visually similar words (chair- > cheer); +/−morphological errors (sleeping- > sleeps)
Pure agraphia		
Impaired access to stored *orthographic* representations for *output*	Word frequency, grammatical word class (nouns better than verbs); +/− orthographic regularity	Phonologically plausible errors (*chair*- > chare; "one"- > *wun*) if POC intact; semantic errors ("one"- > *two*) if POC impaired
Impaired *short-term storage* (buffer)	Word length	Letter substitution, addition, deletion, and transposition in all spelling tasks ("chair"- > *hcap*)
Impaired access to *letter-specific motor plans*	Modality (oral spelling better than written spelling)	Poorly formed letters or substitution of letters that share strokes with the target

OPC: orthography-to-phonology conversion; POC: phonology-to-orthography conversion

skills that are practiced less frequently (both before and after stroke). The nature of reading and spelling deficits will nevertheless vary depending on the site of the stroke as described below.

Strokes responsible for alexia and agraphia

Most of the data regarding the location of damage that results in specific types of reading and spelling impairments comes from patients with ischemic stroke. Cerebral hemorrhage and subarachnoid hemorrhage can also result in alexia or agraphia, but the characteristics of reading and spelling problems after these types of stroke are more variable. Therefore, this chapter will focus on sites of acute or chronic infarct that are associated with damage to specific components of reading and spelling. Much of the data will come from studies of reading and writing impairments associated with regions of hypoperfusion and/or infarct in acute stroke (within 24–48 hours from onset), since structure/function relationships are often clearest before there is opportunity for reorganization of these relationships during recovery and rehabilitation (Hillis *et al.*, 2004). At least in the acute phase of stroke, language deficits and other functional deficits reflect not only the structural lesion, but also the penumbra – the surrounding region of brain that is receiving enough blood to survive, but not enough to function. These regions can be identified using magnetic resonance perfusion weighted imaging (PWI) or CT perfusion (Hillis *et al.*, 2001a,b; Croquelois *et al.*, 2003). Here we discuss regions of infarct and/or hypoperfusion that have been associated with impairment of specific components of reading or spelling, but note that these tasks undoubtedly engage large networks of interacting brain regions.

Right middle cerebral artery (MCA) and posterior cerebral artery (PCA) ischemia

A recent study of 95 patients who had language testing and MRI (including PWI within 48 hours from onset of nondominant hemisphere stroke showed a strong association between viewer-centered (egocentric) neglect dyslexia and hypoperfusion/infarct of right inferior parietal lobule (angular and supramarginal gyri) and visual association cortex (Hillis *et al.*, 2005a). A subsequent, larger study showed that viewer-centered (egocentric) neglect, including neglect dyslexia, was associated with hypoperfusion of BA 44/45 (posterior, inferior frontal gyrus) as well as right inferior parietal hypoperfusion (Hillis, *et al.*, 2005). In both these studies, stimulus-centered neglect dyslexia was associated with hypo-perfusion and/or infarct of right superior temporal cortex. Object-centered neglect dyslexia was characterized by errors on the contralesional side of the canonical representation of the word irrespective of the orientation or format of the word – upside down or right-side up or mirror-reversed or spelled aloud (e.g. the initial letters in patients with right hemisphere lesions or the final letters of the word in patients with left hemisphere lesions). Object-centered neglect dyslexia was distinguished from stimulus-centered neglect dyslexia because patients with left stimulus-centered neglect made errors on the initial letters of words in standard print but the final letters of words in mirror-reversed or upside down print; patients with left object-centered neglect made errors on the initial letters in all tasks. Object-centered neglect was observed only with hypoperfusion and/or infarct of non-dominant superior temporal cortex in left-handed individuals. Single case studies of patients with chronic viewer-centered neglect dyslexia have also implicated right PCA and MCA territory strokes (e.g. Hillis *et al.*, 1998); and single case studies of patients with chronic stimulus-centered neglect dyslexia have implicated right MCA or internal carotid artery (ICA) strokes. For cases of stimulus-centered neglect dyslexia, see Ellis *et al.* (1987), Riddoch *et al.* (1990), Hillis and Caramazza (1991a), Young *et al.* (1991), Arguin and Bub (1993), Nichelli *et al.* (1993), and Subbiah and Caramazza (2000). All previously reported cases of marked object-centered neglect dyslexia have been left-handed and had right (or left, nondominant) hemisphere damage (Baxter and Warrington, 1983; Barbut and Gazzaniga, 1987; Hillis and Caramazza, 1990; 1995a; 1995b; Caramazza and Hillis, 1990a; 1990b; Warrington, 1991).

Left PCA ischemia

Pure alexia (also called "alexia without agraphia," often manifested by letter-by-letter reading), has long been attributed to the combination of lesions in (1) left occipital cortex, which prevents early visual processing in the left hemisphere, and (2) the splenium of the corpus collosum, which prevents visual information from crossing from the right hemisphere visual areas to left hemisphere language areas (Dejerine, 1892; Geschwind, 1965; Damasio and Damasio, 1986; Binder and Mohr, 1992; Chialant and Caramazza, 1998; Miozzo and Caramazza, 1998; Saffran and Coslett, 1998; Cohen et al., 2004). These two lesions are caused by occlusion or stenosis of the left PCA. More recent studies have often emphasized the lesions of the left mid-fusiform gyrus, also in the left PCA territory (or "watershed" region between left PCA and MCA territories), with or without damage to white matter tracks, in causing pure alexia (Binder and Mohr, 1992; Saffran and Coslett, 1998; Cohen et al., 2003; McCandliss et al., 2003). However, a recent study of 80 acute stroke patients indicated that damage to the left mid-fusiform gyrus alone is not associated with impaired reading comprehension, since the right mid-fusiform gyrus seems to be able to carry out the same role in reading, as long as it is not disconnected from left hemisphere language areas by hypoperfusion or infarct of the splenium (Hillis et al., 2005b). Converging evidence from functional imaging studies and lesion studies is consistent with the hypothesis that the left (or right) mid-fusiform gyrus is responsible for computation of a prelexical representation of the string of graphemes that is independent of location, font, or case (Price et al., 1996; Puce et al., 1996; Cohen et al., 2000; 2002; McCandliss et al., 2003; Cohen and Dehaene, 2004; Hillis et al., 2005b). Damage or dysfunction of both mid-fusiform gyri or disconnection of mid-fusiform gyri from visual input or areas important for language processing results in impaired reading.

There is also evidence from both functional imaging studies and lesion studies that the left mid-fusiform gyrus (or a nearby area also in left Brodmann's area 37) has a role in modality-independent lexical output, including writing. Functional imaging studies show activation in this region during a variety of lexical tasks in different modalities (Price et al., 2003; Price and Devlin, 2003; 2004), including spelling (Rapcsak and Beeson, 2004). Damage or dysfunction of this region results in impaired naming (oral and written) as well as impaired oral reading (Raymer et al., 1997; Foundas et al.,

1998; Hillis *et al.*, 2005b). Additional evidence that lesions of left Brodmann's area (BA) 37 can cause spelling impairment has come from studies of chronic stroke patients with impaired access to lexical representations for written output (Patterson and Kay, 1982; Rapcsak *et al.*, 1990; Rapcsak and Beeson, 2004). Lesions to this area have also been implicated in certain cases of selective difficulty in spelling Kanji (equivalent to orthographic word forms) versus Kana (equivalent to sublexical OPC mechanisms; Kawahata *et al.*, 1988; Sakurai *et al.*, 1994; Soma *et al.*, 1989). These results together indicate that BA 37 may be crucial for accessing modality-independent lexical representations for oral reading, writing, and naming.

Left inferior division MCA ischemia

Impaired access to learned spelling of words (orthographic representations), and learned correspondences between spelling and pronunciation, resulting in alexia with agraphia, has long been attributed to damage to the left angular gyrus in studies of chronic stroke (Dejerine, 1891; Benson, 1979; Vanier and Caplan, 1985; Black and Behrmann, 1994) and acute stroke (Hillis *et al.*, 2001a; 2002). Hypoperfusion of left angular gyrus, with or without infarct of this region, was strongly associated with impaired reading comprehension and oral reading of both words and pseudowords in a study of 80 patients within 24 hours of stroke onset (Hillis *et al.*, 2005b). Likewise, acquired dyslexia observed many years after stroke was attributed to hypoperfusion without infarct of left angular gyrus (Love *et al.*, 2002). Impaired access to orthographic representations for spelling has been observed after chronic stroke involving the left angular gyrus (Beauvois and Derouesne, 1981; Dejerine, 1891; Goodman and Caramazza, 1986; Hatfield and Patterson, 1983; Rapcsak and Beeson, 2002; Roeltgen and Heilman, 1984; Vanier and Caplan, 1985) as well as in acute hypoperfusion and/or infarct of left angular gyrus (Hillis *et al.*, 2001a). Some functional imaging studies also show activation in this area during reading (Horwitz *et al.*, 1998; Pugh *et al.*, 2001; Joubert *et al.*, 2004) and spelling (Beeson *et al.*, 2003).

Left superior division MCA ischemia

Lesion studies and functional imaging studies converge in support of the hypothesis that left posterior inferior frontal regions (including Broca's area) is important for modality-specific output in both oral reading and writing (Pugh *et al.*, 2001; Hillis *et al.*, 2002; 2004). Thus, lesions or hypoperfusion in the left Broca's area can result in pure agraphia due to impaired access to lexical orthographic representations (Hillis *et al.*, 1999; 2002; 2004) or impaired

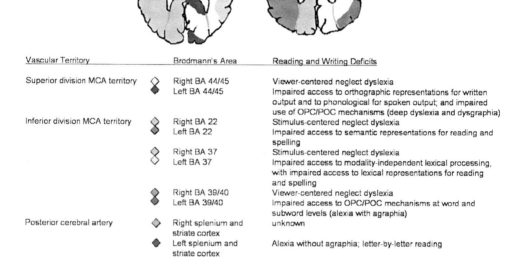

Vascular Territory		Brodmann's Area	Reading and Writing Deficits
Superior division MCA territory	◇	Right BA 44/45	Viewer-centered neglect dyslexia
	◆	Left BA 44/45	Impaired access to orthographic representations for written output and to phonological for spoken output; and impaired use of OPC/POC mechanisms (deep dyslexia and dysgraphia)
Inferior division MCA territory	◇	Right BA 22	Stimulus-centered neglect dyslexia
	◆	Left BA 22	Impaired access to semantic representations for reading and spelling
	◇	Right BA 37	Stimulus-centered neglect dyslexia
	◇	Left BA 37	Impaired access to modality-independent lexical processing, with impaired access to lexical representations for reading and spelling
	◇	Right BA 39/40	Viewer-centered neglect dyslexia
	◆	Left BA 39/40	Impaired access to OPC/POC mechanisms at word and subword levels (alexia with agraphia)
Posterior cerebral artery	◇	Right splenium and striate cortex	unknown
	◆	Left splenium and striate cortex	Alexia without agraphia; letter-by-letter reading

Figure 7.1   Neural regions associated with impairments of specific components of reading and spelling tasks, leading to different profiles of dyslexia and dysgraphia. The sites are shown in neuroradiographic convention, with the left hemisphere on the right side of the figure (OPC: orthography-to-phonology conversion; POC: phonology-to-orthography conversion). For a color version of this figure please see www.cambridge.org/9780521106955.

spoken output in oral reading and other oral tasks. This region may be more important for accessing the orthographic (and phonological) representations of verbs than nouns in word production (see Hillis *et al.*, 2003, for evidence from spelling; see Nadeau *et al.*, 2000, for evidence from reading). Broca's area also has a role in sublexical orthography-to-phonology conversion, probably in the output stage, such that lesions often result in poor oral reading of pseudowords (Rapcsak and Beeson, 2002). Lesions just posterior and superior to Broca's area, in BA 6, can also cause pure agraphia (Exner; 1881; Anderson *et al.*, 1990), probably due to impaired access to letter-specific motor plans (Hillis *et al.*, 2004).

The areas of the brain that are crucial for various aspects of reading and spelling are illustrated in Figure 7.1. The sites of ischemia that result in

Table 7.1. Site of lesion responsible for each type of alexia and agraphia

Reading/writing impairment	Site(s) of lesion or dysfunction
Pure alexia:	
Impaired spatial attention (contralateral to brain damage) to written words	Right BA 18/19 (visual association cortex), BA 22 (superior temporal gyrus), BA 39/40 (inferior parietal lobule)
Impaired computation of a prelexical representations of the sequence of graphemes, independent of location, case, font, or modality	Left BA 17 (occipital) and splenium; left BA 37 (midfusiform gyrus) and splenium; or bilateral midfusiform gyri
Alexia and agraphia:	
Impaired spatial attention (contralateral to brain damage) to abstract, canonical representations of words for reading and spelling	Nondominant BA 22 (superior temporal gyrus)
Impaired access to modality-independent lexical representations for output	Left BA 37 (posterior inferior temporal and fusiform gyri)
Impaired access to learned orthography to phonology correspondence (lexical and sublexical) for input and output	Left BA 39 (angular gyrus)
Impaired use of sublexical OPC and POC mechanisms	Left BA 39 (angular gyrus), Left BA 44/45 (posterior inferior frontal gyrus)
Pure agraphia:	
Impaired access to modality-specific orthographic or phonologic representations for output	Left BA 44/45 (posterior inferior frontal gyrus)
Impaired access to letter-specific motor plans	Left BA 6

Key points Strokes responsible for alexia and agraphia

Stroke type	
Arterial infarct	
Right middle cerebral artery and posterior cerebral artery	Neglect dyslexia
Left posterior cerebral artery	Alexia without agraphia, (letter-by-letter reading)
Left middle cerebral artery: inferior division	Alexia with agraphia (impaired access to orthographic representations)
Left middle cerebral artery: superior division	Pure agraphia (impaired access to lexical orthographic representations)
Hemorrhage	Posterior cortex
Cerebral venous thrombosis	Left lateral sinus?

impairments of specific components of reading and spelling are summarized in Table 7.1.

Assessment of alexia and agraphia in stroke

There are several standardized tests of reading and spelling, and several aphasia batteries that include tests of reading and writing, that are designed for patients with focal brain damage. Some of the commonly used tests are listed in the Key points table. Many of these tests are quite time consuming and are most useful for examining patients at the chronic stage of stroke or for research purposes. Much shorter, bedside assessment of reading and spelling can provide adequate information to characterize reading and spelling problems, in terms of the underlying processes that are impaired (e.g. Hillis *et al.*, 2001a). It is important to examine performance across language tasks to determine if the impairment is specific to reading or spelling, or common to other input or output tasks. For example, comparable impairments in oral reading and oral naming may be due to impaired access to phonological representations for output. It is also important to compare performance across different types of stimuli. Useful tasks include: (1) oral reading of words and pseudo-words; (2) oral and written naming of words matched in frequency and word class to stimulus words used for oral reading; (3) written word/picture matching; (4) matching letters and words in different case or font; (5) converting written words to a different case; (6) spelling to dictation of words and pseudo-words; (7) oral spelling of dictated words; and (8) recognition of orally spelled words. Narrative reading and writing tasks can also be very revealing. Sentence

Key points Tests of reading and writing useful in examining stroke patients

Reading Comprehension Battery for Aphasia (LaPoint and Horner, 1998)

Psycholinguistic Assessments of Language Processing in Aphasia (PALPA) (Kay, Lesser and Coltheart, 1992)

Johns Hopkins Dyslexia Battery (Goodman and Caramazza, unpublished; see Beeson and Hillis, 2001 for stimuli and description)

Johns Hopkins Dysgraphia Battery (Goodman and Caramazza, unpublished; see Beeson and Hillis, 2001 for stimuli and description)

Boston Diagnostic Aphasia Examination III, reading and writing subtests (Goodglass, Kaplan and Barresi, 2001)

Western Aphasia Battery, reading and writing subtests (Kertesz, 1982)

Aachen Aphasia Test (Huber, Poeck and Willmes, 1984)

production deficits can be observed in both reading and writing, but are beyond the scope of this chapter.

Prognosis and management of alexia and agraphia

Recovery from alexia and agraphia, like recovery from other language deficits, likely occurs in separate but overlapping stages (Hillis and Heidler, 2003). The initial stage of recovery, beginning within days to hours of stroke onset, depends on restoration of tissue function. This stage of recovery can be facilitated by interventions that improve blood flow to the ischemic penumbra responsible for some of the acute deficits. Prognosis for recovery at this stage depends on the volume of tissue that is irreversibly infarcted, the availability of treatment, and the mechanism of stroke. The second stage, which begins within days to weeks after onset and may continue for months or years, involves reorganization of structure/function relationships. That is, even if the left angular gyrus is crucial for accessing learned orthographic representations and/or learned orthography-to-phonology correspondences, other regions of the brain may assume this function. Prognosis at this stage probably depends on the volume and site of the lesion, the status of the spared regions of brain, and appropriate stimulation (rehabilitation and practice). The final stage of recovery, which can continue for a lifetime, involves learning strategies to access stored information in new ways, re-learning previously learned spellings and/or pronunciations, and learning compensatory strategies that can be used in place of damaged components.

Most rehabilitation strategies focus either on stimulating reorganization (e.g. Multiple Oral Re-Reading; Moyer, 1979; Beeson, 1998; Beeson and Insalaco, 1998) or on teaching new strategies to compensate for impaired processes. Treatment of reading and writing deficits should begin by identifying the impaired and spared processing components, to enable the clinician to focus on improving the impaired process or on using spared processes to compensate for the damaged ones. For example, many studies have demonstrated the usefulness of re-teaching OPC or POC mechanisms to "sound out" words in reading or writing to compensate for impaired access to learned spelling of words (DePartz, 1986), or to enable self-cuing by providing the initial sound or initial letter of the word (Hillis and Caramazza, 1995d; Nickels, 1992). Detailed descriptions of rehabilitation strategies for impairments involving each cognitive process underlying reading (Friedman, 2002; Hillis, 1993; Hillis and Caramazza, 1994) or spelling (Carlomagno *et al.*, 1994; Beeson and Rapcsak, 2002; Hillis, 1992) or both (Beeson and Hillis, 2001) have been

Key points Examples of rehabilitation strategies for alexia and agraphia

Impaired cognitive process	Strategy
Reading	
Impaired access to orthographic representations from vision; impaired computation of prelexical representations (alexia without agraphia)	1. Speeded reading or lexical decision to encourage "wholistic" word recognition versus letter-by-letter reading (Rothi and Moss, 1992) 2. Tracing letters for cross-modality recognition (Seki, Yajima, Sugishita, 1995)
Impaired access to orthography-to-phonology conversion (at word and subword level)	1. Focus on relearning OPC mechanisms though key words (DePartz, 1986; Hillis, 1993; 2003; Nickels, 1992)
Impaired access to lexical orthographic representations with spared sublexical OPC mechanisms ("surface dyslexia")	1. Training meaning of homophone pairs; e.g., pear/pair (Byng and Coltheart, 1986) or training meanings or pronunciation of words that could be pronounced the same; e.g., bear/beer (Hillis, 2003)
Impaired access to orthography to phonology correspondence (at word and subword level) and impaired access to meaning ("deep dyslexia")	Improving access to meaning through word/picture matching (Hillis, 1994) or trained use of OPC mechanisms to block semantic errors (DePartz, 1986)
Spelling	
Impaired access to phonology-to-orthography conversion (at word and subword level)	Focus on relearning POC mechanisms though key words (Carlomagno *et al.*, 1994; Hillis, 1992)
Impaired accessed to lexical orthographic representations with spared sublexical POC mechanisms ("surface dysgraphia")	1. Training spelling of homophone pairs; e.g., eight/ate (Hillis, 1992) 2. Anagram and Copy Treatment (Beeson, 1999)
Impaired access to orthography-to-phonology conversion (at word and subword level) and impaired access to meaning ("deep dysgraphia")	1. Improving access to semantics by teaching distinct features that distinguish semantic error from target (Hillis, 1991) and/or 2. Teaching POC mechanisms (Hillis and Caramazza, 1995d)

OPC: orthography-to-phonology conversion; POC: phonology-to-orthography conversion

previously reviewed. Some of the representative approaches are summarized in the Key points Table.

The role of pharmacotherapy for treatment of acquired alexia and agraphia has not been well-studied. However, a small series of patients have suggested that a number of medications may be useful in treating other language deficits, either alone or in conjunction with therapy (see Small, 2002; and Chapter 4). These adjuncts to behavioral therapy may also prove to be useful in treatment of alexia and agraphia; this hypothesis requires evaluation with controlled therapeutic trials.

REFERENCES

Anderson, S. W., Damasio, A. R. and Damasio, H. (1990). Troubled letters but not numbers: Domain specific cognitive impairments following focal damage in frontal cortex. *Brain*, **113**, 749–66.

Arguin, M. and Bub, D. N. (1993). Evidence for an independent stimulus-centered spatial reference frame from a case of visual hemineglect. *Cortex*, **29**, 349–57.

Barbut, D. and Gazzaniga, M. S. (1987). Disturbances in conceptual space involve language and speech. *Brain*, **110**, 1487–96.

Baxter, D. M. and Warrington, E. K. (1983). Neglect dysgraphia. *J. Neurol. Neurosurg. Psychiatry*, **46**, 1073–8.

Beauvois, M. F. and Derousne, J. (1981). Lexical or orthographic agraphia. *Brain*, **104**, 21–49.

Beeson, P. M. (1998). Treatment for letter-by-letter reading: A case study. In N. Helm-Estabrooks and A. L. Holland, eds., *Approaches to the Treatment of Aphasia*. San Diego, CA: Singular, pp. 153–77.

Beeson, P. M. (1999). Treating acquired writing impairment. *Aphasiology*, **13**, 367–86.

Beeson, P. M. and Hillis, A. E. (2001). Comprehension and production of written words. In R. Chapey, ed., *Language Intervention Strategies in Aphasia and Related Neurogenic Communication Disorders*, (4th edition). Baltimore: Williams and Wilkens, pp. 572–604.

Beeson, P. M. and Insalaco, D. (1998). Acquired alexia: Lessons from successful treatment. *J. Int. Neuropsychol. Soc.*, **4**, 621–35.

Beeson, P. M. and Rapcsak, S. Z. (2002). Clinical diagnosis and treatment of spelling disorders. In A. E. Hillis, ed., *The Handbook of Adult Language Disorders: Integrating Cognitive Neuropsychology, Neurology and Rehabilitation*. New York: Psychology Press, pp. 101–20.

Beeson, P. M., Rapcsak, S. Z., Plante, E., *et al.* (2003). The neural substrates of writing: A functional magnetic resonance imaging study. *Aphasiology*, **17**, 647–65.

Behrmann, M. and Bub, D. (1992). Surface dyslexia and dysgraphia: Dual routes, single lexicon. *Cogn. Neuropsychol.*, **9**, 209–51.

Benson, D. F. (1979). *Aphasia, Alexia, and Agraphia*. New York: Churchill Livingstone.

Binder, J. R. and Mohr, J. P. (1992). The topography of callosal reading pathways. A case-control analysis. *Brain*, **115**, 1807–26.

Black, S. and Behrmann, M. (1994). Localization in alexia. In A. Kertesz, ed., *Localization and Neuroimaging in Neuropsychology*. San Diego: Academic Press.

Black, S. E., Behrmann, M., Bass, K. and Hacker, P. (1989). Selective writing impairment: Beyond the allographic code. *Aphasiology*, **3**, 265–77.

Bub, D. and Kertesz, A. (1982). Deep agraphia. *Brain Lang.*, **17**, 146−65.

Byng, S. and Coltheart, M. (1986). Aphasia therapy research: Methodological requirements and illustrative results. In E. Hjelmquist and L.-G. Nilsson, eds., *Communication Handicap: Aspects of Psychological Compensation and Technical Aids*, North-Holland: Elsevier Science Publishers B. V.

Caramazza, A. and Hillis, A. E. (1990). Where do semantic errors come from? *Cortex*, **26**, 95−122.

(1990a). Spatial representation of words in the brain implied by studies of a unilateral neglect patient. *Nature*, **346**, 267−9.

(1990b). Levels of representation, coordinate frames, and unilateral neglect. In M. J. Riddoch, ed., *Neglect and the Peripheral Dyslexias, Special Issue of Cognitive Neuropsychology*, 391−445.

Caramazza, A., Miceli, G., Villa, G. and Romani, C. (1987). The role of the graphemic buffer in spelling: Evidence from a case of acquired dysgraphia. *Cognition*, **26**, 59−85.

Carlomagno, S., Iavarone, A. and Colombo, A. (1994). Cognitive approaches to writing rehabilitation. In M. J. Riddoch and G. Humphreys, eds., *Cognitive Neuropsychology and Cognitive Rehabilitation*. London: Lawrence Erlbaum Associates, pp. 485−502.

Chialant, D. and Caramazza, A. (1998). Perceptual and lexical factors in a case of letter-by-letter reading. *Cogn. Neuropsychol.*, **15**, 167−201.

Cohen, L. and Dehaene, S. (2004). Specialization within the ventral stream: The case for the visual word form area. *NeuroImage*, **22**, 466−76.

Cohen, L., Dehaene, S., Naccache, L., *et al.* (2000). The visual word form area: Spatial and temporal characterization of an initial stage of reading in normal subjects and posterior split-brain patients. *Brain*, **123**, 291−307.

Cohen, L., Henry, C., Dehaene, S., *et al.* (2004). The pathophysiology of letter-by-letter reading. *Neuropsychologia*, **42**(13), 1768−80.

Cohen, L., Lehericy, S., Chochon, F., *et al.* (2002). Language-specific tuning of visual cortex? Functional properties of the visual word form area. *Brain*, **125**, 1054−69.

Cohen, L., Martinaud, O., Lemer, C., *et al.* (2003). Visual word recognition in the left and right hemispheres: anatomical and functional correlates of peripheral alexias. *Cerebral Cortex*, **13**, 1313−33.

Coltheart, M., Patterson, K. and Marshall, J. C. (1980). *Deep Dyslexia*. London: Routledge and Kegan Paul.

Croquelois, A., Wintermark, M., Reichhart, M., Meuli, R. and Bogousslavsky, J. (2003). Aphasia in hyperacute stroke: Language follows brain penumbra dynamics. *Ann. Neurol.*, **54**(3), 321−9.

Damasio, A. R. and Damasio, H. (1986). Hemianopia, hemiachromatopsia and the mechanisms of alexia. *Cortex*, **22**, 161−9.

De Partz, M. P. (1986). Re-education of a deep dyslexic patient: Rationale of the method and results. *Cogn. Neuropsychol.*, **3**, 147−77.

Dejerine, J. (1891). Sur un cas de cécité verbale avec agraphie, suivi d'autopsie. *Comptes Rendus Hebdomadaires des Séances et Mémoires de la Société de Biologie*, Ninth series, **3**, 197−201.

Dejerine, J. (1892). Contribution à l'étude anatomo-pathologique et clinique des différentes variétés de cécité verbale. *Memoires Societe Biologique*, **4**, 61–90.

Ellis, A. W., Flude, B. M. and Young, A. W. (1987a). "Neglect Dyslexia" and the early visual processing of letters in words and nonwords, *Cogn. Neuropsychol.*, **4**, 439–64.

(1987b). "Afferent Dysgraphia" in a patient and normal subjects. *Cogn. Neuropsychol.*, **4**, 465–86.

Exner, S. (1881). *Lokalisation des Funcktion der Grosshirnrinde des Menschen*, Wein: Braunmuller.

Foundas, A., Daniels, S. K. and Vasterling, J. J. (1998). Anomia: Case studies with localization. *Neurocase*, **4**, 35–43.

Friedman, R. (2002). Clinical diagnosis and treatment of reading disorders. In A. E. Hillis (ed.) *Handbook of Adult Language Disorders: Integrating Cognitive Neuropsychology, Neurology, and Rehabilitation*, Philadelphia: Psychology Press, pp. 27–43.

Geschwind, N. (1965). Disconnection syndromes in animals and man. *Brain*, **88**, 237–94, 585–644.

Goodglass, H. and Budin, C. (1988). Category and modality specific dissociations in word comprehension and concurrent phonological dyslexia, *Neuropsychologia*, **26**, 67–78.

Goodglass, H., Kaplan, E. and Barresi, B. (2001). *Boston Diagnostic Aphasia Examination 3*. Austin, Tx: Pro-Ed.

Goodman, R. A. and Caramazza, A. (1986). Phonologically plausible errors: Implications for a model of the phoneme-grapheme conversion mechanism in the spelling process. In G. Augst, ed., *Proceedings of the International Colloquium on Graphemics and Orthography*, pp. 300–25.

Hatfield, F. M. and Patterson, K. (1983). Phonological spelling. *Q. J. Exp. Psychol.*, **35a**, 451–68.

Haywood, M. and Coltheart, M. (2000). Neglect dyslexia and the early stages of visual word recognition. *Neurocase*, **6**, 33–44.

Hillis, A. E. (1991). Effects of separate treatments for distinct impairments within the naming process. In T. Prescott, ed., *Clinical Aphasiology*, Vol. **19**. Austin, Texas: Pro-Ed, pp. 255–65.

(1992). Facilitating written language. In R. Peach, ed., *Clinics in Communication Disorders: Approaches to Treatment of Aphasia*, pp. 19–33.

(1993). The role of models of language processing in rehabilitation of language impairments. *Aphasiology*, **7**, 5–26.

(1994). Contributions from cognitive analysis. In R. Chapey, ed., *Language Intervention Strategies in Adult Aphasia*. Baltimore: Williams and Wilkens, pp. 207–19.

(2003). Alexia. In R. Kent, ed., *MIT Encyclopedia of Communication Disorders*. Cambridge, MA: MIT Press, pp. 236–40.

Hillis, A. E. and Caramazza, A. (1990). The effects of attentional deficits on reading and spelling. In A. Caramazza, ed., *Cognitive Neuropsychology and Neurolinguistics: Advances in Models of Cognitive Function and Impairment*. London: Lawrence Erlbaum Associates, pp. 211–75.

(1991a). Spatially-specific deficit to stimulus-centered letter shape representations in a case of "unilateral neglect." *Neuropsychologia*, **29**, 1223–40.

(1991b). Mechanisms for accessing lexical representations for output: Evidence from a category-specific semantic deficit. *Brain Lang.*, **40**, 106–44.

(1994). Theories of lexical processing and theories of rehabilitation. In G. Humphreys and M. J. Riddoch, eds., *Cognitive Neuropsychology and Cognitive Rehabilitation*. Hillsdale, NJ: Lawrence Erlbaum Associates, pp. 449–82.

(1995a). A framework for interpreting distinct patterns of hemispatial neglect. *Neurocase*, 1, 189–207.

(1995b). Spatially-specific deficits in processing graphemic representations in reading and writing. *Brain Lang.*, **48**, 263–308.

(1995c). Converging evidence for the interaction of semantic and phonological information in accessing lexical information for spoken output. *Cogn. Neuropsychol.*, **12**, 187–227.

(1995d). I know it but I can't write it: Selective deficits in long and short-term memory. In R. Campbell, ed., *Broken Memories: Neuropsychological Case Studies*, London: Blackwell, pp. 344–65.

Hillis, A. E., Chang, S. and Breese, E. (2003). The crucial role of posterior frontal regions in modality specific components of the spelling process. *Neurocase*.

Hillis, A. E. and Heidler, J. (2003). Contributions and limitations of the "Cognitive Neuropsychological approach" to treatment: Illustrations from studies of reading and spelling therapy. *Aphasiology*.

Hillis, A. E., Kane, A., Barker, P., Beauchamp, N. and Wityk, R. (2001a). Neural substrates of the cognitive processes underlying reading: Evidence from Magnetic Resonance Perfusion Imaging in hyperacute stroke. *Aphasiology*, **15**, 919–31.

Hillis, A. E., Kane, A., Tuffiash, E., *et al.* (2002). Neural substrates of the cognitive processes underlying spelling: Evidence from MR diffusion and perfusion imaging. *Aphasiology*, **16**, 425–38.

Hillis, A. E., Newhart, M., Heidler, J., Barker, P. B. and Degaonkar, M. (2005). Anatomy of spatial attention: insights from perfusion imaging and hemispatial neglect in acute stroke. *J. Neurosci.*, **25**, 3161–7.

Hillis, A. E., Newhart, M., Heidler, J., *et al.* (2005b). The roles of the "visual word form area" in reading. *NeuroImage*, **24**, 548–59.

Hillis, A. E., Newhart, M., Heidler, J., *et al.* (2005a). The neglected role of the right hemisphere in spatial representation of words for reading. *Aphasiology*, **19**, 225–38.

Hillis, A. E. and Rapp, B. S. (2004). Cognitive and neural substrates of written language comprehension and production. In M. Gazzaniga, ed., *The New Cognitive Neurosciences* (*3rd Edition*). Cambridge, MA: MIT Press, pp. 755–88.

Hillis, A. E., Rapp, B., Benzing, L. and Caramazza, A. (1998). Dissociable coordinate frames of unilateral spatial neglect: Viewer-centered neglect. *Brain Cogn.*, **37**, 491–526.

Hillis, A. E., Rapp, B. C. and Caramazza, A. (1999). When a rose is a rose in speaking but a tulip in writing. *Cortex*, **35**, 337–56.

Hillis, A. E., Wityk, R., Barker, P. B. and Caramazza, A. (2003). Neural regions essential for writing verbs. *Nature Neurosci.*, **6**, 19–20.

Hillis, A. E., Wityk, R. J., Tuffiash, E., *et al.* (2001b). Hypoperfusion of Wernicke's area predicts severity of semantic deficit in acute stroke. *Ann. Neurol.*, **50**, 561–6.

Hillis, A. E., Work, M., Breese, E. L., *et al.* (2004). Re-examining the brain regions crucial for orchestrating speech articulation. *Brain*, **127**, 1479–87.

Horwitz, B., Rumsey, J. M. and Donohue, B. C. (1998). Functional connectivity of the angular gyrus in normal reading and dyslexia. *Proc. Natl. Acad. Sci. USA*, **95**, 8939–44.

Huber, W., Poeck, K. and Willmes, K. (1984). The Aachen Aphasia Test. *Adv. Neurol.*, **42**, 291–303.

Joubert, S., Beauregard, M., Walter, N., *et al.* (2004). Neural correlates of lexical and sublexical processes in reading. *Brain Lang.*, **89**, 9–20.

Kawahata, N., Nagata, K. and Shishido, F. (1988). Alexia with agraphia due to the left posterior inferior temporal lobe lesion: Neuropsychological analysis and its pathogenetic mechanisms. *Brain Lang.*, **33**, 296–310.

Kay, J., Lesser, R. and coltheart, M. (1992). *Psycholinguistic Assessments of Language Processing in Aphasia (PALPA)*. East Sussex, England: Lawrence Erlbaum.

Kinsbourne, M. and Rosenfield, D. B. (1974). Agraphia selective for written spelling. *Brain Lang.*, **1**, 215–25.

Kertesz, A. (1982). *The Western Aphasia Battery*. San Antonio: Psychological Association.

Lapoint, L. L. and Horner, J. (1998). *Reading Comprehension Battery for Aphasia* (2nd edition). Austin, Tx: Pro-Ed.

Love, T., Swinney, D., Wong, E. and Buxton, R. (2002). Perfusion imaging and stroke: A more sensitive measure of the brain bases of cognitive deficits. *Aphasiology*, **16**, 873–83.

McCandliss, B. D., Cohen, L. and Dehaene, S. (2003). The visual word form area: Expertise for reading in the fusiform gyrus. *Trends Cogn. Sci.*, **7**, 293–9.

Miozzo, M. and Caramazza, A. (1998). Varieties of pure alexia: The case of failure to access graphemic representations. *Cogn. Neuropsychol.*, **15**, 203–38.

Moyer, S. B. (1979). Rehabilitation of alexia: A case study. *Cortex*, **15**, 139–44.

Nadeau, S. E., Gonzalez Rothi, L. J. and Crosson, B., (eds.) (2000). *Aphasia and Language: Theory to Practice*. New York: The Guilford Press.

Nichelli, P., Venneri, A., Pentore, R. and Cubelli, R. (1993). Horizontal and vertical neglect dyslexia. *Brain Lang.*, **44**, 264–83.

Nickels, L. (1992). The autocue? Self-generated phonemic cues in the treatment of a disorder of reading and naming. *Cogn. Neuropsychol.*, **9**, 155–82.

Patterson, K. E., Coltheart, M. and Marshall, J. C. (1985). *Surface Dyslexia*. London: LEA.

Patterson, K. E. and Kay, J. (1982). Letter-by-letter reading: Psychological descriptions of a neurological syndrome. *Q. J. Exp. Psychol.*, **34A**, 411–41.

Price, C. J. and Devlin, J. T. (2003). The myth of the visual word form area. *NeuroImage*, **19**, 473–81.

(2004). The pros and cons of labeling a left occipitotemporal region: "The visual word form area." *NeuroImage*, **22**, 477–9.

Price, C. J., Winterburn, D., Giraud, A. L., Moore, C. J. and Noppeney, U. (2003). Cortical localization of the visual and auditory word form areas: A reconsideration of the evidence. *Brain Lang.*, **86**, 272–86.

Price, C. J., Wise, R. J., Warburton, E. A., *et al.* (1996). Hearing and saying. The functional neuro-anatomy of auditory word processing. *Brain*, **119**, 919–31.

Puce, A., Allison, T., Asgari, M., Gore, J. C. and McCarthy, G. (1996). Differential sensitivity of human visual cortex to faces, letterstrings, and textures: A functional magnetic resonance imaging study. *J. Neurosci.*, **16**, 5205–15.

Pugh, K. R., Mencl, W. E., Jenner, A. R., *et al.* (2001). Neurobiological studies of reading and reading disability. *J. Commun. Disord.*, **34**, 479–92.

Rapcsak, S. Z. and Beeson, P. M. (2002). Neuroanatomical correlates of spelling and writing. In A. E. Hillis, ed., *Handbook of Adult Language Disorders: Integrating Cognitive Neuropsychology, Neurology, and Rehabilitation*. Philadelphia: Psychology Press, pp. 71–99.

(2004). The role of posterior inferior temporal cortex in spelling. *Neurology*, **62**, 2221–9.

Rapcsak, S. Z., Rubens, A. B. and Laguna, J. F. (1990). From letters to words: Procedures for word recognition in letter-by-letter reading. *Brain Lang.*, **38**, 504–14.

Rapp, B. C. and Caramazza, A. (1997). From graphemes to abstract letter shapes: Levels of representation in written spelling. *J. Exp. Psychol. [Hum. Percept.]*, **23**, 1130–52.

Raymer, A., Foundas, A. L., Maher, L. M., *et al.* (1997). Cognitive neuropsychological analysis and neuroanatomical correlates in a case of acute anomia. *Brain Lang.*, **58**, 137–56.

Riddoch, M. J., Humphreys, G. W., Cleton, P. and Fery, P. (1990). Levels of coding in neglect dyslexia. *Cogn. Neuropsychol.*, **7**, 479–517.

Roeltgen, D. P. and Heilman, K. M. (1984). Lexical agraphia: Further support for the two strategy hypotheses of linguistic agraphia. *Brain*, **107**, 811–27.

Rothi, L. J. and Heilman, K. M. (1981). Alexia and agraphia with spared spelling and letter recognition abilities. *Brain Lang.*, **12**(1), 1–13.

Rothi, L. J. G. and Moss, S. (1992). Alexia without agraphia: Potential for model-assisted therapy. *Clin. Commun. Disord.*, **2**, 11–18.

Saffran, E. M. and Coslett, H. B. (1998). Implicit vs. letter-by-letter reading in pure alexia: A tale of two systems. *Cogn. Neuropsychol.*, **15**, 141–65.

Sakurai, Y., Sakai, K., Sakuta, M. and Iwata, M. (1994). Naming difficulties in alexia with agraphia for kanji after a left posterior inferior temporal lesion. *J. Neurol., Neurosurg. Psychiatry*, **57**, 609–13.

Seki, K., Yajima, M. and Sugishita, M. (1995). The effect of kinesthetic reading treatment for pure alexia. *Neuropsychologia*, **33**, 595–609.

Shallice, T. (1988). *From Neuropsychology to Mental Structure*, Cambridge: Cambridge University Press.

Small, S. (2002). Biological approaches to the treatment of aphasia. In A. E. Hillis, ed., *The Handbook of Adult Language Disorders: Integrating Cognitive Neuropsychology, Neurology and Rehabilitation*. New York: Psychology Press, pp. 397–411.

Soma, Y., Sugishita, M., Kitamura, K., Maruyama, S. and Imanaga, H. (1989). Lexical agraphia in the Japanese language. Pure agraphia for Kanji due to left posteroinferior temporal lesions, *Brain*, **112**, 1549–61.

Subbiah, I. and Caramazza, A. (2000). Stimulus-centered neglect in reading and object recognition. *Neurocase*, **6**, 13–31.

Vanier, M. and Caplan, D. (1985). CT correlates of surface dyslexia. In K. E. Patterson, J. C. Marshall and M. Coltheart, eds., *Surface Dyslexia: Neuropsychological and Cognitive Studies of Phonological Reading*. London: Laurence Erlbaum.

Warrington, E. K. (1991). Right neglect dyslexia: A single case study. *Cogn. Neuropsychol.*, **8**, 191–212.

Young, A. W., Newcombe, F. and Ellis, A. W. (1991). Different impairments contribute to neglect dyslexia. *Cogn. Neuropsychol.*, **8**, 177–91.

Zangwill, O. L. (1954). Agraphia due to a left parietal glioma in a left-handed man. *Brain*, **77**, 510–20.

8

Acalculia and Gerstmann's syndrome

Laurent Cohen,[1,2] Anna J. Wilson,[2] Véronique Izard,[2] and Stanislas Dehaene[2]

[1]Hôpital de la Salpêtrière, Paris
[2]Cognitive Neuroimaging Unit, Orsay

Introduction

Neurologists' knowledge of number processing impairments is often limited to the notion that acalculia is part of Gerstmann's syndrome (Benton, 1992; Gerstmann, 1940). It may extend to the classical typology proposed by Hécaen, who distinguished aphasic, spatial, and anarithmetic acalculia (Hécaen *et al.*, 1961). Actually, modern research on acalculia (a term coined by Henschen, 1920) has made considerable progress from this point, starting in the 1980s within the expanding framework of cognitive neuropsychology, and soon yielding refined cognitive models (Dehaene, 1992; Deloche and Seron, 1982; McCloskey *et al.*, 1986). Presently, it is an important component of the cognitive neuroscience of numerical abilities, having close links to the methodology used in and theories arising from numerical cognition studies performed in animals, human infants, or normal adults. These methodologies include behavioral measures, functional and anatomical imaging, and electrophysiological techniques (for reviews see Butterworth, 1999; Dehaene and Cohen, 1995; Dehaene *et al.*, 2004).

Beyond its fundamental interest, acalculia constitutes a frequent and incapacitating disorder following acquired, mostly left-hemispheric, brain lesions (Jackson and Warrington, 1986; Rosselli and Ardila, 1989). It interferes with many everyday life activities such as shopping, assessing the balance of a bank account, etc.

In this chapter we will summarize the basic facets of the normal number processing abilities, sketch a simple model of their anatomical implementation, describe an illustrative variety of calculation disorders, briefly discuss the relationships of acalculia, Gerstmann's syndrome and the parietal lobes, and finally propose some guidelines for the assessment and rehabilitation of acalculia in stroke patients.

Acalculia: General presentation

Basic number processing abilities

We will first summarize the main mental operations that we commonly perform when dealing with numbers, and consider their gross cognitive organization. The following inventory also provides the framework for a systematic bedside examination of calculation abilities.

The triple code

Knowledge of a number (e.g. the number 45), comprises three distinct formats under which this number is represented in our brain (Dehaene and Cohen, 1995): A sequence of words ("forty-five"), a string of arabic numerals (45), and as the representation of an abstract quantity independent from conventional symbols. The verbal and Arabic formats are of course specific to adult humans educated within a given language and a given culturally defined numerical system. These symbolic systems in principle allow a perfectly accurate encoding of any number. In contrast, the abstract quantity representation may be shared with preverbal infants (Feigenson *et al.*, 2004), with adults using a language with a minimal number vocabulary (Pica *et al.*, 2004), and with a wide range of animals (Hauser *et al.*, 2003). There is evidence that this quantity representation is approximate, with a precision that decreases as number size increases (Dehaene, 2003). It has been modeled as an oriented mental "number line" on which numerosities are represented as zones of activation (Dehaene and Changeux, 1993). Larger numerosities are represented with an increasing spread of activation, and hence an increased overlap with nearby numerosities. Note that in addition to their main function of referring to quantities, some numerals also have a "nominal" function of referring to pieces of encyclopedic knowledge, such as 52 referring to a bus line, or 1789 to the French Revolution.

Input/output

These three cerebral codes are linked to external objects by appropriate input/output processes. Thus, we can identify verbal numerals (like any other words) upon hearing or reading them, and conversely we can produce them orally or by spelling them out. Similarly, Arabic numerals, which exist only in a visual form, can be identified visually and written down. As for the representation of quantities, this can be activated, for instance, by extracting the numerosity of a set of visual objects (Mandler and Shebo, 1982) or by interpreting finger patterns (Thompson *et al.*, in press). It may also drive hand gestures expressing quantities in a non-verbal form.

Transcoding

The three number codes can also be translated into one another by dedicated processes. For instance, reading aloud the Arabic numeral 45 requires that each digit be identified, together with its position in the string, in order eventually to retrieve from the lexicon the fourth word among those expressing tens ("forty"), and the fifth word expressing units ("five") (Cohen and Dehaene, 1991; McCloskey *et al.*, 1986). Other transcoding processes are involved in writing arabic or verbal numerals to dictation, in naming the numerosity of sets of dots, in accessing the quantity associated with verbal or Arabic numerals, etc.

Calculation

Finally, the three codes are variously involved, often in combination, in the heterogeneous variety of calculation procedures. For instance, familiar multiplication facts have been overlearned at school as rote word associations. Hence, a problem such as 5 × 9 is first translated into a *verbal representation* ("five times nine") which allows for the retrieval of the result in verbal form ("five times nine is forty-five"). More complex calculations, such as 987 × 345, take advantage of the *Arabic representation* of numbers, which is essential for applying the usual multidigit calculation algorithms. As a final example, number comparison (i.e. deciding which of two numbers is larger) relies on the abstract *quantity representation*. Thus, normal adults are faster and more accurate at comparing distant numbers (e.g. 1 vs. 9) than close numbers (e.g. 5 vs. 6), even when targets are presented as verbal or Arabic symbols (Moyer and Landauer, 1967), in agreement with the analogical quantity coding mentioned before. Naturally, coordinating those elementary abilities to solve more complex problems requires effective executive functioning, attentional resources, and working memory.

Anatomical implementation

In order to understand which numerical deficits one might expect in brain-damaged patients, we will delineate the core brain structures that are thought to subserve the above processes (Figure 8.1). Those hypotheses are based upon both lesion studies in brain-damaged patients and activation studies in normal subjects.

Verbal numerals and the language areas

Number words may be viewed as a subset of the general mental lexicon, and their specific combination principles as analogous to morphosyntactic word combination rules. It is therefore plausible that numbers in a verbal form should be processed within the classical set of left-hemispheric language areas, in the

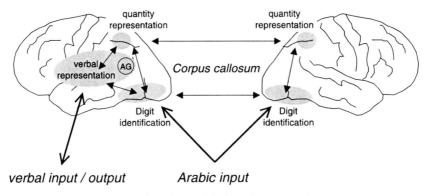

Figure 8.1   Schematic depiction of the triple-code model of number processing.

territory of the left middle cerebral artery. Indeed, impairments of input, output, or transcoding of verbal numerals generally result from the same lesions as aphasia, with which they are generally associated. Within this verbal network, the left angular gyrus seems to be crucial for the retrieval of arithmetic facts stored in a verbal form, first and foremost the familiar multiplication facts ("five times nine is forty-five"), and more generally for the exact calculations afforded by verbal symbols (Cohen *et al.*, 2000a; Delazer *et al.*, 2003; Lampl *et al.*, 1994). The retrieval of rote memories for arithmetical facts may also involve cortico-subcortical loops associated with the language cortex (Dehaene and Cohen, 1997; Delazer *et al.*, 2004).

Arabic numerals and the occipitotemporal cortex

The identification of Arabic numerals, like the categorization of visual objects or printed words, depends on the left ventral occipitotemporal cortex, particularly the fusiform gyrus (Cohen *et al.*, 2000b). There are indications that digits may have a more bilateral representation than letters (Cohen and Dehaene, 1995; Pinel *et al.*, 2001).

Quantities and the HIPS

There is converging evidence that the horizontal segment of the intraparietal sulcus (HIPS) subserves the non-verbal representation of quantities, and is therefore crucial to all semantic manipulations of numbers. This view is supported by functional imaging data, which show activation of the HIPS in most numerical tasks. Importantly, activations increase in experimental conditions with a stronger quantity-related component: approximate versus exact addition; subtraction versus overlearned multiplication problems; novel versus trained arithmetic facts; calculations with large versus small numbers; comparison of close versus distant numbers (for a review see Dehaene *et al.*, 2003). This localization is also compatible with the few studies of patients with acquired semantic deficits in the number domain (see later) (Dehaene and Cohen, 1997; Delazer and Benke, 1997; Lemer *et al.*, 2003), and with data from developmental dyscalculia (Isaacs *et al.*, 2001; Molko *et al.*, 2003).

Connectivity

The cerebral modules implementing the triple-code model are thought to be connected both within and across hemispheres. Language-related mechanisms, which are strongly left-lateralized, are connected to the quantity system in the left intraparietal region and to the digit recognition system in the left fusiform gyrus. Furthermore, we propose that the left and right digit recognition system communicate via the splenium of the corpus callosum, and operate as a single functional unit. Similarly, the left and right quantity systems communicate via a more anterior segment of the corpus callosum. This pattern of connection explains for instance why, in patients with a selective lesion of the callosal splenium, the interhemispheric transfer of exact visual digit identity is impaired, while the transfer of approximate quantities is still possible through the anterior callosum (Cohen and Dehaene, 1996).

Finally, cerebral networks involved in *general functions* of attention, working and long-term memory, executive control, or visuo-spatial processing, contribute to various degrees in essentially all arithmetic tasks.

Varieties of acalculia

We will first consider patients whose lesions shed light on the overall pattern of lateralization of numerical abilities. We then turn to a more analytic description of (1) impairments of number transcoding, which engages mostly verbal/symbolic processes, (2) impairments of non-symbolic quantity manipulation, and (3) impairments of mental arithmetic, which is sensitive to both verbal and quantitative aspects of number processing (Figure 8.2). Finally we will illustrate some meaningful dissociations between acalculia and general language impairments.

Hemispheric specialization

As reviewed above, the left hemisphere is thought to contain a complete number processing system. Accordingly, right-sided lesions generally do not induce acalculia. However this general view requires some qualifications. First, numerical functions may show atypical patterns of lateralization in individual subjects, particularly in left-handers, yielding severe acalculia following right-sided lesions (e.g. Dehaene and Cohen, 1997). Second, the so-called spatial acalculia,

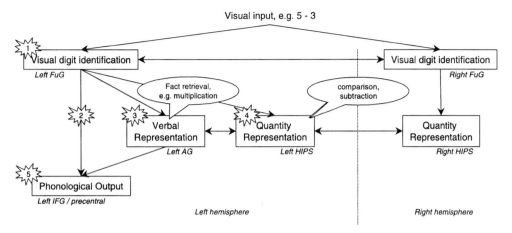

Figure 8.2   Diagram of information-processing pathways involved in processing Arabic digits during various arithmetic tasks. Although still insufficiently specified at both anatomical and functional levels, such diagrams may begin to explain the various neuropsychological dissociations that are observed in human adult lesion cases (functional lesion sites are indicated with stars). Lesion 1, associated with pure alexia, would create an inability to read numbers and to multiply, but not to compare or subtract (Cohen and Dehaene, 1995; 2000). Lesion 2, associated with phonological dyslexia, would create an inability to read numbers, but not to multiply, subtract or compare (Garcia-Orza et al., 2003). Lesions 3 and 4 might explain the frequent double dissociation between multiplication and subtraction in patients who can still read numbers (van Harskamp and Cipolotti, 2001; van Harskamp et al., 2002; Whalen et al., 2002), and the presence or absence of associated deficits in comparison and non-symbolic numerosity processing (Lemer et al., 2003). Lesion 5 might explain residual calculation abilities in patients who fail to produce the solution of arithmetic problems orally, but can still solve them in writing (Whalen et al., 2002). Abbreviations: left AG, left angular gyrus; FuG, fusiform gyrus; HIPS, horizontal segment of intraparietal sulcus; IFG, inferior frontal gyrus. Adapted from (Dehaene et al., 2004).

a side-effect of more diffuse spatial processing impairments, generally results from posterior right-hemispheric lesions (see later). Third, group studies suggest that some numerical tasks are impaired on average in right-damaged patients, such as number comparison (Rosselli and Ardila, 1989) or inferring the principles that underlie numerical series (Langdon and Warrington, 1997).

Moreover, the fact that right lesions generally do not notably affect number use does not imply that the right hemisphere is not endowed with number processing abilities. Indeed, neuropsychological evidence supports the idea that some processes are represented both in the left and in the right hemispheres.

Although rare, isolated callosal lesions are extremely informative on issues of hemispheric specialization. Thus, in a patient with a posterior callosal infarct, Arabic numerals presented selectively to the left hemisphere could successfully be used for any numerical tasks, including comparison, reading aloud, or arithmetic (Cohen and Dehaene, 1996). In contrast, digits presented to the right hemisphere yielded high error rates in reading aloud and in exact arithmetic tasks. However, numbers presented to either hemisphere could be successfully compared to a given standard. This pattern extends observations in callosotomy patients (Gazzaniga and Hillyard, 1971; Gazzaniga and Smylie, 1984; Seymour *et al.*, 1994), and illustrates the ability of the right hemisphere not only to identify Arabic numerals, but also to access and manipulate their quantitative meaning, while verbal output and exact arithmetic is restricted to the left hemisphere. Similar observations were made in patients with pure alexia. Their intact right-hemispheric system allows them to compare numbers (Cohen and Dehaene, 1995), and even to perform some quantity-dependent arithmetic computations (Cohen and Dehaene, 2000), on the basis of Arabic stimuli that they cannot read aloud.

In support of the same ideas, patients with extensive left hemispheric lesions generally show preserved Arabic number comparison abilities, while they may be severely aphasic and acalculic, and unable to read aloud numbers or solve even elementary calculations (Cohen *et al.*, 1994; Dehaene and Cohen, 1991; Grafman *et al.*, 1989; Warrington, 1982). Beyond number comparison, some patients with large left-sided lesions may show more substantial abilities of approximate number manipulation, possibly involving the intact right hemisphere. As an example, patient NAU proposed that there were 350 days in a year, or about 10 eggs in a dozen. He could even reject grossly erroneous addition problems (e.g. $1 + 2 = 9$), while he was unable to discriminate slightly false from exact problems (Dehaene and Cohen, 1991).

Number transcoding deficits

If we consider the three symbolic representations of numbers (Arabic, oral verbal, written verbal), there are six distinct types of transcoding, most of which have been analyzed in detailed cognitive neuropsychological studies (Macaruso *et al.*, 1993; Noël, 2001). Many studies have concentrated on the process of reading aloud Arabic numerals, and we will take this case as an illustrative instance of transcoding deficits.

Reading aloud Arabic numerals entails three successive stages: first, identification of the string of digits, second, translation of the string of digits into a sequence of words according to the appropriate rules, and finally the overt production of this word sequence. These three stages normally take place within the left hemisphere.

Impairments at the initial stage of digit identification correspond to pure alexia, and follow left ventral occipitotemporal lesions. As mentioned before, the corresponding right hemisphere region has roughly equivalent abilities for the identification of Arabic numerals, explaining the fact that patients can paradoxically compare numbers that they cannot read aloud (Cohen and Dehaene, 1995). Impairments at the final stage of spoken or written word output probably depend on general word processing, although dissociations may be observed.

As for the middle stage of translation into a word sequence, this has been analyzed in a number of case studies, including the pioneering study by McCloskey *et al.* (1986) of patients HY and JG. HY produced so-called "lexical" reading errors; i.e. he substituted expected words with other words from the same category (e.g. 54 became "sixty four", or 612 became "six hundred and thirteen"). The patient prepared an adequate word frame (e.g. "a tens name followed by a unit name"), but made errors when selecting specific words to fill that frame. In contrast, patient JG mostly made "syntactic" errors (e.g. 54 became "five hundred and four"). He created erroneous syntactic frames, but selected the appropriate number words (i.e. corresponding to the stimulus digits), in order to fill that erroneous frame. This kind of data allows us to distinguish syntactic from lexical processes within number transcoding, and to clarify the organization of the lexicon of number words, which seems to be in parallel and ordered "stacks" for units ("one", "two", etc), teens ("eleven", "twelve", etc), and tens ("ten", "twenty", etc) (Deloche and Seron, 1984).

It is important to remember that patients with even major transcoding deficits, such as a complete inability to read aloud numbers, may still have a good comprehension of the same numbers. As mentioned before, they may access the quantitative meaning of numbers, and in addition, they may access their encyclopedic meaning. Thus acalculic patients with deep dyslexia, although unable to read them aloud, could readily access and report the historical meaning of the numerals 1789 or 1914 (Cohen *et al.*, 1994; 2000a).

Finally, patients who are unable to map Arabic numerals onto words normally often resort to verbal counting strategies. Thus they may say "one, two, three, four!" when presented with digit 4, or "ten, twenty, thirty!" for the number 30. This strategy requires preserved visual number identification, and preserved automatic counting series. Those two representations can then be matched in order to bypass the impaired direct route to number words: the patient knows that the proposed digit (4) corresponds to the fourth item in the counting series, allowing him to monitor this series and to stop when appropriate. As a further compensation for an impaired verbal output, patients may answer by displaying the appropriate number of fingers. Naturally, alternative output strategies such as counting, using one's fingers, or writing down the answer instead of saying it, are not restricted to transcoding tasks, but can be used in any numeric task requiring a verbal output. For instance, when patient ATH was asked to say how many eggs there are in a dozen, she wrote 12 while saying "sixteen." When presented with $7 + 5$, she said "a dozen ... eleven perhaps" while readily showing 12 (10 and 2) fingers (Cohen *et al.*, 2000a).

Quantity processing deficits

Deficits primarily involving the manipulation of abstract quantities have received much less attention than the more easily diagnosed language-related impairments. Moreover, it is likely that the bilateral representation of quantity-related processes makes them more resistant to focal brain damage.

Core semantic deficits

Only a few patients have been reported who suffered from a core deficit in manipulating abstract quantities, in conjunction with spared language abilities (Dehaene and Cohen, 1997; Delazer and Benke, 1997; Lemer *et al.*, 2003). Such patients are able to read aloud and otherwise transcode all numerical symbols, and to recite automated sequences of number words, such as serial counting or multiplication tables. However, their impairment affects all tasks which require the manipulation of quantities. Thus, patient MAR was mildly impaired at deciding which of two Arabic numbers was larger, and utterly unable to perform a numerical bisection task; i.e. to decide which number fell in the middle of two others. In the arithmetic domain, he was unable to solve even the simplest sub-traction problems, which are typically not stored in rote verbal memory (Dehaene and Cohen, 1997). In the same vein, evaluating the approximate result of additions without going through the exact calculation algorithm is particularly difficult for such patients (Lemer *et al.*, 2003). Importantly, semantic deficits emerge irrespective of the format of input or output. Thus, patient LEC was impaired at deciding which of two 2-digit Arabic numerals was larger, but even more impaired when comparing the numerosity of two sets of dots (Lemer *et al.*, 2003). Both patients MAR and LEC had lesions of their dominant intraparietal region, supporting a crucial role of this area in quantity processing.

Neglect and the "number line"

Beyond core semantic deficits, there is recent evidence that spatial hemineglect may also affect the numerical domain. Thus, in the number bisection task mentioned before, neglect patients systematically selected a number larger than the actual midpoint (e.g. Which number falls in between 11 and 19? Answer: 17) (Zorzi *et al.*, 2002). It is thought that neglect induces an attentional bias in accessing the quasi-spatial "number line" of quantity representation, therefore biasing the selection of responses to simple numerical questions.

Attention to space and the perception of numerosity

Perceiving the numerosity of visual displays may be impaired following visuospatial disorders, without implying an impairment of core numerical representations. Simultagnosia, a classical symptom of Bálint's syndrome following bilateral superior parietal lesions, is an inability to perceive more than one object at a time. When such patients are asked to count a set of random dots, some dots are omitted while others may be counted several times (Luria, 1959). However, Bálint patients are generally quite accurate when estimating the numerosity of sets of one, two or three items (Dehaene and Cohen, 1994). It is thought that perceiving the numerosity of such very small sets, a process known as "subitizing," reflects parallel visual processing and does not require the serial attentional scanning of each object, a process that is compromised in Bálint's syndrome (Rizzo and Robin, 1990). A related phenomenon has been demonstrated in neglect patients, who can estimate the numerosity of sets up to four objects, even when some items fall in the extinguished hemifield and cannot be individually attended to (Vuilleumier and Rafal, 1999).

Impairments of mental calculation

The arithmetic abilities of educated adults (at a basic level the ability to solve addition, subtraction, multiplication, division problems, or combinations thereof) result from a complex interplay of heterogeneous cognitive components. Particularly, as mentioned before, both verbal and quantity-related deficits may interfere with calculation abilities, although in different ways. Stroke may affect those mechanisms in different ways, resulting in a wide variety of arithmetic disorders, all covered under such simplifying terms as anarithmetia or pure acalculia (Hécaen *et al.*, 1961). We will analyze in turn the main cognitive components that may be affected, and the corresponding varieties of acalculia.

Symbolic input and output processes

Deficits affecting the identification of problem operands (i.e. numbers) or the eventual production of responses may induce calculation errors without affecting the core of arithmetic processes. Thus, on the input side, patients with pure alexia make errors in identifying digits visually. Hence they translate digits into erroneous number words, eventually retrieving the wrong multiplication facts from verbal memory (e.g. 2×5 becomes "three times four is twelve") (Cohen and Dehaene, 2000; McNeil and Warrington, 1994). On the output side, patients with impaired oral production may produce erroneous solutions to arithmetic problems orally, but still solve them correctly in writing (e.g. $7 + 7$: spoken answer "twelve" but written answer 14) (Whalen *et al.*, 2002). Also, errors in the identification of *operation symbols* ($+$, $-$, $\times$, $/$) may be a cause of calculation errors, as has been reported in brain-damaged patients (Ferro and Botelho, 1980).

Spatial layout of arithmetic problems

Reading, writing down, or solving multidigit operations on a sheet of paper requires that the component digits and symbols be correctly arrayed in lines and columns. Patients with space processing disorders such as Bálint's syndrome, constructional apraxia, or neglect may be unable to solve such problems as a consequence of their inability to organize calculations properly in space. Spatial acalculia mostly results from posterior right hemisphere lesions (Hécaen *et al.*, 1961; Rosselli and Ardila, 1989).

Executive control and sequencing

All calculations except the simplest ones require some degree of executive processing, and deficits in this broad field may induce numerical impairments.

1. Mentally solving problems that involve several steps and the temporary storage of partial results may be disrupted by working memory impairments (Butterworth *et al.*, 1996).
2. Performing multidigit calculations (e.g. 67×26) involves the scheduling and control of a strictly ordered sequence of elementary steps (e.g. compute 6×7; write down the digit 2; carry 4; compute 6×6; add the carry; etc.). Those overall procedures may be disrupted while elementary calculations are fully preserved (Caramazza and McCloskey, 1987).
3. Patients may read aloud correctly simple problems, including the operation signs, but still select the wrong operation when retrieving the result (e.g. $3 + 3 = 9$) (van Harskamp and Cipolotti, 2001).
4. At a still higher level of executive control, patients with prefrontal lesions may be impaired at working out adequate strategies for the resolution of concrete problems involving numbers, in the absence of acalculia strictly speaking (Fasotti *et al.*, 1992b; Luria, 1966).

Elementary calculation deficits

Patients may master perfectly the sequences of elementary operations involved in multidigit calculations, but fail to recover the elementary arithmetic facts that are required to actually carry out such sequences (Cohen and Dehaene, 1994). Moreover, elementary arithmetic facts themselves are not homogeneous and depend on distinct cognitive abilities, explaining the observation in some patients of clear-cut dissociations between operations. Some facts are learned by rote as automatic verbal associations, and do not require access to the quantitative meaning of numbers. This concerns particularly the most familiar multiplication facts ("five times nine is forty-five"). Other facts must be computed anew using counting and semantic number manipulations such as comparison and estimation. This is typically the case for even simple subtraction problems (e.g. $12 - 7$). Finally, a special set of problems are solved by applying simple algebraic rules (e.g. $n \times 0 = 0$; $n \times 1 = n$; etc.), and may be impaired or preserved independently from other arithmetic facts (McCloskey *et al.*, 1991). This main distinction between a verbal system supporting multiplication and other rote memory-based operations, and a quantity system supporting subtraction and other quantity manipulations, accounts nicely for most cases of dissociations between operations reported in the literature (for a review see e.g. Cohen and Dehaene, 2000). In general, patients with a predominantly verbal deficit are impaired in multiplication more than in subtraction, and frequently have associated language and number transcoding impairments (e.g. Cohen *et al.*, 2000a; Dagenbach and McCloskey, 1992; Pesenti *et al.*, 1994). Conversely, the rarer patients with a predominantly quantitative deficit show the opposite pattern, and may have associated quantity processing deficits, as mentioned above (Dehaene and Cohen, 1997; Delazer and Benke, 1997; Lemer *et al.*, 2003). The strategies used for addition are highly variable across subjects and across tasks in their reliance on verbal and quantitative processes. As a consequence, patients' performances with addition problems may be closer to their performances either in multiplication or in subtraction (Cohen and Dehaene, 2000; Cohen *et al.*, 2000a; Dagenbach and McCloskey, 1992; Dehaene *et al.*, 2003; van Harskamp and Cipolotti, 2001). This view predicts that no patient should show impaired multiplication and subtraction (reflecting impaired verbal and quantity systems), but preserved addition. The opposite pattern (i.e. preserved multiplication and subtraction, reflecting preserved verbal and quantity systems) with impaired addition should also be impossible. This proposal, however, is still open to empirical controversies (van Harskamp and Cipolotti, 2001).

Approximate vs. exact calculation

Quantity manipulation abilities allow the evaluation of the approximate result of simple problems, particularly of addition problems. Patients severely impaired at finding an exact solution to even the simplest problems may still be able to reject grossly erroneous calculations (Warrington, 1982). For instance, patient NAU judged $2 + 2 = 3$ and $2 + 2 = 4$ as equally plausible, but could readily reject $2 + 2 = 9$ (Dehaene and Cohen, 1991). Conversely, patients with preserved exact calculation but impaired quantitative processing may find it difficult to discriminate between slightly and grossly erroneous results. Thus, when presented with problems such as $2 + 3$, patient LEC was unable to choose the more plausible response between two proposed results (4 and 8), without first explicitly computing the exact solution (Lemer *et al.*, 2003).

Algebra and conceptual arithmetic principles

Solving many numerical problems requires the mastery of principles such as $a \times b = b \times a$, $n + 0 = n$, $a \times (b + c) = a \times b + a \times c$, etc. Conceptual processing is thought to involve networks of frontal and parietal areas (Anderson *et al.*, 2004). It is closely related to, and difficult to disentangle from, other previously discussed components of the number processing system, particularly executive control and abstract quantity processing (Delazer *et al.*, 2004; Houde and Tzourio-Mazoyer, 2003). However, it has been shown repeatedly that patients who have forgotten memorized arithmetic facts may show a preserved mastery of algebraic rules (Cohen and Dehaene, 1994; Hittmair-Delazer *et al.*, 1995; Hittmair-Delazer *et al.*, 1994). For instance, when presented with 5×5, a patient spontaneously sketched five rows of five dots and counted them by successive additions (Cohen and Dehaene, 1994). More impressively, one patient could readily reach the forgotten result of 6×8 by successively computing $6 \times 8 = (5 \times 8) + 8$; $5 \times 8 = (10 \times 8)/2$; $10 \times 8 = 80$; $80/2 = 40$; $6 \times 8 = 40 + 8 = 48$ (Hittmair-Delazer *et al.*, 1994). Conversely, although she retained memorized arithmetical facts, a patient with a semantic numerical impairment was unable to apply the simple principle commutativity of multiplication, or to perceive the equivalence between multiplication problems and the corresponding addition series (Delazer and Benke, 1997).

Dissociating numbers and language

The main features of the number processing model could apply to words in general. Thus, the representation of ordinary words, like numbers, associates non-verbal semantic representations with purely verbal information such as oral and written word forms and grammatical features. Nevertheless, many neuropsychological dissociations are observed between numbers and words.

At the semantic level, patients with profound loss of semantics (generally due to frontotemporal dementia) may show a remarkable sparing of calculation as well as number production and comprehension abilities (Butterworth *et al.*, 2001; Cappelletti *et al.*, 2001; Thioux *et al.*, 1998), supporting the idea that numerical semantics rely on parietal regions. Conversely, patients with quantity processing deficits show preserved general semantic abilities (Dehaene and Cohen, 1997; Delazer and Benke, 1997). For instance patient MAR, although unable to decide which number is the mid-point between 4 and 8, could easily determine that Wednesday falls in the middle of Monday and Friday.

At the input level, reports of a possible sparing of Arabic numerals in pure alexia date back to Dejerine, who noted that "the patient recognizes very well all digits," although "he cannot recognize a single letter" (Cohen and Dehaene, 1995; Dejerine, 1892; Holender and Peereman, 1987). This may result from a better compensation by right occipitotemporal regions for the identification of Arabic numerals than of alphabetic stimuli (Pinel *et al.*, 2001).

Dissociations have also been reported at the level of symbolic output. Thus Anderson *et al.* (1990) described a patient with severe agraphia who was unable to trace even single letters, but whose writing of multidigit Arabic numerals was entirely spared (see also Delazer *et al.*, 2002). Similarly, some patients with a phonemic jargon affecting the oral production of ordinary words may produce number words without any phonological errors (Cohen *et al.*, 1997; Geschwind, 1965).

Numbers, Gerstmann's syndrome, and the parietal lobes

Over a series of publications from 1924 to 1957, Josef Gerstmann delineated a syndrome which still carries his name, consisting of acalculia, left–right disorientation, agraphia, and finger agnosia (Gerstmann, 1940). He considered that this association of deficits resulted specifically from lesions affecting the "transitional region of the angular and the middle occipital convolution," and that its four components reflected a common underlying mechanism, namely some form of impairment of the body schema, affecting particularly the hands and fingers. Thus Gerstmann speculated that the link between numbers and body schema stemmed from the "important part [which] is played by the individual fingers and their right and left laterality in acquisition of the functions of writing and calculating."

While the value of Gerstmann's syndrome in localizing lesions to the dominant posterior inferior parietal lobule was largely validated, the hypothesis of a single core deficit was seriously challenged (for a review see Mayer *et al.*, 1999). For instance, Benton (1961; 1992) showed not only that the four cardinal features of the syndrome could be dissociated from one another, but also that "the particular combination of behavioral deficits which form the syndrome show no stronger internal associative bonds than do a score of other combinations of behavioral deficits."

According to this view, Gerstmann's syndrome would reflect the accidental association of deficits affecting distinct systems which all happen to be located in the inferior parietal region. Indeed, functional imaging shows such a functional mosaic in the intraparietal cortex, with regions activated more strongly during calculation, manual tasks, spatial-attentional tasks, or a phonemic language task

(Simon *et al.*, 2002). However, some commonality between the components of Gerstmann's syndrome might still be found in the general spatial and sensorimotor functions implemented by the parietal lobes.

Importantly, as we would predict from the location of Gerstmann lesions and what we know about the role of the intraparietal sulcus in the representation of quantity, the acalculia observed in cases of "pure" Gerstmann's syndrome without aphasia fits with a semantic deficit of quantity processing. Still, the close proximity of the HIPS, the inferior parietal language area, and the superior parietal space-processing cortex, may account for different or more complex patterns of number processing impairments (Figure 8.3).

Key points Main varieties of acalculia

Number transcoding deficits: generally associated with aphasia, engage mostly verbal/symbolic processes (e.g. reading)

Impairment of mental arithmetic: may affect simple problems learned by rote (e.g. 2×3), problems that require some quantity manipulation (e.g. $11-7$), problems that require complex procedures (e.g. 243×76), or various combinations thereof

Impairments of quantity manipulation: spared ability to transcode numerical symbols and to use automated sequences of number words; impairment of tasks requiring the manipulation of quantities irrespective of the format of input or output (deciding which of two numbers is larger, numerical bisection task, simple subtraction problems, evaluating the approximate result of additions. . .)

Peripheral disorders interfering with the use of numerical abilities:

    visuospatial disorders impeding the perception of the numerosity of sets of objects

    alexia and aphasia interfering with the comprehension or production of numerals

    disorders of executive control and sequencing

Acalculia in strokes

To our knowledge no systematic study of numerical abilities in stroke patients has been carried out. Thus the characterization of strokes associated with acalculia is mostly based on single case studies and small series of patients suffering from various conditions, including stroke. Irrespective of the underlying disease, series of patients with focal hemispheric damage have shown that impairments on calculation tests are frequent for a large variety of lesion sites (Grafman *et al.*, 1982; Rosselli and Ardila, 1989), due to the contribution of various mechanisms (e.g. aphasia and visuo-spatial disorders). Selective numerical deficits seem to be relatively specific to left posterior lesions. A follow-up study of 51 acalculic patients (Caporali *et al.*, 2000) has shown that acalculia is frequent in stroke, and that it may improve within the first months; surprisingly the improvement was

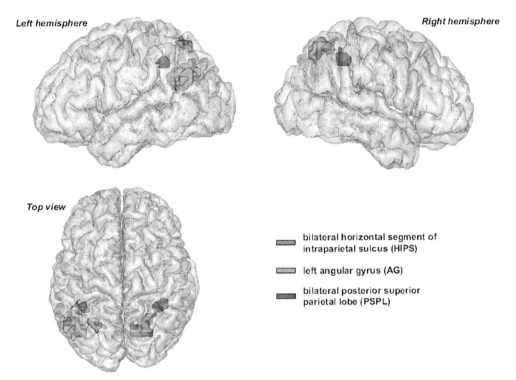

Figure 8.3   Three parietal circuits for number processing. Intersection of activations clusters from a metanalysis of fMRI activation studies. Red: the horizontal segment of the intraparietal sulcus (HIPS) was activated bilaterally in a variety of contrasts sharing a component of numerical quantity manipulation. Green: the left angular gyrus was activated during arithmetic tasks with a strong verbal component. Blue: the posterior superior parietal lobule was activated bilaterally in a few numerical tasks, overlapping with tasks of non-numerical visual attention shift. Reproduced from (Dehaene *et al.*, 2003). For a color version of this figure please see www.cambridge.org/9780521106955.

correlated with recovery of auditory comprehension, but did not depend on the initial severity of acalculia.

Considering the anatomy of numerical processes, as presented in this chapter, acalculia mostly results from infarct in the territory of the dominant middle cerebral artery (especially its inferior/posterior division). Such infarcts may involve the inferior parietal lobule, including the angular gyrus, but frontal lesions may also induce calculation deficits. However, most of these patients are aphasic and acalculia is frequently overlooked. Small infarcts restricted to the interparietal cortex are rare, but may lead to relatively pure disorders of numerical abilities. In the context of agnosic alexia, impaired identification of numerical symbols follows infarct in the territory of the left posterior cerebral artery. Finally, acalculia has also been reported in a few patients with thalamic infarcts, especially in the tuberothalamic territory (Bogousslavsky *et al.*, 1986), and with left lenticulostriate infarcts (Corbett *et al.*, 1986).

Key points Main types of stroke associated with acalculia

Stroke type	Territory/characteristics
Arterial Infarct	Left middle cerebral artery (posterior/inferior division; deep territory)
	Left posterior cerebral artery
	Thalamus (tuberothalamic artery)
Hemorrhage	Left parietal regions

Assessment and rehabilitation of acalculia

The basic examination of numerical abilities in brain-damaged patients should include both verbal and non-verbal aspects of number processing. Guidelines for a bedside examination are proposed in Key points for this section. Naturally, the patient's behavior should be interpreted against the background of a wider assessment of language, vision, attention, and executive functioning. Standardized battery of tests may be useful (e.g. Dellatolas *et al.*, 2001; Delazer *et al.*, 2003a).

Relatively few controlled studies have been devoted to the rehabilitation of acquired acalculia (for recent reviews see Girelli and Seron, 2000; Lochy *et al.*, in press). Most of them have targeted transcoding processes (Deloche *et al.*, 1989), the retrieval of simple arithmetical facts through drill (Girelli *et al.*, 1996)

Key points Suggested tests for the clinical examination of numerical abilities

Forward and backward digit span.

Forward and backward counting.

Symbolic transcoding (reading aloud and taking dictation of simple and multidigit numerals).

Single-digit arithmetic. To reduce the contribution of input and output deficits to the patient's performance, problems may be simultaneously presented in written form and read aloud by the examiner. Familiar multiplication problems and simple subtractions should be tested in priority, as they reflect rote verbal and quantity-based processes, respectively.

Multidigit written calculations.

Concrete arithmetic problems requiring some planning.

Evaluation of the numerosity of sets of dots, presented either briefly to test estimation abilities, or for an unlimited duration to allow for serial counting.

Evaluation to check for other components of Gerstmann's syndrome.

or through conceptual training (Domahs *et al.*, 2003; Girelli *et al.*, 2002), or the creation of strategies for solving concrete problems (Fasotti *et al.*, 1992a).

REFERENCES

Anderson, J. R., Qin, Y., Stenger, V. A. and Carter, C. S. (2004). The relationship of three cortical regions to an information-processing model. *J. Cogn. Neurosci.*, **16**, 637–53.

Anderson, S. W., Damasio, A. R. and Damasio, H. (1990). Troubled letters but not numbers: Domain specific cognitive impairments following focal damage in frontal cortex. *Brain*, **113**, 749–66.

Benton, A. L. (1961). The fiction of the Gerstmann syndrome. *J. Neurol.*, **24**, 176–81.

    (1992). Gerstmann's syndrome. *Arch. Neurol.*, **49**, 445–7.

Bogousslavsky, J., Regli, F. and Assal, G. (1986). The syndrome of unilateral tuberothalamic artery territory infarction. *Stroke*, **17**, 434–41.

Butterworth, B. (1999). *The Mathematical Brain*. London: Macmillan.

Butterworth, B., Cappelletti, M. and Kopelman, M. (2001). Category specificity in reading and writing: the case of number words. *Nat. Neurosci.*, **4**, 784–6.

Butterworth, B., Cipolotti, L. and Warrington, E. K. (1996). Short-term memory impairment and arithmetical ability. *Q. J. Exp. Psychol.*, **49A**, 251–62.

Caporali, A., Burgio, F. and Basso, A. (2000). The natural course of acalculia in left-brain-damaged patients. *Neurol. Sci.*, **21**, 143–9.

Cappelletti, M., Butterworth, B. and Kopelman, M. (2001). Spared numerical abilities in a case of semantic dementia. *Neuropsychologia*, **39**, 1224–39.

Caramazza, A. and McCloskey, M. (1987). Dissociations of calculation processes. In G. Deloche and X. Seron., eds., *Mathematical Disabilities: A cognitive Neuropsychological Perspective*. Hillsdale, NJ: Lawrence Erlbaum Associates, pp. 221–34.

Cohen, L. and Dehaene, S. (1991). Neglect dyslexia for numbers? A case report. Cogn. *Neuropsychol.*, **8**, 39–58.

    (1994). Amnesia for arithmetic facts: A single case study. *Brain and Lang.*, **47**, 214–32.

    (1995). Number processing in pure alexia: the effect of hemispheric asymmetries and task demands. *NeuroCase*, **1**, 121–37.

    (1996). Cerebral networks for number processing: Evidence from a case of posterior callosal lesion. *NeuroCase*, **2**, 155–74.

    (2000). Calculating without reading: Unsuspected residual abilities in pure alexia. *Cogn. Neuropsychol.*, **17**, 563–83.

Cohen, L., Dehaene, S., Chochon, F., Lehéricy, S. and Naccache, L. (2000a). Language and calculation within the parietal lobe: A combined cognitive, anatomical and fMRI study. *Neuropsychologia*, **138**, 1426–40.

Cohen, L., Dehaene, S., Naccache, L., *et al.* (2000b). The visual word form area: Spatial and temporal characterization of an initial stage of reading in normal subjects and posterior split-brain patients. *Brain*, **123**, 291–307.

Cohen, L., Dehaene, S. and Verstichel, P. (1994). Number words and number non-words: A case of deep dyslexia extending to arabic numerals. *Brain*, **117**, 267–79.

Cohen, L., Verstichel, P. and Dehaene, S. (1997). Neologistic jargon sparing numbers: a category specific phonological impairment. *Cogn. Neuropsychol.*, **14**, 1029–61.

Corbett, A. J., McCusker, E. A. and Davidson, O. R. (1986). Acalculia following a dominant-hemisphere subcortical infarct. *Arch. Neurol.*, **43**, 964–6.

Dagenbach, D. and McCloskey, M. (1992). The organization of arithmetic facts in memory: Evidence from a brain-damaged patient. *Brain Cogn.*, **20**, 345–66.

Dehaene, S. (1992). Varieties of numerical abilities. *Cognition*, **44**, 1–42.

(2003). The neural basis of the Weber-Fechner law: a logarithmic mental number line. *Trends Cogn. Sci.*, **7**, 145–7.

Dehaene, S. and Changeux, J. P. (1993). Development of elementary numerical abilities: A neuronal model. *J. Cogn. Neurosci.*, **5**, 390–407.

Dehaene, S. and Cohen, L. (1991). Two mental calculation systems: A case study of severe acalculia with preserved approximation. *Neuropsychologia*, **29**, 1045–74.

(1994). Dissociable mechanisms of subitizing and counting: Neuropsychological evidence from simultanagnosic patients. *J. Exp. Psychol. [Hum. Percept.]*, **20**, 958–75.

(1995). Towards an anatomical and functional model of number processing. *Math. Cogn.*, **1**, 83–120.

(1997). Cerebral pathways for calculation: Double dissociations between Gerstmann's acalculia and subcortical acalculia. *Cortex*, **33**, 219–50.

Dehaene, S., Molko, N., Cohen, L. and Wilson, A. J. (2004). Arithmetic and the brain. *Curr. Opin. Neurobiol.*, **14**, 218–24.

Dehaene, S., Piazza, M., Pinel, P. and Cohen, L. (2003). Three parietal circuits for number processing. *Cogn. Neuropsychol.*, **20**, 487–506.

Dejerine, J. (1892). Contribution à l'étude anatomo-pathologique et clinique des différentes variétés de cécité verbale. *Mémoires de la Société de Biologie*, **4**, 61–90.

Delazer, M. and Benke, T. (1997). Arithmetic facts without meaning. *Cortex*, **33**, 697–710.

Delazer, M., Domahs, F., Bartha, L., *et al.* (2003). Learning complex arithmetic – an fMRI study. *Brain Res. Cogn.*, **18**, 76–88.

Delazer, M., Domahs, F., Lochy, A., *et al.* (2004). Number processing and basal ganglia dysfunction: a single case study. *Neuropsychologia*, **42**, 1050–62.

Delazer, M., Girelli, L., Grana, A. and Domahs, F. (2003a). Number processing and calculation – normative data from healthy adults. *Clin. Neuropsychol.*, **17**, 331–50.

Delazer, M., Lochy, A., Jenner, C., Domahs, F. and Benke, T. (2002). When writing 0 (zero) is easier than writing O (o): a neuropsychological case study of agraphia. *Neuropsychologia*, **40**, 2167–77.

Dellatolas, G., Deloche, G., Basso, A. and Claros-Salinas, D. (2001). Assessment of calculation and number processing using the EC301 battery: cross-cultural normative data and application to left- and right-brain damaged patients. *J. Int. Neuropsychol. Soc.*, **7**, 840–59.

Deloche, G. and Seron, X. (1982). From one to 1: An analysis of a transcoding process by means of neuropsychological data. *Cognition*, **12**, 119–49.

(1984). Semantic errors reconsidered in the procedural light of stack concepts. *Brain Lang.*, **21**, 59–71.

Deloche, G., Seron, X. and Ferrand, I. (1989). Reeducation of number transcoding mechanisms: A procedural approach. In X. Seron and G. Deloche, eds., *Cognitive Approach in Neuropsychological Rehabilitation*. Hillsdale, NJ: Lawrence Erlbaum.

Domahs, F., Bartha, L. and Delazer, M. (2003). Rehabilitation of arithmetic abilities: Different intervention strategies for multiplication. *Brain Lang.*, **87**, 165–6.

Fasotti, L., Bremer, J. J. C. B. and Eling, P. A. T. M. (1992a). Influence of improved test encoding on arithmetical word problem solving after frontal lobe damage. *Neuropsychol. Rehabil.*, **2**, 3–20.

Fasotti, L., Eling, P. A. T. M. and Bremer, J. J. C. B. (1992b). The internal representation of arithmetical word problem sentences: Frontal and posterior patients compared. *Brain Cogn.*, **20**, 245–63.

Feigenson, L., Dehaene, S. and Spelke, E. (2004). Core systems of number. *Trends Cogn. Sci.*, **8**, 307–14.

Ferro, J. M. and Botelho, M. A. S. (1980). Aphasia for arithmetical signs: A cause of disturbed calculation. *Cortex*, **16**, 175–80.

Garcia-Orza, J., Leon-Carrion, J. and Vega, O. (2003). Dissociating arabic numeral reading and basic calculation: a case study. *Neurocase*, **9**, 129–39.

Gazzaniga, M. S. and Hillyard, S. A. (1971). Language and speech capacity of the right hemisphere. *Neuropsychologia*, **9**, 273–80.

Gazzaniga, M. S. and Smylie, C. E. (1984). Dissociation of language and cognition: A psychological profile of two disconnected right hemispheres. *Brain*, **107**, 145–53.

Gerstmann, J. (1940). Syndrome of finger agnosia disorientation for right and left agraphia and acalculia. *Arch. Neurol. Psychiat.*, **44**, 398–408.

Geschwind, N. (1965). Disconnection syndromes in animals and man. *Brain*, **88**, 237–94.

Girelli, L., Bartha, L. and Delazer, M. (2002). Strategic learning in the rehabilitation of semantic knowledge. *Neuropsychol. Rehabil.*, **12**, 41–61.

Girelli, L., Delazer, M., Semenza, C. and Denes, G. (1996). The representation of arithmetical facts: evidence from two rehabilitation studies. *Cortex*, **32**, 49–66.

Girelli, L. and Seron, X. (2000). La revalidation des troubles du calcul et du traitement des nombres. In X. Seron and M. van der Linden, eds., *Traité de Neuropsychologie Clinique*. Vol. **2**. Marseille: Solal, 215–25.

Grafman, J., Kampen, D., Rosenberg, J., Salazar, A. and Boller, F. (1989). Calculation abilities in a patient with a virtual left hemispherectomy. *Behav. Neurol.*, **2**, 183–94.

Grafman, J., Passafiume, D., Faglioni, P. and Boller, F. (1982). Calculation disturbances in adults with focal hemispheric damage. *Cortex*, **18**, 37–49.

Hauser, M. D., Tsao, F., Garcia, P. and Spelke, E. S. (2003). Evolutionary foundations of number: spontaneous representation of numerical magnitudes by cotton-top tamarins. *Proc. R. Soc. Lond. B. Biol. Sci.*, **270**, 1441–6.

Hécaen, H., Angelergues, R. and Houillier, S. (1961). Les variétés cliniques des acalculies au cours des lésions rétro-rolandiques: Approche statistique du problème. *Rev. Neurol.* **105**, 85–103.

Henschen, S. E. (1920). *Klinische und anatomische Beitraege zur Pathologie des Gehirns.* Stockholm: Nordiska Bokhandeln.

Hittmair-Delazer, M., Sailer, U. and Benke, T. (1995). Impaired arithmetic facts but intact conceptual knowledge — a single case study of dyscalculia. *Cortex*, **31**, 139–47.

Hittmair-Delazer, M., Semenza, C. and Denes, G. (1994). Concepts and facts in calculation. *Brain*, **117**, 715–28.

Holender, D. and Peereman, R. (1987). Differential processing of phonographic and logographic single-digit numbers by the two hemispheres, In G. Deloche and X. Seron, eds., *Mathematical Disabilities: A Cognitive Neuropsychological Perspective.* Hillsdale, NJ: Lawrence Erlbaum Associates, pp. 43–86.

Houde, O. and Tzourio-Mazoyer, N. (2003). Neural foundations of logical and mathematical cognition. *Nat. Rev. Neurosci.*, **4**, 507–14.

Isaacs, E. B., Edmonds, C. J., Lucas, A. and Gadian, D. G. (2001). Calculation difficulties in children with a very low birthweight. A neural correlate. *Brain*, **124**, 1701–7.

Jackson, M. and Warrington, E. K. (1986). Arithmetic skills in patients with unilateral cerebral lesions. *Cortex*, **22**, 611–20.

Lampl, Y., Eshel, Y., Gilad, R. and Sarova-Pinhas, I. (1994). Selective acalculia with sparing of the subtraction process in a patient with left parietotemporal hemorrhage. *Neurology*, **44**, 1759–61.

Langdon, D. W. and Warrington, E. K. (1997). The abstraction of numerical relations: a role for the right hemisphere in arithmetic? *J. Int. Neuropsychol. Soc.*, **3**, 260–8.

Lemer, C., Dehaene, S., Spelke, E. and Cohen, L. (2003). Approximate quantities and exact number words: Dissociable systems. *Neuropsychologia*, **41**, 1942–58.

Lochy, A., Domahs, F. and Delazer, M. (in press). Rehabilitation of acquired calculation and number processing disorders. In J. Campbell, ed., *The Handbook of Mathematical Cognition.*

Luria, A. R. (1959). Disorders of simultaneous perception in a case of bilateral occipito-parietal brain injury. *Brain*, **82**, 437–49.

(1966). *The Higher Cortical Functions in Man.* New York: Basic Books.

Macaruso, P., McCloskey, M. and Aliminosa, D. (1993). The functional architecture of the cognitive numerical-processing system: Evidence from a patient with multiple impairments. *Cogn. Neuropsychol.*, **10**, 341–76.

Mandler, G. and Shebo, B. J. (1982). Subitizing: An analysis of its component processes. *J. Exp. Psychol. [Gen.]*, **111**, 1–21.

Mayer, E., Martory, M. D., Pegna, A. J., *et al.* (1999). A pure case of Gerstmann syndrome with a subangular lesion. *Brain*, **122** (Pt 6), 1107–20.

McCloskey, M., Aliminosa, D. and Sokol, S. M. (1991). Facts rules and procedures in normal calculation: Evidence from multiple single-patient studies of impaired arithmetic fact retrieval. *Brain Cogn.*, **17**, 154–203.

McCloskey, M., Sokol, S. M. and Goodman, R. A. (1986). Cognitive processes in verbal-number production: Inferences from the performance of brain-damaged subjects. *J. Exp. Psychol. Gen.*, **115**, 307–30.

McNeil, J. E. and Warrington, E. K. (1994). A dissociation between addition and subtraction within written calculation. *Neuropsychologia*, **32**, 717–28.

Molko, N., Cachia, A., Riviere, D., *et al.* (2003). Functional and structural alterations of the intraparietal sulcus in a developmental dyscalculia of genetic origin. *Neuron*, **40**, 847−58.

Moyer, R. S. and Landauer, T. K. (1967). Time required for judgements of numerical inequality. *Nature*, **215**, 1519−20.

Noël, M. P. (2001). Numerical cognition. In B. Rapp, ed., *The Handbook of Cognitive Neuropsychology*. Philadelphia: Psychology Press.

Pesenti, M., Seron, X. and Van Der Linden, M. (1994). Selective impairment as evidence for mental organisation of arithmetical facts: BB, a case of preserved subtraction? *Cortex*, **30**, 661−71.

Pica, P., Lemer, C., Izard, V. and Dehaene, S. (2004). Exact and approximate arithmetic in an Amazonian indigene group. *Science* (in press).

Pinel, P., Dehaene, S., Riviere, D. and LeBihan, D. (2001). Modulation of parietal activation by semantic distance in a number comparison task. *Neuroimage*, **14**, 1013−26.

Rizzo, M. and Robin, D. A. (1990). Simultanagnosia: A deficit of sustained attention yields insights on visual information processing. *Neurology*, **40**, 447−55.

Rosselli, M. and Ardila, A. (1989). Calculation deficits in patients with right and left hemisphere damage. *Neuropsychologia*, **27**, 607−17.

Seymour, S. E., Reuter-Lorenz, P. A. and Gazzaniga, M. S. (1994). The disconnection syndrome: basic findings reaffirmed. *Brain*, **117**, 105−15.

Simon, O., Mangin, J. F., Cohen, L., Le Bihan, D. and Dehaene, S. (2002). Topographical layout of hand, eye, calculation, and language-related areas in the human parietal lobe. *Neuron*, **33**, 475−87.

Thioux, M., Pillon, A., Samson, D., *et al.* (1998). The isolation of numerals at the semantic level. *Neurocase*. **4**.

Thompson, J. C., Abbott, D. F., Wheaton, K. J., Syngeniotis, A. and Puce, A. (in press). Digit representation is more than just hand waving. *Cogn. Brain Res.*

van Harskamp, N. J. and Cipolotti, L. (2001). Selective impairments for addition, subtraction and multiplication. Implications for the organisation of arithmetical facts. *Cortex*, **37**, 363−88.

van Harskamp, N. J., Rudge, P. and Cipolotti, L. (2002). Are multiplication facts implemented by the left supramarginal and angular gyri? *Neuropsychologia*, **40**, 1786−93.

Vuilleumier, P. and Rafal, R. (1999). Both means more than two: localizing and counting in patients with visuospatial neglect. *Nat. Neurosci.*, **2**, 783−4.

Warrington, E. K. (1982). The fractionation of arithmetical skills: A single case study. *Q. J. Exp. Psychol.*, **34A**, 31−51.

Whalen, J., McCloskey, M., Lindemann, M. and Bouton, G. (2002). Representing arithmetic table facts in memory: Evidence from acquired impairments. *Cogn. Neuropsychol.*, **19**, 505−22.

Zorzi, M., Priftis, K. and Umilta, C. (2002). Brain damage: neglect disrupts the mental number line. *Nature*, **417**, 138−9.

9

Hemispatial neglect

Patrik Vuilleumier

University Medical Center & University Hospital, Geneva, Switzerland

Introduction

Hemispatial neglect is among the most frequent and most disabling consequences of focal brain lesions. It entails a complex constellation of neuropsychological deficits in perception and action towards the side of space opposite to a focal brain lesion, which can occur in various combinations and with various degrees of severity. These deficits may persist in the chronic stages many years beyond the acute neurological insult. Moreover, the presence of hemispatial neglect has a major impact on functional recovery and on the burden for caregivers. Although some manifestations of neglect may be very striking, especially in acute stroke patients, some deficits are frequently missed by physicians during a general neurological examination and must therefore be specifically looked for, since they can provide valuable localization signs.

Hemispatial neglect has also attracted much interest in cognitive neuroscience research because it has important implications for understanding the neurobiological substrates of important human cognitive functions, intimately connected with conscious awareness, selective attention, and the mental representation of space. Many aspects of spatial neglect are still poorly understood and debated, but recent advances in our knowledge of the neurophysiology and functional anatomy of attention have begun to shed new light on some of the possible neuropsychological underpinnings (Driver and Vuilleumier, 2001b; Corbetta and Shulman, 2002). However, this chapter will mainly concentrate on the clinical presentation and evolution of spatial neglect and related deficits, while it will only briefly describe the current hypotheses concerning the neural mechanisms of this complex disorder (for more complete reviews, see Driver *et al.*, 2004; Kerkhoff, 2001; Halligan *et al.*, 2003).

General clinical manifestations of spatial neglect

Hemispatial neglect is generally defined as a failure to detect and orient to stimuli in the space contralateral to a focal brain lesion (i.e. the contralesional side), which cannot be explained by primary sensory or primary motor disturbances, nor by any general intellectual loss or confusion. Neglect can be apparent in responses to external stimulation as well as during spontaneous behavior. Typically, across a variety of situations and tasks, these patients behave as if a portion of the contralesional space did not exist and could not be conceived any longer. Thus, a patient with right hemisphere damage and left spatial neglect will not turn towards the examiner or visitors who approach or call them from the contralesional left side. They will instead always tend to orient their head and gaze towards the ipsilesional right side, even when eventually answering questions asked by the examiner standing on their left. Such patients may eat only from the right side of their plate but neglect the left half; read only the right side of pages or columns in books and newspapers; shave or make-up only one half of their face; and even dress up only half of their body, while forgetting to slip on their left-arm sleeve. They may also fail to use their contralesional hand to grasp objects, despite the hand not being weak, or fail to move their contralesional leg to get out of the bed, despite the leg not being paralyzed.

Importantly, neglect patients do not complain of their failures. Rather, they typically do not realize that they are missing information, and sometimes even deny that their contralesional limb is impaired (so-called "anosognosia" – see Chapter 10). This apparent loss of awareness and interest for all contralesional events seems to reflect their general inability to build a full representation of the contralesional hemispace, sometimes including the contralesional hemibody (see Chapter 10), and to direct attention towards this side, either voluntarily or reflexively.

In the clinic, spatial neglect is not only diagnosed by observation of the spontaneous behavior of patients (i.e. contralesional deviation of eyes and head, etc.), but also demonstrated by a variety of simple paper-and-pencil tests (see also later). The most characteristic tests are different variants of *cancellation tasks*, in which patients have to search for one or more visual targets among an array of distracters, randomly distributed on a sheet of paper, and to cross out the specified targets (Figure 9.1A). For example, when required to put a mark on all of the lines spread over a page, or to circle all exemplars of a given letter presented together with other letters on a page, neglect patients will typically perform quite accurately for items located on the ipsilesional side of the page, but fail to detect and mark those on the left side – thus neglecting to explore and orient their attention to the contralesional items. Likewise, in *line bisection tasks*, where patients are required to indicate the midpoint of horizontal lines (or other stimuli), their mark will consistently deviate towards the ipsilesional side – as if ignoring or compressing the contralesional extent of these lines (Figure 9.1B). Further, when drawing from memory or copying, neglect patients

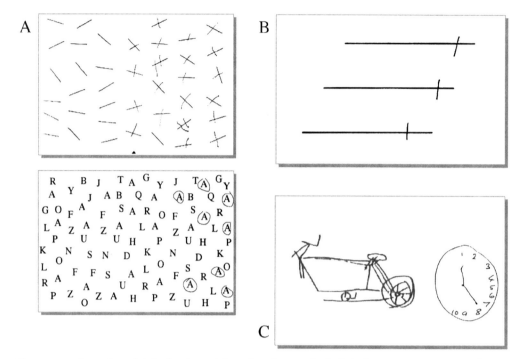

Figure 9.1   Examples of left visual spatial neglect in standard clinical tests. (A) Two cancellation tasks, in which the patient must find and mark lines (top) or the letter A (bottom) across the whole visual array. (B) Line bisection task, in which the patient has to mark the midpoint of long lines placed at different spatial position. (C) Drawing of a bike and a clock.

usually show striking omissions of important features on the contralesional side (Figure 9.1C), even for single objects with characteristic spatial layouts (e.g. a clockface, silhouette, or bike).

Neglect deficits can be distinguished along different dimensions, for instance in terms of perceptual input and motor output functions, sensory modalities, sectors of space, frames of reference or spatial scale, as well as other related cognitive subcomponents. However, it remains unclear to what extent these different aspects may rely on distinct neural systems that can be affected together or sometimes dissociate, depending on the location or size of brain lesions. Many aspects of neglect cannot easily be classified as perceptual only, or motoric only, but rather seem to involve some failures at the interface between perception and action, where sensory inputs can access conscious awareness to control motor plans and behavior (e.g. orienting to a stimulus present in the world), and vice versa, where goal-directed behavior and actions can influence sensory processing and awareness (e.g. exploring the world for the presence of a stimulus). It is likely that such an interface is dependent on the function of a network of cortical and subcortical regions, centered on association areas in the parietal and frontal cortex that are critically implicated in the representation of space, as well as in the control of attention and intention processes (Mesulam, 1999). Neglect typically follows lesions in parietal and frontal areas, as well as interconnected subcortical regions, while primary sensory and motor pathways may remain relatively intact (Vallar *et al.*, 2003; Kumral and Evyapan, 1999). Thus, impaired detection of contralesional stimuli in neglect is typically not due to elementary sensory losses, but is thought to reflect a failure to direct attention in contralesional space, whereas impaired exploration is not caused by a simple oculomotor disturbance or weakness, but rather seems to result from a failure to generate intentions directed towards the contralesional space. However, these attentional and intentional aspects appear intimately connected at the brain level and may engage similar populations of neurons in the parietal cortex, essentially computing the relative location and saliency of stimuli in space (Driver and Vuilleumier, 2001b; Andersen and Buneo, 2003). Nevertheless, it is useful to distinguish the clinical manifestations of neglect along different lines of deficits as observed in different task conditions.

Perceptual deficits

Neglect is clearly different from a simple sensory disorder. In particular, signs of visual neglect must be distinguished from those associated with a visual field defect (e.g. hemianopia), and cannot be explained by such elementary losses. Patients who have hemianopia only (without neglect) do not exhibit the same contralesional failures in drawing or cancellation tasks. Although they are blind in one hemifield, they can still normally explore and orient towards the contralesional side. Conversely, some patients may show severe spatial neglect even though they have no hemianopia. Moreover, whereas visual field defects are typically characterized by a sharp demarcation between the impaired and intact side along the vertical midline (due to the projection of each hemiretina to the contralateral occipital cortex), spatial neglect does not respect this retinotopic midline and typically shows a more graded pattern of deficit from the impaired to the intact side.

However, in some patients with neglect, it may be difficult to determine with certainty whether a concomitant visual field cut is also present or not. Spatial neglect may be so severe that it can mimic hemianopia and produce a "pseudo-hemianopia" (Kooistra and Heilman, 1989), with an apparent blindness to all stimulation presented in the contralesional visual field despite the demonstration of preserved visual pathways (e.g. using visual evoked potentials). Two clinical features may help distinguish "pseudo-hemianopia" from real hemianopia by demonstrating its non-sensory nature. First, reducing the demands to fixate on a central stimulus during visual perimetry or confrontation testing will improve pseudo-hemianopia, but not real field cuts – a phenomenon showing that contralesional impairments in vision in the former case are primarily caused by a limitation in the ability to direct attention to the contralesional side, but not by a true scotoma (Walker *et al.*, 1991). Second, unlike retinotopic field cuts that remain unchanged with different gaze directions, pseudo-hemianopia will improve when the patient turns the eyes more to the right side, such that the retinal midline (and part of the left visual field) now falls on the right side relative to the head or body midline, indicating the contralesional visual impairment is not determined by purely retinal coordinates but by spatial coordinates (Vuilleumier *et al.*, 1999).

On the other hand, patients who have hemianopia in addition to spatial neglect may show worse performance in some visuomotor tasks, suggesting that field defects can interact with neglect and exacerbate some clinical manifestations (Doricchi and Angelelli, 1999; Ferber and Karnath, 2001b) as well as long-term prognosis (Cassidy *et al.*, 1999), although many other visual tasks are not necessarily affected (Halligan *et al.*, 1990). In particular, line bisection and estimation of the horizontal size of visual objects can be impaired in patients with hemianopia, even without spatial neglect (Ferber and Karnath, 2001b). Furthermore, patients with spatial neglect often show an ipsilesional deviation when pointing straight ahead to indicate their subjective body midline, but this bias is reversed in patients with hemianopia, and absent in patient with both disorders (Ferber and Karnath, 1999). Accordingly, deviations in the subjective straight ahead have been found not to correlate reliably with neglect severity (Bartolomeo and Chokron, 1999; Chokron *et al.*, 2002), unlike what was previously thought (Karnath *et al.*, 1991).

Perceptual extinction is another deficit associated with neglect showing that sensory disturbances alone cannot explain the deficits found in these patients. Such extinction is observed during double simultaneous stimulation, such that one stimulus delivered on the contralesional side is not perceived when paired with a concurrent stimulus on the ipsilesional side, even though the same contralesional stimulus is correctly perceived when presented alone (Figure 9.2). Extinction can be observed in all sensory modalities, either in isolation or in various combinations including vision (Ladavas, 1990; Di Pellegrino and De Renzi, 1995; Vuilleumier and Rafal, 2000), touch (Aglioti *et al.*, 1998; Olson *et al.*, 2003), hearing (Deouell and Soroker, 2000; Bellmann *et al.*, 2001), and smell

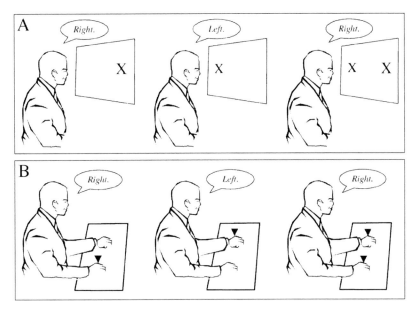

Figure 9.2   Illustration of perceptual extinction on double simultaneous stimulation. (A) Left visual extinction. (B) Left tactile extinction.

(Bellas *et al.*, 1988), but not for taste due to the predominantly ipsilateral projections of gustatory inputs (Berlucchi *et al.*, 2004). Extinction differs from primary sensory loss, where contralesional deficits are found even with a single unilateral stimulation, although some sensory loss may also be associated and then exacerbate extinction on double stimulation. However, the presence of "trimodal extinction" (affecting vision, touch, and hearing in the same patient) is highly suggestive of a *supramodal* spatial deficit, rather than *unimodal* sensory loss (Heilman *et al.*, 1970). Extinction is interpreted as a deficit in spatial attention, with a failure to orient contralesionally arising specifically in the presence of a competing stimulation on the ipsilesional side, while elementary perceptual abilities are relatively intact (e.g. allowing detection of single stimuli on the contralesional side). Moreover, extinction is not an all-or-none phenomenon, but can vary from trial to trial or from day to day, also reflecting its attentional nature. Furthermore, the role of non-sensory factors is demonstrated by observations that extinction is not simply determined by the body part being stimulated, but also by the location in space of such body parts. For instance, tactile extinction on the contralesional left hand can be reduced by changing the position of the hand (Moscovitch and Behrmann, 1994) or crossing the patient's arms (Aglioti *et al.*, 1999; Bartolomeo *et al.*, 2004), while extinction on the intact hand can sometimes be obtained when the ipsilesional hand is placed in the contralesional space (Bartolomeo et al., 2004; Valenza et al., 2004). Similar effects of gaze direction have been found for visual extinction (Vuilleumier and Schwartz, 2001). These effects highlight that neglect deficits arise at the level of some higher-level representation of stimuli in space, rather than at the purely perceptual processing stages.

Extinction may also be observed when double simultaneous stimuli are presented in different modalities, such as for a *tactile* stimulus on the contra-lesional side paired with a *visual* stimulus in the ipsilesional side (Mattingley et al., 1997; Di Pellegrino et al., 1997; Ladavas et al., 1998). Such crossmodal extinction suggests that competition for spatial attention may involve mech-anisms responsible for a supramodal representation of space (but see also Olson et al., 2003). These supramodal effects seem also to interact with motor and proprioceptive information, because extinction between touch and vision may depend on whether the visual stimulus is perceived at a location close to the non-touched hand and hence integrated within a single bimodal (visuotactile) representation of this hand (Di Pellegrino et al., 1997; Ladavas et al., 1998; see also Farne and Ladavas, 2000; Maravita et al., 2001).

Motor deficits

Many tasks used to assess neglect involve both perceptual and motor components. For instance, line bisection or cancellation tasks require not only perception of the presence and extent of visual stimuli in contralesional space, but also direction of the eyes and the hand towards the appropriate location in contralesional space. Thus, failures to respond to contralesional targets might reflect not only spatial biases in *attentional* processes, but also biases in *intentional* processes responsible for planning or executing movements towards the contralesional side, even with the ipsilesional limb.

Several studies have tried to disentangle motor and perceptual components in spatial neglect, using a variety of experimental procedures to uncouple the direction of sensory information and motor action, such as with pulley-systems (Bisiach et al., 1990), videos (Coslett et al., 1990), mirrors (Tegner and Levander, 1991) or different hand start-position for responding to the same targets (Mattingley et al., 1992; 1998; Husain et al., 2000). Taken together, the findings from these studies converge to suggest that the performance of neglect patients may be determined not only by an impairment in perceiving contralesional visual stimuli, but also by some impairment in initiating movements in a contralesional direction. This combined perceptual–motor deficit may accord with a role of integrated sensorimotor representation of space within the parietal and frontal cortices (Andersen *et al.*, 1997; Colby, 1998). Such motoric aspects have variably been termed "directional hypokinesia" (Coslett *et al.*, 1990; Mattingley *et al.*, 1992; Heilman *et al.*, 1985) or "premotor neglect" (Bisiach *et al.*, 1990; Harvey *et al.*, 2002), sometimes with a further distinction between manual biases (melokinetic) and oculomotor biases (ophthalmokinetic) during spatial exploration tasks (Bisiach *et al.*, 1995).

Premotor and perceptual factors have also been distinguished using a variant of line bisection, the "landmark task" (Milner *et al.*, 1993; Harvey *et al.*, 1995), in which patients have to report which is the longer (or the shorter) of the two portions of a pre-bisected horizontal line. Given that both portions of the line have an equal length in this situation, pointing to the left end of the line when asked to report the *shorter* segment would indicate perceptual neglect, whereas pointing to the right end would indicate motor neglect. In addition, computing difference scores relative to performance on the same task but when asked to report the *longer* segment can provide some measure of perceptual and motor/response biases in the same patient (Toraldo *et al.*, 2002; Bisiach *et al.*, 1998a). A task requiring patients to extend a line to double its length may also show an overextension of the line towards the left side, consistent with misperception or compression of the left portion of the line rather than directional neglect (Bisiach *et al.*, 1994), although a similar behavior may be seen in right brain-damaged patients without neglect (Ferber and Karnath, 2001b; Bisiach *et al.*, 1998b).

Spatial neglect can also be manifest during exploration in the absence of any external sensory stimulation. Eye movement recordings show that when patients are asked to find a (non-existing) target in an otherwise dark and empty room, their search is limited to the ipsilesional side of space but rarely directed towards the contralesional side (Karnath and Fetter, 1995), even though their saccades show normal speed and amplitude, and are still directed equally often to the left and right *within* the ipsilesional sector of explored space (Niemeier and Karnath, 2000). Manual search in the dark or blindfolded (e.g. to find an object on the desk) shows a similar bias towards the ipsilesional side, and a failure to explore the contralesional space. Taken together, these findings highlight the existence of a disturbed representation of contralesional space in neglect patients, affecting their motor behavior even without any sensory targets.

Finally, a different type of motor neglect can often be observed, characterized by a failure to use or move the contralesional limb, even though the limb is not paralyzed or only minimally weak (Laplane and Degos, 1983; Castaigne *et al.*, 1972). Such motor neglect or under-use of a limb has also been termed "unilateral hypokinesia" (Valenstein and Heilman, 1981; Watson and

Heilman, 1981) and can sometimes affect the arm or leg separately. It is typically seen in spontaneous behavior, concerning both voluntary and more automatic actions, but can be fully reversed by verbal instructions (Laplane et al., 1986). This can also be associated with motor extinction – a failure (or difficulty) to execute a contralesional movement at the same time as a similar ipsilesional movement, even though contralesional movement can be performed alone (Valenstein and Heilman, 1981; Watson and Heilman, 1981). Although this form of unilateral motor neglect is commonly present in patients with other signs of hemispatial neglect, it can also be seen in a relatively pure form without any evidence of perceptual neglect (Laplane et al., 1986; Laplane, 1990).

Frames of reference

One of the most striking aspects of spatial neglect is that it can arise at different spatial scales within the same patient, and also differentially affect distinct parts of external space. As well as ignoring stimuli at the extreme left in their environment, patients may neglect a left page when reading a small book, omit some words to the left of the right page, or even miss a few letters at one end of each word. Thus, the portion of space defined as "contralesional" and being eventually "neglected" may vary as a function of the stimulus or the task, and sometimes vary between different patients.

For example, distinct frames of reference can define spatial neglect with respect to different left–right coordinates. Some aspects of neglect can affect stimuli presented in the left hemispace as determined by "egocentric" coordinates, relative to the midline of the body, head, or eyes of the patient (Vuilleumier et al., 1999; Ladavas, 1987; Vallar et al., 1995; Karnath et al., 1998; Mennemeier et al., 1994). Other aspects of neglect involve "allocentric" coordinates, affecting the left side of each individual stimulus, irrespective of its location with respect to the patient's body (Driver and Halligan, 1991; Chatterjee, 1994; Behrmann and Tipper, 1999). To determine the role of these different spatial coordinates in neglect, several studies have manipulated the position of the patient, for instance by turning or tilting the head or the body (e.g. Ladavas, 1987; Karnath et al., 1998; Mennemeier et al., 1994), such that the same stimulus is presented at the same retinal location but occupies different locations in space with respect to egocentric coordinates. These experiments have typically shown that spatial neglect is much more affected by the relative egocentric position of a stimulus than by its position on the retina or on the limb, in accord with a spatial rather than a sensory deficit (see also Vuilleumier et al., 1999; Behrmann et al., 2002). This is similar to the effects of crossing or rotating the arms in studies of tactile extinction (see Moscovitch and Behrmann, 1994; Aglioti *et al.*, 1999; Bartolomeo *et al.*, 2004). Ispilesional deviations in line bisection are also typically increased when the line is placed further to the left of the patient's body (Butter *et al.*, 1988a).

Other studies have manipulated the orientation or the nature of the stimulus (e.g. Driver and Halligan, 1991; Behrmann and Moscovitch, 1994; Driver *et al.*, 1994; Marshall and Halligan, 1994; Farah *et al.*, 1990), such that the left side of an object is presented on the right side of the patient, and vice versa, for instance by rotating or tilting the main axis of letters and shapes. In such cases, neglect patients may show worse detection for the left side of an object presented in their right visual field, than for the right side of an object presented in their left visual field, indicating that neglect can operate in allocentric or "object-centered" coordinates. Some of these effects may result from a preserved perceptual analysis of the global shape of objects, with contralesional neglect arising for the contralesional half of the shape to which attention is more focally directed (Halligan and Marshall, 1991a; Driver and Pouget, 2000). Moreover, many patients show an effect of both egocentric and allocentric factors (Behrmann and Tipper, 1999), but some dissociations have been reported (Chatterjee, 1994; Humphreys and Riddoch, 1995).

In addition, "object-based" effects can occur during *reading* and *spelling* of single words, with some letters being omitted irrespective of the modality and order of presentation (Caramazza and Hillis, 1990; Hillis and Caramazza, 1991). Difficulties in reading are common in neglect patients and are characterized by omissions and transformations of the initial letters in individual words ("neglect dyslexia"), but these errors are strongly modulated by lexical and semantic factors, typically worse for non-words than real words (Di Pellegrino *et al.*, 2001; Ladavas *et al.*, 1997; Behrmann *et al.*, 1990). These effects suggest that preserved word recognition processes can influence the spatial extent of attention and neglect during word reading.

A combination of object-based and space-based neglect is also frequently seen in the *drawings* of patients. For example, when copying a scene with different objects (Figure 9.3), a patient may fail to draw some items on the extreme left side of the scene (i.e. egocentric or space-based neglect), but also fail to draw some features on the left side of objects situated on the right side of the scene (i.e. allocentric or object-based neglect). Note however that, in many situations, as in drawing tasks, different frames of reference are typically aligned and cannot be unambiguously disentangled without further tests. For instance, it could be possible that the spatial layout of objects in the scene to copy is not strictly coded in an egocentric frame of reference, but rather coded in allocentric coordinates

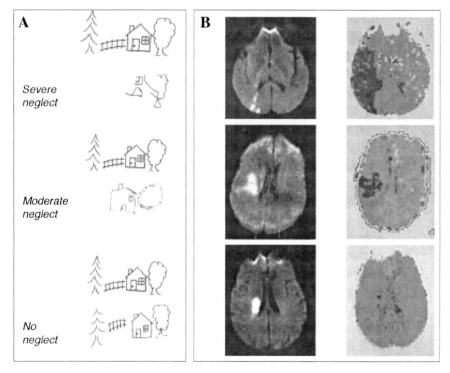

Figure 9.3   Differences in symptoms and lesions in three patients with acute right hemisphere stroke. (A) Copy of Ogden's multi-element scene from each patient, showing different degrees of severity in left spatial neglect, from severe (top) through to moderate neglect (middle) and no neglect (bottom). Performance in top row reveals both space-based/egocentric and object-based/allocentric omissions on the left side. (B) Abnormalities in diffusion weighted MRI (DWI, left column) and perfusion MRI (PWI, right column) in each patient, showing that stroke with similar volume of infracted tissue can be associated with different degrees of hypoperfusion in the right hemisphere (blue colored areas), corresponding with the different degrees of neglect severity. For a color version of this figure please see www.cambridge.org/9780521106955.

centered on the page or the desktop, which by themselves constitute larger objects in space.

Sectors of space

Neglect can differentially affect extra-personal, peri-personal, and personal sectors of space. Neglect of *personal space* refers to the inability of patients to reach towards contralesional parts of their own body (Bisiach *et al.*, 1986; Beschin and Robertson, 1997) or towards objects or marks (e.g. cotton balls or threads) attached to their contralesional body (Cocchini *et al.*, 2001;

Buxbaum *et al.*, 2004), while using the intact ipsilesional hand. Although reaching to distal body parts may also be impaired due to proprioceptive disturbances, such failures to localize and reach for more proximal regions of the body may result from a loss in the representation of the personal hemibody. However, such deficit is rarely present alone (Beschin and Robertson, 1997; Guariglia and Antonucci, 1992) and more often associated with other manifestations of neglect (Buxbaum *et al.*, 2004).

Neglect of *peri-personal* space is much more usual and refers to all deficits seen for stimuli presented within reaching distance, but not on the patient's own body. Peri-personal neglect therefore concerns most of the typical bedside and paper-and-pencil tests (see above), both perceptual and motor, as well as the cross-modal interactions between different sensory stimuli presented close to body parts (e.g. Ladavas *et al.*, 1998; Ladavas *et al.*, 2000).

Neglect of *extra-personal* space concerns stimuli presented outside reach, for instance in far distance (Cowey *et al.*, 1994; Pizzamiglio *et al.*, 1989). Dissociations have been observed between patients showing neglect for near but not far visual space (Halligan and Marshall, 1991b), and vice versa, patients showing neglect for far but not near space (Vuilleumier *et al.*, 1998). These distance effects can be modulated when patients use a tool or laser-pointer (Farne and Ladavas, 2000; Berti and Frassinetti, 2000; Pegna *et al.*, 2001), which may induce an extension of the peri-personal or near extra-personal deficits to the far space, while such deficits are not present without a tool in the same patient. Some distance effects might also arise in peri-personal space during tactile exploration (Beschin *et al.*, 1996), and potentially in auditory space (Vallar *et al.*, 1995).

In some cases, impairments in spatial attention have been distinguished along the radial axis (Mennemeier *et al.*, 1992) or vertical axis (altitudinal neglect, cf. Rapcsak *et al.*, 1988; Shelton *et al.*, 1990) within peri-personal space (using line bisection and sometimes cancellation tasks), but the mechanisms of such biases remain unclear and potentially interact with other functional asymmetries in the upper/lower visual field.

Imaginal representation

Remarkably, neglect can also arise in *memory* or *mental imagery tasks* testing for so-called "representational" aspects. When asked to describe from memory the settings of a familiar place, neglect patients may fail to describe elements that would be situated on the contralesional side (Bisiach and Luzzatti, 1978; Bartolomeo *et al.*, 1994), even though they may correctly report the same elements when asked to adopt a different perspective in their mind's eye, such that previously omitted details are now reported and previously reported details are now neglected (Bisiach and Luzzatti, 1978; Ortigue *et al.*, 2001). Similar neglect may arise for the mental representation of single objects such as a clockface (Grossi *et al.*, 1989) or for items in visual scenes that were previously correctly seen or learned by verbal description (Beschin *et al.*, 1997; Denis *et al.*, 2002). Such deficits may sometimes arise in isolation (Ortigue *et al.*, 2001; Beschin *et al.*, 1997; Guariglia *et al.*, 1991; Coslett, 1997) but more frequently co-occur with other perceptual deficits (Bartolomeo *et al.*, 1994).

A somewhat related phenomenon has been observed during *numerical tasks* that may require some form of spatial code, such as imaging numbers aligned along a mental line with a left-to-right progression for increasing quantities (Zorzi *et al.*, 2002; Vuilleumier *et al.*, 2004; Fischer, 2001). For instance, neglect patients may show a systematic "rightward" deviation in their bisection of numerical intervals (e.g. stating that 5 is halfway between 2 and 6) (Zorzi *et al.*, 2002). They may also be unable to shift "leftward" from a point on such mental number line when judging quantities smaller than a fixed number (e.g., 6 relative to 7), but not impaired in judging larger quantities (e.g., 8 relative to 7, or 6 relative to 5), and these numerical effects are reversed when the patients are asked to judge hours on a clockface (where small numbers can now be imagined on the right side) (Vuilleumier *et al.*, 2004).

Dissociations between neglect subtypes

Several of the manifestations described have been found to arise to different degrees in different patients, suggesting that they may implicate partly distinct cognitive systems and have distinct neuroanatomical substrates. Such dissociations may exist between perceptual and premotor neglect (Buxbaum *et al.*, 2004; Brighina *et al.*, 2002), perceptual and representational neglect (Guariglia *et al.*, 1991; Coslett, 1997), as well as between personal and peri-personal or extra-personal space (Buxbaum *et al.*, 2004; Azouvi *et al.*, 2002), and between near and far sectors of space (Halligan and Marshall, 1991b; Vuilleumier *et al.*, 1998; Weiss *et al.*, 2000). Moreover, although egocentric coordinates may play a predominant role in many aspects of spatial neglect, object-centered deficits can also dissociate (Ota *et al.*, 2001; Hillis *et al.*, 2005). Some patients with *bilateral brain lesions* may exhibit left neglect for parts of individual objects together with neglect of all objects on the opposite *right* side of space (Humphreys and Riddoch, 1995; Halligan and Marshall, 1998), or different degrees of body-centered and object-centered neglect after successive strokes (Ota *et al.*, 2003). Finally, while perceptual extinction is often found without other florid signs of spatial neglect in chronic stages, spatial neglect has also occasionally been reported without perceptual extinction (Cocchini *et al.*, 1999).

Nevertheless, in many more patients, different aspects of spatial neglect are all present together to some extent. This may reflect damage to a common neural network coding for space in different coordinate systems, and controlling attention for both perception and action simultaneously; or this could result from large lesions destroying many different spatial systems in the same patient (Driver *et al.*, 2004). In addition, besides lateralized neglect deficits, several aspects of neglect might result from non-spatial or non-lateralized deficits associated with right hemisphere damage, including an abnormal tendency to focus attention on local parts of the scene (Halligan and Marshall, 1998), impairments in sustained attention and arousal (Robertson *et al.*, 1998; Samuelsson *et al.*, 1998), reduced processing speed even for stimuli presented at fixation (Husain *et al.*, 1997), or impaired working memory of spatial locations across short time delays and/or saccades (Ellis *et al.*, 1996; Husain *et al.*, 2001; Pisella *et al.*, 2004). Future research on cognitive mechanisms of neglect should determine whether such deficits simply tend to co-occur with neglect after right brain lesions, or rather interact with abnormal spatial biases in attention and intention in order to produce the typical clinical symptoms of neglect.

Implicit processing

Another striking aspect of spatial neglect is that, despite inattention and unawareness, some stimuli presented in the contralesional space may still be processed without consciousness and sometimes influence the behavior of patients (Marshall and Halligan, 1988). This unconscious or "implicit" processing has been demonstrated using a variety of different tasks and in different sensory modalities, especially for vision (e.g. Berti and Rizzolatti, 1992; Berti *et al.*, 1994; McGlinchey-Berroth *et al.*, 1993; Volpe *et al.*, 1979; Vuilleumier *et al.*, 2001b) but also for touch (Aglioti *et al.*, 1998; Vallar *et al.*, 1991; Maravita, 1997; Berti *et al.*, 1999) and hearing (Deouell and Soroker, 2000). Such implicit effects are thought to result from some residual processing still taking place in early sensory cortices spared by the lesion, prior to the stages where spatial neglect or perceptual extinction may arise (for reviews, see Driver and Vuilleumier, 2001a; Berti, 2003). In some cases, implicit processing may proceed up to involve a relatively elaborate stimulus analysis, including access to semantic associations (Berti and Rizzolatti, 1992; McGlinchey-Berroth *et al.*, 1993) or response selection stages (Rafal *et al.*, 2002). Residual processing can also produce long-lasting effects on implicit memory tests (Vuilleumier *et al.*, 2001b).

Furthermore, besides these unconscious effects, residual processing may contribute to modulate neglect and extinction, explaining why pictures of salient and real objects are less severely extinguished than nonsense objects

(Ward and Goodrich, 1996; Vuilleumier *et al.*, 2001c), and why contralesional stimuli are often better detected when they form a common perceptual "gestalt" with simultaneous ipsilesional stimuli (grouping effects) (Ward *et al.*, 1994; Vuilleumier, 2000). These effects may, however, vary between patients, depending on whether their brain lesions spare the early sensory cortical areas that are presumably responsible for such residual implicit processing (Vuilleumier, 2000; Vallar *et al.*, 2000) (see also Rees *et al.*, 2000; Vuilleumier *et al.*, 2001a).

Key points Main characteristics of spatial neglect

Attentional deficits

Impaired detection of events or stimuli on the side of space contralateral to a focal brain lesion

Spontaneous deviation of head or eyes towards the ipsilesional side

Lack of spontaneous or reflexive orienting to the contralesional side

Impairments arising for stimuli in personal, peripersonal, or extrapersonal space (near or far)

Misses for objects or words located in the contralesional space relative to the body (egocentric)

Misses for contralesional parts of single objects or words (allocentric)

Omissions of contralesional words or contralesional letters during reading

Omissions of contralesional features in drawing or copying

Deviation to the ipsilesional side in line bisection

Extinction of contralesional stimuli on double simultaneous stimulation

Unimodal or multimodal (vision, touch, audition)

Not explained by a primary sensory or motor disorder ($\neq$ hemianopia)

Intentional deficits

Lack of voluntary exploration or search directed into the contralesional space (oculomotor or manual)

Lack or slowing of movements in contralesional direction (directional hypokinesia)

Lack of spontaneous or reflexive use of contralesional limbs (unilateral hypokinesia)

Extinction of contralesional movement during bilateral simultaneous action

Other related spatial deficits

Impaired description of contralesional information in mental imagery

Lack of awareness or denial of contralesional hemiplegia (anosognosia), hemiasomatognosia

Focal attentional bias towards local visual features (zooming-in), impaired global attention (zooming-out)

Other common non-spatial deficits

General slowing

Impaired sustained attention

Limitation in processing many simultaneous stimuli in time or space (simultanagnosia)

Occurrence of spatial neglect in stroke

In one form or another, neglect is very common following hemispheric strokes, particularly after lesions on the non-dominant (right) side (for a meta-analysis, see Bowen *et al.*, 1999). Ischemic and hemorrhagic lesions are equally responsible, since the anatomical site more than the etiological cause of damage plays a determinant role in the occurrence of the disorder. However, neglect is generally more prevalent and more severe with cortical than with purely subcortical damage, and typically does not occur with lacunar stroke, but lesions in the basal ganglia or thalamus are not uncommon (see later).

Across all stroke types, the reported frequency of spatial neglect varies widely, ranging from 15% to 85% during the acute stage (<20 days) in patients who have had a first right hemisphere stroke (Azouvi *et al.*, 2002; Bowen *et al.*, 1999; Stone *et al.*, 1998; Stone *et al.*, 1991; Pedersen *et al.*, 1997). Neglect signs are still present in 30–40% of these patients three months after the stroke (Bowen *et al.*, 2002; Tatemichi *et al.*, 1994), and some deficits may persist for several years after the initial insult (Cassidy *et al.*, 1998; Samuelsson *et al.*, 1997). Critically, both the tests used to assess neglect and the time of assessment relative to stroke onset can affect the reported rate of occurrence, since clinical manifestations can show a large variability (see above) and recovery rate is rapid during the early weeks (see later) (Bowen *et al.*, 1999; Farne *et al.*, 2004). When acute patients with right hemisphere damage (RHD) are screened with a detailed battery examining a wide range of deficits, more than 80% of them may present some degree of neglect on at least one measure, whereas only 36% are considered to show moderate to severe neglect across several tasks (Azouvi *et al.*, 2002). Using a systematic battery is therefore usually more sensitive than using any single test alone. Hemiplegia and hemianopia are frequently associated (in more than two-thirds of cases, cf. Cassidy *et al.*, 1999; Azouvi *et al.*, 2002).

A major hemispheric asymmetry has long been recognized, with neglect being not only more frequent but also more severe and more persistent after right- than left-side lesions, at least in right-handed patients (Bowen *et al.*, 1999; Vallar, 1993; Stone *et al.*, 1992). Results from a meta-analysis of 17 studies including both left and right hemisphere strokes (Bowen *et al.*, 1999) indicate a frequency of right neglect ranging from zero to 76% after left hemisphere damage (LHD), with a median of 21%, in contrast to a frequency ranging from 13% to 82% after RHD, and a median of 43%. Similarly, when screened with a detailed battery examining a range of deficits, patients with acute LHD showed some degree of right neglect in about 40% of the cases, but fewer than 10% showed severe neglect across several different tasks

(Beis *et al.*, 2004), which is at most half the frequency found with the same battery in patients with RHD (Azouvi *et al.*, 2002). One possible exception, however, concerns the occurrence of personal neglect and motor neglect, which might be equally frequent after hemispheric strokes on either side (Beis *et al.*, 2004). Moreover, right neglect after left hemisphere lesions may affect anterior more often than posterior regions, unlike left neglect after RHD (Ogden, 1985b), and also show some qualitative differences (Beis *et al.*, 2004). In particular, the severity of deficits is less reliably correlated between different tests in LHD than RHD patients, suggesting that these deficits are more elusive and less consistent after LHD than RHD (Beis *et al.*, 2004). These hemispheric differences do not seem to be accounted for by language disturbances or differences in the selection of patients. Furthermore, right spatial neglect due to LHD has also been found to show a more rapid recovery than left neglect after RHD. Thus, in one study using the same tests at two different times after stroke onset, right and left neglect were almost equally frequent during the first 3 days (62% and 72%, respectively) (Stone *et al.*, 1991b), but the presence of right neglect was significantly reduced after 3 months whereas left neglect was not significantly improved (33% and 75%, respectively) (Stone *et al.*, 1992).

This hemispheric asymmetry in the occurrence of spatial neglect is usually attributed to a right hemisphere dominance for the distribution of attention in space (Mesulam, 1999; Heilman and Abell, 1979). A common hypothesis is that the right hemisphere can control attention in both sides of space, while the left hemisphere can control attention in the contralateral right hemispace only. Hence, unilateral LHD might still leave the right hemisphere capable of representing space bilaterally, whereas unilateral RHD might result in a complete loss of the representation of left space (Heilman and Van Den Abell, 1980; Weintraub and Mesulam, 1987). Accordingly, many studies using functional brain imaging in healthy subjects have shown a right hemisphere dominance in activation produced during various attentional tasks (Gitelman *et al.*, 1999; LaBar *et al.*, 1999). Moreover, in reflexive spatial orienting tasks, such hemispheric asymmetry might be more pronounced in inferior than in the superior parietal cortical regions (Corbetta and Shulman, 2002).

Rarely, however, patients with atypical hemispheric dominance may present with "crossed" symptoms. This may take various forms or various degrees, such as severe right neglect without aphasia following a left hemisphere lesion, or a combination of neglect and aphasia after damage in the same (right or left) hemisphere, even in the presence of right-handedness (Cambier *et al.*, 1985; Posteraro and Mara vita, 1996; Paghera *et al.*, 2003; Marchetti *et al.*, 2005).

Key points Strokes responsible for spatial neglect

Acute infarct
Anterior circulation:
Middle cerebral artery: *most common*
    superficial: cortical damage in inferior parietal, superior parietal, inferior frontal regions
    deep: lenticulostriate territory basal ganglia (putamen > caudate)
Anterior choroid artery: *Uncommon*: lesion of posterior internal capsule
Anterior cerebral artery: *rare*: mesial prefrontal region
Posterior circulation:
    Posterior cerebral artery: *uncommon*: combination of superficial and deep infarcts
    Thalamic lesions: *occasional*: anterior tuberothalamic syndrome, paramedian, pulvinar
Watershed infarcts: posterior, anterior, both

Acute hemorrhage
Lobar: parieto-frontal region

Deep: large subcortical hemorrhage

Chronic stroke
Multiple strokes, vascular dementia
Diffuse white matter diseases: Binswanger, MELAS

Anatomical correlates and subtypes of spatial neglect

Spatial attention is known to implicate a distributed network of cortical and subcortical regions in the brain, interconnecting parietal and frontal areas together with anterior cingulate cortex, basal ganglia and specific thalamic nuclei, as well as some lower structures in the brainstem such as the superior colliculus and reticular formation (Mesulam, 1981; 1999; Heilman *et al.*, 2003). This network was initially identified by the neuroanatomical analysis of neglect disorders and neurophysiological work in animals, but has been confirmed and refined by recent functional neuroimaging studies (PET and fMRI) in healthy human subjects (Corbetta and Shulman, 2002; Gitelman *et al.*, 1999). Some areas within this network overlap with neural systems involved in the control of saccadic eye movements, including in particular the superior parietal regions within the intraparietal sulcus (IPS) and the frontal eye field (FEF) region in the posterior middle frontal gyrus, reflecting the close functional relationships between mechanisms for spatial attention and oculomotor control (Corbetta *et al.*, 1998).

It is usually thought that damage anywhere in this widespread network, particularly in the right hemisphere (see above), can result in neglect for contralesional space (Mesulam, 1981; 1999; Heilman *et al.*, 2003). However, it is likely that some variability in the severity, persistence, and perhaps type of neglect symptoms might arise as a function of the different sites of lesion, although there is still considerable uncertainty and controversy as to which brain areas might be more specifically responsible for different clinical aspects of spatial neglect. Results from functional neuroimaging studies in healthy subjects suggest that different attentional functions might be subserved by partially segregated neural networks (Corbetta and Shulman, 2002), with areas in intraparietal cortex and superior frontal cortex being particularly important for the voluntary (endogenous) direction of attention, while a more inferior network in the temporoparietal junction (TPJ) and inferior frontal cortex might be more important for the reflexive (exogenous) orientation of attention in response to salient or unexpected stimuli (Figure 9.4). It is conceivable that both of these "dorsal" and "ventral" attention systems might be disrupted in neglect, either differentially or jointly (especially in the right hemisphere). However, the exact anatomical–clinical relationships for these two networks still remain largely speculative. Interestingly, factorial analyses of neglect symptoms have also suggested the existence of two main component contributing to the clinical syndrome (Azouvi *et al.*, 2002; Kinsella *et al.*, 1993), but related to scanning or exploratory functions and to spatial representional functions, respectively.

Anatomical–clinical correlations of spatial neglect in stroke might be compli-cated by the fact that structurally intact areas can be dysfunctional due to ischemia in salvageable tissue distant from an infarcted territory (e.g. penumbra; Perani *et al.*, 1987; Hillis *et al.*, 2002) or due to functional effects or disconnection secondary to the lesion (e.g. diaschisis; Perani *et al.*, 1987; Bogousslavsky *et al.*, 1988; Vuilleumier, 2005). Using functional measures such as fMRI and EEG in addition to structural anatomical imaging can also provide a better under-standing of the functional mechanisms involved in spatial neglect and related deficits (Vuilleumier *et al.*, 2001a; Leibovitch *et al.*, 1999; Leibovitch *et al.*, 1998; Vuilleumier *et al.*, 2002; Driver *et al.*, 2001; Rees *et al.*, 2002; Marzi *et al.*, 2000).

Cerebrovascular topographic associations

Left hemispatial neglect is typically associated with lesions in the right middle cerebral artery (MCA) territory (Figure 9.5). It is particularly common with cortical damage in the inferior parietal region after infarction of the inferior MCA division (Caplan *et al.*, 1986; Hier *et al.*, 1983a). A severe but relatively pure and multimodal form of neglect, with perceptual and exploratory symptoms but no hemiparesis, can also occur after watershed infarcts involving

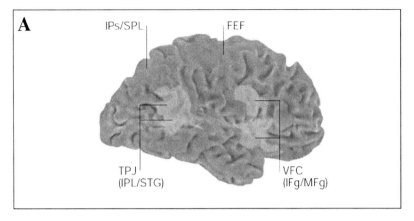

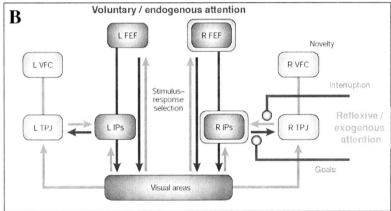

Figure 9.4   A recent neurocognitive model of visual spatial attention, proposed by Corbetta and Shulman (2002). (A) Two "superior" (blue) and "inferior" (yellow) networks of areas in parietal and prefrontal cortex have been identified by functional neuroimaging in normal subjects, and are also the most commonly damaged in neglect patients. (B) These two interconnected networks might be responsible for different attentional subcomponents, related to more intentional/endogenous (blue) and more reflexive/exogenous (yellow) aspects of spatial orienting. Abbreviations: FEF = frontal eye field (superior frontal gyrus), IFG = inferior frontal gyrus, MFG = middle frontal gyrus IPL = inferior parietal lobule, IPS = intraparietal sulcus, SPL = superior parietal lobule, TPJ = temporo-parietal junction, VFC = ventral pre-frontal cortex, L = left, R = right. For a color version of this figure please see www.cambridge.org/9780521106955.

both the anterior and posterior cortical borderzones but sparing the central sensorimotor areas (Kumral and Evyapan, 1999). Larger infarcts extending to the subcortical white matter or restricted to the deep subcortical MCA territory usually result in variable degrees of neglect, in combination with severe weakness and somatosensory loss (Levine *et al.*, 1988; Ferro *et al.*, 1987).

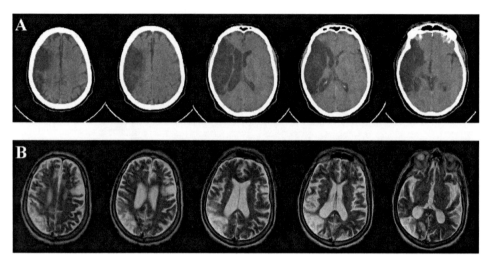

Figure 9.5   Examples of typical brain lesions associated with persistent left spatial neglect after focal strokes. (A) Chronic CT scan in a patient with a complete infarction of the MCA territory. (B) Sub-acute MRI in a patient with a focal infarction in superficial MCA territory, involving the posterior-inferior parietal cortex. Both patients showed persistent signs of neglect after one year of follow up.

Lacunar infarcts do not produce neglect or perceptual extinction (Tanaka *et al.*, 2001). In subcortical cases, the basal ganglia region is often implicated (Buxbaum *et al.*, 2004; Damasio *et al.*, 1987; Maguire and Ogden, 2002), more frequently at the level of the putamen than caudate (Karnath *et al.*, 2002; Kumral *et al.*, 1999). Much more rarely, small infarcts restricted to the anterior choroidal artery and affecting the posterior limb of the internal capsula may cause a severe syndrome with neglect, sensorimotor hemiplegia, and hemianopia (Cambier *et al.*, 1983; Decroix *et al.*, 1986; Ferro and Kertesz, 1984). However, in these subcortical cases, spatial neglect might potentially arise either through the disruption of specific corticosubcortical networks (Karnath *et al.*, 2002; Fimm *et al.*, 2001) or through the concomitant hypoperfusion of distant parietal cortical areas, as can be shown by SPECT (Bogousslavsky *et al.*, 1988) or perfusion MRI (Hillis *et al.*, 2002).

Strokes in the anterior cerebral artery (ACA) territory are less common but can produce contralesional neglect with predominant motor symptoms such as unilateral hypokinesia and deficits in bimanual movements (Chamorro *et al.*, 1997), associated with damage to medial premotor areas and cingulate cortex. Perceptual neglect has also been observed (Klatka *et al.*, 1998). Generally, neglect due to frontal lesions may be particularly exacerbated by the presence of distracters, which tend to capture attention and exploration of the patient (Husain and Kennard, 1997), sometimes even without severe contralesional deficits in perceptual tasks nor extinction. Thus, frontal patients may reflexively orient and make saccades towards ipsilesional more than contralesional stimuli but still detect the contralesional stimuli (Butter *et al.*, 1988b).

Lesions in the posterior cerebral artery (PCA) territory usually produce visual field defects without spatial neglect when limited to the occipital lobe, but may rarely mimic MCA symptoms (Cals *et al.*, 2002; Maulaz *et al.*, 2005). Some signs of neglect are present in 20–40% of patients when there is an involvement of both the superficial and deep/thalamic territories. Moreover, one recent study found a higher occurrence of lesions in the parahippocampal gyrus in patients with chronic neglect (Mort *et al.*, 2003). On the other hand, focal lesions restricted to the thalamus are also associated with transient signs of neglect, including strokes in the anterior/tuberothalamic territory (Bogousslavsky *et al.*, 1986; Ghika-Schmid and Bogousslavsky, 2000; Schmahmann, 2003), the posterior/pulvinar territory (Karnath *et al.*, 2002; Rafal and Posner, 1987), and more rarely the central/paramedian region (Schmahmann, 2003; Carrera *et al.*, 2004).

A few rare cases of spatial neglect have been observed after vascular lesions restricted to connection pathways in the white matter, without any visible cortical damage, including Binswanger's disease (Mayer *et al.*, 1993) and anterior callosal infarction after bilateral carotid occlusion (Kumral *et al.*, 1995), suggesting a role for disconnection mechanisms (see also Goldenberg, 1986; Heilman and Adams, 2003; Gaffan and Hornak, 1997).

Functional neuroanatomy and subtypes of spatial neglect

Several studies have attempted to identify brain areas most specifically implicated in disorders of spatial attention by comparing the lesion site in large groups of patients with persistent neglect relative to control groups without neglect (e.g. Mort *et al.*, 2003; Vallar and Perani, 1986; Karnath *et al.*, 2001; 2004). The most consistent finding from early studies based on correlations with anatomical CT or MRI is a common involvement of the right inferior parietal lobule (Figure 9.6), at the temporoparietal junction (TPJ), as well as frequent lesions in frontal lobe, basal ganglia and thalamus (Damasio *et al.*, 1987; Maguire and Ogden, 2002; Karnath *et al.*, 2002; 2004; Mort *et al.*, 2003; Vallar and Perani, 1986), consistent with the anatomy of brain networks implicated inspatial representation and attention (Mesulam, 1985; 1999). However, a recent study including only neglect patients without hemianopia found the greatest area of lesion overlap in the superior temporal gyrus (Karnath *et al.*, 2001), but this finding remains controversial since this area was not damaged in at least half of the neglect patients

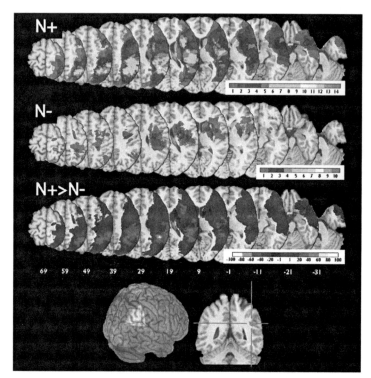

Figure 9.6   Overlap of lesions associated with neglect. Color bars indicate the number of patients with neglect (N+) and without neglect (N−) in the study of Mort *et al.* (2003). For a color version of this figure please see www.cambridge.org/9780521106955.

and other studies suggest that lesions in this area do not always cause neglect (Buxbaum *et al.*, 2004; Mort *et al.*, 2003). One study also found a higher frequency of lesion in the right parahippocampal gyrus (Mort *et al.*, 2003) but this awaits replication (see Maulaz *et al.*, 2005). Another common finding is that patients with neglect typically have larger lesions and a greater number of different areas damaged compared with non-neglect patients (e.g. Buxbaum *et al.*, 2004; Samuelsson *et al.*, 1997; Maguire and Ogden, 2002), consistent with the idea that this syndrome may entail several distinct subcomponents (Driver *et al.*, 2004; Kinsella *et al.*, 1993).

As already mentioned, a potential limitation of these previous anatomical studies is that they were often performed in subacute rather than chronic patients, and some symptoms might be related to areas of hypoperfusion beyond the visible infarct as shown by structural brain imaging. A series of recent studies using a combination of perfusion and diffusion weighted MRI has convincingly demonstrated that neglect symptoms (as well as aphasia) in patients with acute stroke correlate with perfusion anomalies shown by PWI better than with areas of early infarction shown by DWI, and also correlate well with improvements of neglect symptoms following reperfusion interventions (Hillis *et al.*, 2002; 2000; 2003 Worrall *et al.*, 2001). Both neglect and aphasia deficits found in the acute setting were only moderately associated with site and size of cortical infarct identified on the follow-up CT scans (Hillis *et al.*, 2000; 2002; 2003; Worrall *et al.*, 2001). This is particularly the case for subcortical stroke in the MCA territory where neglect symptoms were associated with dysfunction in the superficial cortical areas (Figure 9.3). However, consistent with previous anatomical studies, the most common regions of cortical hypoperfusion were typically found in inferior parietal/supramarginal and frontal areas (Hillis *et al.*, 2000; 2005).

Additional effects of subcortical lesions might be caused by functional disconnection or diaschisis (Perani *et al.*, 1987; Bogousslavsky *et al.*, 1988; Leibovitch *et al.*, 1998; 1999). Moreover, in chronic stages, patients with persistent neglect show more frequent involvement of white matter tracts in the paraventricular region, possibly involving the superior longitudinal fascicle connecting parietal and frontal cortex (Samuelsson *et al.*, 1997; Doricchi and Tomaiuolo, 2003). Note also that the addition of other deficits (e.g. hemianopia) may affect both the clinical manifestations and prognosis of neglect (Ferber and Karnath, 1999; 2001b; Cassidy *et al.*, 1999; Doricchi and Angelelli, 1999; Doricchi *et al.*, 2005).

Another limitation of these clinical–anatomical correlation studies is that most relied on a single global score of neglect in order to distinguish between affected patients and controls, such as by summing up contralesional omissions made by the patient across a range of different neuropsychological tests. Given the diversity of neglect symptoms and the frequency of dissociations, this approach might result in mixing patients with relatively different clinical symptoms in the same group since they will show the same "global score," but due to failures in different tests and different spatial domains. Although some studies found that neglect deficits across different tests tend to correlate well with each other (Buxbaum *et al.*, 2004; Halligan *et al.*, 1989), other studies found poor correlations (Hier *et al.*, 1983a; Agrell *et al.*, 1997). Therefore, a number of studies have attempted to relate specific components or subtypes of neglect to distinct neuroanatomical correlates.

One of the earlier attempt of this sort was to distinguish between *perceptual* aspects associated with parietal lesions and *premotor* aspects associated with frontal or subcortical lesions (Bisiach *et al.*, 1990; 1995; Heilman and Valenstein, 1972; Binder *et al.*, 1992). Recent studies have cast some doubt on this distinction by showing that patients with focal parietal lesions can exhibit motor biases unexplained by their perceptual biases (Mattingley *et al.*, 1998;

Husain *et al.*, 2000). Patients with frontal neglect may be particularly impaired on tasks with many distractors (Husain and Kennard, 1997) or requiring a strategic exploration of space (e.g. cancellation or search tasks) as opposed to purely perceptual spatial judgments (e.g. line bisection) (Binder *et al.*, 1992). Furthermore, frontal neglect has been variably associated with damage to the superior frontal cortex (including frontal eye field region) (Mesulam, 1999; Maguire and Ogden, 2002) as well as the inferior frontal gyrus (Stein and Volpe, 1983; Husain and Kennard, 1996), but it is unclear whether this correlates with different types of deficit (see Corbetta and Shulman, 2002).

A lesion involving the basal ganglia may cause neglect (Karnath *et al.*, 2002), but when restricted to this region may also impair visual search for contralesional targets without producing any deficits in the detection of visual stimuli in the contralesional visual field (Fimm *et al.*, 2001), or without significant deviation in line bisection (Binder *et al.*, 1992).

Pure *motor neglect* affecting the contralesional arm or leg can arise without other signs of perceptual neglect, and often follows focal lesion in the antero-lateral thalamus (Laplane *et al.*, 1986; Laplane, 1990; Fiorelli *et al.*, 1991) or medial prefrontal cortex (Chamorro *et al.*, 1997). Motor neglect and motor extinction have also been associated with basal ganglia lesions (Watson and Heilman, 1981).

By contrast, *perceptual extinction* may arise without other signs or persist after recovery from acute spatial neglect (Lundervold *et al.*, 2005), and seems more critically associated with lesions in the inferior parietal cortex (Karnath *et al.*, 2003), relative to patients who have more extensive deficits in spatial exploration and more severe signs of neglect. This might be consistent with a major role of the inferior parietal cortex in the control of exogenous stimulus-driven spatial attention (Corbetta and Shulman, 2002; Schwartz *et al.*, 2005), which may be particularly impaired in patients with persistent neglect (Bartolomeo and Chokron, 2002).

A recent study using perfusion MRI in acute patients also suggested distinct neural correlates for "egocentric" and "allocentric" deficits in spatial neglect (Hillis *et al.*, 2005). Omissions of objects in egocentric contralesional space were found to correlate with hypoperfusion in the inferior parietal cortex (angular and supramarginal gyrus) as well as the posterior inferior frontal gyrus and occipital cortex, whereas allocentric neglect for the contralesional side of the objects (irrespective of their position) correlated with hypoperfusion in the superior and inferior temporal cortex. Furthermore, there was no correlation between the severity of egocentric and allocentric deficits (Hillis *et al.*, 2005). Functional neuroimaging studies in healthy subjects also revealed that partly distinct neural networks involved egocentric and allocentric spatial processing, although some areas overlap in the superior parietal cortex (Vallar et al., 1999).

Neuroanatomical dissociations might also exist between neglect for *near* and *far space*, reported in patients with more superior/parietal lesions (Halligan and Marshall, 1991b; Berti and Frassinetti, 2000) versus more inferior/temporal lesions (Vuilleumier et al., 1998). Such a distinction is consistent with functional imaging studies in healthy subjects (Weiss et al., 2000; Weiss et al., 2003). Furthermore, studies in the monkey have shown that different areas in the parietal (Bremmer et al., 1996) and frontal (Rizzolatti et al., 1983) cortex might code for space within and beyond reaching distance.

Representational neglect in mental imagery can be observed without other signs of perceptual or motor neglect, sometimes associated with frontal, frontomesial, or parieto-occipital lesions (Guariglia et al., 1991; Coslett, 1997), or more rarely thalamic lesions (Ortigue et al., 2001), with sparing of the inferior parietal lobe.

Personal neglect, hemi-asomatognosia, and *anosognosia* for hemiplegia may also have distinct neuroanatomical correlates, variably associated with the inferior parietal cortex (Feinberg et al., 1990) or the mid insula/basal ganglia region (Baier and Karnath, 2005).

Other non-spatial or non-lateralized deficits associated with neglect may also result from lesions outside the parietal cortex but contribute to neglect (Husain and Rorden, 2003). For instance, *non-spatial attentional* deficits are present in RHD patients with and without acute neglect, independent of parietal or frontal damage (Farne et al., 2004), but can nonetheless exacerbate spatial biases caused by the parietal or frontal lesion. *Local biases* in attention are also seen after right temporoparietal lesions without neglect (Lamb et al., 1989) but may worsen attentional capture by details on the ipsilesional side (Halligan and Marshall, 1998).

Clinical assessment of spatial neglect

Given the variety of neglect symptoms, the frequent dissociations between symptoms and patients, and the common fluctuations of performance in single patients in the same task, it is obvious that no single test can provide a reliable diagnosis of spatial neglect, even in the acute stage of stroke. Moreover, the correlation between the severity of neglect in different tests may vary considerably (Hier et al., 1983a; Agrell et al., 1997), although there is some consistency for left spatial neglect deficits in RHD patients (Buxbaum et al., 2004; Azouvi et al., 2002; Halligan et al., 1989) that seems better than for *right* spatial neglect in LHD (Beis et al., 2004). A comprehensive assessment of neglect therefore often requires a systematic battery to examine different spatial domains, and a total score derived from such a battery seems more sensitive than any single test alone (Azouvi et al., 2002; Stone et al., 1992). Moreover, in subacute and chronic stages of neglect, behavioral measures derived from everyday life may prove as reliable or even better than some paper-and-pen tests (Azouvi et al., 2003).

Common neglect batteries include the BIT (Behavioral Inattention Test; Wilson et al., 1987; Stone, et al., 1991a) and GEREN (Groupe d'Etude sur la Rééducation et l'Evaluation de la Négligence; Azouvi et al., 2002; 2003; Rousseaux et al., 2001), which both provide quantitative measures for various aspects of neglect, in paper-and-pen tests as well as in more naturalistic situations of everyday life. Other comprehensive batteries are described by Buxbaum and colleagues (Buxbaum et al., 2004), Hillis and colleagues (Hillis et al., 2000; 2003), and Maguire and Ogden (2002). However, a limitation of most of these batteries is their relatively long time to administer (minimum 30−45 minutes), which is clearly inconvenient in the acute stroke setting. Shorter tests with good sensitivity still need to be developed in order to make quick and reliable diagnosis of neglect in patients with acute stroke (Merrino and Heilman, 2003). Treatment by thrombolysis is half as frequent in right than left hemisphere stroke, simply because the presence of cognitive deficits such as neglect is underestimated by the current measures of neurological functions used in the acute stages of stoke (Di Legge et al., 2005). For instance, a short series of tests of spatial neglect provide a much better estimate of perfusion abnormalities as well as reperfusion changes than NIHSS scores in acute right hemisphere strokes (Hillis et al., 2003).

In acute clinical settings, spatial neglect can often be demonstrated by *spontaneous deviation* of the head and gaze towards the ipsilesional side, which may be reducible with or without incentive, or not reducible. Such deviation can sometimes be inferred also by the eye position seen on an acute CT scan of the head, prior to any visible ischemic lesion in brain tissue (Simon et al., 2003). Asking the patients to provide a *verbal description* of complex visual scenes (such as the Cookie Theft picture) will also often reveal spatial neglect.

Extinction on double simultaneous stimulation (DSS) is a rapid and simple test that can easily be done at the bedside, by comparing detection of contralesional stimuli in single versus double trials. In vision, each quadrant can be examined separately. Extinction is sometimes found within the same hemifield. For touch, different limbs can be tested at homologous or non-homologous locations (e.g. face and hand) and different types of stimulation can be used. Auditory extinction is sometimes difficult to distinguish from presby-acusia. Testing extinction in different egocentric positions (e.g. changing gaze direction or crossing arms) or using crossmodal stimulation (e.g. vision and touch, vision and hearing) can be useful to test to confirm a non-sensory deficit and demonstrate the spatial attentional nature of the deficit.

Cancellation tasks are generally the most sensitive tests (Agrell *et al.*, 1997; Ferber and Karnath, 2001a), in both RHD and LHD (Azouvi *et al.*, 2002; Beis *et al.*, 2004), but their sensitivities vary greatly with the attentional demands of the task (Rapcsak *et al.*, 1989). Targets are randomly spread on a sheet of paper (e.g. letters A), with or without distracters (e.g. other letters or shapes), and all targets must be marked by the patient, generally until he/she decides that his/her search is complete. Typically, neglect patients start on the ipsilesional side and omit more contralesional than ipsilesional targets. Adding a time-out limit can increase sensitivity and reduce the duration of such test. The Albert test (Albert, 1973), in which all items are lines and must be cancelled, has a poor sensitivity, since many neglect patients can succeed when given enough time. The star cancellation test (Wilson *et al.*, 1987), letter cancellation test (Mesulam, 1985) and bells cancellation test (Gauthier *et al.*, 1989) all are more sensitive but also more difficult, as they contain an increasing number of targets and distracters (in this given order). Letters and bells tests miss fewer than 6% of patients with spatial neglect apparent in other situations (Ferber and Karnath, 2001a). Furthermore, in RHD patients with left-to-right reading habits, a tendency to start their search on the right side of the page is the most sensitive test of spatial neglect (Azouvi *et al.*, 2002), and often persists in more chronic stages when the patient eventually finds all targets (but different biases may exist in people with right-to-left reading habits; (Chokron *et al.*, 1998)).

Some variants of cancellation tasks are useful to combine tests for different *frames of reference*, such as egocentric (body-centered) versus allocentric (object-centered) neglect (Driver and Halligan, 1991; Ota *et al.*, 2001) (Figure 9.7). For instance, in Ota's task (Ota *et al.*, 2001), open-circle targets to be cancelled are defined by the presence of a gap on either their right or left side, and mixed with full-circle distracters without any gap. In one simple version, patients have to mark all open circles: omissions of targets on the contralesional part of the page will measure egocentric neglect, while omissions of targets with a gap on their contralesional side (irrespective of location on the page) will measure allocentric neglect. Alternatively, patients can be asked to encircle the full-circle targets and put an "x" into the open-circle targets (Hillis *et al.*, 2005). In another cancellation task with *double arrays* (Driver and Halligan, 1991), similar targets (e.g. lines) can be clustered into two distinct groups on the page (or printed in two distinct colors), thus constituting two large "objects" made of smaller objects.

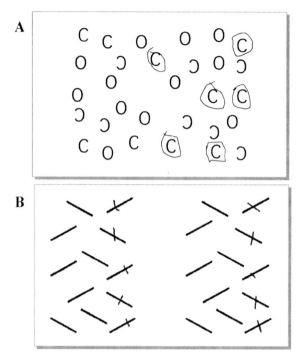

Figure 9.7   Cancellation tasks with space-based/egocentric and object-based/allocentric components. (A) Version of Ota's task in which targets are open circles: omissions on the left side of the display indicate "egocentric neglect" and omissions on the left side of items indicate "allocentric neglect". (B) Version of Driver & Halligan's task in which omissions of lines of the left side of each group of indicate "allocentric neglect".

Omissions of the contralesional group will measure egocentric neglect, while omissions of targets on the contralesional side of each group will measure allocentric neglect. Cancellation tests can also be compared when performed on the right or left side of the patient's body.

Performance on a cancellation task can be determined by both a failure to direct attention to contralesional space and a capture of attention on the ipsilesional side. Thus, cancellation tests requiring *erasure of targets* will lead to more complete exploration contralesionally and more hits (Mark *et al.*, 1988); whereas cancellation tests using *invisible marks* will exacerbate iterative exploration ipsilesionally and reduce hits (Wojciulik *et al.*, 2001).

Drawing tasks also provide a sensitive measure, especially when requiring a copy of complex objects in complex layouts, such as Gainotti's (Gainotti *et al.*, 1972) or Ogden's (Ogden, 1985a) scene (with a house, a fence, and trees). Drawing deficits are more frequently impaired in acute than in chronic patients

(Johannsen and Karnath, 2004) and must be distinguished from constructional apraxia. Drawing or copying a clock typically shows a clustering of all numbers on the ipsilesional half of the clockface, but this clock test is less sensitive to neglect than the drawing of more complex objects and is modulated by the presence of hemianopia (Agrell *et al.*, 1997). Interestingly, performance in clock drawing can improve when patients have to draw separate features (or numbers) each in turn, under instructions from the examiner, as compared with spontaneous drawing or copying without a prescribed sequence (Di Pellegrino, 1995), suggesting that a deficit in disengaging attention from right-sided elements also plays an important role in neglect during drawing.

Reading can reveal omissions of words on the contralesional end of lines, particularly when words are arranged in indented paragraphs (Bellas *et al.*, 1988), as well as omissions and transformations of initial letters, particularly with non-word letter-strings (Chatterjee, 1995).

Another useful and sensitive test is the *Baking Tray task* (Tham and Tegnér, 1996), in which patients are asked to place a series of 16 items on an empty sheet of paper in front of them. The number of items on each half of the sheet provides a sensitive measure of spatial biases in perception and action. *Tactile exploration* without vision can also be tested by asking patients to find an object placed in front of them, while blindfolded or in the dark (Karnath and Perenin, 1998). Neglect patients will typically show a lack or reduced exploration of their contralesional space.

By contrast, *line bisection* is frequently used but has a relatively poor sensitivity and correlates poorly with other tests (Agrell *et al.*, 1997; Ferber and Karnath, 2001a). Longer lines are more sensitive. Ipsilesional deviations may reverse into contralesional deviations when line length is shorter, an effect called "crossover" that might be related to visual field defects more than to spatial or attentional disturbances (Doricchi *et al.*, 2005). Accordingly, performance on line bisection is markedly influenced by hemianopia (Ferber and Karnath, 2001b; Doricchi and Angelelli, 1999). Deviation in line bisection should therefore be generally treated with caution in clinical diagnosis. Line bisection can be influenced also by many other factors such as the relative egocentric position in right or left space, the presence of cues at the right or left end of the line, the direction of visual scanning, the hand used, or the "cognitive content" of the line (e.g. if it is made of small or large numbers (Fischer, 2001), words (Lee *et al.*, 2004), etc.). Other interesting variants include the *Landmark task* (Milner *et al.*, 1993; Harvey *et al.*, 1995), which requires the patient to point to the longer (or the shorter) of the two portions of a pre-bisected horizontal line. Comparing judgments in the "longer" versus "shorter" condition can provide some measure of perceptual versus motor/response biases in the same patient

(Toraldo *et al.*, 2002; Bisiach *et al.*, 1998a), but this test often requires many trials to obtain reliable results. Bisection can be performed also on vertical or radial lines.

Motor or premotor components are usually difficult to assess reliably at the bedside, except by clinical observations. *Motor extinction* can be tested by bilateral simultaneous movements (tapping with fingers, raising arms, clicking on golf counters held in each hand, etc.), but this is often hampered by hemiparesis. However, testing more proximal movements (e.g. shoulder elevation on one or both sides) can provide a measure of motor initiation and intentional function even in the presence of distal weakness (Coslett, 1989). Patients can also be required to hold a grip force dynamometer in the contralesional hand, either in the presence or in the absence of simultaneous movements with the ipsilesional limb. Using *crossed responses* (e.g. responding to right stimuli by left movements, and vice versa) can also be used to uncouple sensory and premotor components (Heilman *et al.*, 2003), but such a test can be difficult to perform due to disinhibition of reflexive behavior after a frontal lesion (Butter *et al.*, 1988b). Alternatively, speeded lateralized motor responses can be measured for central visual targets, using two right/left lateralized button-keys (Buxbaum *et al.*, 2004) or a single central button-key reached from two right/left starting positions (Mattingley *et al.*, 1998), but such tests require a computerized apparatus.

Personal neglect is tested by asking the patient to reach with their ipsilesional hand towards a contralesional part of their own body (Beschin and Robertson, 1997) or towards objects or marks (e.g. cotton balls or threads) attached to their contralesional body (the "fluff test"; Cocchini *et al.*, 2001; Buxbaum *et al.*, 2004). Clinically, signs of personal neglect can also be observed when patients put on their glasses and incorrectly adjust the distance and position of the left-sided branch. Performance in *near or far extra-personal space* can be tested in some cases by performing the same tasks at different distances (cancellation, bisection, reading, etc.), using a laser pointer, stick, or computer mouse.

Representational neglect is often difficult to evaluate with standardized tests that can be performed by all patients since they heavily rely on personal memory and knowledge. The most useful tests include the *description of familiar squares or routes* in the city (i.e. walking a street one way and then returning; Bisiach *et al.*, 1993) *naming cities* or states as imagined on a canonical map of the country (Figure 9.8) (Rode *et al.*, 1995; Bartolomeo *et al.*, 2005); or judging the angle made between the hour-hand and minute-hand on an *imagined clockface* (Grossi *et al.*, 1989).

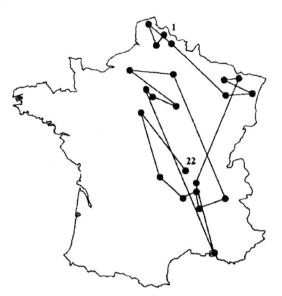

Figure 9.8   Map description. Example of left "representational" or "imaginal" neglect in which the patient provides names of cities situated only on the right-side of the imagined map of France. Connected lines indicate the order of report. From Rode *et al.* (2001).

A variety of other computerized tests of spatial attention can be used, including the classic *visual cuing* paradigm developed by Posner and colleagues (Bartolomeo and Chokron, 2002; Posner *et al.*, 1987), in which patients are required to respond to lateralized targets (in right or left visual field), preceded by a cue indicating the correct (valid) or incorrect (invalid) location of the target. Neglect patients show a disproportionate increase in their response times and misses for contralesional targets that are preceded by an invalid cue on the ipsilesional side (so-called "disengagement deficit" or "pseudo-extinction"), reflecting a failure to overcome the initial capture of attention on the ipsilesional side (Bartolomeo and Chokron, 2002). This deficit is typically more severe with stimulus-driven or exogenous cuing (e.g. a brief flash in visual periphery), than with symbolically driven or endogenous cuing (e.g. a central arrow).

Other tasks can be useful to test non-spatial or non-lateralized deficits that are commonly associated with neglect, in particular tests of *sustained attention* (e.g. continuous auditory target monitoring) (Robertson *et al.*, 1997) or *divided attention* (dual vs single tasks [Buxbaum *et al.*, 2004]). Other tasks may also test for near and far space, local perceptual biases, spatial working memory, and so forth (see above), but these tasks are rarely used in clinical practice.

Key points Assessment of spatial neglect

Orientation of head and gaze (spontaneous and after stimulation)

Perceptual extinction on double stimulation	in 3 modalities (vision, touch, hearing) across modalities (crossmodal extinction) with different postures of gaze and arms (e.g. crossed)

Description of scenes (near or far)

Drawing	multi-element visual scenes, multi-element objects (e.g., clock, bicycle, face) spontaneous and/or copy
Cancellation tasks	standard versions (lines, star, letters, bells, shapes, etc.), performed in central, right, or left hemispace variants for egocentric and allocentric indices (Ota's task, double arrays) other variants: with invisible marks, with erasure of targets
Line bisection task	horizontal, vertical, or radial lines different length performed in central, right, or left hemispace

Landmark task (pre-bisected lines)
Reading: real words, non-words, compound words, text with indented paragraphs
Baking tray task
Tactile exploration while blindfolded
Distant extrapersonal space (far vs near): same as in peri-personal space (above) but with laser pointer, stick

Personal space: reach for contralesional body parts, fluff test

Motor neglect of contralesional limb(s)	observation of spontaneous use extinction or slowing during bilateral movement grip force in single vs bilateral condition shoulder elevation
Motor neglect in contralateral space	crossed responses, directional responses

Mental imagery: route and scene description, map description, imagined clockface
Posner cueing task
Sustained attention task (continuous monitoring task, sustained auditory response task)
Divided attention task (dual visual + auditory detection, vs. single task)
Local vs. global perception: hierarchical Navon stimuli, embedded figures, overlapping shapes

Anosognosia (for hemiplegia, hemianopia, and neglect)
Impaired spatial working memory, impaired spatial remapping

Recovery and prognosis

Spatial neglect disorders following acute strokes usually show a substantial but quite variable degree of spontaneous recovery. Such improvement depends on the size and site of lesions, etiology, severity of initial symptoms, as well as age, concomitant brain atrophy, and other premorbid factors (Pedersen *et al.*, 1997; Cassidy *et al.*, 1998; Hier *et al.*, 1983b; Levine *et al.*, 1986). However, it remains difficult to predict for individual patients (Lundervold *et al.*, 2005; Cherney and Halper, 2001). Recovery can be particularly rapid with subcortical strokes, where neglect symptoms are probably associated with transient cortical dysfunction (Worrall *et al.*, 2001; Hillis *et al.*, 2003), whereas longlasting neglect is typically associated with large MCA infarction, frontoparietal cortical lesions, or extensive white matter damage in periventricular regions (Samuelsson *et al.*, 1997; Farne *et al.*, 2004).

Recovery is often most rapid during the first 10 days and then reaches a plateau after 2–3 months (Stone *et al.*, 1992; Lundervold *et al.*, 2005; Kinsella and Ford, 1980), but some progress can still be achieved up to one year post-onset. Approximately half of the patients show satisfactory recovery after 3 months, but persistent signs are still often found many months later in other cases (Farne *et al.*, 2004; Appelros *et al.*, 2004). Severe anosognosia during the first days is usually associated with poorer outcome (Stone *et al.*, 1992). Signs of neglect for both personal and far extra-personal space tend to recover quicker and more completely than other common signs of peripersonal neglect (Appelros *et al.*, 2004).

Importantly, the presence of spatial neglect has repeatedly been shown to be associated with significantly poorer functional outcome in the long term, in terms of both elementary motor functions and independence in everyday life activities (Farne *et al.*, 2004; Cherney and Halper, 2001; Jehkonen *et al.*, 2000; Gillen *et al.*, 2005). Rehabilitation strategies are usually effective, though with several limitations and relatively poor generalization to novel tasks (Bowen *et al.*, 2002; Mark, 2003). Cognitive and behavioral training need to be tailored to individual patients' deficits (Gillen *et al.*, 2005; Pachalska *et al.*, 2004).

Different therapeutic approaches have been proposed (Pierce and Buxbaum, 2002; Rode *et al.*, 2001; Robertson *et al.*, 1995). Most often, patients undergo intensive training to direct search and attention towards their contralesional side (Kerkhoff, 1998). Such training can produce useful benefits, but often with little generalization to daily life (Pierce and Buxbaum, 2002). Another approach is to modulate arousal, but again the challenge is also to generalize this successfully to self-arousal during daily life (Robertson *et al.*, 1995). Drug treatment using dopaminergic substances produces variable effects, by modulating both arousal and spatial orienting biases (Fleet *et al.*, 1987; Grujic *et al.*, 1998).

Caloric stimulation of the vestibular organs (e.g. via iced water in the left ear) is another technique to ameliorate perceptual and exploratory neglect (and even other deficits such as imaginal neglect, or anosognosia), presumably by inducing some shift in the internal representation of space (Cappa *et al.*, 1987). However, such effects are typically transient. Similar benefits can be obtained by vibratory stimulation of neck muscles, again only transiently (Karnath, 1995). Patch occlusion of the ipsilesional eye or ipsilesional temporal hemifield may sometimes reduce abnormal capture of attention on the intact side, but is not always tolerated by the patient (Beis *et al.*, 1999). Remarkably, longer-term improvements have been reported following brief periods of prism adaptation during reaching tasks (Rossetti *et al.*, 1998; Frassinetti *et al.*, 2002). Patients are trained to reach to targets while they wear prisms shifting visual inputs towards the ipsilesional side, such that their reaches to visual targets will initially err to the ipsilesional side; but following a single or a few sessions, such a procedure can then trigger some automatic adaptation process that redirects spatial behavior further to the contralesional side (Rode *et al.*, 2003). As prism adaptation does not appear successful in every case, it remains to be determined which patients might benefit from this procedure. Future successful rehabilitation might also use different combinations of approaches in different patients.

Key points Management and treatment of spatial neglect

Sensory stimulation of contralesional space	
Incentive for exploration of contralesional space	
Training spontaneous scanning and orienting to contralesional space	
Active and passive stimulation of left arm (motor and proprioceptive)	
Vestibular manipulations	caloric ear stimulation
	transcutaneous neck-muscle vibration
Drug treatments	dopaminergic, bromocriptine
	(cholinergic?)
Eye patching (ipsilesional eye, ipsilesional hemifield)	
Prism adaptation	
(TMS?)	

REFERENCES

Aglioti, S., Smania, N. and Moro, V. (1998). Tactile salience influences extinction. *Neurology*, **50**(4), 1010–14.

Aglioti, S., Smania, N. and Peru, A. J. (1999). Frames of reference for mapping tactile stimuli in brain-damaged patients. *J. Cogn. Neurosci.*, **11**(1), 167–79.

Agrell, B. M., Dehlin, O. I. and Dahlgren, C. J. (1997). Neglect in elderly stroke patients: A comparison of five tests. *Psychiatry Clin. Neurosci.*, **51**(5), 295—300.

Albert, M. (1973). A simple test of visual neglect. *Neurology*, **23**, 658—64.

Andersen, R. A. and Buneo, C. A. (2003). Sensorimotor integration in posterior parietal cortex. *Adv. Neurol.*, **93**, 159—77.

Andersen, R., Snyder, L. H., Bradley, B. C., *et al.* (1997). Multimodal representation of space in the posterior parietal cortex and its use in planning movement. *Ann. Rev. Neurosci.*, **20**, 303—30.

Appelros, P., Nydevik, I., Karlsson, G. M., *et al.* (2004). Recovery from unilateral neglect after right-hemisphere stroke. *Disabil. Rehabil.*, **26**(8), 471—7.

Azouvi, P., Samuel, C., Louis-Dreyfus, A., *et al.* (2002). Sensitivity of clinical and behavioural tests of spatial neglect after right hemisphere stroke. *J. Neurol. Neurosurg. Psychiatry*, **73**(2), 160—6.

Azouvi, P., Oliver, S., de Montety, G., *et al.* (2003). Behavioral assessment of unilateral neglect: Study of the psychometric properties of the Catherine Bergego Scale. *Arch. Phys. Med. Rehabil.*, **84**(1), 51—7.

Baier, B. and Karnath, H. O. (2005). Neuroanatomical correlates of anosognosia for hemiparesis. *J. Neurosci.*, **25**, 7134—8.

Bartolomeo, P., Bachoud-Levi, A. C., Azouvi, P., *et al.* (2005). Time to imagine space: A chronometric exploration of representational neglect. *Neuropsychologia*, **43**(9), 1249—57.

Bartolomeo, P. and Chokron, S. (1999). Egocentric frame of reference: its role in spatial bias after right hemisphere lesions. *Neuropsychologia*, **37**(8), 881—94.

(2002). Orienting of attention in left unilateral neglect. *Neurosci. Biobehav. Rev.*, **26**(2), 217—34.

Bartolomeo, P., D'Erme, P. and Gainotti, G. (1994). The relationship between visuospatial and representational neglect. *Neurology*, **44**(9), 1710—14.

Bartolomeo, P., Perri, R. and Gainotti, G. (2004). The influence of limb crossing on left tactile extinction. *J. Neurol. Neurosurg. Psychiatry*, **75**(1), 49—55.

Behrmann, M., Ghiselli-Crippa, T., Sweeney, J. A., *et al.* (2002). Mechanisms underlying spatial representation revealed through studies of hemispatial neglect. *J. Cogn. Neurosci.*, **14**(2), 272—90.

Behrmann, M. and Moscovitch, M. (1994). Object-centered neglect in patients with unilateral neglect: Effects of left-right coordinates of objects. *J. Cogn. Neurosci.*, **6**, 1—16.

Behrmann, M., Moscovitch, M., Black, S. E., *et al.* (1990). Perceptual and conceptual mechanisms in neglect dyslexia. *Brain*, **113**, 1163—83.

Behrmann, M. and Tipper, S. P. (1999). Attention accesses multiple reference frames: Evidence from visual neglect. *J. Exp. Psychol. [Hum. Percept.]*, **25**(1), 83—101.

Beis, J. M., Andre, J. M., Baumgarten, A., *et al.* (1999). Eye patching in unilateral spatial neglect: Efficacy of two methods. *Arch. Phys. Med. Rehabil.*, **80**(1), 71—6.

Beis, J. M., Keller, C., Morin, N., *et al.* (2004). Right spatial neglect after left hemisphere stroke: Qualitative and quantitative study. *Neurology*, **63**(9), 1600—5.

Bellas, D. N., Novelly, R. A., Eskenazi, B., *et al.* (1988). The nature of unilateral neglect in the olfactory sensory system. *Neuropsychologia*, **26**(1), 45—52.

Bellmann, A., Meuli, R. and Clarke, S. (2001). Two types of auditory neglect. *Brain*, **124**(Pt 4), 676–87.

Berlucchi, G., Moro, V., Guerrini, C., *et al.* (2004). Dissociation between taste and tactile extinction on the tongue after right brain damage. *Neuropsychologia*, **42**(8), 1007–16.

Berti, A. (2003). Unconscious processing in neglect. In *The Cognitive and Neural Bases of Spatial Neglect*, ed. H. O. Karnath *et al.*, Oxford University Press.

Berti, A. and Frassinetti, F. (2000). When far becomes near: Remapping of space by tool use. *J. Cogn. Neurosci.*, **12**(3), 415–20.

Berti, A. and Rizzolatti, G. (1992). Visual processing without awareness: Evidence from unilateral neglect. *J. Cogn. Neurosci.*, **4**, 345–51.

Berti, A., Frassinetti, F. and Umilta, C. (1994). Nonconscious reading? Evidence from neglect dyslexia. *Cortex*, **30**, 181–97.

Berti, A., Oxbury, S., Oxbury, J., *et al.* (1999). Somatosensory extinction for meaningful objects in a patient with right hemispheric stroke. *Neuropsychologia*, **37**(3), 333–43.

Beschin, N. and Robertson, I. H. (1997). Personal versus extrapersonal neglect: a group study of their dissociation using a reliable clinical test. *Cortex*, **33**(2), 379–84.

Beschin, N., Cazzani, M., Cubelli, R., *et al.* (1996). Ignoring left and far: An investigation of tactile neglect. *Neuropsychologia*, **34**, 41–2.

Beschin, N., Cocchini, G., Della Sala , S., *et al.* (1997). What the eyes perceive, the brain ignores: A case of pure unilateral representational neglect. *Cortex*, **33**(1), 3–26.

Binder, J., Marshall, R., Lazar, R., *et al.* (1992). Distinct syndromes of hemineglect. *Arch. Neurol.*, **49**(11), 1187–94.

Bisiach, E., Brouchan, M., Poncet, M., *et al.* (1993). Unilateral neglect in route description. *Neuropsychologia*, **31**(11), 1255–62.

Bisiach, E., Geminiani, G., Berti, A., *et al.* (1990). Perceptual and premotor factors of unilateral neglect. *Neurology*, **40**, 1278–81.

Bisiach, E. and Luzzatti, C. (1978). Unilateral neglect of representational space. *Cortex*, **14**, 129–33.

Bisiach, E., Perani, D., Vallar, G., *et al.* (1986). Unilateral neglect: Personal and extrapersonal. *Neuropsychologia*, **24**, 759–67.

Bisiach, E., Ricci, R., Lualdi, M., *et al.* (1998a). Perceptual and response bias in unilateral neglect: Two modified versions of the Milner landmark task. *Brain Cogn.*, **37**(3), 369–86.

Bisiach, E., Ricci, R. and Madona, M. N., *et al.* (1998b). Visual awareness and anisometry of space representation in unilateral neglect: A panoramic investigation by means of a line extension task. *Conscious Cogn.*, **7**(3), 327–55.

Bisiach, E., Rusconi, M. L., Peretti, V. A., *et al.* (1994). Challenging current accounts of unilateral neglect. *Neuropsychologia*, **32**, 1431–4.

Bisiach, E., Tegner, R., Ladavas, E., *et al.* (1995). Dissociation of ophthalmokinetic and melokinetic attention in unilateral neglect. *Cereb. Cortex*, **5**(5), 439–47.

Bogousslavsky, J., Miklossy, J., Regli, F., *et al.* (1988). Subcortical neglect: Neuropsychological, SPECT, and neuropathological correlations with anterior choroidal artery territory infarction. *Ann. Neurol.*, **23**(5), 448–52.

Bogousslavsky, J., Regli, F., and Assal, G., *et al.* (1986). The syndrome of unilateral tuberothalamic artery territory infarction. *Stroke*, **17**(3), 434–41.

Bowen, A., Lincoln, N. B., and Dewey, M. E. (2002). Spatial neglect: Is rehabilitation effective? *Stroke*, **33**(11), 2728–9.

Bowen, A., Mckenna, K. and Tallis, R. C. (1999). Reasons for variability in the reported rate of occurrence of unilateral spatial neglect after stroke. *Stroke*, **30**(6), 1196–202.

Bremmer, F., Duhamel, J.-R., Ben Hamed, S., *et al.* (1996). The representation of movement in near extrapersonal space in the macaque ventral intraparietal area. In *Parietal Lobe Contributions to Orientation in 3D Space*, ed. P. Thier and H.-O. Karnath. Heidelberg: Springer-Verlag, pp. 619–30.

Brighina, F., Bisiach, E., Piazza, A., *et al.* (2002). Perceptual and response bias in visuospatial neglect due to frontal and parietal repetitive transcranial magnetic stimulation in normal subjects. *Neuroreport*, **13**(18), 2571–5.

Butter, C. M., Mark, V. W. and Heilman, K. M. (1988a). An experimental analysis of factors underlying neglect in line bisection. *J. Neurol. Neurosurg. Psychiatry*, **51**(12), 1581–3.

Butter, C. M., Rapcsak, S. Z., Watson, R. T., *et al.* (1988b). Changes in sensory inattention, directional akinesia, and release of fixation reflex following a unilateral frontal lesion: A case report. *Neuropsychologia*, **26**, 533–45.

Buxbaum, L. J., Ferraro, M. K., Veramonti, T., *et al.* (2004). Hemispatial neglect: Subtypes, neuroanatomy, and disability. *Neurology*, **62**(5), 749–56.

Cals, N., Devuyst, G., Afsa, N., *et al.* (2002). Pure superficial posterior cerebral artery territory infarction in The Lausanne Stroke Registry. *J. Neurol.*, **249**(7), 855–61.

Cambier, J., Graveleau, P., Decroix, J. P., *et al.* (1983). Anterior choroidal artery syndrome. Neuropsychological study of 4 cases. *Rev. Neurol. (Paris)*, **139**(10), 553–9.

Cambier, J., Masson, M., Guillot, M., *et al.* (1985). Right neglect with hemiasomatognosia, mental confusion, apraxia and agraphia without aphasia. *Rev. Neurol. (Paris)*, **141**(12), 802–5.

Caplan, L. R., Kelly, M., Kase, C. S., *et al.* (1986). Infarcts of the inferior division of the right middle cerebral artery: Mirror image of Wernicke's aphasia. *Neurology*, **36**(8), 1015–20.

Cappa, S., Sterzi, R., Vallar, G., *et al.* (1987). Remission of hemineglect and anosognosia during vestibular stimulation. *Neuropsychologia*, **25**(5), 775–82.

Caramazza, A. and Hillis, A. E. (1990). Spatial representation of words in the brain implied by studies of a unilateral neglect patient. *Nature*, **346**(6281), 267–9.

Carrera, E., Michel, P. and Bogousslavsky, J. (2004). Anteromedian, central, and posterolateral infarcts of the thalamus: Three variant types. *Stroke*, **35**(12), 2826–31.

Cassidy, T. P., Bruce, D. W., Lewis, S., *et al.* (1999). The association of visual field deficits and visuo-spatial neglect in acute right-hemisphere stroke patients. *Age Ageing*, **28**(3), 257–60.

Cassidy, T. P., Lewis, S. and Gray, C. S. (1998). Recovery from visuospatial neglect in stroke patients. *J. Neurol. Neurosurg. Psychiatry*, **64**, 555–7.

Castaigne, P., Laplane, D. and Degos, J. D. (1972). 3 cases of motor neglect due to prerolandic frontal lesion. *Rev. Neurol. (Paris)*, **126**(1), 5–15.

Chamorro, A., Marshall, A. S., Volls-Sole, J., *et al.* (1997). Motor behavior in stroke patients with isolated medial frontal ischemic infarction. *Stroke*, **28**(9), 1755–60.

Chatterjee, A. (1994). Picturing unilateral spatial neglect: Viewer versus object centred reference frames. *J. Neurol. Neurosurg. Psychiatry*, **57**(10), 1236–40.

(1995). Cross-over, completion and confabulation in unilateral spatial neglect. *Brain*, **118**, 455–65.

Cherney, L. R. and Halper, A. S. (2001). Unilateral visual neglect in right-hemisphere stroke: A longitudinal study. *Brain Inj.*, **15**(7), 585–92.

Chokron, S., Bartolomeo, P., Perenin, M. T., *et al.* (1998). Scanning direction and line bisection: A study of normal subjects and unilateral neglect patients with opposite reading habits. *Brain Res. Cogn.*, **7**(2), 173–8.

Chokron, S., Colliot, P., Bartolomeo, P., *et al.* (2002). Visual, proprioceptive and tactile performance in left neglect patients. *Neuropsychologia*, **40**(12), 1965–76.

Cocchini, G., Beschin, N. and Jehkonen, M. (2001). The fluff test: A simple task to assess body representation neglect. *Neuropsychol. Rehabil.*, **11**, 17–31.

Cocchini, G., Cubelli, R., Della Sala, S., *et al.* (1999). Neglect without extinction. *Cortex*, **35**(3), 285–313.

Colby, C. (1998). Action-oriented spatial reference frames in cortex. *Neuron*, **20**(1), 15–24.

Corbetta, M., Akbudak, E., Conturo, T. E., *et al.* (1998). A common network of functional areas for attention and eye movements. *Neuron*, **21**(4), 761–73.

Corbetta, M. and Shulman, G. L. (2002). Control of goal-directed and stimulus-driven attention in the brain. *Nat. Rev. Neurosci.*, **3**(3), 201–15.

Coslett, H. B. (1989). Hemihypokinesia after right hemisphere stroke. *Brain Cogn.*, **9**, 267–78.

Coslett, H. B. (1997). Neglect in vision and visual imagery: A double dissociation. *Brain*, **120**(7), 1163–71.

Coslett, H. B., Bowers, D., Fitzpatrick, E., *et al.* (1990). Directional hypokinesia and hemispatial inattention in neglect. *Brain*, **113**, 475–86.

Cowey, A., Small, M. and Ellis, S. (1994). Left visuospatial neglect can be worse in far than in near space. *Neuropsychologia*, **32**, 1059–66.

Damasio, A. R., Damasio, H. and Chui, H. C., *et al.* (1987). Neglect following damage to frontal lobe or basal ganglia. *Neuropsychologia*, **18**(2), 123–32.

Decroix, J. P., Graveleau, P., Masson, M., *et al.* (1986). Infarction in the territory of the anterior choroidal artery. A clinical and computerized tomographic study of 16 cases. *Brain*, **109**(Pt 6), 1071–85.

Denis, M., Beschin, N., Logie, R. H., *et al.* (2002). Visual perception and verbal descriptions as sources for generating mental representations: Evidence from representational neglect. *Cogn. Neuropsychol.*, **19**(2), 97–112.

Deouell, L. Y. and Soroker, N. (2000). What is extinguished in auditory extinction? *Neuroreport*, **11**(13), 3059–62.

Di Legge, S., Fang, J., Saposnik, G., *et al.* (2005). The impact of lesion side on acute stroke treatment. *Neurology*, **65**(1), 81–6.

Di Pellegrino, G. (1995). Clock-drawing in a case of left visuo-spatial neglect: a deficit of disengagement? *Neuropsychologia*, **33**(3), 353–8.

Di Pellegrino, G. and De Renzi, E. (1995). An experimental investigation on the nature of extinction. *Neuropsychologia*, **33**, 153–70.

Di Pellegrino, G., Ladavas, E. and Farne, A. (1997). Seeing where your hands are. *Nature*, **388**, 370.

Di Pellegrino, G., Ladavas, E. and Galletti, C. (2001). Lexical processes and eye movements in neglect dyslexia. *Behav. Neurol.*, **13**(1–2), 61–74.

Doricchi, F. and Angelelli, P. (1999). Misrepresentation of horizontal space in left unilateral neglect: Role of hemianopia. *Neurology*, **52**(9), 1845–52.

Doricchi, F., Guariglia, P., Figliozzi, F., *et al.* (2005). Causes of cross-over in unilateral neglect: Between-group comparisons, within-patient dissociations and eye movements. *Brain*, **128**(Pt 6), 1386–406.

Doricchi, F. and Tomaiuolo, F. (2003). The anatomy of neglect without hemianopia: A key role for parietal-frontal disconnection? *Neuroreport*, **14**(17), 2239–43.

Driver, J., Baylis , G. C, Goodrich, S. J., *et al.* (1994). Axis-based neglect of visual shapes. *Neuropsychologia*, **32**, 1353–65.

Driver, J. and Halligan, P. W. (1991). Can visual neglect operate in object-centered coordinates? An affirmative single case study. *Cogn. Neuropsychol.*, **8**, 475–94.

Driver, J. and Pouget, A. (2000). Object-centered visual neglect, or relative egocentric neglect? *J. Cogn. Neurosci.*, **12**(3), 542–5.

Driver, J. and Vuilleumier, P. (2001a). Unconscious processing in neglect and extinction. In *Out of Mind: Varieties of Unconscious Processing*, ed. B. DeGelder *et al.*. Oxford University Press, pp. 107–39.

Driver, J. and Vuilleumier, P. (2001b). Perceptual awareness and its loss in unilateral neglect and extinction. *Cognition*, **79**, 39–88.

Driver, J., Vuilleumier, P., Eimer, M., *et al.* (2001). Functional MRI and evoked potential correlates of conscious and unconscious vision in parietal extinction patients. *Neuroimage*, **14**, 68–75.

Driver, J., Vuilleumier, P. and Husain, M. (2004). Spatial neglect and extinction. In *The New Cognitive Neurosciences*, ed. M. Gazzaniga. MIT Press.

Ellis, A. X., Della Salla, S. and Logie, R. H. (1996). The Bailiwick of visuo-spatial working memory: Evidence from unilateral spatial neglect. *Cogn. Brain Res.*, **3**(2), 71–8.

Farah, M. J., Brunn, J. L., Wong, A. B., *et al.* (1990). Frames of reference for allocating attention to space: Evidence from the neglect syndrome. *Neuropsychologia*, **28**, 335–47.

Farne, A., Buxbaun, L. J., Feraro, M., *et al.* (2004). Patterns of spontaneous recovery of neglect and associated disorders in acute right brain-damaged patients. *J. Neurol. Neurosurg. Psychiatry*, **75**(10), 1401–10.

Farne, A. and Ladavas, E. (2000). Dynamic size-change of hand peripersonal space following tool use. *Neuroreport*, **11**(8), 1645–9.

Feinberg, T. E., Haber, L. S. and Leeds, N. E. (1990). Verbal asomatognosia. *Neurology*, **40**, 1391–4.

Ferber, S. and Karnath, H. O. (1999). Parietal and occipital lobe contributions to perception of straight ahead orientation. *J. Neurol. Neurosurg. Psychiatry*, **67**(5), 572–8.

(2001a). How to assess spatial neglect̶line bisection or cancellation tasks? *J. Clin. Exp. Neuropsychol.*, **23**(5), 599–607.

(2001b). Size perception in hemianopia and neglect. *Brain*, **124**(Pt 3), 527–36.

Ferro, J. M. and Kertesz, A. (1984). Posterior internal capsule infarction associated with neglect. *Arch. Neurol.*, **41**(4), 422−4.

Ferro, J. M., Kertesz, A. and Black, S. E. (1987). Subcortical neglect: Quantitation, anatomy, and recovery. *Neurology*, **37**(9), 1487−92.

Fimm, B., Zahn, R., Mull, M., *et al.* (2001). Asymmetries of visual attention after circumscribed subcortical vascular lesions. *J. Neurol. Neurosurg. Psychiatry*, **71**(5), 652−7.

Fiorelli, M., Blin, J., Bakchine, S., *et al.* (1991). PET studies of cortical diaschisis in patients with motor hemi-neglect. *J. Neurol. Sci.*, **104**(2), 135−42.

Fischer, M. H. (2001). Number processing induces spatial performance biases. *Neurology*, **57**, 822−6.

Fleet, W. S., Valenstein, E., Watson, R. T., *et al.* (1987). Dopamine agonist therapy for neglect in humans. *Neurology*, **37**(11), 1765−70.

Frassinetti, F., Angeli, V., Meneghello, F., *et al.* (2002). Long-lasting amelioration of visuospatial neglect by prism adaptation. *Brain*, **125**(Pt 3), 608−23.

Gaffan, D. and Hornak, J. (1997). Visual neglect in the monkey: Representation and disconnection. *Brain*, **120**(9), 1647−57.

Gainotti, G., Messerli, P. and Tissot, R. (1972). Qualitative analysis of unilateral spatial neglect in relation to laterality of cerebral lesions. *J. Neurol. Neurosurg. Psychiatry*, **35**(4), 545−50.

Gauthier, L., Dehaut, F., and Joanette, Y., (1989). The Bells Test: A quantitative and qualitative test for visual neglect. *Int. J. Clin. Neuropsychol.*, **11**, 49−54.

Ghika-Schmid, F. and Bogousslavsky, J. (2000). The acute behavioral syndrome of anterior thalamic infarction: A prospective study of 12 cases. *Ann. Neurol.*, **48**(2), 220−7.

Gillen, R., Tennen, H., and McKee, T., (2005). Unilateral spatial neglect: Relation to rehabilitation outcomes in patients with right hemisphere stroke. *Arch. Phys. Med. Rehabil.*, **86**(4), 763−7.

Gitelman, D. R., Nobre, A. C., Parrish, T. B., *et al.* (1999). A large-scale distributed network for covert spatial attention: Further anatomical delineation based on stringent behavioural and cognitive controls. *Brain*, **122**, 1093−106.

Goldenberg, G. (1986). Neglect in a patient with partial callosal disconnection. *Neuropsychologia*, **24**(3), 397−403.

Grossi, D., Modafferi, A., Pelosi, L., *et al.* (1989). On the different roles of the cerebral hemispheres in mental imagery: The "O'Clock Test" in two clinical cases. *Brain Cogn.*, **10**(1), 18−27.

Grujic, Z., Mapstone, M., Gitelman, D. R., *et al.* (1998). Dopamine agonists reorient visual exploration away from the neglected hemispace. *Neurology*, **51**(5), 1395−8.

Guariglia, C. and Antonucci, G. (1992). Personal and extrapersonal space: A case of neglect dissociation. *Neuropsychologia*, **30**, 1001−10.

Guariglia, C., Padovani, A., Partano, P., *et al.* (1991). Unilateral neglect restricted to visual imagery. *Nature*, **364**, 235−7.

Halligan, P. W., Fink, G. R. Marshall, J. C., *et al.* (2003). Spatial cognition: Evidence from visual neglect. *Trends Cogn. Sci.*, **7**(3), 125−33.

Halligan, P. W. and Marshall, J. C. (1991a). Figural modulation of visuo-spatial neglect: A case study. *Neuropsychologia*, **29**, 619−28.

(1991b). Left neglect for near but not far space in man. *Nature*, **350**, 498–500.

(1998). Visuospatial neglect: The ultimate deconstruction? *Brain Cogn.*, **37**(3), 419–38.

Halligan, P. W., Marshall, J. C., Wade, D. T., (1989). Visuospatial neglect: Underlying factors and test sensitivity. *Lancet*, **2**(8668), 908–11.

(1990). Do visual field deficits exacerbate visuo-spatial neglect? *J. Neurol. Neurosurg. Psychiatry*, **53**(6), 487–91.

Harvey, M., Kramer McCaffery, T., Dow, L., *et al.* (2002). Categorisation of 'perceptual' and 'premotor' neglect patients across different tasks: Is there strong evidence for a dichotomy? *Neuropsychologia*, **40**(8), 1387–95.

Harvey, M., Milner, A. I., and Roberts, R. C., *et al.* (1995). An investigation of hemispatial neglect using the Landmark Task. *Brain Cogn.*, **27**(1), 59–78.

Heilman, K. M. and Van Den Abell, T. (1979). Right hemisphere dominance for mediating cerebral activation. *Neuropsychologia*, **17**, 315–21.

Heilman, K. M. and Adams, D. J. (2003). Callosal neglect. *Arch. Neurol.*, **60**(2), 276–9.

Heilman, K. M., Boweres, B., Coslett, H. B., *et al.* (1985). Directional hypokinesia: Prolonged reaction times for leftward movements in patients with right hemisphere lesions and neglect. *Neurology*, **35**, 855–9.

Heilman, K. M., Pandya, D. M. and Geschwind, N. (1970). Trimodal inattention following parietal lobe ablations. *Trans. Am. Neurol. Assoc.*, **95**, 259–68.

Heilman, K. M. and Valenstein, E. (1972). Frontal lobe neglect in man. *Neurology*, **22**, 660–4.

Heilman, K. M. and Van Den Abell, T. (1980). Right hemisphere dominance for attention: The mechanisms underlying hemispheric asymmetries of inattention (neglect). *Neurology*, **30**, 327–30.

Heilman, K. M., Watson, R. T. and Valenstein, E. (2003). Neglect and related disorders. In *Clinical Neuropsychology*, ed. K. M. Heilman and E. Valenstein. Oxford University Press, pp. 279–336.

Hier, D. B., Mondlock, J. and Caplan, I. R. (1983a). Behavioral abnormalities after right hemisphere stroke. *Neurology*, **33**(3), 337–44.

(1983b). Recovery of behavioral abnormalities after right hemisphere stroke. *Neurology*, **33**(3), 345–50.

Hillis, A. E., Barker, P. B., Beauchamp, N. J., *et al.* (2000). MR perfusion imaging reveals regions of hypoperfusion associated with aphasia and neglect. *Neurology*, **55**(6), 782–8.

Hillis, A. E. and Caramazza, A. (1991). Deficit to stimulus-centered, letter shape representations in a case of "unilateral neglect". *Neuropsychologia*, **29**(12), 1223–40.

Hillis, A. E., Newhart, M., Heidler, J., *et al.* (2005). Anatomy of spatial attention: Insights from perfusion imaging and hemispatial neglect in acute stroke. *J. Neurosci.*, **25**(12), 3161–7.

Hillis, A. E., Wityk, R. J., Barker, P. B., *et al.* (2002). Subcortical aphasia and neglect in acute stroke: The role of cortical hypoperfusion. *Brain*, **125**(Pt 5), 1094–104.

(2003). Change in perfusion in acute nondominant hemisphere stroke may be better estimated by tests of hemispatial neglect than by the National Institutes of Health Stroke Scale. *Stroke*, **34**(10), 2392–6.

Humphreys, G. W. and Riddoch, M. J. (1995). Separate coding of space within and between perceptual objects: Evidence from unilateral visual neglect. *Cogn. Neuropsychol.*, **12**, 283–311.

Husain, M. and Kennard, C. (1996). Visual neglect associated with frontal lobe infarction. *J. Neurol.*, **243**, 652–7.

(1997). Distractor-dependent frontal neglect. *Neuropsychologia*, **35**, 829–41.

Husain, M., Mannan, S., Hodgson, T., *et al.* (2001). Impaired spatial working memory across saccades contributes to abnormal search in parietal neglect. *Brain*, **124**(Pt 5), 941–52.

Husain, M., Mattingley, J. B, Rorden, C., *et al.* (2000). Distinguishing sensory and motor biases in parietal and frontal neglect. *Brain*, **123**(Pt 8), 1643–59.

Husain, M. and Rorden, C. (2003). Non-spatially lateralized mechanisms in hemispatial neglect. *Nat. Rev. Neurosci.*, **4**(1), 26–36.

Husain, M., Shapiro, K., Martin, J., *et al.* (1997). Abnormal temporal dynamics of visual attention in spatial neglect patients. *Nature*, **385**(6612), 154–6.

Jehkonen, M., Ahonen, J. P, Dastidar, P., *et al.* (2000). Visual neglect as a predictor of functional outcome one year after stroke. *Acta. Neurol. Scand.*, **101**(3), 195–201.

Johannsen, L. and Karnath, H. O. (2004). How efficient is a simple copying task to diagnose spatial neglect in its chronic phase? *J. Clin. Exp. Neuropsychol.*, **26**(2), 251–6.

Karnath, H. O. (1995). Transcutaneous electrical stimulation and vibration of neck muscles in neglect. *Exp. Brain Res.*, **105**(2), 321–4.

Karnath, H. O., Ferber, S. and Himmelbach, M. (2001). Spatial awareness is a function of the temporal not the posterior parietal lobe. *Nature*, **411**(6840), 950–3.

Karnath, H. O. and Fetter, M. (1995). Ocular space exploration in the dark and its relation to subjective and objective body orientation in neglect patients with parietal lesions. *Neuropsychologia*, **33**(3), 371–7.

Karnath, H. O., Fetter, M. and Niemeier, M. (1998). Disentangling gravitational, environmental, and egocentric reference frames in spatial neglect. *J. Cogn. Neurosci.*, **10**(6), 680–90.

Karnath, H. O., Fruhmann Berger, M., Kuker, *et al.* (2004). The anatomy of spatial neglect based on voxelwise statistical analysis: A study of 140 patients. *Cereb. Cortex*, **14**(10), 1164–72.

Karnath, H. O., Himmelbach, M. and Kuker. (2003). The cortical substrate of visual extinction. *Neuroreport*, **14**(3), 437–42.

Karnath, H. O., Himmelbach, M. and Rorden, C. (2002). The subcortical anatomy of human spatial neglect: Putamen, caudate nucleus and pulvinar. *Brain*, **125**(Pt 2), 350–60.

Karnath, H. O. and Perenin, M. T. (1998). Tactile exploration of peripersonal space in patients with neglect. *Neuroreport*, **9**(10), 2273–7.

Karnath, H. O., Schenkel, P. and Fischer, B. (1991). Trunk orientation as the determining factor of the 'contralateral' deficit in the neglect syndrome and as the physical anchor of the internal representation of body orientation in space. *Brain*, 1997–2014.

Kerkhoff, G. (1998). Rehabilitation of visuospatial cognition and visual exploration in neglect: A crossover study. *Restor. Neurol. Neurosci.*, **12**(1), 27–40.

(2001). Spatial hemineglect in humans. *Prog. Neurobiol.*, **63**(1), 1–27.

Kinsella, G. and Ford, B. (1980). Acute recovery from patterns in stroke patients: Neuropsychological factors. *Med. J. Aust.*, **2**(12), 663–6.

Kinsella, G., Olver, J., Ng, K.,, *et al.* (1993). Analysis of the syndrome of unilateral neglect. *Cortex*, **29**(1), 135–40.

Klatka, L. A., Depper, M. H. and Marini, A. M. (1998). Infarction in the territory of the anterior cerebral artery. *Neurology*, **51**(2), 620–2.

Kooistra, C. A. and Heilman, K. M. (1989). Hemispatial visual inattention masquerading as hemianopia. *Neurology*, **39**, 1125–72.

Kumral, E. and Evyapan, D. (1999). Associated exploratory-motor and perceptual-sensory neglect without hemiparesis. *Neurology*, **52**(1), 199–202.

Kumral, E., Evyapan, D. and Balkir, K. (1999). Acute caudate vascular lesions. *Stroke*, **30**(1), 100–8.

Kumral, E., Kocaer, T., Sagduyu, A., *et al.* (1995). Infarctus calleux après occlusion bilatérale des artères carotides internes. *Rev. Neurol.*, **151**, 202–5.

LaBar, K. S., Gitelman, D. R., Parrish, T. B., *et al.* (1999). Neuroanatomic overlap of working memory and spatial attention networks: A functional MRI comparison within subjects. *Neuroimage*, **10**, 695–704.

Ladavas, E. (1987). Is the hemispatial deficit produced by right parietal damage associated with retinal or gravitational coordinates? *Brain*, **110**, 167–80.

Ladavas, E. (1990). Selective spatial attention in patients with visual extinction. *Brain*, **113**, 1527–38.

Ladavas, E., di Pellegrino, G., Farne, A., *et al.* (1998). Neuropsychological evidence of an integrated visuotactile representation of peripersonal space in humans. *J. Cogn. Neurosci.*, **10**(5), 581–9.

Ladavas, E., Farne, A., Zeloni, G., *et al.* (2000). Seeing or not seeing where your hands are. *Exp. Brain Res.*, **131**(4), 458–67.

Ladavas, E., Shallice, T. and Zanella, M. T. (1997). Preserved semantic access in neglect dyslexia. *Neuropsychologia*, **35**(3), 257–70.

Lamb, M. R., Robertson, L. C. and Knight, R. T. (1989). Attention and interference in the processing of global and local information: Effects of unilateral temporal-parietal junction lesions. *Neuropsychologia*, **4**, 471–83.

Laplane, D. (1990). Is there a correlation between motor neglect and unilateral sensory neglect. *Rev. Neurol.(Paris)*, **146**(10), 635–8.

Laplane, D., Baulac, M. and Carydakis, C. (1986). Motor neglect of thalamic origin. *Rev. Neurol. (Paris)*, **142**(4), 375–9.

Laplane, D. and Degos, J. D. (1983). Motor neglect. *J. Neurol. Neurosurg. Psychiatry*, **46**, 152–8.

Lee, B. H., Kang, S. J., Park, J. M., *et al.* (2004). The Character-line Bisection Task: A new test for hemispatial neglect. *Neuropsychologia*, **42**(12), 1715–24.

Leibovitch, F. S., Black, S. E., Caldwell, C. B., *et al.* (1998). Brain-behavior correlations in hemispatial neglect using CT and SPECT: The Sunnybrook Stroke Study. *Neurology*, **50**(4), 901–8.

(1999). Brain SPECT imaging and left hemispatial neglect covaried using partial least squares: The Sunnybrook Stroke study. *Hum. Brain Mapp.*, **7**(4), 244–53.

Levine, D. N., Warach, J. D., Benowitz, L., *et al.* (1986). Left spatial neglect: Effects of lesion size and premorbid brain atrophy on severity and recovery following right cerebral infarction. *Neurology*, **36**(3), 362–6.

Levine, R. L., Lagreze, H. L., Dobkin, J. A., *et al.* (1988). Large subcortical hemispheric infarctions. Presentation and prognosis. *Arch. Neurol.*, **45**(10), 1074−7.

Lundervold, A. J., Bergmann, N. and Wootton, C. (2005). Visual neglect in the first weeks after a stroke in the right hemisphere. *Scand. J. Psychol.*, **46**(3), 297−303.

Maguire, A. M. and Ogden, J. A. (2002). MRI brain scan analyses and neuropsychological profiles of nine patients with persisting unilateral neglect. *Neuropsychologia*, **40**(7), 879−87.

Maravita, A. (1997). Implicit processing of somatosensory stimuli disclosed by a perceptual after-effect. *NeuroReport*, **8**(7), 1671−4.

Maravita, A., Husain, M., Clarke, K., *et al.* (2001). Reaching with a tool extends visual-tactile interactions into far space: Evidence from cross-modal extinction. *Neuropsychologia*, **39**(6), 580−5.

Marchetti, C., Carey, D. and Della Salla, S. (2005). Crossed right hemisphere syndrome following left thalamic stroke. *J. Neurol.*, **252**(4), 403−11.

Mark, V. W. (2003). Acute versus chronic functional aspects of unilateral spatial neglect. *Front. Biosci.*, **8**, e172−189.

Mark, V. W., Kooistra, C. A. and Heilman, K. M. (1988). Hemispatial neglect affected by non-neglected stimuli. *Neurology*, **38**, 1207−11.

Marshall, J. C. and Halligan, P. W. (1988). Blindsight and insight in visuo-spatial neglect. *Nature*, **336**, 766−7.

(1994). The yin and the yang of visuospatial neglect: A case study. *Neuropsychologia*, **32**, 1037−57.

Marzi, C., Girelli, M., Miniussi, C., *et al.* (2000). Electrophysiological correlates of conscious vision: Evidence from unilateral extinction. *J. Cogn. Neurosci.*, **12**(5), 869−77.

Mattingley, J. B., Bradshaw, J. G. and Phillips, J. C. (1992). Impairments of movement initiation and execution in unilateral neglect: Directional hypokinesia and bradykinesia. *Brain*, **115**, 1849−74.

Mattingley, J. B., Driver, J., Beschin, N., *et al.* (1997). Attentional competition between modalities: Extinction between touch and vision after right hemisphere damage. *Neuropsychologia*, **35**(6), 867−80.

Mattingley, J. B., Husain, M., Rorden, L., *et al.* (1998). Motor role of human inferior parietal lobe revealed in unilateral neglect patients. *Nature*, **392**(6672), 179−82.

Maulaz, A. B., Bezerra, J. C. and Bogousslavsky (2005). Posterior cerebral artery infarction from middle cerebral artery infarction. *Arch. Neurol.*, **62**(6), 938−41.

Mayer, S. A., Tatemichi, T. K., Hair, L. S., *et al.* (1993). Hemineglect and seizures in Binswanger's disease: Clinical-pathological report. *J. Neurol. Neurosurg. Psychiatry*, **56**(7), 816−19.

McGlinchey-Berroth, R., Milberg, W. P., Verfaellie, M., *et al.* (1993). Semantic processing in the neglected visual field: Evidence from a lexical decision task. *Cogn. Neuropsychol.*, **10**, 79−108.

Mennemeier, M., Chatterjee, A. and Heilman, K. M. (1994). A comparison of the influences of body and environment centred reference frames on neglect. *Brain*, **117**, 1013−21.

Mennemeier, M., Wertman, E. and Heilman, K. M. (1992). Neglect of near peripersonal space: Evidence for multidirectional attentional systems in humans. *Brain*, **115**, 37−50.

Merrino, J. G. and Heilman, K. M. (2003). Measurement of cognitive deficits in acute stroke. *Stroke*, **34**, 2396−7.

Mesulam, M. M. (1981). A cortical network for directed attention and unilateral neglect. *Ann. Neurol.*, **4**, 309−25.

(1985). Attention, confusional states and neglect. In *Principles of Behavioral Neurology*, ed. M. M. Mesulam. F. A. Davis, pp. 125−68.

(1999). Spatial attention and neglect: Parietal, frontal and cingulate contributions to the mental representation and attentional targeting of salient extrapersonal events. *Philos. Trans. R. Soc. Lond. B. Biol. Sci.*, **354**(1387), 1325−46.

Milner, A. D., Harvey, M., Roberts, R. C., *et al.* (1993). Line bisection errors in visual neglect: Misguided action or size distortion? *Neuropsychologia*, **31**(1), 39−49.

Mort, D. J., Malhotra, P., Mannan, S. K., *et al.* (2003). The anatomy of visual neglect. *Brain* **126**(9), 1986−97.

Moscovitch, M. and Behrmann, M. (1994). Coding of spatial information in the somatosensory system: Evidence from patients with neglect following parietal lobe damage. *J. Cogn. Neurosci.*, **6**, 151−5.

Niemeier, M. and Karnath, H. O. (2000). Exploratory saccades show no direction-specific deficit in neglect. *Neurology*, **54**(2), 515−18.

Ogden, J. A. (1985a). Contralesional neglect of constructed visual images in right and left brain-damaged patients. *Neuropsychologia*, **23**(2), 273−7.

(1985b). Anterior-posterior interhemispheric differences in the loci of lesions producing visual hemineglect. *Brain Cogn.*, **4**, 59−75.

Olson, E., Stark, M. and Chatterjee, A. (2003). Evidence for a unimodal somatosensory attention system. *Exp. Brain Res.*, **151**, 15−23.

Ortigue, S., Viaud-Delmon, I., Annoni, J. M., *et al.* (2001). Pure representational neglect after right thalamic lesion. *Ann. Neurol.*, **50**(3), 401−4.

Ota, H., Fujii, T., Suzuki, K., *et al.* (2001). Dissociation of body-centered and stimulus-centered representations in unilateral neglect. *Neurology*, **57**(11), 2064−9.

Ota, H., Fujii, T., Tabuchi, M., *et al.* (2003). Different spatial processing for stimulus-centered and body-centered representations. *Neurology*, **60**(11), 1846−8.

Pachalska, M., Franczuk, B., MacQueen, B. J., *et al.* (2004). Reintegrating space and object representations in patients with hemispatial neglect: Two case studies. *Disabil. Rehabil.*, **26**(9), 549−61.

Paghera, B., Marien, P. and Vignolo, L. A. (2003). Crossed aphasia with left spatial neglect and visual imperception: A case report. *Neurol. Sci.*, **23**(6), 317−22.

Pedersen, P. M., Jorgensen, H. S., Nakayama, H., *et al.* (1997). Hemineglect in acute stroke − incidence and prognostic implications. The Copenhagen Stroke Study. *Am. J. Phys. Med. Rehabil.*, **76**(2), 122−7.

Pegna, A. J., Petit, L., Caldara-Schnetzer, A. S., *et al.* (2001). So near yet so far: Neglect in far or near space depends on tool use. *Ann. Neurol.*, **50**(6), 820−2.

Perani, D., Vallar, G., Cappa, S., *et al.* (1987). Aphasia and neglect after subcortical stroke. A clinical/cerebral perfusion correlation study. *Brain*, **110**(2), 1211−29.

Pierce, S. R. and Buxbaum, L. J. (2002). Treatments of unilateral neglect: A review. *Arch. Phys. Med. Rehabil.*, **83**(2), 256–68.

Pisella, L., Berberovic, N., and Mattingley, J. B. (2004). Impaired working memory for location but not for colour or shape in visual neglect: A comparison of parietal and non-parietal lesions. *Cortex*, **40**(2), 379–90.

Pizzamiglio, L., Cappa, S., Vallar, G., *et al.* (1989). Visual neglect for far and near extrapersonal space in humans. *Cortex*, **25**, 471–7.

Posner, M. I., Walker, J. A., Friedrich, F. J., *et al.* (1987). How do the parietal lobes direct covert attention? *Neuropsychologia*, **25**, 135–46.

Posteraro, L. and Maravita, A. (1996). A new case of atypical cerebral dominance. *Ital. J. Neurol. Sci.*, **17**(3), 237–40.

Rafal, R., Danziger, S., Grossi, G., *et al.* (2002). Visual detection is gated by attending for action: Evidence from hemispatial neglect. *Proc. Natl. Acad. Sci. USA*, **99**(25), 16371–5.

Rafal, R. D. and Posner, M. I. (1987). Deficits in human visual spatial attention following thalamic lesions. *Proc. Natl. Acad. Sci. USA*, **84**, 7349–53.

Rapcsak, S. Z., Cimino, C. R. and Heilman, K. M. (1988). Altitudinal neglect. *Neurology*, **38**(2), 277–81.

Rapcsak, S. Z., Verfaellie, M., Fleet, W. S., *et al.* (1989). Selective attention in hemispatial neglect. *Arch. Neurol.*, **46**(2), 178–82.

Rees, G., Wojciulik, E., Clarke, K., *et al.* (2000). Unconscious activation of visual cortex in the damaged right hemisphere of a parietal patient with extinction. *Brain*, **123**(8), 1624–33.

(2002). Neural correlates of conscious and unconscious vision in parietal extinction. *Neurocase*, **8**(5), 387–93.

Rizzolatti, G., Matelli, M. and Pavesi, C. (1983). Deficits in attention and movement following the removal of postarcuate (area 6) and prearcuate (area 8) cortex in macaque monkeys. *Brain*, **106**, 655–73.

Robertson, I. H., Manly, T., Beschin, N., *et al.* (1997). Auditory sustained attention is a marker of unilateral spatial neglect. *Neuropsychologia*, **35**(12), 1527–32.

Robertson, I. H., Mattingley, J. B., Rorden, A., *et al.* (1998). Phasic alerting of neglect patients overcomes their spatial deficit in visual awareness. *Nature*, **395**, 169–72.

Robertson, I. H., Tegner, R., Tham, K., *et al.* (1995). Sustained attention training for unilateral neglect: Theoretical and rehabilitation implications. *J. Clin. Exp. Neuropsychol.*, **17**(3), 416–30.

Rode, G., Perenin, M. T. and Boisson, D. (1995). Neglect of the representational space: Demonstration by mental evocation of the map of France. *Rev. Neurol. (Paris)*, **151**(3), 161–4.

Rode, G., Pisella, L., Rossetti, Y., *et al.* (2003). Bottom-up transfer of sensory-motor plasticity to recovery of spatial cognition: Visuomotor adaptation and spatial neglect. *Prog. Brain Res.*, **142**, 273–87.

Rode, G., Rossetti, Y., Badan, M., *et al.* (2001). Role of rehabilitation in hemineglect syndromes. *Rev. Neurol. (Paris)*, **157**(5), 497–505.

Rossetti, Y., Rode, G., Pisella, L., *et al.* (1998). Prism adaptation to a rightward optical deviation rehabilitates left hemispatial neglect. *Nature*, **395**(6698), 166–9.

Rousseaux, M., Beis, J. M., Pradat-Diehl, P., *et al.* (2001). Presenting a battery for assessing spatial neglect. Norms and effects of age, educational level, sex, hand and laterality. *Rev. Neurol. (Paris)*, **157**(11 Pt 1), 1385–400.

Samuelsson, H., Hjelmquist, E. K., Jensen, C., *et al.* (1998). Nonlateralized attentional deficits: An important component behind persisting visuospatial neglect? *J. Clin. Exp. Neuropsychol.*, **20**(1), 73–88.

Samuelsson, H., Jensen, C., Ekholm, S., *et al.* (1997). Anatomical and neurological correlates of acute and chronic visuospatial neglect following right hemisphere stroke. *Cortex*, **33**(2), 271–85.

Schmahmann, J. D. (2003). Vascular syndromes of the thalamus. *Stroke*, **34**(9), 2264–78.

Schwartz, S., Vuilleumier, P., Hutton, C., *et al.* (2005). Attentional load and sensory competition in human vision: Modulation of fMRI responses by load at fixation during task-irrelevant stimulation in the peripheral visual field. *Cereb. Cortex*, **15**(6), 770–86.

Shelton, P. A., Bowers, D. and Heilman, K. M. (1990). Peripersonal and vertical neglect. *Brain*, **113**, 191–205.

Simon, J. E., Morgan, S. C., Pexman, J. H., *et al.* (2003). CT assessment of conjugate eye deviation in acute stroke. *Neurology*, **60**(1), 135–7.

Stein, S. and Volpe, B. T. (1983). Classical "parietal" neglect syndrome after subcortical right frontal lobe infarction. *Neurology*, **33**(6), 797–9.

Stone, S. P., Halligan, P. W., Marshall, J. C., *et al.* (1998). Unilateral neglect: A common but heterogeneous syndrome. *Neurology*, **50**(6), 1902–5.

Stone, S. P., Halligan, P. W., Wilson, B., *et al.* (1991a). Performance of age-matched controls on a battery of visuo-spatial neglect tests. *J. Neurol. Neurosurg. Psychiatry*, **54**(4), 341–4.

Stone, S. P., Patel, P., Greenwood, R. J., *et al.* (1992). Measuring visual neglect in acute stroke and predicting its recovery: The visual neglect recovery index. *J. Neurol. Neurosurg. Psychiatry*, **55**(6), 431–6.

Stone, S. P., Wilson, B., Wroot, A., *et al.* (1991b). The assessment of visuo-spatial neglect after acute stroke. *J. Neurol. Neurosurg. Psychiatry*, **54**(4), 345–50.

Tanaka, Y., Minematsu, K., Hara, H., *et al.* (2001). Sensory extinction phenomenon of double simultaneous stimulation: The analysis of consecutive stroke series with acute and unilateral lesions. *Rinsho Shinkeigaku*, **41**(9), 569–73.

Tatemichi, T. K., Desmond, D. W., Stern, Y., *et al.* (1994). Cognitive impairment after stroke: Frequency, patterns, and relationship to functional abilities. *J. Neurol. Neurosurg. Psychiatry*, **57**(2), 202–7.

Tegner, R. and Levander, M. (1991). Through a looking glass: A new technique to demonstrate directional hypokinesia in unilateral neglect. *Brain*, **113**, 1943–51.

Tham, K. and Tegnér, R. (1996). The Baking Tray task: A test of spatial neglect. *Neuropsychol. Rehab.*, **6**, 19–25.

Toraldo, A., McIntosh, R. D., Dijkerman, H. C., *et al.* (2002). Disentangling perceptual and response bias in unilateral neglect: A methodological proposal. *Brain Cogn.*, **48**(2–3), 593–7.

Valenstein, E. and Heilman, K. M. (1981). Unilateral hypokinesia and motor extinction. *Neurology*, **31**, 445–8.

Valenza, N., Seghier, M. L., Schwarz, S., *et al.* (2004). Tactile awareness and limb position in neglect: Functional magnetic resonance imaging. *Ann. Neurol.*, **55**(1), 139–43.

Vallar, G. (1993). The anatomical basis of spatial neglect in humans. In *Unilateral Neglect: Clinical and Experimental Studies,* ed. I. H. Robertson and J. C. Marshall. Lawrence Erlbaum Associates, pp. 27–62.

Vallar, G., Bottini, G. and Paulesu, E. (2003). Neglect syndromes: The role of the parietal cortex. In *The Parietal Lobes Vol. 93*, ed. A. M. Siegel *et al.*, Lippincott, Williams & Wilkins, pp. 219–315.

Vallar, G., Bottini, G., Sterzi, R., *et al.* (1991). Hemianesthesia, sensory neglect, and defective access to conscious experience. *Neurology*, **41**(5), 650–2.

Vallar, G., Daini, R. and Antonucci, G. (2000). Processing of illusion of length in spatial hemineglect: A study of line bisection. *Neuropsychologia*, **38**(7), 1087–97.

Vallar, G., Guariglia, C., Nico, D., *et al.* (1995). Spatial hemineglect in back space. *Brain*, **118**(2), 467–72.

Vallar, G., Lobel, E., Galati, G., *et al.* (1999). A fronto-parietal system for computing the egocentric spatial frame of reference in humans. *Exp. Brain Res.*, **124**(3), 281–6.

Vallar, G. and Perani, D. (1986). The anatomy of unilateral neglect after right-hemisphere stroke lesions: A clinical/CT correlation study in man. *Neuropsychologia*, **24**, 609–22.

Volpe, B. T., Ledoux, J. E. and Gazzaniga, M. S. (1979). Information processing in an "extinguished" visual field. *Nature*, **282**, 722–4.

Vuilleumier, P. (2000). Faces call for attention: Evidence from patients with visual extinction. *Neuropsychologia*, **38**(5), 693–700.

(2005). Visual extinction and hemispatial neglect after brain damage: Neurophysiological basis of residual processing. In *Neurobiology of Attention,* ed. L. Itti *et al.*, Elsevier, pp. 351–7.

Vuilleumier, P., Armony, J., Clarke, K., *et al.* (2002). Neural response to emotional faces with and without awareness: Event-related fMRI in a parietal patient with visual extinction and spatial neglect. *Neuropsychologia*, **40**, 2156–66.

Vuilleumier, P., Ortigue, S. and Brugger, P. (2004). The number space and neglect. *Cortex*, **40**(2), 399–410.

Vuilleumier, P. and Rafal, R. (2000). A systematic study of task-dependent visual extinction: Between and within-field deficits of attention in hemispatial neglect. *Brain*, **123**, 1263–79.

Vuilleumier, P., Sagiv, N., Hazeltine, E., *et al.* (2001a). Neural fate of seen and unseen faces in unilateral spatial neglect: A combined event-related fMRI and ERP study of visual extinction. *Proc. Nat. Acad. Sci. USA*, **98**(6), 3495–500.

Vuilleumier, P. and Schwartz, S. (2001). Modulation of visual perception by eye gaze direction in patients with spatial neglect and extinction. *Neuroreport*, **12**(10), 2101–4.

Vuilleumier, P., Schwartz, S., Clarke, K., *et al.* (2001b). Implicit processing and learning of visual stimuli in parietal extinction and neglect. *Cortex*, **37**, 741–4.

Vuilleumier, P., Valenza, N. and Landis, T. (2001c). Explicit and implicit perception of illusory contours in unilateral spatial neglect: Behavioural and anatomical correlates of preattentive grouping mechanisms. *Neuropsychologia*, **39**, 597–610.

Vuilleumier, P., Valenza, N., Mayer, E., *et al.* (1998). Near and far visual space in unilateral neglect. *Ann. Neurol.*, **43**, 406–10.

Vuilleumier, P., Valenza, N., Perrig, S., *et al.* (1999). To see better to the left when looking more to the right: Effects of gaze direction and frame of spatial coordinates in unilateral neglect. *J. Int. Neuropsychol. Soc.*, **5**, 75–82.

Walker, R., Findlay, J. M., Young, A. W., *et al.* (1991). Disentangling neglect and hemianopia. *Neuropsychologia*, **29**(10), 1019–27.

Ward, R. and Goodrich, S. (1996). Differences between objects and nonobjects in visual extinction: A competition for attention. *Psychological Science*, **7**, 177–80.

Ward, R., Goodrich, S. and Driver, J. (1994). Grouping reduces visual extinction: Neuropsychological evidence for weight-linkage in visual selection. *Visual Cognition*, **1**, 101–29.

Watson, T. and Heilman, K. M. (1981). Unilateral hypokinesia and motor extinction. *Neurology*, **31**, 445–8.

Weintraub, S. and Mesulam, M. M. (1987). Right cerebral hemisphere dominance in spatial attention. *Arch. Neurol.*, **44**, 621–5.

Weiss, P. H., Marshall, J. C., Wunderlich, G., *et al.* (2000). Neural consequences of acting in near versus far space: A physiological basis for clinical dissociations. *Brain*, **123**(Pt 12), 2531–41.

Weiss, P. H., Marshall, J. C., Zilles, K., *et al.* (2003). Are action and perception in near and far space additive or interactive factors? *Neuroimage*, **18**(4), 837–46.

Wilson, B. A., Cockburn, J. and Halligan, P. W., *et al.* (1987). *Behavioural Inattention Test*, Thames Valley Test Company.

Wojciulik, E., Husain, M., Clarke, K., *et al.* (2001). Spatial working memory deficit in unilateral neglect. *Neuropsychologia*, **39**(4), 390–6.

Worrall, B. B., Farace, E., Hillis, A. E., *et al.* (2001). Correlation of aphasia and/or neglect with cortical infarction in a subpopulation of RANTTAS. *Cerebrovasc. Dis.*, **11**(3), 257–64.

Zorzi, M., Priftis, K. and Umilta, C. (2002). Brain damage: Neglect disrupts the mental number line. *Nature*, **417**(6885), 138–9.

10

Anosognosia and denial after right hemisphere stroke

Anne Peskine and Philippe Azouvi

University of Versailles-Saint-Quentin, France

General presentation of anosognosia

Anosognosia is a puzzling condition. It refers to patients suffering from various neurological impairments who deny or lack awareness of their deficits, although these deficits may have serious consequences in their everyday life. Studying anosognosia is important for two reasons. The first one is a practical reason. Indeed, as pointed out by Heilman (1991), anosognosia is not a trivial problem. It may impair patients' motivation to engage in a rehabilitation program, and anosognosia has repeatedly been found associated with poor functional recovery from stroke. But studying anosognosia is also of great theoretical importance, as it may help our understanding of the complex relationships between brain injury and various forms of consciousness. However, despite this, anosognosia remains one of the least studied of the major neuropsychological symptoms after stroke, and its pathophysiology is still very poorly understood.

Detailed historical review of anosognosia have been published recently (Bisiach and Geminiani, 1991; Prigatano and Schacter, 1991). First observations of patients with impaired awareness of neurological deficits were reported in the late nineteenth century by von Monakow in 1885 and by Anton in 1889 in cases of cortical blindness. It seems that Pick, in 1898, was actually the first to report unawareness of left hemiplegia, but it was Joseph Babinski who first coined the term "anosognosia," and his contribution, at a meeting held by the French Neurological Society on June 11, 1914, remains a landmark in the field (Babinski, 1914).

Anosognosia may be associated with many disorders. Perhaps the most dramatic is unawareness of hemiplegia. However, there are many other defects of which patients may be unaware. These include: cortical blindness, hemianopia, cortical deafness, aphasia, memory loss, and the dysexecutive syndrome (Prigatano and Schacter, 1991). Whether common neuropsychological mechanisms produce anosognosia for different types of deficit remains undetermined.

In this review, we will focus on anosognosia associated with right-hemisphere stroke, that is mainly anosognosia for hemiplegia, and/or hemianopia.

Key points Main characteristics of anosognosia

Anosognosia: denial or lack of awareness of a clear neurological deficit
— concerns deficits in the motor (hemiplegia), visual (hemianopia, cortical blindness), auditory (cortical deafness) or cognitive (aphasia, dysexecutive syndrome) domains
— may be dissociated (anosognosia concerns only one of the multiple deficits of the patient)
— may be associated with misoplegia (patients express hatred towards the contralesional limb) or somatoparaphrenia (bodily delusions)

Anosognosia after right hemisphere stroke: Clinical features

Babinski (1914), in his seminal report, described a patient who, although "her intellectual and affective functions seemed grossly preserved (...) seemed to ignore the existence of a nearly complete hemiplegia (...). She never complained of it, she even never mentioned it (...). When asked to move her left arm, she remained immobile, silent, just as if the request concerned someone else." Babinski also introduced the term "anosodiaphoria" to refer to some hemiplegic patients who, without ignoring their hemiplegia, seemed indifferent and did not appear to be affected by their paralysis (Babinski, 1914). Other clinical manifestations have been described later, such as misoplegia (Critchley, 1974), where patients express hatred towards the contralesional limb, or somatoparaphrenia (Gerstmann, 1942), corresponding to a variety of bodily delusions, where patients fail to acknowledge ownership of their own contralesional limbs, or attribute them to someone else, or treat the limb(s) as a separate person or object.

Anosognosia is a complex disorder, and surprising dissociations and contradictions have been reported in anosognosic patients. This leads some authors to distinguish between different types or degrees of anosognosia (Marcel *et al.*, 2004; Vuilleumier, 2000; 2004). Specificity — the degree to which lack of awareness is restricted to a particular deficit — is an important issue of anosognosia for hemiplegia (Marcel *et al.*, 2004). For example, an individual might not mention his flaccid hemiparesis but complain elaborately about some trivial discomfort of infirmity. One of the first anosognosic patients reported by Babinski (1914) complained of an old phlebitis, while being unaware of hemiplegia. Even within the domain of neurological deficits, patients may deny weakness while retaining full awareness of language or visual impairments. In addition, different levels of awareness can be observed within a specific modality regarding different ipsilateral body parts (e.g. some patients acknowledge leg weakness while failing to appreciate their paretic arm). Bisiach *et al.* (1986) found that a few patients with severe anosognosia for visual field defect had minimal, if at all, anosognosia for motor impairment. In a study of 206 subacute−chronic neglect patients, Azouvi *et al.* (2002) found that anosognosia for hemiplegia, for visual impairments, and for neglect behavior in everyday life were weakly correlated, suggesting that they may dissociate one with each other. Marcel *et al.* (2004) systematically studied specificity of anosognosia for hemiplegia. They found that unawareness of hemiplegia, somatosensory loss, and visual field defects were all doubly dissociated.

In addition, anosognosia is not an all-or-nothing phenomenon. There are various degrees of severity of anosognosia, which may range from uncritical underestimation to explicit, intractable denial of neurological deficits. A distinction has been made between awareness of a deficit, awareness of its consequences and concurrent awareness of instances of failures entailed by the deficit (Marcel *et al.*, 2004). Several terms have been used to distinguish between these different degrees of anosognosia, such as complete versus incomplete anosognosia, systematic versus partial denial, or verbal versus behavioral anosognosia (Gerstmann, 1942; Willanger *et al.*, 1981). Anton (1889; quoted by Bisiach and Geminiani, 1991) pointed out that a patient may admit his or her hemiplegia and nonetheless set about walking or knitting. Marcel *et al.* (2004) suggested that unawareness of hemiplegia is frequently encountered at the acute phase of stroke, while only unawareness of its consequences commonly persists late after stroke. Moreover, the degree of awareness may wax and wane across the course of a single day. Some patients may temporarily acknowledge their paresis during the demonstration of the motor impairment by the examiner, but deny again their problems just a few minutes later.

Also, dissociations have been repeatedly reported between explicit, verbal awareness and patient's behavior, suggesting that some degree of implicit knowledge may persist in anosognosic patients. Patients may deny any motor impairment but accept to stay in hospital without ever trying to leave their chair on their own. This may be taken as informal evidence of partial knowledge, or as a dissociation of knowledge (McGlynn and Schacter, 1989; Bisiach and Geminiani, 1991; Marcel *et al.*, 2004). Marcel *et al.* (2004) found that some patients who overestimated their current task ability did not overestimate when asked how well the examiner, if he was in their current condition, could do each task. This suggests some form of implicit awareness.

Another peculiar characteristic of anosognosia for hemiplegia is the patient's response to confrontation by the examiner. Some anosognosic patients, when asked why they failed to move their paretic limb, claim that they are too tired or lack interest. Even when faced with obvious contradictions between their statements and their actions, they appear indifferent to these discrepancies.

Characteristics of strokes responsible for anosognosia

Incidence of anosognosia after stroke: Right–left asymmetry

There is a wide consensus that anosognosia is more frequent after right than after left hemisphere stroke. A selection bias due to the difficulty of testing left brain-damaged patients with aphasia cannot account for this asymmetry, which has also been found in studies using intracarotid barbiturate injection (the Wada procedure) (Gilmore *et al.*, 1992; Adair *et al.*, 1995). For example, Adair *et al.* (1995) questioned subjects both during and three minutes after barbiturate injection, and found that 30 of 31 individuals (97%) denied left hemiparesis after right carotid injection, while 15 of 31 (48%) denied right hemiparesis after left carotid injection. The proportion of subjects with anosognosia during or after the procedure was similar.

Studies of anosognosia after stroke yielded similar results. Table 10.1 shows the results from several representative studies. Differences in the reported rate of incidence might be related to different times and/or different methods of assessment. In some studies, anosognosia was assessed on unselected patients at the acute stage of stroke. Stone *et al.* (1993) studied 171 consecutive patients at 2–3 days post-stroke, and found an incidence rate of anosognosia of 28% after

Table 10.1. Frequency of anosognosia for hemiplegia in a sample of representative studies

	n (number of assessable patients)	% RBD (right brain damage)	% LBD (left brain damage)
Nathanson *et al.* (1952)	100	68	32
Cutting (1978)	70	58	14
Hier *et al.* (1983a)	41	36	
Bisiach *et al.* (1986)	36	33	
Levine *et al.* (1991)	13	46	
Starkstein *et al.* (1992)	80	51	16
Stone *et al.* (1993)	171	28	5
Pedersen *et al.* (1996)	566	36	9
Azouvi *et al.* (2002)	206	17	
Beis *et al.* (2004)	78		6
Marcel *et al.* (2004)	64	12–29	0–9

right hemisphere stroke and 5% after left hemisphere stroke. Interestingly, they also found an asymmetric pattern for anosodiaphoria (27% vs. 2% respectively). Similar findings were reported by Pedersen *et al.* (1996), who used a standardized questionnaire (Bisiach *et al.*, 1986) to assess 566 consecutive, unselected acute stroke patients included in a large community-based study (the Copenhagen Stroke Study). Incidence of anosognosia after right and left hemisphere stroke was respectively 36% and 9%. A somewhat lower incidence was reported more recently by Appelros *et al.* (2002; 2003), who studied 349 acute stroke patients (1–4 days post-onset) in a population-based stroke-incidence study. Out of 276 (79%) patients able to complete an anosognosia questionnaire (Starkstein *et al.*, 1992), 48 (17%) showed signs of anosognosia, 26 after right hemisphere damage, 19 after left hemisphere damage and 3 after unknown or bilateral damage.

Studies on subacute/chronic patients also found a right hemisphere prevalence for anosognosia. A recent French multicentre study included subacute stroke patients in rehabilitation units, after a right ($n = 206$) or a left ($n = 78$) hemisphere stroke (Azouvi *et al.*, 2002; Beis *et al.*, 2004). The Bisiach *et al.* (1986) questionnaire was used to assess anosognosia for motor and for visual impairments. Anosognosia for hemiplegia was found in 17% of cases after right hemisphere stroke versus 6% after left hemisphere stroke. Anosognosia for visual impairments was more frequent, but also with a marked right–left asymmetry (incidence respectively 46% and 10%). Marcel *et al.* (2004) systematically assessed different forms of anosognosia in subacute stroke patients (22 left and 42 right). For all questions, unawareness was more common in the right hemisphere damaged group, but the difference was statistically significant only with respect to anosognosia for arm paresis (29% vs. 0%), for touch sensation impairments in the leg (66% vs. 19%), and for dependence in daily-life activities (52% vs. 14%). However, unawareness of somatosensory loss in the arm and of hemianopia was almost as common in left- and in right-brain damaged groups. Finally, in a meta-analysis, Pia *et al.* (2004) selected four studies published over the time period 1938–2001 reporting the prevalence of anosognosia for hemiplegia in relation to the lesion side, on a total of 280 patients. Anosognosia was found in 54.1% of cases after right brain damage and 9.2% after left brain damage, a difference that was highly significant.

Key points Main types of stroke associated with anosognosia for hemiplegia

Stroke type	Territory/characteristics
Arterial Infarct	middle cerebral artery: posterior-inferior and deep branches; anterior choroidal artery
Hemorrhage	Fronto-parietal, lenticular, and thalamus

Recovery

Typically, anosognosia for hemiplegia develops immediately after brain injury and resolves within two weeks, persisting in less than 10% of the patients. In 1953, Critchley (1953) maintained that anosognosia lasting more than "some days" is a disorder associated with "psychiatric features, ranging from a mere confusional to an actual demential state" (pp. 232–4). Hier *et al.* (1983a,b) found that 36% of patients were anosognosic at the acute stage, and the median time to recovery was 11 weeks. Persisting anosognosia late after stroke is uncommon, although a few cases have been reported (Berti *et al.*, 1996; Cocchini *et al.*, 2002; Venneri and Shanks, 2004). Several authors have suggested that chronic anosognosia is always associated with intellectual disorders and/or prefrontal dysfunction. However, case reports of chronic anosognosia without overt intellectual and reasoning deficits have been reported. Venneri and Shanks (2004) recently reported the case of an 85-year-old right-handed woman who showed persistent anosognosia for hemiplegia following a hemorrhagic stroke. Anosognosia was associated with left visuospatial neglect, but there were no global reasoning, memory, or language problems, except for poor performance on verbal fluency tasks. The patient confabulated extensively on themes of active excursions and bizarre acts of persecution. SPECT examination showed an area of hypoperfusion in the right frontal lobe extending beyond the precentral cortex into lateral and orbital associative cortex. Persisting anosognosia was tentatively attributed by the authors to an inability to monitor and check the "real" and especially to assess the truth of mental contents (Venneri and Shanks, 2004).

Anosognosia as a marker of prognosis after right hemisphere stroke

Clinicians often claim that lack of awareness prevents the patients from actively engaging in a rehabilitation program and may be a cause of rehabilitation failure. Early non-systematic observations suggested that left hemiplegic patients have less or slower recovery and less social adjustment than right hemiplegics (Hurwitz and Adams, 1972; Held *et al.*, 1975). Several authors have studied the influence of neglect on functional recovery after stroke. However, as recently outlined by Appelros *et al.* (2003), many of these studies did not use multivariate analysis, thus leaving open the intervention of confounding factors. Denes *et al.* (1982) found that neglect was the worst prognostic factor for functional recovery in hemiplegia, when compared to other cognitive disorders, such as aphasia, intellectual deterioration, or disturbed emotional reactions. This finding has been subsequently largely reproduced by other authors, who showed that neglect has an unfavorable influence upon functional outcome, improvement on rehabilitation, length of hospital stay, and discharge to home (Wade *et al.*, 1983; Fullerton *et al.*, 1986a,b; Paolucci *et al.*, 1996a,b; Kalra *et al.*, 1997;

Katz *et al.*, 1999; Jehkonen *et al.*, 2000). This remains nevertheless a matter of debate, and several recent large and well-designed studies, using multivariate analysis to control for confounding variables, found contradictory results. Pedersen *et al.* (1997) found no independent influence of neglect on recovery, while two other studies reported that neglect had a significant negative impact on functional outcome after controlling for other confounding variables, such as age or stroke severity (Paolucci *et al.*, 1996a,b; Appelros *et al.*, 2002; 2003).

The influence of anosognosia has been less frequently studied. Gialanella and Mattioli (1992) studied patients one and six months post-stroke. They found that extrapersonal neglect alone was not associated with poor recovery, while patients with neglect and anosognosia had the worst motor and functional outcome. However, they only used univariate analyses. Jehkonen *et al.* (2000) reported that hemiparesis and unawareness of illness lengthened the duration of hospital stay, while the presence of a relative reduced it. These three factors were the best predictors of the time from right hemisphere stroke to discharge to home. Sundet *et al.* (1988) found the presence of pathological emotional reactions, including denial of illness, to be a more important predictor of self-reported functional status than other cognitive variables in a multivariate analysis. In a large community-based study, Pedersen *et al.* (1996) found that, although neglect by itself was not a significant independent predictor of poor recovery, anosognosia did have a profound influence on prognosis. Multivariate analyses showed that, after controlling for the influence of other variables, the presence of anosognosia per se predicted 11.5 points less in discharge Barthel index, increased the likelihood of death during hospital stay by a factor of 4.4, and reduced the likelihood of discharge to independent living by 0.43. Appelros *et al.* (2002; 2003), however, found contrasting results in another population-based study. At the acute stage, neglect and anosognosia were both found to influence disability in a multiple logistic regression analysis. Moreover, anosognosia was a stronger predictor than neglect (Appelros *et al.*, 2002). The level of disability was established in survivors after one year, and the authors looked for correlations with cognitive impairments at the acute stage. At that time, only neglect was still significantly associated with dependency (Appelros *et al.*, 2003).

Anatomy of anosognosia for hemiplegia after right brain damage

It is difficult to find an agreement between different studies relative to the intrahemispheric localization of lesions associated with anosognosia for hemiplegia. As recently outlined by Pia *et al.* (2004), it seems that there is no specific brain area involved in causing the denial behavior. Indeed, many different regions, either cortical or subcortical, have been found associated with anosognosia. Bisiach *et al.* (1986) found that, for lesions involving the cortical convexity, anosognosia was associated with inferoposterior parietal damage, while in the case of deep lesions, the more likely anatomical correlates of anosognosia were damage to the thalamus and/or the lenticular nucleus. Quite similar results were reported by Starkstein *et al.* (1992). Other authors emphasized the role of the basal ganglia (Small and Ellis, 1996; Ellis and Small, 1997). They found that the majority (70–79%) of anosognosic patients had a lesion involving this region, while this was observed in only 30% of non-anosognosic patients (Small and Ellis, 1996; Ellis and Small, 1997). The size of the lesion may be an important factor to consider. Hier *et al.* (1983) found that denial of illness occurred consistently only after larger strokes, a finding similar to that of Levine *et al.* (1991). Pedersen *et al.* (1996) also failed to find any particular association of anosognosia with localization of the stroke lesion in any of the cerebral lobes, but found that anosognosia was associated with larger strokes.

Pia *et al.* (2004) conducted a meta-analysis on the anatomy of anosognosia for hemiplegia. When considering lesions restricted to a single cortical structure, anosognosia was equally frequent after damage to frontal, parietal, or temporal lobes. If considering lesions involving more than one lobe, the combination of fronto-parietal and fronto-temporo-parietal lesions seemed to be the most frequent cause of anosognosia. The fronto-parietal combination of lesions was significantly more frequent than all the others. A number of patients (41%) presenting with anosognosia had a lesion involving subcortical structures, that was purely subcortical in 44% of cases. In these patients, there was a slight tendency for a more frequent involvement of the basal ganglia. Pia *et al.* (2004) concluded that anosognosia could be the consequence of a lesion in a fronto-parietal circuit related to space and motor representation.

Assessment of anosognosia

Only a few well standardized and/or semi-quantitative assessment methods for anosognosia have been reported, most of which are of unknown reliability (see Key points). Some of them have been designed specifically to assess anosognosia after right hemisphere stroke. Cutting (1978) was probably one of the first authors to design a standardized anosognosia questionnaire. This questionnaire includes three different levels. The first level uses general questions focusing on awareness of hemiplegia, starting with open questions such as "Why are you here? What is the matter with you?", then using more precise terms such as "is it weak, paralysed or numb?". Then, if denial has been elicited on general questions, two procedures are used: the examiner picks up the patient's arm and requests the patient to lift his arms by himself, while asking him questions such as "What is this? Can you lift it? Can't you see that the two arms are not at the same level?". The third level includes questions addressing anosognosic phenomena, such as anosodiaphoria, non-belongings, misoplegia, and kinesthetic hallucinations.

The scale proposed by Bisiach *et al.* (1986) is probably the most widely used. It includes two parts, one related to anosognosia for motor impairment, and one for visual-field defect. A four-level score is used. A score of 0 is given if the disorder is spontaneously reported by the patient following a general question about his complaints. A score of 1 is given if the disorder is reported only following a specific question about the left limbs' strength. If the disorder is acknowledged only after its demonstration by the examiner, the score is 2. A score of 3 corresponds to no acknowledgement at all of the disorder.

A standardized questionnaire has also been designed by Starkstein *et al.* (1992), with a four-level score ranging from 0 (normal score, the patient is able to spontaneously report the disorder following a general question) to 3 (severe anosognosia).

The Catherine Bergego Scale (Bergego *et al.*, 1995; Azouvi *et al.*, 1996; Azouvi *et al.*, 2003) permits an assessment of awareness of neglect behavior in daily life. Neglect behavior is assessed by an examiner from a direct observation of the patient in ten everyday life situations such as grooming, dressing, eating, spatial orientation, or finding personal belongings. A parallel self-assessment version is given to the patient. Scores range from zero (no neglect) to three for each item. An anosognosia score can be computed from the difference between the examiner's score and the patient's self-assessment. This anosognosia score has been found significantly correlated with neglect severity (Azouvi *et al.*, 1996; 2003).

Other scales have been designed to assess various forms of unawareness. An awareness interview has been designed by Anderson and Tranel (1989) to assess awareness of various cognitive and motor impairments in patients with stroke, head trauma, or dementia. It includes seven question related to different problems (reason for hospitalization, motor impairments, thinking ability, orientation, memory, language, and visual perceptual problems), and a post-test question addressing awareness of quality of test performance and ability to return to normal activities. For each question, a three-level score is used. Unawareness was operationally defined as a discrepancy between the subject's description of abilities and measurement of those abilities by the examiner. The Patient Competency Rating Scale, designed by Prigatano and his colleagues (Prigatano and Altman, 1990; Prigatano *et al.*, 1990), is a standardized questionnaire focusing on ability on various practical skills. The subject's scoring is compared to staff or family ratings. This questionnaire is, however, more specifically designed to assess anosognosia after head trauma rather than anosognosia for hemiplegia.

Key points Assessment of anosognosia after right hemisphere stroke

Source	Methodology
Cutting (1978): standardized questionnaire	Starts with general questions, then focuses on specific impairments; includes assessment of "anosognosic phenomena"
Bisiach *et al.* (1986): standardized questionnaire	Awareness of motor and visual impairments; score uses a 4-level scale (range: 0–3)
Azouvi *et al.* (2003): Catherine Bergego scale	Awareness of behavioral neglect in daily life situations; score based on the difference between therapist's and patient's assessment (range: 0–30)
Prigatano *et al.* (1990): patient competency rating scale	Questionnaire asking the patient and a relative (or staff member) to rate the subject's ability on a variety of practical skills
Anderson & Tranel (1989): awareness interview	Awareness of various cognitive and motor impairments after brain injury; based on a comparison of examiner's and subject's report; three-level score for each question

Pathogenesis

The pathogenesis of anosognosia remains unsettled. The role of *concomitant cognitive or neurological disorders* has been emphasized by some investigators who suggested that disorientation or frontal lobe type deficits could be more frequent in anosognosic patients (Cutting 1978; Levine *et al.*, 1991; Starkstein *et al.*, 1992). A frontal lobe dysfunction could cause a deficit in reality monitoring. However, global mental confusion or major intellectual disturbances seem insufficient to explain anosognosia. Indeed, there are numerous observations of patients with anosognosia and with normal mentation and orientation. Recently, Marcel *et al.* (2004) failed to find an association between anosognosia and scores in frontal lobe tests. Moreover, the fractionation of anosognosia into function-specific forms argues against the explanation of anosognosia in terms of general confusion. In a similar way, there does not seem to be any significant relationship of anosognosia with sensory and/or motor loss (Bisiach *et al.*, 1986; Starkstein *et al.*, 1992; Marcel *et al.*, 2004). So, it is unlikely that anosognosia could simply result from the lack of direct feedback about the affected limb's state (Vuilleumier, 2004).

The relationship of anosognosia with unilateral neglect represents a more complex issue. Patients with neglect, particularly with personal neglect, lack regard for their contralesional limbs and sometimes fail to acknowledge the existence of their left arm or leg (asomatognosia). Logically, an individual without an adequate concept of half the body might not make reliable judgments about the function of these limbs. The frequent association of neglect and anosognosia for motor loss is a common finding in most studies. For example, in the Pedersen *et al.* (1996) study, anosognosia was present in 73% of patients with hemineglect and in 6% of those without hemineglect, a difference that was highly significant. Azouvi *et al.* (2002) also reported statistically significant, albeit moderate, correlations between three measures of anosognosia and unilateral neglect. However, several studies showed that neglect and anosognosia can be doubly dissociated one from each other, thus making unlikely the explanatory power of neglect as a cause of anosognosia. Adair *et al.* (1995) tested personal neglect and anosognosia for hemiplegia after selective anesthesia of the right hemisphere using the Wada procedure, and found that both disorders could be dissociated. Bisiach *et al.* (1986) found clear examples of dissociation between both personal and extrapersonal neglect and anosognosia for hemiplegia, in 97 patients with right hemisphere lesions. Similar findings have been reported by Cutting (1978) who observed that, although personal neglect was rare in patients without anosognosia for hemiplegia, it occurred in only one-third of the anosognosic patients. Extrapersonal neglect was more common than personal neglect, but was present in only half of patients with anosognosia. Dauriac-Le Masson *et al.* (2002) recently reported a double dissociation between unilateral neglect and anosognosia in two patients with a subacute right hemisphere stroke. These different studies permit us to conclude unambiguously that, although anosognosia for hemiplegia is frequently associated with neglect, it is not simply a manifestation of inattention to the left side of egocentric space.

The link between neglect and anosognosia has, however, recently been revisited by Vallar *et al.* (2003) who suggested that one mechanism underlying anosognosia for hemiplegia is unawareness of a deficit of intention, or movement planning component, rather than or in addition to unawareness of a primary motor deficit. They founded their assumption on the results of vestibular stimulation. Indeed, temporary remission of anosognosia after vestibular stimulation may represent recovery from a neglect-related component of which the patient is typically unaware.

Psychological motivation can induce denial for severe and/or disabling medical illnesses, such as heart disease, cancer or AIDS. Refusal to acknowledge illness or putting it out of one's mind is a quite common defense or coping mechanism in such conditions. Healthy persons may also show a natural tendency to use denial mechanisms to deal with environmental stress. Weinstein and Kahn (1953) studied the premorbid personality of patients with anosognosia and found that anosognosic patients used denial mechanisms before their strokes more frequently than did controls. However, this finding has not been reproduced, and such mechanisms could not account for the observation that anosognosia for hemiplegia is more frequent after right then left hemisphere stroke. Moreover, several studies found that anosognosic patients do not seem to show a tendency to deny illness of just any kind (Bisiach and Geminiani, 1991). Nevertheless, emotional changes have been reported in patients with anosognosia, such as apathy, inappropriate cheerfulness, and depression (Cutting, 1978; Levine *et al.*, 1991; Starkstein *et al.*, 1992). It has been suggested that anosognosia might involve a deficient affective drive to respond to uncertainties about current bodily states or current cognitive abilities (Vuilleumier, 2000).

Anosognosia has sometimes tentatively been attributed to a *disconnection mechanism* (Geschwind, 1965a; 1965b). Within this theory, anosognosia for hemiplegia would be related to the isolation of right hemisphere processes from language centers in the left hemisphere. Anosognosic patients could not verbally report transactions within the injured right hemisphere, a structure lacking direct connection to language centers. Without input from the right hemisphere, the "eloquent" brain "confabulates" a response to questions regarding function subserved by the injured brain. However, such a theory could not explain why patients who verbally deny their deficit would not be able to express deficit awareness non-verbally. Moreover, informal observation indicates that bringing the paralyzed extremity into the right visual field does not enhance recognition of deficit. The disconnection hypothesis has been more recently revisited, and it has been suggested that disconnection of a parietal conscious awareness system from particular input modules may result in specific forms of anosognosia (McGlynn and Schacter, 1989; Berti *et al.*, 1998).

The discovery theory has been proposed by Levine *et al.* (1991). This theory rests upon a main premise: deficits are not passively experienced in the same way as other environmental stimuli. In Levine *et al.*'s (1991) words, neurological deficit is not "phenomenally immediate," creating an ambiguous experience for the patient. Hence, patients must learn of dysfunction through a process of self-observation and inference. Levine *et al.* (1991) assert that two broad forms of deficiency preclude that discovery: sensory loss and some cognitive impairment. Recent studies (Marcel *et al.*, 2004) do not support this hypothesis.

Many explanations of anosognosia for hemiplegia view the primary problems in terms of inadequate information or "feedback" from the paralyzed limb to a hypothetical monitor of bodily function. This theory has roots in the sensory loss theory and the discovery theory. According to Heilman (1991), these theories cannot explain denial of hemiplegia when the arm is brought into a normal visual and attentional field and the patient is explicitly asked to monitor the arm's function. Heilman (1991) suggests then a *feedforward or intentional theory:* the intention system would not be able to set the monitor. Under this assumption, anosognosia is a failure of monitoring and may be related to (1) an impaired monitor, (2) the absence of feedback, (3) false feedback, or (4) the improper setting of the monitor.

In summary, there is to date no univocal account for anosognosia. What emerges from the empirical studies is that anosognosia might reflect the impairment of a specific monitoring process, rather than being produced by a combination of somatosensory and cognitive deficits. In addition, as pointed out by Marcel *et al.* (2004), there may be more than one kind of awareness and awareness may differ according to its object. Accordingly, anosognosia could be a non-unitary phenomenon.

Therapy for anosognosia

We are not aware of any controlled study of therapy for anosognosia for hemiplegia. When patients have a complete syndrome of impaired self-awareness, it is futile to try to argue with them. Rather, patients should be examined to determine the extent and the nature of their complete syndrome of impaired awareness. Inevitably, these patients will experience a number of failures that they do not understand. Resistance to rehabilitation emerges usually when their syndrome recovers from complete to partial. Therapists should try to evaluate the method of coping the patient is using when partially aware of something wrong.

Caloric vestibular stimulation may produce a temporary remission of unilateral neglect and of anosognosia. Rode *et al.* (1992) reported a 69-year-old woman who had sustained a right hemisphere stroke and subsequently presented with a complete hemiplegia and delusions concerning her left hemibody when referred to rehabilitation 6 months later. The patient showed a severe extrapersonal and personal neglect as well as a complete anosognosia for both motor and visual deficits. After the first vestibular stimulation, the patient was totally aware of her hemiplegia while unilateral neglect also dramatically improved. The delayed post-stimulation state showed that the anosognosia was less severe as the patient

Key points Management and treatment of anosognosia for hemiplegia

---

Anosognosia: impairs motivation to engage a rehabilitation program
Rehabilitation of anosognosia: further trials required
Compensatory approach
Vestibular Stimulation: temporary remission

---

acknowledged that she could not walk like everybody else. This finding has been subsequently reproduced in a group study (Rode *et al.*, 1998). However, these effects are short-lasting and cannot readily be recommended as a therapy method for anosognosia.

In conclusion, anosognosia remains an unresolved issue, which has major implications for prognosis and functional recovery after right hemisphere stroke. As recently outlined by Vuilleumier (2004) and Marcel *et al.* (2004), there is a need for new experimental approaches and new therapeutic tools to better understand the cognitive and neural mechanisms underlying both awareness of normal functioning and anosognosia of neurological impairments.

REFERENCES

Adair, J. C., Na, D. L., *et al.* (1995). Anosognosia for hemiplegia: Test of the personal neglect hypothesis. *Neurology*, **45**, 2195–9.

Anderson, S. W. and Tranel, D. (1989). Awareness of disease states following cerebral infarction, dementia, and head trauma: Standardized assessment. *The Clinical Neuropsychologist*, **3**, 327–39.

Appelros, P., Karlsson, G. M., *et al.* (2002). Neglect and anosognosia after first-ever stroke: incidence and relationship to disability. *J. Rehabil. Med.*, **34**(5), 215–20.

Appelros, P., Karlsson, G. M., *et al.* (2003). Prognosis for patients with neglect and anosognosia with special reference to cognitive impairment. *J. Rehabil. Med.*, **35**(6), 254–8.

Azouvi, P., Marchal, F., *et al.* (1996). Functional consequences and awareness of unilateral neglect: Study of an evaluation scale. *Neuropsychol. Rehabil.*, **6**, 133–50.

Azouvi, P., Olivier, S., *et al.* (2003). Behavioral assessment of unilateral neglect: Study of the psychometric properties of the Catherine Bergego Scale. *Arch. Phys. Med. Rehabil.*, **84**, 51–7.

Azouvi, P., Samuel, C., *et al.* (2002). Sensitivity of clinical and behavioral tests of spatial neglect after right hemisphere stroke. *J. Neurol. Neurosurg. Psychiatry*, **73**, 160–6.

Babinski, J. (1914). Contribution à l'étude des troubles mentaux dans l'hémiplégie organique cérébrale (Anosognosie). *Rev. Neurol.*, **27**, 845–8.

Beis, J., Keller, C., *et al.* (2004). Right spatial neglect after left hemisphere stroke: Qualitative and quantitative study. *Neurology*, **63**, 1600–5.

Bergego, C., Azouvi, P., *et al.* (1995). Validation d'une échelle d'évaluation fonctionnelle de l'héminégligence dans la vie quotidienne: l'échelle CB. *Annales de Réadaptation et de Médecine Physique*, **38**, 183–9.

Berti, A., Ladavas, E., *et al.* (1996). Anosognosia for hemiplegia, neglect dyslexia, and drawing neglect: clinical findings and theoretical considerations. *J. Int. Neuropsychol. Soc.*, **2**(5), 426–40.

Berti, A., Ladavas, E., *et al.* (1998). Anosognosia for motor impairment and dissociations with patients' evaluation of the disorder: Theoretical considerations. *Cogn. Neuropsychiatry*, **3**, 21–44.

Bisiach, E. and Geminiani, G. (1991). Anosognosia related to hemiplegia and hemianopia. In *Awareness of Deficit after Brain Injury*, ed. G. P. Prigatano and D. L. Schacter. New York: Oxford University Press, pp. 17–39.

Bisiach, E., Vallar, G., *et al.* (1986). Unawareness of disease following lesions of the right hemisphere: anosognosia for hemiplegia and anosognosia for hemianopia. *Neuropsychologia*, **24**, 471–82.

Cocchini, G., Beschin, N., *et al.* (2002). Chronic anosognosia: a case report and theoretical account. *Neuropsychologia*, **40**(12), 2030–8.

Critchley, M. (1953). *The Parietal Lobes*. London: Hafner Press.

(1974). Misoplegia or hatred of hemiplegia. *M. Sinai J. Med.*, **41**, 82–7.

Cutting, J. (1978). Study of anosognosia. *J. Neurol., Neurosurg. Psychiatry*, **41**, 548–55.

Dauriac-Le Masson, V., Mailhan, L., *et al.* (2002). Double dissociation entre négligence unilatérale gauche et anosognosie. *Rev. Neurol.*, **158**, 427–30.

Denes, G., Semenza, C., *et al.* (1982). Unilateral spatial neglect and recovery from hemiplegia. *Brain*, **105**, 543–52.

Ellis, S. and Small, M. (1997). Localization of lesion in denial of hemiplegia after acute stroke. *Stroke*, **28**(1), 67–71.

Fullerton, K. J., McSherry, D., *et al.* (1986). Albert's test: A neglected test of perceptual neglect." *Lancet*, **1**, 430–2.

Gerstmann, J. (1942). Problems of imperception of disease and of impaired body territories with organic lesions. *Arch. Neurol. Psychiatry*, **48**, 890–913.

Geschwind, N. (1965a). Disconnexion syndromes in animals and man. I. *Brain*, **88**(2), 237–94.

(1965b). Disconnexion syndromes in animals and man. II. *Brain*, **88**(3), 585–644.

Gialanella, B. and Mattioli, F. (1992). Anosognosia and extrapersonal neglect as predictors of functional recovery following right hemisphere stroke. *Neuropsychol. Rehabil.*, **2**, 169–78.

Gilmore, R. L., Heilman, K. M., *et al.* (1992). Anosognosia during Wada testing. *Neurology*, **42**(4), 925–7.

Heilman, K. M. (1991). Anosognosia: Possible neuropsychological mechanisms. In *Awareness of Deficit after Brain Injury*, ed. G. P. Prigatano and D. L. Schacter. New York: Oxford University Press, pp. 53–62.

Held, J. P., Pierrot-Deseilligny, E., *et al.* (1975). Devenir des hémiplégies vasculaires par atteinte sylvienne en fonction du côté de la lésion. *Annales de Réadaptation et de Médecine Physique*, **18**, 592–604.

Hier, D. B., Mondlock, J., *et al.* (1983a). Behavioral abnormalities after right hemisphere stroke. *Neurology*, **33**, 337–344.

Hier, D. B., Mondlock, J., *et al.* (1983b). Recovery of behavioral abnormalities after right hemisphere stroke. *Neurology*, **33**, 345–50.

Hurwitz, L. J. and Adams, G. F. (1972). Rehabilitation of hemiplegia: indices of assessment and prognosis. *Br. Med. J.*, **1**(792), 94–8.

Jehkonen, M., Ahonen, J. P., *et al.* (2000). Visual neglect as a predictor of functional outcome one year after stroke. *Acta Neurol. Scand.*, **101**(3), 195–201.

Kalra, L., Perez, I., *et al.* (1997). The influence of visual neglect on stroke rehabilitation. *Stroke*, **28**, 1386–91.

Katz, N., Hartman-Maeir, A., *et al.* (1999). Functional disability and rehabilitation outcome in right hemisphere damaged patients with and without unilateral spatial neglect. *Arch. Phys. Med. Rehabil.*, **80**(4), 379–84.

Levine, D. N., Calvanio, R., *et al.* (1991). The pathogenesis of anosognosia for hemiplegia. *Neurology*, **41**, 1770–81.

Marcel, A. J., Tegner, R., *et al.* (2004). Anosognosia for plegia: specificity, extension, partiality and disunity of bodily unawareness. *Cortex*, **40**(1), 19–40.

McGlynn, S. M. and Schacter, D. L. (1989). Unawareness of deficits in neuropsychological syndromes. *J. Clin. Exp. Neuropsychol.*, **11**(2), 143–205.

Paolucci, S., Antonucci, G., *et al.* (1996a). Predicting stroke in patient rehabilitation outcome: The prominent role of neuropsychological disorders. *Eur. Neurol.*, **36**, 385–90.

Paolucci, S., Antonucci, G., *et al.* (1996b). Facilitatory effect of neglect rehabilitation on the recovery of left hemiplegic stroke patients: A cross-over study. *J. Neurol.*, **243**, 308–14.

Pedersen, P. M., Jorgensen, H. S., *et al.* (1996). Frequency, determinants, and consequences of ansosognosia in acute stroke. *J. Neurol. Rehabil.*, **10**, 243–50.

Pedersen, P. M., Jorgensen, H. S., *et al.* (1997). Hemineglect in acute stroke. Incidence and prognostic implications. The Copenhagen stroke study. *Am. J. Phy. Med. Rehabil.*, **76**, 122–7.

Pia, L., Neppi-Modona, M., *et al.* (2004). The anatomy of anosognosia for hemiplegia: a meta-analysis. *Cortex*, **40**(2), 367–77.

Prigatano, G. P. and Altman, I. M. (1990). Impaired awareness of behavioral limitations after traumatic brain injury. *Arch. Phys. Med. Rehabil.*, **71**, 1058–64.

Prigatano, G. P., Altman, I. M., *et al.* (1990). Behavioral limitations that traumatic-brain-injured patients tend to underestimate. *Clinical Neuropsychologist*, **4**, 163–76.

Prigatano, G. P. and Schacter, D. L. (1991). *Awareness of Deficit after Brain Injury: Clinical and Theoretical Issues*. New York: Oxford University Press.

Rode, G., Charles, N., *et al.* (1992). Partial remission of hemiplegia and somatoparaphrenia through vestibular stimulation in a case of unilateral neglect. *Cortex*, **28**, 203–8.

Rode, G., Perenin, M. T., *et al.* (1998). Improvement of the motor deficit of neglect patients through vestibular stimulation: evidence for a motor neglect component. *Cortex*, **34**(2), 253–61.

Small, M. and Ellis, S. (1996). Denial of hemiplegia: an investigation into the theories of causation. *Eur. Neurol.*, **36**(6), 353–63.

Starkstein, S. E., Fedoroff, J. P., *et al.* (1992). Anosognosia in patients with cerebrovascular lesions: A study of causative factors. *Stroke*, **23**, 1446−53.

Stone, S. P., Halligan, P. W., *et al.* (1993). The incidence of neglect phenomena and related disorders in patients with an acute right or left hemisphere stroke. *Age Ageing*, **22**, 46−52.

Sundet, K., Finset, A., *et al.* (1988). Neuropsychological predictors in stroke rehabilitation. *J. Clin. Exp. Neuropsychol*, **10**(4), 363−79.

Vallar, G., Bottini G., *et al.* (2003). Anosognosia for left-sided motor and sensory deficits, motor neglect, and sensory hemiinattention: is there a relationship? *Prog. Brain Res.*, **142**, 289−301.

Venneri, A. and Shanks M. F. (2004). Belief and awareness: reflections on a case of persistent anosognosia. *Neuropsychologia*, **42**(2), 230−8.

Vuilleumier, P. (2000). Anosognosia. In *Behavior and Mood Disorders in Focal Brain Lesions*. ed. J. Bogousslavsky and J. L. Cummings. Cambridge, UK: Cambridge University Press, pp. 465−519.

(2004). Anosognosia: the neurology of beliefs and uncertainties. *Cortex*, **40**(1), 9−17.

Wade, D. T., Skilbeck, C. E., *et al.* (1983). Predicting Barthel ADL score at 6 months after an acute stroke. *Arch. Phys. Med. Rehabil.*, **64**, 24−8.

Weinstein, E. A. and Kahn, R. L. (1953). Personality factors in denial of illness. *AMA Arch. Neurol. Psychiatry*, **69**(3), 355−67.

Willanger, R., Danielsen, U. T., *et al.* (1981). Denial and neglect of hemiparesis in right-sided apoplectic lesions. *Acta Neurol. Scand.*, **64**(5), 310−26.

11

Asomatognosia

Sebastian Dieguez,[1] Fabienne Staub,[2] and Julien Bogousslavsky[3]

[1]Swiss Federal Institute of Technology, Lausanne, Switzerland
[2]Centre Hospitalier Universitaire Vaudois, Lausanne, Switzerland
[3]Swiss Medical Network, Montreux, Switzerland

General presentation of the disorders of bodily awareness

The sense we have of our own bodies is of a very complex nature. French psychiatrist Henri Ey (1973) wrote: "In this sector of sensibility, neither the primary sensorial organ, neither the specific modality, neither especially the distinction of the subject and the object, are clear notions." In fact, it is through its pathologies that our bodily sense came to be known as a useful theoretical construct.

In this chapter we will use the term *asomatognosia* as the general heading for the disorders of bodily awareness, where one's body may be perceived in an unusual manner, or not perceived as having changed in its functions. Following neurological damage, the body can be entirely or partly forgotten, ignored, denied, disowned, or misperceived. These disorders have proven notoriously difficult to organize and classify. What is more, the topic of asomatognosia is confounded with those of hemineglect, anosognosia, delusions, and more generally all disorders of the awareness of the self. A framework will be proposed in order to see things clearer in this multifaceted topic that draws its unity from phenomenological resemblance, organic overlap, and presumably common mechanisms ranging from sensorimotor functions to higher cognition. Hence, we will state that asomatognosia, roughly defined as the disturbances of the body schema, encompasses a wide array of clinical pictures under a unitary conceptual framework.

The body: Insights from neurology

Maybe the most striking feature of the normal perception of our body is paradoxically that we *do not* notice it. Under normal circumstances, we do not have the slightest idea of the extraordinary complex mechanisms smoothly operating under our skulls to give us a complete and ongoing picture of our corporeal self. This "background" feeling of embodiment has been theorized successively as cenesthesis, somatopsyche and schema. Henry Head (1920)

215

famously described it as the frame of reference by which the brain keeps track of our movements and postural changes, a complex percept of multisensory afferences he called "body schema." A few years after Head's insights, Paul Schilder (1935) proposed another view about the human knowledge of the body, which he conceptualized as the "body image." The distinction between the body schema of Head and the body image of Schilder can be roughly seen as a distinction between implicit—unconscious—automatic processes and explicit—conscious—wilful body knowledge, respectively (Gallagher, 1986; Paillard, 1999).

On assessing the body schema

Testing for disorders of corporeal awareness has always been a problem. Body knowledge involves multiple systems; in fact there is hardly one single cognitive domain that does not intervene at some point, and it has proven very difficult to quantify these disorders, which are inherently subjective. Sometimes it is better to rely on behavioral observation, at other times on verbal accounts. Proposals for assessment have included verbal questionnaires, observational rating scales, self-rating scales, normal mirrors, skewed mirrors, self-drawings, use of dolls and manikins, tests of motor imagery, etc. For a review, see McCrea *et al.* (1982).

Our approach

We will focus on what we see as disorders of the body schema; that is, the ongoing, direct *phenomenal experience* of one's own body. That means we will leave aside disturbances of higher order processes involving one's *body knowledge*, like finger agnosia, autotopoagnosia, ideomotor or visuo-imitative apraxia, which appear as a distortion of the phenomenal body landscape only when the patient is required to achieve very specific and unusual tasks.

What place for asomatognosia? Relationship to anosognosia and related disorders

Usually, the topic of asomatognosia is taken as a subsubject of anosognosia or neglect. Here we propose to do the reverse; that is, to start from asomatognosia as a disorder of the phenomenology and awareness of one's body, and to see where anosognosia and related phenomena fit. This is going back to the way in which these questions were organized early on in the French tradition of neuropsychiatry. For Jean Lhermitte (1939), and then Hécaen and de Ajurriaguerra (1952), it seemed clear that anosognosia was part hemiasomatognosia. The body was the centre of focus. Near the middle of the century, in the USA, perhaps thanks to the popularization of psychoanalysis in the after-war, authors like Weinstein, Goldstein, and Critchley saw hemiasomatognosia as a subtype of the general topic of denial of illness. A hemiasomatognosic patient simply became synonymous with one presenting anosognosia for hemiplegia, the so-called Anton—Babinski syndrome (see Chapter 10). Perceptual, attentional, motivational, and personality factors became the central perspective from which all kind of disorders were seen. In the early 1980s, in Italy, Bisiach, unearthing an obscure but seminal work by Zingerle (1913; see also Benke *et al.*, 2004), made a new step by grouping hemiasomatognosia, anosognosia, unilateral neglect, and delusions under a unified supra-modal center whose disruptions received the general heading of "dyschiria." After that, hemineglect became the focus of a massive industry of behavioral researches, anosognosia gave rise to regular efforts both epidemiological and theoretical, and hemiasomatognosia per se became a neglected issue. More recently, asomatognosia has been seen as a specific disorder of the self (e.g. Feinberg, 2001; Keenan, 2003). Of course, considerations on the anatomical substrate of such symptoms were made all along, with a clear emphasis on a key role for the right parietal lobe and underlying structures.

It now seems clear that to understand asomatognosia we would have to adopt a multidimensional approach which takes into account the respective roles of associated neurological and cognitive signs, levels of general awareness, emotional reactions, as well as psychological factors like personality and contextual factors.

A framework proposal

We propose a comprehensive framework for the disorders of the body schema (Table 11.1). This framework involves two axes that we believe can serve to grossly encompass most of those conditions:

1. the general attitude of the patient, and
2. the breadth of their phenomenal experience.

We also distinguish between specifically unilateral disorders of the body schema, which are usually the result of acute insults to the right hemisphere, and disorders involving the whole body or bilateral parts of it, these being mostly psychiatric or paroxystic in nature and which will be dealt with only briefly in this chapter.

What we call *general attitude* is the way the patient reacts to their damaged new self after a stroke or another neuropsychiatric event. They may be:

1. *indifferent* to the obvious changes they suffer and simply behave like nothing has happened to them;
2. *delusional* about their new feelings and make weird rationalizations to explain them in a factual mode ("This hand *is* not mine, it *is* my mother's"); or
3. *critical* of (or lucid about) whatever strange feelings he may be experiencing, and therefore explain them in a comparative mode ("It is *as if* my hand was not mine anymore").

Table 11.1. A comprehensive framework for disorders of the body schema

		Indifferent	Delusional	Critical
Defective	Unilateral	Hemiasomatognosia (disownership) Motor and personal neglect	Somatoparaphrenia: disownership (limb or half body lost, gone, stolen)	Feeling of absence (illusion of amputation) Hemi-depersonalisation Alien hand syndromes
	Non-unilateral	Pain asymbolia Akinetic mutism	Cotard's syndrome Koro Conversion hysteria	Depersonalisation
Productive	Unilateral	Hallucinatory movements	Somatoparaphrenia: misownership Reduplication of limbs	Supernumerary phantom limb (kinesthetic illusion)
		Allochiria	Personification Misoplegia Hemiconcern	Feelings of transformation, micro/ macrosomatognosia
	Non-unilateral	Bilateral hallucinated movements	Possession Lycanthropy Self-mutilation Ekbom syndrome Body dysmorphic disorder Anorexia nervosa	Alice in wonderland syndrome Heautoscopy, out-of-body experience

Thus, general attitude refers to the manner in which a change in the body schema or the actual body (or both), is perceived: in the first case it is simply not perceived, in the second it is a form of hallucination, and in the third it is an illusion (or hallucinosis).

If *indifferent* and *critical* are general attitudes that seem quite straight-forward and do not need further elaboration, *delusional* maybe needs to be clarified. We will state that a delusion is a false belief that is "firmly sustained despite ... incontrovertible and obvious proof or evidence to the contrary" (DSM-IV, 1994, p. 765; in Davies *et al.*, 2005). In this chapter we deal with delusions specifically concerning the body schema, often restricted to isolated body parts (that is, these patients may sound perfectly reasonable in all other domains).

What we call *breadth of phenomenal experience* is more difficult to define. We follow Metzinger (2003) in his view that the brain creates a phenomenal model of reality, which encompasses the self and the world and that pretty much creates the vivid impression for us human creatures to be someone and to be there. According to this view, our whole life is like a grandiose simulation elaborated by a complex machinery evolved to do just that. This rich multimodal display could arguably be transformed, reduced, or enhanced following a stroke. We propose to subdivide these pathological modifications of phenomenal space into "defective" and "productive" (or "negative" and "positive"). In *defective* forms, something is missing. In *productive* forms, something appears. The distinction between defective and productive disorders may sometimes be quite artificial, but it is useful to distinguish very different clinical pictures. Indeed, the distinction between defective and productive forms of somatognosic disorders was long ago superbly captured in the title of the Hécaen and de Ajuriaguerra masterwork on the subject, *Méconnaissances et Hallucinations Corporelles* (1952), and is now accepted in the literature on hemineglect (Vallar, 1998). Negative and positive symptoms are also seen as plausibly linked by some authors (Gerstmann, 1942; Davies *et al.*, 2005).

Some additional comments on this classification are warranted before we proceed to describe the disorders. First, it has to be emphasized that our framework is not inflexible. Intermediary forms do exist (Hécaen and de Ajuriaguerra, 1952). Second, fluctuations are the norm in somatognosic disturbances, as a single patient may shift on both axes in a matter of minutes or hours, or more slowly as part of the illness course. Third, our framework delineates three modes of general attitude of the patient regarding their disturbed body schema (indifferent, delusional, critical), but it must be emphasized that this does not exhaust the full range of possible emotional nuances and contextual effects that could be involved. Independently of their symptoms, patients may be irritated, angry, fearful, depressed, or even amused. Fourth, one should always bear in mind that these patients may show very different and sometimes dissociated levels of awareness; for example they might perfectly understand the nature of their illness but still make delusional claims about body parts. And last, for all disorders of the body schema, we do not know much about the difference between upper and lower limbs. Bisiach and his colleagues (1986) found that when both upper and lower limbs show sensorimotor impairment, about 20% of patients show dissociated degrees of awareness, and they tend to be less aware of the motor impairment regarding the lower limb. However, clinical impression tells us that hemiasomatognosia and delusions occur more frequently for the upper limb, which seems coherent with the notion that the latter occupies a far more important place in the daily life and higher symbolic activities of humans.

Unilateral disorders

"Indifferent" disorders

"Indifferent" disorders of the body schema refer to patients who are either unaware of the existence or of an impairment of a distal part of their body (defective disorders), or are unaware of the fallacious nature of their perception of it (productive disorders). The attitude of these patients entails an extreme disinterest for the body parts involved.

[Defective] Hemiasomatognosia, personal and motor neglect

The most common use of the term hemiasomatognosia[1] usually refers to patients who behave as if half of their body simply does not exist. This is in fact quite intermingled with what modern authors refer to as anosognosia for hemiplegia, personal neglect, or motor neglect. Nevertheless, this term persists in the literature and from the beginning has suffered from some inconsistencies. It was Jean Lhermitte (1939) who first introduced the word, specifically referring to the phenomenon of "unilateral misperception of one's own body." "Misperception" was to be understood as an ill-defined feeling ranging from unawareness to total estrangement. A patient may behave as if they've never possessed one half of their body, for example denying ownership of their left hand when shown it by the doctor, or attributing it to someone else. They may also manifest perplexity or disgust with their paralyzed limb and even hit it aggressively or try to throw it out of the bed.

Confronted by the over-encompassing content of the notion, authors have tried to further segregate hemiasomatognosia into various dichotomies. Frederiks (1963a) distinguished between conscious and non-conscious forms. "Conscious hemiasomatognosia" refers to cases where a part of the body seems to simply have vanished from one's experiential content, with the experiencer fully and lucidly noticing this "absence" (see critical disorders section). So called "non-conscious hemiasomatognosia," on the other hand, is closely related to anosognosia and neglect after stroke, and this is what most authors commonly refer to as hemiasomatognosia.

---

[1] Other even more disgraceful terms have blossomed to refer to this disorder: autosomatamnesia and autosomatagnosia (Gerstmann), hemisomatagnosia (Semenza), hemisomatoagnosia (Denes), somato-agnosia (Alajouanine), arnesomelia (Critchley).

We would simply say that hemiasomatognosia applies to such instances where a patient shows marked indifference to contralesional distal body parts, behaving as if they didn't exist and had never existed before. When confronted through the visual or tactile modality to these ignored body parts, the patient may show varied reactions, ranging from lucid acceptation of ownership to claims that would put them into the delusional category (and hence would receive the label "somatoparaphrenia" – see later).

In fact, it is not clear whether hemiasomatognosia should be considered as anything other than the most extreme form of personal or motor neglect. Personal neglect refers to a subtype of the neglect syndrome which involves mainly inattention to one's contralesional body. This is the classic textbook depiction of the patient forgetting to comb, shave or make up the left side of his/her head/face. It is very rarely dissociated from the other forms of extrapersonal neglect (Guariglia and Antonucci, 1992; Peru and Pinna, 1997; Buxbaum *et al.*, 2004). Somatosensory hemineglect, a defective awareness of contralesional tactile or proprioceptive stimuli (Vallar, 1998), mostly found under extinction paradigms and rarely dissociated from neglect in other modalities, is also somehow conflated with hemiasomatognosia. The term "motor neglect" has been proposed for patients who fail to use their contralesional limbs in the absence of obvious primary sensorimotor deficits (Castaigne *et al.*, 1970). This has been influential on theories of hemispatial neglect based on brain mechanisms for action, and is diversely accounted for as a motor-intentional or feed-forward disturbance, a hemispatial limb akinesia, or a directional akinesia (Heilman and Adams, 2003). Again, this forgetfulness could well be an important part of the defective, "indifferent" view of hemiasomatognosia we are holding here, and is perfectly compatible with what we see as a profound unilateral disturbance of the body schema.

[Productive] Hallucinatory movements (kinesthetic hallucinations), allochiria

In this section we will only address the cases where a patient experiences a feeling or a movement that did not happen, and clearly fails to notice the aberrant nature of their experience. It is important to distinguish these hallucinations from the illusory forms that will be addressed in the "critical"/ productive section. Nevertheless, a common denomination of these kinesthetic hallucinations is "illusory limb movements," and this term may be somewhat valid insofar as the patient is able to spontaneously criticize their actually mistaken experience. The observation is not rare in the neurological ward: when asked to raise their left arm, the patient says they are done, when in fact nothing happened. Feinberg *et al.* (2000) studied these "illusory limb movements" in patients with left hemiplegia, and found that they are strongly associated with the degree of anosognosia and to a lesser extent with hemispatial neglect. These authors explicitly argued against viewing these manifestations as phantoms, in favor of a confabulatory explanation (in this view, anosognosic patients do not really experience a movement, they just unconsciously make up a story to comply with the experimenter, thereby protecting their self-integrity). However, we see no reason to deny that at least some of these patients really believe and feel they have actually moved, and that such a strong feeling is likely to denote the presence of a phantom phenomenon (see Bakheit, 2000). Some patients seem to border on the delusional, as when they claim to actually *see* their arm moving, *hear* their hands clapping or *feel* the nose of the experimenter. These cases do not preclude the presence of a phantom, but additional disturbances are clearly involved and may include mechanisms similar to other confabulatory manifestations (Hirstein, 2005).

We wish to advance here a third explanation of kinesthetic hallucinations, different from the phantom and confabulation accounts just given. We find very plausible that some remarkable responses of right-damaged patients may be explained by a transfer of the experiential content from the contralesional side to the ipsilesional, as is sometimes the case with extrapersonal hemineglect (Manly *et al.*, 2002). This is known diversely as allochiria, alloesthesia or allo-kinesia, and could be a mechanism for certain forms of hemiasomatognosia. This may manifest itself on request, when the patient raises the right arm when asked to raise the left one, or in the spontaneous grasping and exploratory movements of the right hand. Maybe the movements the patient intends genuinely to do with their left arm are unconsciously "transposed" to the right side. Marcel *et al.* (2004a) demonstrated that about 25% of normals are suscep-tible to migration and fusion of tactile stimuli from one hand to the other. During simultaneous stimulation on both hands, using slightly different stimuli, these persons have a tendency to fuse or replace the stimuli on an attended hand with that which was felt on the other unattended hand. The authors speculate that this might be a premorbid tendency analogous to the disorders of bodily spatial mislocations in brain-damaged patients, as seen especially in right-hemisphere damaged patients. It is possible that this premorbid suscept-ibility also participates in the development of hemiasomatognosia and may account for some aberrant motor responses these patients make.

"Delusional" disorders

"Loss of awareness of one's body, asomatognosia is an acquired disorder observed in victims of right hemisphere stroke who may perceive all or part of a body half as being strange, transformed, or even totally alien." This definition of asomatognosia given by Paysant *et al.* (2004) perfectly shows the lack of conceptual care with which the subject is usually handled. How could one have no *awareness* of one's half-body and yet *perceive* it as alien, strange, and or transformed? This is why we thought it useful to distinguish between defective and productive forms of asomatognosia. Furthermore, we wanted to restore the original meaning of the term *somatoparaphrenia*, as it was clearly intended by Gerstmann (1942), to denote delusional manifestations. Hence, as soon as a patient makes overtly bizarre claims about his experience, we are in the realm of somatoparaphrenia (Table 11.2).

[Defective] Somatoparaphrenia: Disownership[2]

Some patients are clearly delusional in their claim that some part of their body is missing, and it is in this sense that we label these forms as defective. However, it is obvious that from a phenomenological point of view, many of these patients are clearly overproductive in their claims about the purported "loss." We fully acknowledge that any delusion is by definition "productive," and therefore this may be one conceptual inconsistency of our framework. These patients may claim that a limb has been simply lost or gone, but also stolen or chopped, sometimes as a result of some elaborated paranoid scheme. But importantly, no further productive elaboration on the nature of the contralesional half is provided, so we feel that there is a sense in delineating a category of delusional/defective disorders, as those patients seem to absurdly rationalize a unilateral narrowing of their phenomenal bodily experience.

The milder form of this kind of delusion may simply manifest itself in the patient who repetitively holds, despite evidence to the contrary, that their left hand does not pertain to them. This is of course very close to hemiasomatognosia and it may indeed be difficult to decide whether the claim derives from a really delusional belief or not. One case reported by Hécaen and de Ajurriaguerra (1952, observation 13, pp. 60–70) illustrates this difficulty: this patient spontaneously denied ownership of his left hand, but without attributing it to someone else (he only said "It's not mine" when shown it). However, he attributed to himself (or "appropriated") one hand of the examiner ("There is mine, now I have two of them!'). The patient clung to that idea even when the examiner made movements with his hand or walked backwards. However when the doctor was two meters away, he said: "I'm beginning to wonder if it's not mine."

---

[2] The term "disownership" is taken from Starobinski (1982), who introduced the word "désappartenance" in French to denote the delusional loss of one's body in Cotard's syndrome. Here we use it in contrast to "misownership," which would not only be a loss of ownership of one's body part, but also a delusional replacement of it by some other entity. *Dis*ownership is a defective experience, *mis*ownership is a productive one.

Table 11.2. Diverse manifestations of somatoparaphrenia

Content of delusion	Limb considered lost or stolen	Hoff and Potzl, 1935; Halligan *et al.*, 1995
	Own limb attributed to someone else's same body part (doctor, nurse, niece, husband)	Bottini *et al.*, 2002
	Someone else's limb appropriated by the patient (family, medical staff, neighboring patients)	Hécaen and de Ajuriaguerra, 1952
	A whole body felt on one's side with negative content: an old man, a cadaver, a little "nigger" with sexual content ("erotoplegia"), sometimes incestuous: a woman, one's daughter a child	von Hagen and Ives, 1937; Assal, 1983; Zingerle, 1913; Ehrenwald, 1930; Morin *et al.*, 2003
	Limb perceived as horrible: disfigured, deformed, rotten, strange	Lhermitte, 1939
	Limb claimed to have been replaced (Capgras arm)	Ives and Nielsen, 1937
	Limb perceived as different: size, weight, length, colour, texture (macro-microsomatognosia). Rarely delusional.	Frederiks, 1963b
	Delusional reduplication of body parts	Weinstein *et al.*, 1954
	Limb perceived as an animal, dead, alive, part of it or entire (usually snake)	Potzl, 1924
	Limb perceived as "some flesh"	Lhermitte, 1939
	Limb perceived as an object: a prosthesis, stilts, a plank	Hécaen and Ajuriaguerra, 1952; Ehrenwald, 1930
	Half-body perceived as a "presence," a "ghost"	Critchley, 1953
	Limb felt as possessed by a dead relative or the devil	Nightingale, 1982
	Unspecified: "a strange," "a mass," "a plaque"	Marcel *et al.*, 2004b
	Whatever is covered by the use of nicknames for the plegic limb	Critchley, 1955
Emotional reactions	Disgust, aversion, hostility for limb, not necessarily misperceived (misoplegia). Very rarely mutilations	Critchley, 1974, Personal observation
	Mild or severe paranoid content - staff or other patient suspected of making cruel jokes - limb felt as one's own, but fear that somebody might steal it	Hécaen *et al.*, 1954, Personal observation
	Sexual content	Critchley, 1953

Table 11.2. (*Cont.*)

Indifference, no affective reaction	Assal, 1983
Other reactions: depression, anxiety, amusement, irritation	Critchley, 1955
Patient spontaneously asks to get rid of the misperceived limb or vehemently complains to the staff	Ehrenwald, 1930; Hécaen *et al.*, 1954
Delusion appears only on confrontation	Assal, 1983
Excessive concern for the plegic limb (hemiconcern, "philoplegia"), sometimes delusional (personification)	Bogousslavski *et al.*, 1995; Critchley, 1955

[Productive] Somatoparaphrenia: Misownership, delusional reduplication of body parts, personification of the plegic limb, misoplegia, hemiconcern

The most common form of productive somatoparaphrenia is as follows: when shown their own left hand, the patient claims it is not theirs, but the doctor's. This is already a full step further from the mere claim that the hand shown is not one's hand. The patient has moved from a defective delusion to a productive one. However, we wish to caution against jumping too fast to the conclusion that this is necessarily delusional. Indeed, attributing the hand emerging from the neglected left visual field to the closest person around may be the only logical solution to the left hemiplegic patient, for they see a hand that they don't feel. The same can be said in cases where the patient appropriates someone else's hand as their own, which is another form of somatoparaphrenia. Nevertheless, little doubt remains as to the delusional nature of the claim when the patient attributes their hand to someone who is clearly *not* present (a nurse, another doctor, some relative), or indeed to a *dead* person (Assal, 1983; Feinberg, 2001). These types of delusion may appear spontaneously or only on demand. Some patients may even act on their delusional belief, like the one described by Hécaen and colleagues (1954) who wrote a letter to a nurse complaining about her robbed arm.

Delusional claims about parts of one's body are reminiscent of the mis-identification syndromes. For instance, Ives and Nielsen (1937) observed a case of delusional replacement of the left arm. The patient said: "Someone is substituting this arm [pointing to the left, paralyzed one] for my left arm," "my wife rubbed this arm, but it wasn't my arm." These are claims that one cannot help but compare to the Capgras syndrome.

When encouraged to seek their left hand from the shoulder downwards, somatoparaphrenic patients, in contrast to "mild" hemiasomatognosics, may still deny ownership of their upper limb (Assal, 1983). One patient put it this way, after being clearly shown that her left arm merged with her shoulder, so that it *must* be hers: "But my eyes and my feelings don't agree, and I must believe my feelings. I know they look like mine, but I can feel they are not, and I can't believe my eyes" (quoted in Nielsen, 1938a). As is the case with anosognosia, fluctuations are the norm in these patients, especially when confronted. They may be forced to acknowledge the irrationality of their claims, but soon after, they show a strange amnesia for the lucid episode and go back to their delusion.

Occasionally, one can encounter very prolific patients that defy understanding and attempts at classification. Ehrenwald (1930) described such a case. When asked to show his left hand, this patient searched for it everywhere and when he finally found it, he maintained that it was not the good one, the one found being different from the real one. He then argued that, in fact, he left his real hand at home. Totally anosognosic for his hemiplegia, he claimed that there was a "nest of hands" in his bed and wanted the doctor to get rid of them. This is reminiscent of the "delusional reduplication of body parts" that some patients may display in a state of confusion. They may claim to have several new limbs or any body part and to be able to see, touch, and manipulate them. They also frequently have other reduplicative delusions involving people, places, or events (Bechterev, 1926; Weinstein *et al.*, 1954).

Sometimes it appears that the delusional content is directly related to the patient's life experience, as in a former slaughterhouse employee described by Lhermitte (1939) who complained that his left arm had been turned into a large chunk of dead flesh separated from him and suspended near his bed. The affected limb is sometimes felt as possessed by an external entity, like a dead relative or the devil (Nightingale, 1982). Other times, it is the patient who gives it an identity of its own, a manifestation called "personification" by Critchley (1955). In his words: "The crippled and useless limbs are referred to as though invested with a personality or identity of their own, but in a semi-facetious proprietary fashion, as one might look upon a plaything or a pet." The simplest manifestations are when the limb is addressed in the third person: "she," "it," "he," or "him." Some patients even give a nickname to their plegic limb. Critchley also coined the term "misoplegia" to denote the behavior displayed by some hemiplegic patients, who seem to profoundly hate or dislike their paretic limb: "The hemiplegic patient develops a morbid dislike directed towards the offending immobile limbs. It is not a hostile or paranoid reaction towards the actual fact of his being crippled or paralyzed" (Critchley, 1974). These cases are by definition aware of their hemiparesis, therefore they are not anosognosic. The patient feels an estrangement regarding their half-body and displays a behavior that can range from a simple feeling of disgust to organized self-inflicted harm (Figure 11.1).

It is sometimes hard to say if it is a full-blown delusion or not. Misoplegia usually emerges after a period of anosognosia and may represent a form of emotional response when the cruel reality is faced. Interestingly, however, both conditions have been observed to cohabit alternatively in the same patient (Moss and Turnbull, 1996).

Another mode of reaction in some patients may be considered the opposite of misoplegia. This has been called "hemiconcern" and refers to patients who over-focus on the left part of their body (Bogousslavsky *et al.*, 1995). They can look at it for long periods of time, rub it, cuddle it, pinch it, and manipulate it. This peculiar behavior concerned only their own bodies and resolved in a few days when the hemisensory loss improved. Maybe critically, none of these patients had hemispatial neglect or anosognosia.

"Critical" disorders

We now turn to unilateral "critical" disorders of the body schema. Situations where the patient is lucid about the unusual nature of their experience, and therefore is neither indifferent nor delusional, correspond partially to what Frederiks (1963a) labeled "conscious hemiasomatognosia." These include patients who distinctly feel as if half of their body has vanished or who experience it as dramatically diminished from their conscious bodily representations.

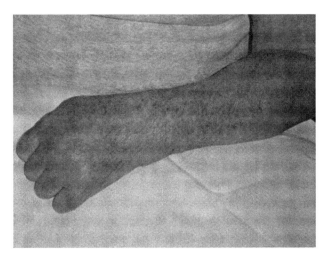

Figure 11.1 Self inflicted lesions in a misoplegic patient. This patient claimed that he wanted to take revenge on his paralysed left arm by physically mistreating it. He actually did so by striking it violently on the table, scratching it, inserting needles in it, and even by self-inflicting cigarette burns. He kept repeating his auto-aggressions so much that his wife had to constantly monitor him (personal case).

Alien hand syndromes will also be discussed in this section, although with some conceptual caveats.

[Defective] feeling of absence (true feeling of amputation), hemi-depersonalization, phantom amputation, alien hand syndromes

To get an idea of what it is like to feel one's body as incomplete, we have to turn to the rare phenomenon of the "feeling of absence," which is also called "true feeling of amputation," and usually involves a lateralized part of the body. It might be seen as the reverse of the classic "phantom limb" of the amputated, as most amputated subjects do not feel like a body part is missing but instead live with the strong illusion that the missing part is still there (for a fictional account, see Weir-Mitchell, 1905). In the "feeling of absence" a part of the body seems to be missing, or in other words the body is oddly felt as complete *without* a lateralized part. Sometimes, a part of the body is experienced as if it had been separated from the rest of the body. A limb may seem to be floating in the air, a few centimeters away from the trunk. Those feelings are mainly the result of short-term paroxystic fits or migraine (Hécaen and de Ajuriaguerra, 1952; Frederiks, 1963a), though illusions such as the impression that a part of the body is lost have also been described after strokes, usually of subcortical localization (Cambier *et al.*, 1984; Peru and Pinna, 1997). There is no necessary hemiplegia, ansosognosia or unilateral spatial neglect associated with these feelings.

The term "hemi-depersonalization" refers to a similar disorder, though here the part of the body is not perceived as absent but as alien or bizarre, somehow less rich in phenomenal content (Ehrenwald, 1931; Lhermitte, 1939; Critchley, 1953). The patient is aware of their strange experience, which is usually of short duration, and is often able to provide full details of it. Visual feedback may relieve the unpleasant sensation, but usually is not enough to restore the feeling of completeness. Frederiks (1969) suggests that such feelings of absence are of subcortical origin, but evidence is clearly still insufficient in this area.

Even rarer in the stroke unit is the very special case of "phantom amputation." This should be investigated whenever a previously amputated individual suffers a stroke. Such patients sometimes feel modifications of an already existing phantom, including the disappearance thereof. In amputated subjects, phantoms are thought to partly arise from some cortical remapping that occurs when deafferented somato-sensory areas are taken over by adjacent areas (Ramachandran and Hirstein, 1998). If these reorganized cortices are further damaged, one may think that the phantom would equally be challenged at the phenomenal level. Indeed, there is evidence that this occurs (Bornstein, 1949; Appenzeller and Bicknelle, 1969; Yarnitsky *et al.*, 1988).

Alien hand phenomena seem difficult to situate in our scheme. We feel they are of a very different nature from the other disorders just described. Here, one's hand is not felt to be controlled by oneself, but seems to have a life of its own. The patient is usually not delusional and is fully aware that something is going wrong. Phenomenal space seems to be broken down (loss of a feeling of agency) and enhanced (something "alien" has taken control) at the same time. The feeling of ownership seems ambiguous and the emotional reaction of the patient is very much present, mostly charged with negative affects (though positive cases have been described by Groom *et al.*, 1999). Only in certain rare cases, the patient with an alien hand manifests a full-blown delusion of disownership (Feinberg *et al.*, 1998). What authors have meant by "alien hand" is enormously diverse. It was initially introduced to refer to the elaborate goal-directed movements of the left hand that the callosotomized subject feels are out of his control (Bogen, 1979). The French term "main étrangère" seems closer to hemiasomatognosia in that the patient mistakes his left hand for that of someone else (Brion and Jedynack, 1972). French authors have also the expression "main capricieuse," which is analogous to Bogen's alien hand, to refer to the fact that the hand, usually the left one, seems to disobey the intentions of the patient. "Intermanual conflict," "compulsive utilization of objects," "anarchic hand," "wayward hand," "callosal apraxia," "diagonistic dyspraxia," "agonistic dyspraxia," "repulsive/magnetic apraxia," "levitation" are other colorful terms, often overlapping in their meaning, that refer to disorders in the awareness of manual motor control (Bakchine *et al.*, 1999; Scepkowski and Cronin-Golomb, 2003; Biran and Chatterjee, 2004). Feinberg *et al.* (1992) have argued for the existence of two kinds of alien hand phenomena, which they called callosal and frontal. The callosal type manifests itself mostly as intermanual conflict, with the nondominant left hand acting out of control and often mirroring, or getting in the way of, the intentional right-hand movements. The frontal type would affect the dominant hand and presents itself as compulsive tool manipulation, a kind of elaborated grasp reflex. Another more recent dichotomy has been made between anterior and posterior forms, with the former being more of the frontal type, and the latter manifesting itself as purposeless anarchic or levitating movements (Scepkowski and Cronin-Golomb, 2003). Recent publications have proposed a somewhat different view, arguing that posterior lesions account for the intermanual conflict and anterior ones, added to the former, produce a kind of intra-cognitive conflict, whereby a patient may suffer from interminable doubts, hesitations, and changes of intentions (Nishikawa *et al.*, 2001; Barbeau *et al.*, 2004).

Table 11.3. Comparison of illusory and delusional supernumerary limbs

Supernumerary phantom limb	Delusional reduplication of body part
Illusion	Delusion–hallucination
No confusion	Confusion
Installation often delayed	Acute phenomenon
Can be persistent	Limited in time
Central or peripheral lesion	Central lesion only
Lesion can be limited	Large brain lesion/dysfunction
Right or left hemisphere damage	Right hemisphere damage
Subcortical lesion more frequent	Cortical involvement (especially parietal)
Duplication always concerns the affected limb	Duplication can involve any body part

[Productive] Feelings of transformation, illusory supernumerary limb

When made in similitic mode, often using the qualifier "as if," unusual claims about one's body parts can be included in the present category. This happens in other instances, mostly paroxystic or of subcortical etiology, where the fully lucid patient complains that unilateral parts of his body now feel changed in many possible respects. These include changes in sensation, as in mild somatosensory numbing or severe thalamic painful syndrome, but also in varied qualities of the limb, like weight, form, length, volume, speed of movement, temperature, etc. These are not delusions, but could be theorized as the starting point of aberrant elaborations if higher cognitive mechanisms are also disturbed (Davies *et al.*, 2005). Frederiks (1963b), for instance, made clear that what he called micro- and macrosomatognosia were not delusions. In these cases, the patient perceives parts of his body (or indeed the entire body) as abnormally small or large, respectively.

Damage to the central nervous system can sometimes produce illusory limbs, called supernumerary phantoms because they are experienced as an additional part of the body, in most cases a third limb. These patients are fully aware of the illusory nature of their perception, but they may nevertheless suffer considerable anxiety from their strange experience (Table 11.3). Observations of supernumerary phantom limbs are scarce in the literature, but different forms of the phenomenon seem to exist. Most cases experience their extra limb as a somesthetic illusion replacing the plegic limb in an immobile manner. Voluntary control of the supernumerary phantom limb is exceptional, but we have recently described such a case (Staub and Bogousslavsky, 2005; see Figure 11.2). Finally, the supernumerary phantom can merely be a kind of "trace" left by a normal limb, where the phantom occupies the previous position of the real limb after a short delay (McGonigle *et al.*, 2002).

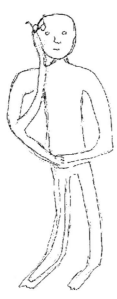

Figure 11.2 Patient self-drawing showing her supernumerary phantom limb. This phantom only "appeared" when the patient commanded her right plegic arm to move.

Non-unilateral disorders of the body scheme

To conclude this review, we will provide a quick overview of disorders involving misperception of the whole body or of non-lateralized parts of it. Most of them are rather seldom found in the stroke unit, but as they all may plausibly be conceived as disorders of the body schema, they may therefore be linked to an impairment of the cerebral structures underlying somatognosia.

"Indifferent" disorders
Defective

Akinetic mutism and catatonia. Akinetic mutism (see Chapter 22) has been conceptualized as a potential form of bilateral motor neglect by Heilman and Adams (2003). These patients give the impression of simply ignoring their own existence as a whole, or at least of dramatically under-using their body when they would in fact be perfectly able to do so. This neurological disorder is strongly reminiscent of the classic manifestations of catatonia, and both have been related to a profound disorder of willed action due to the disruption of cortico-sub-cortical midline structures involving the anterior cingulate gyrus (Northoff, 2002; Nagaratnam *et al.*, 2004).

Pain asymbolia. Schilder and Stengel introduced this term in 1931 to denote "patients who are able to perceive the presence of a painful stimulus, but show a lack of concern about it" (Nagasako *et al.*, 2003). Although described as a disorder involving mainly the left hemisphere by Hécaen and de Ajurriaguerra (1952), it actually seems to rely on lesions of the depth of the primary somatosensory areas, mostly the insula and the cingulum, irrespective of side, and has been theorized as a sensori-limbic disconnection (Berthier *et al.*, 1988; Ramachandran, 1998).

Productive

Whole-body hallucinations. This would involve hallucinatory movements extended bilaterally and could include, quite speculatively, full immersion in daily dreaming, non-critical out-of-body experiences, and hypnagogic/hypnopompic hallucinations. In such cases, the brain manages to produce a virtual healthy body of a sort, a hallucinated self unaware of the actual state of the real body (Metzinger, 2003). We are unsure if brain damage could produce such states.

"Delusional" disorders
Defective

Cotard's syndrome. "Délire des négations" was the term initially proposed by Jules Cotard for the disorder that now bears his name (Cotard, 1880; 1882). Lhermitte (1939) interpreted this delusion as a "total asomatognosia." It is often described as the delusion of being dead; however, the cases initially described presented many other features and some patients claimed in fact not to be dead at all, but immortal (Starobinski, 1982). The syndrome includes deeply negativist ideas, self-deprecatory delusions, a distorted view of the outside world, perceptual anomalies, and delusions about the body. A profound disturbance of the body schema has been advanced as the key mechanism (Ferro, 2003), plausibly involving a right hemisphere disturbance (Young and Leafhead, 1996).

Conversion hysteria. Somatoform conversion, the classic manifestation of hysteria, manifests itself as various disturbances of the body schema. A decrease in subcortical regional blood-flow has been shown to correlate with hysterical sensorimotor loss (Vuilleumier *et al.*, 2001).

Koro syndrome. Koro syndrome is mostly a culture-bound syndrome, initially described in Southwest Asia, in which the victim experiences a sudden and intense fear that his penis is going to shrink and to retract in the abdomen, or indeed has already done so. It has been occasionally linked to unspecified organic brain damage (Durst and Rosca-Rebaudengo, 1991).

Productive

Eating disorders. Patients with eating disorders are well known to suffer from a defective body image. They often have a very distorted idea of what they look like. This is especially the case with anorexia nervosa where, among other symptoms, the patient feels overweight despite obvious evidence to the contrary. Anorexia has been described following temporal lobe epilepsy (Signer and Benson, 1990) or tumors involving the ventromedial hypothalamus (Herzog and Copeland, 1985). It has also been observed to resolve after a left thalamic stroke (Dusoir *et al.*, 2005).

Ekbom syndrome. Also called delusional parasitosis or presenile dermatozoic delusion, Ekbom's syndrome is the delusion that one's body is infested with bugs. It mainly affects depressed elderly women, who sometimes go as far as to try extracting the parasites they feel under their skin. Organic factors like dementia, drug psychosis, real dermatological infections, and cerebrovascular disease are present in most cases (Flynn *et al.*, 1989; Benattar *et al.*, 2004).

Body dysmorphic disorder. Dysmorphophobia, or body dysmorphic disorder, is a disabling preoccupation with a nonexistent or slight defect in one's physical appearance, an irrational disgust with one's whole body or non-lateralized parts of it. These patients have a poor insight and are often delusional. Their major concern is with their face, but virtually all surfaces and parts of their body can be the focus of excessive worry. It has been linked in one case to an inflammatory process inducing a left frontotemporal atrophy (Gabbay *et al.*, 2003).

Self-induced harm. Self-injurious behaviors in the general sense encompass all deliberate, non-accidental, and repetitive infliction of self-harm without suicidal intent. Such behaviors are not infrequent in the psychiatric population and could be related to a compulsive need for bodily physiological tension reduction (Brain *et al.*, 1998). The neuroanatomical underpinnings of self-harm are unknown, but clues could be obtained from Gilles de la Tourette syndrome, in which it is quite common (Mathews *et al.*, 2004).

Possession and lycanthropy. Two rather spectacular forms of productive delusions are cases of demoniacal possession and lycanthropy. These patients respectively behave and feel as if they were inhabited by some malevolent entity or as if they have just shape-shifted into some animal. These disorders have historically been linked to the development of neuropsychiatry, and one can still sometimes observe these colorful clinical pictures following acute psychosis or brain damage (Assal, 1985; McCormick and Goff, 1992; Noll, 1992). They have been interpreted as extreme delusional manifestations of depersonalization.

"Critical" disorders
Defective

Depersonalization. Depersonalization is the feeling that one is not quite oneself anymore. It is usually a stressful sudden event, and is accompanied by hypochondriac feelings, difficulties thinking, disturbed perception and recognition of the external world, as well as the sensation of not inhabiting one's body (Dugas and Moutier, 1911). It is the key component of the now called dissociative disorders. A link with anosognosia, asomatognosia, somatopara-phrenia and Cotard's syndrome has been made long ago (Ehrenwald, 1931; Lhermitte, 1939). There is recent evidence that it is primarily the result of a right hemisphere disturbance (Simeon *et al.*, 2000; Sierra *et al.*, 2002; Duggal, 2003).

Productive

Alice in Wonderland syndrome. This elegant eponym refers to the illusion that one's body or parts of it are shrinking or enlarging (Todd, 1955), similarly to what Frederiks (1963b) called micro- and macrosomatognosia. These per-ceptual distortions can also involve other persons or objects (metamorphopsia), and feelings of levitation. They are mostly found during seizures or migraine.

Heautoscopy and out-of-body experience. Under the general heading of "auto-scopic phenomena," heautoscopy and out-of-body experiences refer to the illusion that one is leaving one's body, usually with a preserved awareness of the situation, as the "real body" is often reported to be seen at a distance. Evidence is accumulating for a plausible neurological account of these phenomena, involving subnormal activity at the temporo-parieto-occipital junction (Metzinger, 2005; Blanke *et al.*, 2004).

Anatomical correlates and mechanisms

Many of the neurological disorders just described are still in need of an explanation, and there is no clear distinction on the etiology and mechanisms that lead to their many clinical presentations (see Table 11.4).

Neither the prevalence nor the precise stroke location of these disorders has been systematically studied in large series of consecutive stroke patients to our knowledge.

Lesions of the right hemisphere are overwhelmingly the norm for these disorders. Though the obvious matter of aphasia precluding the demonstration of such symptomatology, following left-sided lesions, has been raised, this argument is not sufficient to contradict the dominance of the right hemisphere for asomatognosia. Many facets of asomatognosia would anyway be visible only by observing the patient without requiring verbal reports, and the comparison of right- and left-brain damaged subjects reveals a right hemisphere dominance concerning aspects of bodily representation, somatic attention, and evaluation

Table 11.4. Lesion location of disorders of the body schema

Hemiasomatognosia	Right gyrus supramarginalis and underlying structures
Somatoparaphrenia	Posterior right hemisphere, right insula, subcortical structures (right or left)
Misoplegia	Right hemisphere
Alien hand syndrome	Corpus callosum (mostly anterior part), medial frontal lobe, right posterior structures
Supernumerary phantom limb	Subcortical structures (right or left), right frontomesial
Feeling of amputation	Subcortical structures (right or left)
Hemiconcern	Right postcentral gyrus, upper and middle temporal gyri, anterior and inferior areas of the parietal gyrus and supramarginal gyrus.

of (and concern for) plausibility, all of which are largely relevant for asomatognosia disorders (Marcel *et al.*, 2004b). Furthermore, intracarotid amytal studies fail to find asomatognosic disorders following left hemisphere inactivation. After right hemisphere inactivation, however, subjects very often manifest hemiasomatognosia, which they do not remember after recovery (Adair *et al.*, 1995; Meador *et al.*, 2000). On a more anecdotal level, Feinberg (2001, pp. 11–12) wrote: "I have examined over one hundred patients with asomatognosia and not a single case was caused by damage to the left hemisphere with nonrecognition of the right arm or leg. One reason the left arm is more commonly affected with the condition than the right may be due to the association between asomatognosia and hemispatial neglect." Indeed, Feinberg *et al.* (1990) found that neglect was a necessary condition for the occurrence of "verbal asomatognosia" in the group of patients they studied. The relationship between hemiasomatognosia and anosognosia, another right hemisphere disorder, has been poorly investigated, although the existence of dissociations has been recognized a long time ago (Lhermitte, 1939). Indeed, in most patients with anosognosia, the cardinal sign of hemiasomatognosia – not recognizing one's own hand – cannot be evidenced (Heilman *et al.*, 1998). Furthermore, cases with hemiasomatognosia have also been reported without anosognosia, albeit perhaps more rarely (Morin *et al.*, 2002; Halligan *et al.*, 1995). At the moment, it seems reasonable to state that anosognosia may be a sufficient but not necessary candidate to induce at least defective forms of hemiasomatognosia, whereas hemineglect seems to be necessary, but not sufficient.

Somatoparaphrenia usually also involves neglect and is overwhelmingly caused by damage to the right hemisphere. This is part of the general idea that the right hemisphere is more prone to delusions when damaged (Cutting, 1990; Kumral and Öztürk, 2004). Misoplegia and personification have not received sufficient attention to draw definitive conclusions about their anatomical substrate, but they were always found in right-sided strokes.

Widespread damage to the right hemisphere leads to reduced attention and vigilance, and this might compromise general awareness and lead to imperception of impairment (anosognosia). To the extent that anosognosia for hemiplegia is related to asomatognosia by lesion location, symptom overlap, and phenomenological similarity, one may assume that disorientation and confusion also are frequent but unnecessary factors for the latter to manifest itself. Indeed, anosognosia for hemiplegia has been repeatedly said to arise in states of general confusion or when arousal and vigilance are at their lowest (Nathanson *et al.*, 1952; Cutting, 1978; Anderson and Tranel, 1989), although counterexamples have been found from the beginning (Babinski, 1914) and more recent studies have shown that, as a group, anosognosic patients do not differ from non-anosognosic hemiplegic patients on measures of intellectual ability (Berti *et al.*, 1996; Small and Ellis, 1996; Marcel *et al.*, 2004b). Authors have insisted, on the basis of their personal impression, that delusional claims about the half-body always seem to be caused by widespread and acute cortical damage to the right hemisphere, which would always be accompanied by profound intellectual disturbances (Gerstmann, 1942; Sandifer, 1946; Hécaen and de Ajuriaguerra, 1952; Weinstein *et al.*, 1954). However, the extremely deluded patient reported by Halligan *et al.* (1995), for instance, was shown *not* to have generalized mental deterioration. In any case, general intellectual impairment cannot be a sufficient factor for asomatognosia, since many confused, disoriented, or demented patients do not show such disturbances. What remains clear is that dissociations are expected, and it is hard to maintain accounts in terms of general cognitive impairment for unawareness, denial, disownership, or delusions regarding one's body when these manifestations concern only certain symptoms but not others, only certain body parts but not others, only certain levels of awareness but not others, only certain associated signs but not others, only certain phenomenological content but not others, and which can in any case fluctuate from hour to hour or even entirely resolve momentarily through caloric vestibular stimulation (Bisiach *et al.*, 1991; Rode *et al.*, 1992). The same can be argued against general accounts of anosognosia and asomatognosia in terms of psychological denial (Bisiach and Geminiani, 1991).

As we learn more about the specific clinical and phenomenological aspects of the disorders of body schema, the question of their precise anatomical substrate seems increasingly unsatisfactory. Feinberg *et al.* (1990) studied patients with right hemisphere damage showing what they call "verbal asomatognosia," meaning that they denied or misattributed ownership of their left hand when the latter was shown to them by the experimenter. They found a frequent involvement of the supramarginal gyrus and the underlying deep structure of the posterior corona radiata. These areas were spared in a control group of neglect patients without asomatognosia. Less frequently involved regions were the insular cortex and the lentiform nucleus. The angular gyrus was rarely involved. This study confirmed the earlier findings of Nielsen (1938b), which also insisted on the importance of the right supramarginal gyrus and underlying structures in the genesis of hemiasomatognosia.

Hemiconcern was related to strokes involving the territory of the right anterior parietal artery, which includes the postcentral gyrus, the upper and middle temporal gyri, the anterior and inferior areas of the parietal gyrus, and the supramarginal gyrus (Bogousslavsky et al., 1995).

There is, however, no precise anatomo-clinical correlate that could dissociate the disorders of the body schema reviewed in this chapter from other right hemisphere syndromes like unilateral neglect and anosognosia for hemiplegia. Besides, it is important to add that delusional claims about the right half of the body have also been recorded following left-sided strokes (Nielsen, 1938b; Miura et al., 1996; Cereda et al., 2002). Nevertheless, we feel confident to say that these cases are exceptions to the rule.

The anatomical basis and mechanisms involved in alien hand syndrome seem to be more thoroughly understood. The general picture is that of an interhemispheric disconnection, involving primarily the corpus callosum and related anterior or posterior structures. Etiology may be very diverse, and we will restrict the following lines to cases induced by strokes. In the anterior forms, the medial prefrontal cortex and supplementary motor area are usually damaged, following infarcts of the callosal, anterior cerebral, or anterior communicating arteries. The posterior forms are often the result of infarcts of the posterior artery and damage to structures underlying the parieto-temporo-occipital junction (Scepkowski and Cronin-Golomb, 2003; Billard et al., 2004).

Accounts of disorders like illusory phantom limb and feelings of absence or transformation of body parts usually follow a subcortical stroke, regardless of lateralization.

Assessing asomatognosia

We would recommend seeing the patient as soon as possible, as the most interesting aspects of the body schema disorders are very often transient and

Table 11.5. Methods to assess asomatognosia

Direct observation
Interview with caregivers and visiting relatives
Guided interview with the patient (see Appendix)
Enlist associated disorders
Bisiach's scale for personal neglect
Ownership of plegic hand (verbal asomatognosia)
Self drawing
Use of mirrors

---

rarely persist more than a few days. They are sometimes fairly easy to detect through direct observation. However, this requires that the clinician knows what to look for and how to do it best (Table 11.5). Besides, one must be prepared to hear or observe things that are not necessarily expected. As is the case for anosognosia, there is no standard assessment procedure for asomatognosia. The approach must be tailored to each individual case and thus requires creativity from the examiner (Bisiach and Geminiani, 1991). For cases where the patient is critical, one has to count on their willingness to report their strange feelings. Patients sometimes do so spontaneously, but often one has to specifically ask if certain symptoms are present, and therefore a trustful relationship needs to be established, otherwise the patient may be reluctant to speak up, fearing that they may be labeled as "crazy." As the clinician cannot spend much of the day with the patient, interviewing staff caregivers and visiting relatives is also helpful in order to gain additional insight.

General approach to the investigation of body schema disorders

While listening to the patient describing a part of their body, it is important to distinguish between metaphorical statements like "My arm is *like* a dead animal" and firm beliefs in the presence of an elaborated delusion ("Someone put a disgusting dead arm in my bed tonight"). Halligan *et al.* (1995) insist on this distinction between use of *simile* (which they prefer to "metaphor") and *factive* mode. In the same conversation, a patient may easily slip from one to another. In any case, one should not jump to conclusions on the basis of a first impression. The patient's claims should always be further investigated by asking for details, and a first error should be further explored at least by giving the patient a chance to correct themselves. This is the only way to probe the exact nature of the claim. The clinician should not fear to directly confront the patient. In our experience, use of confrontational style during the interview does not lead to catastrophic reactions in such patients (quite the contrary, they are most of the time curiously willing to answer the weirdest requests from the clinician).

It is very important that the interview be made without suggesting responses to the patient. All observations are far more interesting if they are made in the patient's own words, as spontaneously as possible (Halligan *et al.*, 1995). Therefore, the goal of the clinician is to carefully orient the patient towards some general aspects of their experience, and only then, depending on their responses, to progressively focus on more specific aspects. Social psychologists use a "funneled debriefing procedure" to ensure that their experimental subjects have no idea of the specific hypotheses held by the experimenter, in order to exclude any possible biases (Bargh and Chartrand, 2000). We propose to do just the same with neurological patients, a funneled interview for assessing disorders of the body schema (see Appendix). While assessing the patient, one should keep in mind that asomatognosic disorders observed at the bedside are often a fluctuating phenomenon, so one should not hesitate to ask the same questions at different times. Just because a patient recognizes from the beginning that they have had a stroke and that their left side is plegic does not mean they won't present signs of asomatognosia upon narrower questioning. Also, delusions may flourish as the patient–clinician relationship and the conversation becomes friendlier and less formal, and this may vary from one examiner to another (Jaffe and Slote, 1958). The immediate spatio-temporal context should also be taken into account, as major variations can be observed depending on multiple contextual factors. For instance, the mere fact of standing on the left or on the right of the patient during the interview may alter their participation and responses (Weinstein, 1969).

Specific tests of asomatognosia

A thorough bedside interview should be straightforward enough to detect disorders of the body schema, as the very nature of these disorders seems to preclude a more quantifiable approach.

As we have equated some forms of hemiasomatognosia with personal neglect, we propose to follow Bisiach *et al.*'s proposal (1986) to score this:
Ask patient to grasp his/her [contralesional] hand with the other.
0 = grasp without hesitation or cuing
1 = crossing the midline but failure to contact the contralesional hand
2 = movement towards but failure to cross the midline
3 = no movement toward the target.
Another method is the so-called "fluff test" (Cocchini *et al.*, 2001). A simplified version of this is to spread cotton balls on the left side of the patient blindfolded,

and upon removal of the blindfold simply ask them to locate and remove all the cotton balls (Buxbaum *et al.*, 2004). Observation of how the patient behaves in their daily activities is perhaps the best way to detect inattention to their own half-body. A patient may also be asked to pantomime self-directed gestures like combing or shaving.

Feinberg and his colleagues operationalized "verbal asomatognosia" with a simple test of ownership: "The normal right arm was lifted, and the patient was asked, 'What is this?' [...] The examiner then lifted, by the elbow, the limb contralateral to the lesion and moved the patient's hand and forearm into the hemispace ipsilateral to the lesion. The patient was again asked, 'What is this?' A patient was judged to have verbal asomatognosia if the limb was misidentified. Care was taken to keep the examiner's hand and arm out of the patient's ipsilateral hemispace" (quoted from Feinberg *et al.*, 1990; see also Feinberg *et al.*, 2000; Meador *et al.*, 2000). It was not precisely stated in those papers whether the visual aspect of the arm should be considered, but we would like to advise against the presence of distinctive features, like rings, colored or artificial nails, bracelets, or IV tubes. The patient's right and left hand should be exempted from recognizable or distractible details and the experimenter's hand should be as out of view as possible. Seeing one's ring can help to acknowledge that the hand being shown is one's own;[3] conversely, seeing IV tubes, bandages, etc, could exacerbate an anosognosic patient's belief that the hand shown cannot be theirs, since they think everything is all right with them anyway. Testing for ownership of a body part should also be made in the tactile modality, which is the "signe de la main étrangère" of Brion and Jedynak (1972): out of view, the experimenter puts the left hand into the right one and asks "What do you have in your hand?". The "sign" is present if the patient answers anything other than "my hand."

Another easy test, which clinicians tend to overlook, consists in showing another's hand to the patient. Interestingly, specific delusions can adapt to the type of hand shown: a male hand can be attributed to a husband, and a feminine hand to a female relative (Assal, 1983; see also Garçin *et al.*, 1938).[4] Hands can be presented from the left and from the right (no delusion is usually elicited when

---

[3] In fact, the opposite may also be true. A patient described by Aglioti *et al.* (1996) denied the ownership of her ring *only* when she wore it on her left hand, which she steadfastly denied being hers. When shown on the examiner's finger, she immediately recognized the ring as hers!

[4] In the same vein, Bottini and his colleagues(2002) have made the following observation: their somatoparaphrenic patient FB could not report any stimuli to her left hand, which she tenaciously attributed to her niece, however, when told it was her niece's hand being touched, she could reliably report those same stimuli.

a hand is presented from the right). We suggest also doing this in the tactile modality.

To quantify asomatognosia, Morin *et al.* (2002) adaptated Bisiach's scale for anosognosia (Bisiach *et al.*, 1986) in the following manner:

Shown their left hand and asked "What am I showing you?", the patient answers:

0 = "It's my hand"

1 = "It's a hand" or "it's your hand", but admits it's their hand when asked directly

2 = patient accepts hand shown as theirs only if the contiguity between the hand and the body is demonstrated

3 = patient refuses this last demonstration.

For ongoing research purposes, we slightly adapted Cutting's questionnaire (Cutting, 1978), which could be a shorter way to assess for somatognosic disorders, but is obviously more susceptible to bias the patient's responses than the funneled interview we propose (see Appendix):

1. *Anosodiaphoria:* Is it a nuisance? How much trouble does it cause you? What caused it?
2. *Nonbelonging:* Do you ever feel that it doesn't belong to you? Do you feel that it belongs to someone else?
3. *Strange feelings:* Do you feel the arm is strange or odd?
4. *Misoplegia:* Do you dislike the arm? Do you hate it?
5. *Personification:* Do you ever call it names?
6. *Somesthetic/kinesthetic hallucinations:* Do you ever feel it moves without your moving it yourself? How big or strong is it? How is the other arm?
7. *Phantom supernumerary illusion:* Do you ever feel as if there was more than one arm/hand? Do you ever feel a strange arm lying beside you? Do you ever feel your arm as separate from the real one/from you?

Another interesting approach may be to ask the patient to make a drawing of how he perceives himself (Morin *et al.*, 2002; see also McCrea *et al.*, 1982). This should be tried whenever possible, but we would warn against over-interpreting the results as it is impossible to segregate the many factors involved in such a task (premorbid ability to draw, emotional context, visuo-spatial disorders, etc.).

One last approach we would like to suggest is the use of mirrors with these patients. In 1978, Verret and Lapresle described a woman with right-hemisphere damage who denied ownership of her left arm upon direct visual contact. However, she would acknowledge that it was hers when viewing it reflected in a mirror or when touching it out of view. A recent study by Paysant *et al.* (2004) showed a reverse pattern of that found by Verret and Lapresle. They called this new clinical entity "mirror asomatognosia." They investigated right-brain damaged patients at least two months after stroke, when clinically their body schema seemed to be corrected. In the acute phase, most of them had features of asomatognosia, loosely defined (feelings of transformation, strangeness, or alienation of the left upper limb). At the time of testing, "asomatognosia" had resolved in all patients. However, when placed in front of a mirror, strange feelings in their arm reappeared in most of them (the effect was stronger with an inverted mirror). Hence, in this research, a corrected body schema was shown to be fragile when confronted with the displayed body image in the mirror. It can thus be said that exposure to a mirror can either *correct* or *induce* disorders of the body schema. A mirror can also be used to generate illusory movements in a plegic limb, a method inspired by Ramachandran's work on phantom limbs (Ramachandran, 1998). When the mirror is placed in a vertical parasagittal position, one has the illusion that the reflected moving hand is the plegic one. This has been shown to elicit illusory movements in patients with disorders of the body schema (Zampini *et al.*, 2004), and even to be helpful for rehabilitation of hemiparesis (Altschuler *et al.*, 1999).

Course and outcome

Although disorders of the body schema are usually an acute and transient manifestation of stroke, virtually all time courses have been described. These range from an acute episode lasting a few hours, sometimes even less in ictal or paroxystic cases, to chronic cases lasting from months to years. Presentation may vary on a single time course, with changes in somatognosia not necessarily paralleling those in sensorimotor functions, arousal, cognitive impairment, type of phenomenological experience, and level of awareness. There are some reported cases of longstanding somatoparaphrenia following stroke (Ehrenwald, 1930; Rode *et al.*, 1992). Misoplegia and supernumerary phantom limbs can also remain chronic (personal observations). It is not clear what conditions exactly are involved in the resolution or chronicization of these disorders. Even though the influence of general factors like vigilance and confusion on the emergence of different types of asomatognosic phenomena remains unresolved, the clinical impression is that usually most of the acute disorders of somatognosia resolve as vigilance improves. Other candidates for an improvement are the shrinking of the ischemic penumbra, mechanisms of early plasticity, and repeated confrontation with medical staff, neighboring patients and relatives. All these may not be sufficient however, and much remains to be known on the possible effects of lesion location and extent, demographic factors, disconnection of functional regions, misfiring cortical reorganization, personality and motivational factors, and unstable socio-cultural adjustments. It is sufficient to add here that we do not know much about the functional significance of acute disorders of somatognosia for either the outcome or for the success of rehabilitation. Initial and persistent anosognosia has been said to be a negative factor in recovery, though associated disorders also result in poor outcome (Jehkonen *et al.*, 2000). However there are no data concerning asomatognosic disorders per se.

Rehabilitative pathways

As asomatognosia is usually only a transient disorder after stroke, it has not been the subject of efforts towards rehabilitation. Besides, such patients generally suffer from other neurological and cognitive disorders that are the main target of rehabilitation. Therefore, the attitude with these patients does not differ in any remarkable way from that adopted with all right-brain damaged patients. Physiotherapeutic interventions for the plegic limb, like constraint-induced movement therapy (Mark and Taub, 2004), have been proved to be efficient even for associated non-motoric disorders; however, we are not aware of any rehabilitative study specifically aimed at disorders of the body schema.

We would like to briefly outline four other approaches that are not strictly speaking rehabilitative methods, but which nevertheless seem important pathways to a better understanding of the nature of asomatognosia and could ultimately lead to specific rehabilitative proposals.

1. Vestibular caloric stimulation has been shown to momentarily disrupt hemineglect and somatoparaphrenia. This procedure consists in irrigating the contralesional external ear canal with cold water for one minute (60 mL, 20°C). The effects are often dramatic, as this can entirely eliminate for a few minutes a longstanding anosognosia, hemineglect, or somatoparaphrenia (Bisiach *et al.*, 1991; Rode *et al.*, 1992; Vallar *et al.*, 1997; Ramachandran, 2000).

2. Adaptation to prismatic deviation has also been demonstrated to be a promising approach to hemineglect. In this procedure, the patient has to wear special lenses that induce a deviation of the whole visual field towards the ipsilesional side. During this time, they progressively adapt to the deviation by correcting motor movements in a pointing task towards the contralesional side. After the goggles are removed, an aftereffect occurs in which the pointing errors are directed toward the contralesional side, thereby alleviating unilateral spatial neglect for a few hours or even days (Maravita *et al.*, 2003). Such a procedure can also relieve representational neglect (Rode *et al.*, 2001) and somatosensory function, like sensitivity and proprioception (Dijkerman *et al.*, 2004), thereby showing the malleability of a supra-modal body-centered spatial frame that could be explored in further studies for asomatognosia.

3. Using mirrors can be a way to investigate the effects of indirect visual feedback on one's body schema. Such an approach may improve or impair somatognosia, for reasons not yet understood. It is nevertheless known that indirect visual feedback can improve hemiparesis (Altschuler *et al.*, 1999) and lower sensory thresholds (Schaefer *et al.*, 2005).

4. Researchers on the body schema have often shown its considerable plasticity, which in some circumstances may enable the incorporation of external objects in it. This has been experimentally shown in normal subjects (Armel and Ramachandran, 2003; Ehrsson *et al.*, 2004; Tsakiris and Haggard, 2005) and in brain-damaged patients (Maravita and Iriki, 2004). The phenomenon has been linked to somatoparaphrenia, as these patients seem to incorporate objects or other persons' body parts into their left side (Botvinick, 2004).

These approaches, together with behavioral neurology, psychopathology and cognitive neuroscience, will hopefully shed new lights on this permanent, yet so fugitive, sense we have of our own body, and ultimately of our intimate self.

REFERENCES

Adair, J. C., Gilmore, R. L., Fennell, E. B., Gold, M. and Heilman, K. M. (1995). Anosognosia during intracarotid barbiturate anesthesia: Unawareness or amnesia for weakness. *Neurology*, **45**, 241–43.

Aglioti, S., Smania, N., Manfredi, M. and Berlucchi, G. (1996). Disownership of left hand and objects related to it in a patient with right brain damage. *Neuroreport*, **8**, 293–6.

Altschuler, E. L., Wisdom, S. B., Stone, L., *et al.* (1999). Rehabilitation of hemiparesis after stroke with a mirror. *Lancet*, **353**, 2035–6.

Anderson, S. W. and Tranel, D. (1989). Awareness of disease states following cerebral infarction, dementia, and head trauma: Standardized assessment. *The Clinical Neuropsychologist*, **3**, 327–39.

Appenzeller, O. and Bicknelle, J. M. (1969). Effects of nervous system lesions on phantom experience in amputees. *Neurology*, **19**, 141–6.

Armel, K. C. and Ramachandran, V. S. (2003). Projecting sensations to external objects: Evidence from skin conductance response. *Proc. R. Soc. Lond. B*, **270**, 1499–506.

Assal, G. (1983). Non, je ne suis pas paralysée, c'est la main de mon mari. *Arch. Suisses Neurol. Psychiatrie*, **133** (fascicule 1), 151–7.

(1985). Transformation en animal, métamorphose ou métaphore? *Arch. Suisses Neurol. Neurochir. Psychiatrie*, **136**, 33–42.

Babinski, J. (1914). Contribution à l'étude des troubles mentaux dans l'hémiplégie organique cérébrale (anosognosie). *Revue Neurologie*, **27**, 845–8.

Bakchine, S., Slachevsky, Tourbah, A., Serres, I. and Abdelmounni, H. (1999). Quatre mains "étranges" pour deux mains après une lésion calleuse. *Rev. Neurol.*, **155**, 929–34.

Bakheit, A. M. (2000). Illusory movements of the paralysed upper limb in stroke. *J. Neurol. Neurosurg. Psychiatry*, **69**, 837.

Barbeau, E., Joubert, S. and Poncet, M. (2004). A single case-study of diagonistic dyspraxia. *Brain and Cognition*, **54**, 215–17.

Bargh, J. A. and Chartrand, T. (2000). The mind in the middle. In H. T. reis and C. M. Judd, eds., *Handbook of Research Methods in Social and Personality Psychology*. Cambridge, pp. 253–85.

Bechterev, V. M. (1926). Partial cortical and subcortical paralyses of psychoreflexive functions. *Obozr Psykhiatr*, 31–41.

Benattar, B., Le Roux, A., Van Amerongen, P., Hanon, C. and Pascal, J. C. (2004). À propos du syndrome d'Ekbom. *Ann. Méd. Psychol.*, **162**, 755–61.

Benke, T., Luzzatti, C. and Vallar, G. (2004). Hermann Zingerle's "Impaired perception of the own body due to organic brain disorders". 1913. An introductory comment, and an abridged translation. *Cortex*, **40**, 265–74.

Berthier, M., Starkstein, S. and Leiguarda, R. (1988). Asymbolia for pain: A sensori-limbic disconnection syndrome. *Ann. Neurol.*, **24**, 41–9.

Berti, A., Làdavas, E. and Della Corte, M. (1996). Anosognosia for hemiplegia, neglect dyslexia, and drawing neglect: Clinical findings and theoretical considerations. *Journal of the International Neuropsychological Society*, **2**, 426–40.

Billard, T., Osseby, G. V., Minier, D., Couvreur, G., Rouaud, O., Moreau, T. and Giroud, M. (2004). Le syndrome de la main étrangère par infarctus du corps calleux: à propos d'un cas. *Rev. Neurol. (Paris)*, **160**, 563–7.

Biran, I. and Chatterjee, A. (2004). Alien hand syndrome. *Arch. Neurol.*, **61**, 292–4.

Bisiach, E. and Geminiani, G. (1991). Anosognosia related to hemiplegia and hemianopia. In G. P. Prigatano and D. L. Schacter, eds., *Awareness of Deficit after Brain Injury*. Oxford.

Bisiach, E., Rusconi, M. L. and Vallar, G. (1991). Remission of somatoparaphrenic delusion through vestibular stimulation. *Neuropsychologia*, **29**, 1029–31.

Bisiach, E., Vallar, G., Perani, D. and Berti, A. (1986). Unawareness of disease following lesions of the right hemisphere: Anosognosia for hemiplegia and anosognosia for hemianopia. *Neuropsychologia*, **24**, 471–82.

Blanke, O., Landis, T., Spinelli, L. and Seeck, M. (2004). Out-of-body experience and autoscopy of neurological origin. *Brain*, **127**, 243–58.

Bogen, J. E. (1979). The callosal syndrome. In K. M. Heilman and E. V. Valenstein, eds., *Clinical Neuropsychology*. New York: Oxford University Press, pp. 295–338.

Bogousslavsky, J., Kumral, E., Regli, F., Assal, G. and Ghika, J. (1995). Acute hemiconcern: a right anterior parietotemporal syndrome. *J. Neurol. Neurosurg. Psychiatry*, **58**, 428–32.

Bornstein, B. (1949). Sur le phénomène du membre fantôme. *L'Encéphale*, **38**, 32–46.

Bottini, G., Bisiach, E., Sterzi, R. and Vallar, G. (2002). Feeling touches in someone else's hand. *Neuroreport*, **13**, 249–52.

Botvinick, M. (2004). Probing the neural basis of body ownership. *Science*, **305**, 782–3.

Brain, K. L., Haines, J. and Williams, C. L. (1998). The psychophysiology of self-mutilation: Evidence of tension reduction. *Arch. Suicide Res.*, **4**, 227–42.

Brion, S. and Jedynak, C. P. (1972). Troubles du transfert interhémisphérique. A propos de trois observations de tumeurs du corps calleux. le signe de la main étrangère. *Rev. Neurol. (Paris)*, **126**, 257–66.

Buxbaum, L. J., Ferraro, M. K., Veramonti, T., *et al.* (2004). Hemispatial neglect. Subtypes, neuroanatomy, and disability. *Neurology*, **62**, 749–56.

Cambier, J., Elghozi, D., Graveleau, P. and Lubetzki, C. (1984). Right hemiasomatognosia and sensation of amputation caused by left subcortical lesion. Role of callosal disconnection. *Rev. Neurol. (Paris)*, **140**, 256–62.

Castaigne, P., Laplane, D. and Degos, J.-D. (1970). Trois cas de négligence motrice par lésion rétro-rolandique. *Rev. Neurol. (Paris)*, **122**, 234–42.

Cereda, C., Ghika, J., Maeder, P. and Bogousslavsky, J. (2002). Strokes restricted to the insular cortex. *Neurology*, **59**, 1950–5.

Cocchini, G., Beschin, N. and Jehkonen, M. (2001). The fluff test: A simple task to assess body representation neglect. *Neuropsychol. Rehabil.*, **11**, 17–31.

Cotard, J. (1880). Du délire hypocondriaque dans une forme de mélancolie anxieuse. *Ann. Méd. Psychol. (Paris)*, **4**, 168–74.

    (1882). Du délire des négations. *Arch. Neurol.*, **4**, 152–70, 282–96.

Critchley, M. (1953). *The Parietal Lobes*, New York: Hafner Press.

    (1955). Personification of paralysed limbs in hemiplegics. *BMJ*, July 30, 284–286.

    (1974). Misoplegia, or hatred of hemiplegia. *M. Sinai J. Med.*, **41**, 82–7.

Cutting, J. (1978). Study of anosognosia. *J. Neurol. Neurosurg. Psychiatry*, **41**, 548–55.

    (1990). *The Right Cerebral Hemisphere and Psychiatric Disorders*, Oxford University Press.

Davies, M., Aimola Davies, A. and Coltheart, M. (2005). Anosognosia and the Two-factor Theory of Delusions. *Mind and Language*, **20**, 209–36.

Dijkerman, H. C., Webeling, M., ter Wal, J. M., Groet, E. and van Zandvoort, M. J. (2004). A long-standing improvement of somatosensory function after prism adaptation, a case study. *Neuropsychologia*, **42**, 1697–702.

Dugas, L. and Moutier, F. (1911). *La dépersonnalisation*, Paris: Alcan.

Duggal, H. S. (2003). A lesion approach to neurobiology of dissociative symptoms. *J. Neuropsychiatry Clin. Neurosci.*, **15**, 245–6.

Durst, R. and Rosca-Rebaudengo, P. (1991). The disorder named Koro. *Behav. Neurol.*, **4**, 1–14.

Dusoir, H., Owens, C., Forbes, R. B., *et al.* (2005). Anorexia nervosa remission following left thalamic stroke. *J. Neurol. Neurosurg. Psychiatry*, **76**(1), 144–5.

Ehrenwald, H. (1930). Verändertes Erleben des Körperbildes mit konsekutiver Wahnbildung bei linksseitiger Hemiplegie. *Monatsschrift fur Psychiatrie une Neurologie*, **75**, 89–97.

    (1931). Anosognosie une depersonalisation. Ein Beitrag zur Psychologie der linksseitig Hemiplegischen. *Nervenartz*, **4**, 681–8.

Ehrsson, H. H., Spence, C. and Passingham, R. E. (2004). That's my hand!Activity in premotor cortex reflects feeling of ownership of a limb. *Science*, **305**, 875–7.

Ey, H. (1973). Les hallucinations corporelles. In H. Ey, ed., *Traité des Hallucinations*. Paris: Masson.

Feinberg, T. E. (2001). *Altered Selves: How the Brain Creates the Self*. Oxford: Oxford University press.

Feinberg, T. E., Haber, L. D. and Leeds, N. E. (1990). Verbal asomatognosia. *Neurology*, **40**, 1391–4.

Feinberg, T. E., Schindler, R. J., Flanagan, N. G. and Haber, L. D. (1992). Two alien hand syndromes. *Neurology*, **42**, 19–24.

Feinberg, T. E., Roane, D. M. and Ali, J. (2000). Illusory limb movements in anosognosia for hemiplegia. *J. Neurol. Neurosurg. Psychiatry*, **68**, 511–13.

Feinberg, T. E., Roane, D. M. and Cohen, J. C. (1998). Partial status epilepticus associated with asomatognosia and alien hand-like behaviors. *Arch. Neurol.*, **55**, 1574–6.

Ferro, F. M. (2003). Le corps en fragment dans le syndrome de Jules Cotard. *Evolution Psychiatrique*, **68**, 579–89.

Flynn, F. G., Cummings, J. L., Scheibel, J. and Wirshing, W. (1989). Monosymptomatic delusion of parasitosis associated with ischemic cerebrovascular disease. *J. Geriatr. Psychiatry Neurol.*, **2**, 134–9.

Frederiks, J. A. M. (1963a). Anosognosie et hémiasomatognosie. *Rev. Neurol. (Paris)*, **109**, 585–97.

  (1963b). Macrosomatognosia and microsomatognosia. *Psychiat. Neurol. Neurochir.*, **66**, 531–6.

  (1969). Disorders of the body schema. In P. J. Vinken and G. W. Bruyn, eds., *Handbook of Clinical Neurology*. Vol. **4**, pp. 207–40.

Gabbay, V., Asnis, G. M., Bello, J. A., *et al.* (2003). New onset of body dysmorphic disorder following frontotemporal lesion. *Neurology*, **61**, 123–5.

Gallagher, S. (1986). Body image and body schema: A conceptual clarification. *J. Mind Behav.*, **7**, 541–54.

Garçin, R., Varay, A. and Dimo, H. (1938). Document pour servir à l'étude des troubles du schéma corporel. *Rev. Neurol.*, **69**, 498–510.

Gerstmann, J. (1942). Problem of imperception of disease and of impaired body territories with organic lesions. *Arch. of Neurol. Psychiatry*, **48**, 890–913.

Groom, K. N., Ng, W. K., Kevorkian, C. G. and Levy, J. K. (1999). Egosyntonic alien hand syndrome after right posterior cerebral artery stroke. *Arch. Phys. Med. Rehabil.*, **80**, 162–5.

Guariglia, C. and Antonucci, G. (1992). Personal and extrapersonal space: A case of neglect dissociation. *Neuropsychologia*, **30**, 1001–10.

Halligan, P. W., Marshall, J. C. and Wade, D. T. (1995). Unilateral somatoparaphrenia after right hemisphere stroke: A case description. *Cortex*, **31**, 173–82.

Head, H. (1920). *Studies in Neurology*, Vol. II. London.

Hécaen, H. and de Ajuriaguerra, J. (1952). *Méconnaissances et Hallucinations Corporelles. Intégration et désintégration de la somatognosie.* Paris: Masson.

Hécaen, H., de Ajuriaguerra, J., Le Guillant and Angelergues, R. (1954). Délire centré sur un membre fantôme chez une hémiplégique gauche par lésion vasculaire avec anosognosie. *Evolution Psychiatrique*, **19**, 273–9.

Heilman, K. M. and Adams, D. J. (2003). Callosal neglect. *Arch. Neurol.*, **60**, 276–9.

Heilman, K. M., Barrett, A. M. and Adair, J. C. (1998). Possible mechanisms of anosognosia: A defect in self-awareness. *Phil. Trans. R. Soc. Lond. B.*, **353**, 1903–9.

Herzog, D. B. and Copeland, P. M. (1985). Eating disorders. *N. Engl. J. Med.*, **313**, 295–303.

Hirstein, W. (2005). *Brain Fiction*. MIT Press.

Hoff, H. and Potzl, O. (1935). Ueber ein neues parieto-occipitales syndrom. Seelenlähmung des Schauens, Störung des Körperschemas, Wegfall des zentralen Seehens. *Jahrb. f. Psychiat. Neurol.*, **52**, 173–218.

Ives, E. and Nielsen, J. (1937). Disturbances of body scheme: Delusion of the absence of part of body in two cases with autopsy verification of lesion. *Bull. Los Angeles Neurol. Soc.*, **2**, 120–5.

Jaffe, J. and Slote, W. H. (1958). Interpersonal factors in denial of illness. *AMA. Arch. Neurol. Psychiat.*, **80**, 653.

Jehkonen, M., Ahonen, J.-P., Dastidar, P., Laippala, P. and Vilkki, J. (2000). Unawareness of deficits after right hemisphere stroke: Double-dissociations of anosognosia. *Acta Neurol. Scand.*, **102**, 378–84.

Keenan, J. P. (2003). *The Face in the Mirror: The Search for the Origins of Consciousness*, New York: Harper Collins.

Kumral, E. and Öztürk, O. (2004). Delusional state following acute stroke. *Neurology*, **62**, 110–13.

Lhermitte, J. (1939). *L'Image de Notre Corps*, Paris: Nouvelle Revue Critique.

Manly, T., Woldt, K., Watson, P. and Warburton, E. (2002). Is motor perseveration in unilateral neglect "driven" by the presence of neglected left-sided stimuli? *Neuropsychologia*, **40**, 1794–803.

Maravita, A. and Iriki, A. (2004). Tools for the body (schema). *Trends Cogn. Sci.*, **8**, 79–85.

Maravita, A., McNeil, J., Malhotra, P., *et al.* (2003). Prism adaptation can improve contralesional tactile perception in neglect. *Neurology*, **60**, 1829–31.

Marcel, A. J., Postma, P., Gillmeister, H., *et al.* (2004a). Migration and fusion of tactile sensation – premorbid susceptibility to allochiria, neglect and extinction? *Neuropsychologia*, **42**, 1749–67.

Marcel, A. J., Tegnér, R. and Nimmo-Smith, I. (2004b). Anosognosia for plegia: Specificity, extension, partiality and disunity of bodily awareness. *Cortex*, **40**, 19–40.

Mark, V. W. and Taub, E. (2004). Constraint-induced movement therapy for chronic stroke hemiparesis and other disabilities. *Restor. Neurol. Neurosci.*, **22**, 317–36.

Mathews, C. A., Waller, J., Glidden, D. V., *et al.* (2004). Self injurious behavior in Tourette syndrome: Correlates with impulsivity and impulse control. *J. Neurol. Neurosurg. Psychiatry*, **75**, 1149–55.

McCormick, S. and Goff, D. C. (1992). Possession states: Approaches to clinical evaluation and classification. *Behav. Neurol.*, **5**, 161–7.

McCrea, C. W., Summerfield, A. B. and Rosen, B. (1982). Body image: A selective review of existing measurement techniques. *Br. J. Med. Psychol.*, **55**, 225–33.

McGonigle, D. J., Hänninen, R., Salenius, S., *et al.* (2002). Whose arm is it anyway? An fMRI case study of supernumerary phantom limb. *Brain*, **125**, 1265–74.

Meador, K. J., Loring, D. W., Feinberg, T. E., Lee, G. P. and Nichols, M. E. (2000). Anosognosia and asomatognosia during intracarotid amobarbital inactivation. *Neurology*, **55**, 816–20.

Metzinger, T. (2003). *Being No One. The Self-Model Theory of Subjectivity*, Cambridge, MA: MIT Press.

(2005). Out-of-Body Experiences as the origin of the concept of a "soul". *Mind and Matter*, **3**, 57–84.

Miura, N., Takeda, A., Terao, S., *et al.* (1996). Somatoparaphrenia caused by the lesion in the dominant cerebral hemisphere – a case report. *No To Shinkei*, **48**, 275–9. (Abstract in English)

Morin, C., Durand, E., Marchal, F., *et al.* (2002). Asomatognosie et troubles de l'oralité. Une lecture psychanalytique. *Annales de Réadaptation et de Médecine Physique*, **46**, 12–23.

Morin, C., Pradat-Diehl, P., Mazevet, D., *et al.* (2003). Un enfant dans le bras. Un trouble féminin de l'image du corps en neurology? *Bull. Assoc. Lacan. Int.*, **101**, 13–22.

Moss, A. D. and Turnbull, O. H. (1996). Hatred of hemiparetic limbs (misoplegia) in a 10 year old child. *JNNP*, **61**, 210–11.

Nagaratnam, N., Nagaratnam, K., Ng, K. and Diu, P. (2004). Akinetic mutism following stroke. *J. Clin. Neurosci.*, **11**, 25–30.

Nagasako, E. M., Oaklander, A. L. and Dworkin, R. H. (2003). Congenital insensitivity to pain: An update. *Pain*, **101**, 213–19.

Nathanson, M., Bergman, P. S. and Gordon, G. G. (1952). Denial of illness: Its occurrence in one hundred cases of hemiplegia. *Arch. Neurol. Psychiatry*, **68**, 380–7.

Nielsen, J. M. (1938a). Gerstmann syndrome; finger agnosia, agraphia, confusion of right and left, acalculia. Comparison of this syndrome with disturbances of body scheme resulting from lesions of right side of brain. *Arch. Neurol. Psychiat.*, **39**, 536–60.

(1938b). Disturbances of the body scheme: Their physiological mechanism. *Bull. Los Angeles Neurol. Soc.*, **3**, 127–35.

Nightingale, S. (1982). Somatoparaphrenia: A case report. *Cortex*, **18**, 463–7.

Nishikawa, T., Okuda, J., Mizuta, I., *et al.* (2001). Conflict of intentions due to callosal disconnection. *J. Neurol. Neurosurg. Psychiatry*, **71**, 462–71.

Noll, R. (1992). *Vampires, Werewolves and Demons: Twentieth Century Reports in the Psychiatric Literature*, New York: Brunner/Mazel.

Northoff, G. (2002). What catatonia can tell us about "top-down modulation": A neuropsychiatric hypothesis. *Behav. Brain Sci.*, **25**, 555–77.

Paillard, J. (1999). Body schema and body image: A double dissociation in deafferented patients. In G. N. Gantchev, S. Mori, and J. Massion, eds., *Motor Control, Today and Tomorrow*. Sofia: Academic Publishing House, "Prof. M. Drinov".

Paysant, J., Beis, J. M., Le Chapelain, L. and André, J. M. (2004). Mirror asomatognosia in right lesions stroke victims. *Neuropsychologia*, **42**, 920–5.

Peru, A. and Pinna, G. (1997). Right personal neglect following a left hemisphere stroke. A case report. *Cortex*, **33**, 585–90.

Potzl, O. (1924). Ueber Störungen der Selbstwahrnehmung bei linksseitiger Hemiplegie. *Z. ges. Neurol. Psychiat.*, **93**, 117–68.

Ramachandran, V. S. (1998). Consciousness and body image: Lessons from phantom limbs, Capgras syndrome and pain asymbolia. *Phil. Trans. R. Soc. London B.*, **353**, 1851–9.

(2000). Memory and the brain: New lessons from old syndromes. In D. L. Schacter and E. Scarry, eds., *Memory, Brain, and Belief.* Cambridge: Harvard University Press, pp. 87–114.

Ramachandran, V. S. and Hirstein, W. (1998). Perception of phantom limbs: The D. O. Hebb lecture. *Brain*, **121**, 1603—30.

Rode, G., Charles, N., Perenin, M.-T., *et al.* (1992). Partial remission of hemiplegia and somatoparaphrenia through vestibular stimulation in a case of unilateral neglect. *Cortex*, **28**, 203—8.

Rode, G., Rossetti, Y. and Boisson, D. (2001). Prism adaptation improves representational neglect. *Neuropsychologia*, **39**, 1250—4.

Sandifer, P. H. (1946). Anosognosia and disorders of the body scheme. *Brain*, **69**, 122—37.

Scepkowski, L. A. and Cronin-Golomb, A. (2003). The alien hand: Cases, categorizations, and anatomical correlates. *Behav. Cogn. Neurosci. Rev.*, **2**, 261—77.

Schaefer, M., Heinze, H.-J. and Rotte, M. (2005). Viewing touch improves tactile sensory threshold. *NeuroReport*, **16**, 367—70.

Schilder, P. (1935). *L'Image de Notre Corps*, Paris: Gallimard.

Schilder, P. and Stengel, E. (1931). Das Krankheitsbild der Schmerzasymbolie. *Ztchr. Neurol. Psych.*, **129**, 250—79.

Sierra, M., Lopera, F., Lambert, M. V., Phillips, M. L. and David, A. S. (2002). Separating depersonalisation and derealisation: The relevance of the "lesion method". *J. Neurol. Neurosurg. Psychiatry*, **72**, 530—2.

Signer, S. F. and Benson, D. F. (1990). Three cases of Anorexia Nervosa associated with temporal lobe epilepsy. *Am. J. Psychiatry*, **147**, 235—7.

Simeon, D., Guralnik, O., Hazlett, E. A., *et al.* (2000). Feeling unreal: A PET study of depersonalisation disorder. *Am. J. Psychiatry*, **157**, 1782—8.

Small, M. and Ellis, S. (1996). Denial of hemiplegia: An investigation into the theories of causation. *Eur. Neurol.*, **36**, 353—63.

Starobinski, J. (1982). L'immortalité mélancolique. *Le Temps de la Réflexion*, **3**, 231—51.

Staub, F. and Bogousslavsky, J. (2005). Identité et appartenance corporelle: Fantômes et membres surnuméraires. *Arch. Suisses Neurol. Psychiatrie*, **156**, 189—95.

Todd, J. (1955). The syndrome of Alice in Wonderland. *Can. Med. Assoc. J.*, **73**, 701—6.

Tsakiris, M. and Haggard, P. (2005). The rubber hand illusion revisited: Visuotactile integration and self-attribution. *J. Exp. Psychol. [Hum. Percept.]*, **31**, 80—91.

Vallar, G. (1998). Spatial hemineglect in humans. *Trends Cogn. Sci.*, **2**, 87—97.

Vallar, G., Guariglia, C. and Rusconi, M. L. (1997). Modulation of the neglect syndrome by sensory stimulation. In P. Their and H.-O. Karnath, eds., *Parietal Lobe Contribution to Orientation in 3D Space*. Heidelberg: Springer-Verlag, pp. 555—78.

Verret, J. M. and Lapresle, J. (1978). Syndrome d'Anton Babinski avec reconnaissance du membre supérieur gauche lors de sa vision dans un miroir. *Rev. Neurol. (Paris)*, **134**, 709—13.

von Hagen, K. and Ives, E. R. (1937). Anosognosie (Babinski), Imperfection of hemiplegia. Report of 6 cases, one with autopsy. *Bull. Los Angeles Neurol. Soc.*, **2**, 95—103.

Vuilleumier, P., Chicherio, C., Assal, F., *et al.* (2001). Functional neuroanatomical correlates of hysterical sensorimotor loss. *Brain*, **124**, 1077—90.

Weinstein, E. A. (1969). Disorders of the body schema in organic mental syndromes. In P. J. Vinken and G. W. Bruyn, eds., *Handbook of Clinical Neurology*, Vol. **4**, pp. 241—7.

Weinstein, E. A., Kahn, R. L., Malitz, S. and Rozanski, J. (1954). Delusional reduplications of parts of the body. *Brain*, **77**, 45–60.

Weir-Mitchell, S. (1905). The case of George Dedlow. In S. Weir-Mitchell, ed, *The Autobiography of a Quack*, New York: The Century, pp. 83–109.

Yarnitsky, D., Barron, S. A. and Bental, E. (1988). Disappearance of phantom pain after focal brain infarction. *Pain*, **32**, 285–7.

Young, A. W. and Leafhead, K. M. (1996). Betwixt life and death: Case studies of the Cotard delusion. In P. W. Halligan and J. C. Marshall, eds., *Method in Madness: Case Studies in Cognitive Neuropsychiatry*, London: Psychology Press, pp. 147–171.

Zampini, M., Moro, V. and Aglioti, S. M. (2004). Illusory movements of the contralesional hand in patients with body image disorders. *JNNP*, **75**, 1626–8.

Zingerle, H. (1913). Ueber Störungen des Wahrnehmung des eigenen Körpers bei organischen Gehirnerkrankungen. *Mschr. Psychiat. Neurol.*, **34**, 13–36.

Appendix

A funneled guideline for the bedside interview

1) Begin with questions on general awareness: "Is everything ok? Is there something wrong you would like to mention?" In case of delusional manifestations, ask the patient if they think that what they are saying makes sense; if they think that what they are saying corresponds to reality or is plausible in the real world.

2) Slightly more directed questions may prompt the patient to elaborate on their feelings and knowledge of the situation: "What is wrong with you, what happened to you? Where are we now? Why are you here?" If they answer correctly ("I have had a stroke" or "Something happened in my brain"), continue in a general mode: "So how do you feel now?" If they answer anything other than stroke or hemiplegia ("I'm tired," "could be better," "good," "hungry," "my knee hurts," etc.), ask "is there anything else that bothers you?"

3) Before going on with specific questions about the body schema, continue asking general questions which may help the patient to develop some insight about their condition: "How's your mood?", "Do you think that what happened to you was serious?", "Do you think you could have died?", "What did the doctors tell you about your condition?" Testing for general insight into the condition can also be made with general promptings like: "Do you want to take a walk with me?", "Do you think you could go home right now?", "When do you think you'll be able to work again? Tomorrow?" This is generally an efficient way to elicit confabulations.

4) At this moment, if the patient does not make specific comments, one should begin to progressively focus the interview: "Is there a weaker side?", "What's wrong with the left side?", "What do you think of your left side?", "How does

it feel?" One could further investigate the patient's insight by asking the following: "Do you know the meaning of the word hemiplegia? And paralysis? Can you please define it for me?"

5) Then confront the patient with requests that require some performance on their part: "Can you raise your left arm for me?", "Are you done?", "Tell me where your left arm is right now", "Try to touch my hand here [or nose]", "Can you feel my hand [nose]?" If they raise the wrong hand, one should ask the patient what hand they think they have moved, and then ask them again to move the left one: "No, try again with the other hand please." Lhermitte liked to ask the following "Please raise your right hand *and then* the other", which is an excellent request often overlooked by clinicians. A bilateral task like asking the patient to clap his hands is very good to reveal the extent of unawareness of hemiplegia and to prompt rationalisations.

6) After having established the presence or absence of unawareness of hemiplegia, denial of hemiplegia and delusional claims or rationalisations, one can specifically check if the plegic hand is recognized or disowned. The examiner takes the plegic arm at shoulder level, brings it in the ipsilesional visual space and asks "What is this?", and only then, depending on the answer given, "Who's hand is it?" Usually, errors refer to the examiner's arm, but sometimes the answer is weirder (daughter, niece, wife, father, another doctor, nurse, a neighboring patient). If the patient attributes his hand to the examiner, one should confront the patient by showing one's hands and asking "Are you sure? How many hands do I have then?" If he attributes his hand to someone else, confront him by asking "Is your [niece, father, husband, etc.] here right now? Where is your [niece, father, husband, etc] right now?" The reverse test can also be made, consisting in presenting to the patient a hand which is not his. The questions remain the same: "What is this?", and then "Who's hand is that?"

7) Even if no delusion or severe anosognosia are present, one should ask specific questions about how the patient feels about certain body parts, especially the upper contralesional limb (arm and hand). This may help to reveal misoplegia, personification or feelings of transformation of the plegic limb. Examples of questions are: "How do you feel about your [usually left] arm?", "Take a look at your left hand. How does it appear to you?", "Touch it, how does it feel?", "Tell me about your left side/hand/arm/leg/foot", "To what could you compare your left hand? (maybe prompt with the following categories: an animal, an object, a person, or an event)", "Is it mean? Or do you like it?", "Do you have a name for it?", "Tell me about its size/temperature/matter/weight/speed of movement/strength/smell/color", "Is there someone near or behind you at times?", "Do you *feel* someone near or behind you at times?"

8) Finally, depending on the general clinical picture that appeared after the preceding steps, directly confront the patient with their true condition or further explore the confabulatory process. A good procedure is to make the patient palpate the continuity of their arm, from the trunk and shoulder to the hand. One can also ask the patient to count their hands or all of their fingers, and orient their attention on specific details, like rings, nails, scars, etc. Extreme confabulation can be sought with deliberately aberrant stories, for example: "I just saw someone leaving the ward with an arm, could it be yours? Do you want me to call security? In the meantime, do you wish a new arm to replace your missing one?"

12

Disorders of visuoconstructive ability

Diane Dupuy and Olivier Godefroy

University Hospital, Amiens, France

General presentation of visuoconstructive disorders

This chapter deals with the inability to assemble the elements of a two- or three-dimensional object, respecting their orientations and spatial relationships. This disorder is generally known as "constructional apraxia," a term introduced by Kleist (1934) and frequently used in clinical practice. According to Benton's definition (1967), "constructional apraxia denotes an impairment in combinatory or organizing activity, in which details must be clearly perceived and in which the relationships among the component parts of the entity must be apprehended if the desired synthesis of them is to be achieved." Since the term apraxia introduces some confusion with other varieties of apraxia, the term "disorders of visuo-constructive ability" is frequently preferred and will be used here.

Impairment of visuoconstructive ability is easily demonstrated in a patient with abnormalities in drawings (either free or copied) not explained by low visual acuity or motor disorders. Drawing difficulties related to purely motor, cerebellar, proprioceptive or extrapyramidal disorders are not considered to be apraxic. In addition, gestural apraxia per se does not induce visuoconstructive impairment (Ajuriaguerra et al., 1960). Drawing disturbances related to visual agnosia, simultagnosia and Bálint's syndrome are usually considered to be secondary to perceptual disorders and are not classified as apraxic. From a practical point of view, the examiner must ensure that the patient's ability to identify the figure to be copied is spared before concluding a disorder of visuoconstructive ability. Finally, visuoconstructive disorders are frequently associated with hemineglect, especially in right brain damage. However, disturbances of drawing purely related to hemineglect, such as deviation of the drawing to one side (usually right) of the sheet of paper and omission of one side (usually left) of the drawing, are usually not considered per se to be visuoconstructive disorders.

Copying simple drawings (simple geometric drawings, daisy, star...) is easy to administer at the bedside and is frequently used in clinical practice. The diagnosis of a subtle deficit is difficult on the basis of simple tests and requires the use of more complex tests, such as the clock drawing test, copy of the complex

Rey's figure or three-dimensional block constructions. However, complex tasks also involve executive processes (Lhermitte *et al.*, 1972; Shallice, 1989) and this interferes with the interpretation of impaired performance. In clinical practice, this indicates that when the deficit is observed only on complex tests, especially when it is not severe, interpretation must consider the possibility of disorders of executive functions before concluding a subtle deficit of visuoconstructive ability.

Impairment of visuoconstructive ability may totally prevent drawing, but more frequently leads to characteristic disturbances such as oversimplification, global disorganization, fragmentation, errors in the orientation of components, spatial arrangement and the relations between each component of the drawing (see Figures 12.1–12.5). In unilateral lesions, asymmetry of the disturbances of the drawing is frequently observed: it is usually prominent on the contralesional side. This asymmetry is more frequent and more marked in right-brain damaged patients, a finding attributed to the higher frequency and severity of hemineglect in right-sided lesion. The closing-in phenomenon (i.e. the patient tries to draw directly in the figure to be copied) is observed more frequently in diffuse damage, especially when it includes the frontal lobes (Ajuriaguerra *et al.*, 1960; Gainotti, 1972).

Disorders of visuoconstructive ability were initially considered to be specific to parietal lesions, but they may also be observed in frontal, subcortical, and diffuse brain damage. They have been reported in early studies with a frequency ranging from 15% to 40% of patients with unilateral brain damage (for a review, see Gainotti, 1985), regardless of the side of the lesion. Several studies have suggested that qualitative differences exist between constructional disturbances of right- and left-brain damaged patients (e.g. Arrigoni and De Renzi, 1964; Warrington *et al.*, 1966; for a review, see Gainotti, 1985). It is usually claimed that drawing disturbances differ according to lesion side, a finding which would reflect the different contributions of each hemisphere, as the right hemisphere is especially important for visual–spatial processes and the left hemisphere is important for execution (Hécaen, 1951; Duensing, 1953). Left-brain damaged patients draw slowly, produce an increased number of angles (especially on the copy of a star and a cube) and oversimplification of the whole drawing is frequently observed. The presence of a model facilitates the drawings. Conversely, the characteristics of drawing impairment in right brain damage include preservation of the overall complexity (at least in some parts of the drawing), maintenance of the number of angles (compared to the model), failure to reproduce spatial relations between different parts of the drawing, and left prominence of disturbances (especially omissions related to an associated hemineglect). The presence of a model does not improve drawing. Group studies have reported simplistic drawings with fewer lines and details of left-sided lesions

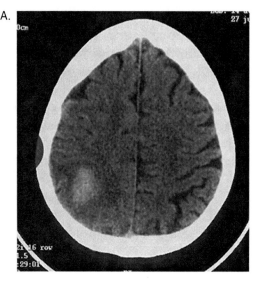

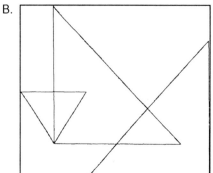

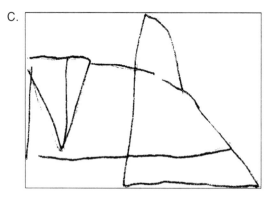

Figure 12.1 Visuoconstructive disorders due to right parietal hematoma. (A) 52-year-old with a right parietal hematoma. (B) Mini Mental State Examination: 20/30 copy of the embedded triangles. (C) Failure to reproduce spatial relations despite relative sparing of angle numbers and complexity.

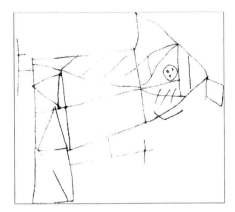

Figure 12.2 Visuoconstructive disorders due to postaneurysmal frontal damage. Copy of the Complex Rey's figure with errors (total score: 18/36) and relative sparing of the global structure.

and spatial distortion with hemineglect of right-sided lesions (Hécaen and Assal, 1970; Binder, 1982; Swindell *et al.*, 1988; Kirk and Kertesz, 1989; Suhr *et al.*, 1998). However, these characteristics have not been replicated in all studies and appear to concern only some patients (Gainotti *et al.*, 1985).

Disorders of visuoconstructive ability are usually considered to be indicative of lesions of the posterior cortex, an interpretation supported by the frequent association with hemianopia or fluent aphasia (De Renzi and Faglioni, 1967; Arena and Gainotti, 1978). Mechanisms of drawing disturbances may differ according to the site of the lesion. The relation with hemineglect has only been observed in patients with right posterior stroke, suggesting that visual–spatial disorders contribute to the visuoconstructive disorders due to right parietal lesion (Marshall *et al.*, 1994). Drawing difficulties may also be observed in patients with a frontal lesion, especially when complex figures or block design are used (Luria and Tsvetkova, 1964; Benton, 1968; Pillon, 1981). In frontal damage, the copy of Rey's Complex Figure (Rey, 1959) was found to improve when the examiner provided a decomposition of the copy into successive stages (Lhermitte *et al.*, 1972; Pillon, 1981) and when the examiner stressed that the patient verify that the objective has been achieved (Dérouesné *et al.*, 1975). These results indicate that the copying of complex figures involves some executive processes, such as planning and verification (i.e. comparison of the results with the preliminary intention) that are impaired in frontal damage, as proposed by Luria and Tsvetkova (1964). Finally, visuoconstructive ability may also be impaired in subcortical lesions (Kirk and Kertesz, 1993). This deficit is likely to be due to interruption of white matter tracts and, in some patients, to small associated cortical lesions.

A detailed cognitive approach to visuoconstructive ability has yet to be developed. Studies in the late twentieth century proposed that visuoconstructive ability requires visual–spatial analysis and representation (thought to depend mainly on the right posterior cortex), precise gestural and motor control

A.

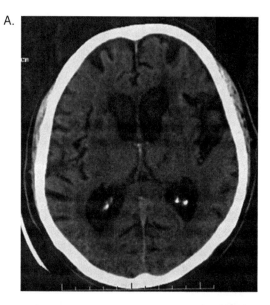

B.

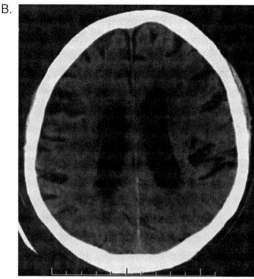

Figure 12.3 Visuoconstructive disorders in vascular dementia. (A, B) 76-year-old man with vascular dementia due to small vessels disease. Mini Mental State Examination: 13/30. (C) Spatial disorganization of the copy of embedded triangles.

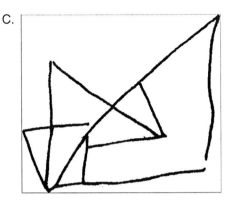

C.

Figure 12.3 *(Cont.)*

(thought to depend mainly on the left posterior cortex), and planning (at least in complex constructive tasks), which is mainly mediated by the prefrontal cortex. Such a view is useful for clinical practice, but is clearly an oversimplification of this complex human ability.

Key points Main characteristics of visuoconstructive disorders

Inability to assemble the elements of a multidimensional object, respecting their
    orientations and spatial relations
Characteristic disturbances: oversimplification, global disorganization, fragmentation, errors
    in the orientation of components, in the spatial arrangement and relation between
    each component; closing-in phenomenon
Differences according to lesion location (concern only some patients):
left lesion: oversimplification, increased number of angles, facilitation by copy
right lesion: "left prominence of disturbances" related to associated hemineglect,
    spatial distortion, preservation of the overall complexity, maintenance
    of angles number
frontal lesion: complex figure, improvement by decomposition into successive stages

Visuoconstructive disorders observed in stroke

Frequency of visuoconstructive impairment

Only a few series of consecutive stroke patients have been subjected to systematic neuropsychological assessment including visuoconstructive ability. These assessments were performed several months post-stroke and used tests such as Rey's complex figure test (Rey, 1959), the Rosen drawing test (Rosen, 1983) or the block design subtest of the Wechsler Adult Intelligence Scale. In ischemic stroke, significant impairment was observed in 17–26% of patients (Tatemichi *et al.*, 1994; Hochstenbach *et al.*, 1998; Sachdev *et al.*, 2004). Despite minor improvement (Hochstenbach *et al.*, 2003), a significant deficit was still observed in long-term stroke survivors (Engstad *et al.*, 2003). In patients suffering from a ruptured aneurysm, visuoconstructive disorders were observed in 21–39% of patients (Ogden *et al.*, 1993; Kreiter *et al.*, 2002; Mayer *et al.*, 2002), the upper range being observed using the Rey's figure test. The use of very simple tests, such as the Clock Drawing test or the drawing subtest of the Mini Mental State Examination, in a sample of stroke patients, revealed a higher frequency of disturbances (25–47% of impaired patients) within 14 days post-stroke (Friedman, 1991).

Visuoconstructive disorders in stroke

Most characteristics of visuoconstructive disorders indicated in the introduction have been described in mixed series of patients with a high proportion of cerebrovascular disease and are applicable to stroke. Several studies focusing on stroke patients have examined the effect of lesion side and site on quantitative and qualitative aspects of drawing disturbances, temporal course, and prognostic value.

Studies assessing global score on various drawing tests have reported controversial results (Arrigoni and De Renzi, 1964; De Renzi and Faglioni, 1967; Binder, 1982; Swindell *et al.*, 1988; Kirk and Kertesz, 1989; Suhr *et al.*, 1998). The global score of the Clock Drawing test was found to be impaired to the same extent regardless of the site of the stroke (Suhr *et al.*, 1998). Even in studies not demonstrating any effect of lesion side on global score, the types of error were found to differ according to lesion side, with a higher rate of neglect errors, spatial distortion, and graphic difficulties in right-sided strokes, and with simplified drawings with fewer lines and fewer details in left-sided strokes (Binder, 1982; Swindell *et al.*, 1988; Kirk and Kertesz, 1989; Suhr *et al.*, 1998).

Recovery from constructional disorders has been examined in several studies. In patients with a first unilateral stroke of the right hemisphere, complete recovery of constructive disorders (assessed using the Rey's figure and block design subtest) was observed in about 70% of patients and occurred within 20 weeks post-stroke (Hier *et al.*, 1983). Comparisons according to side of stroke have shown better and more complete recovery in left hemisphere stroke (Sunderland *et al.*, 1994), a finding also observed in groups of mixed brain lesions (Swindell *et al.*, 1988).

A.

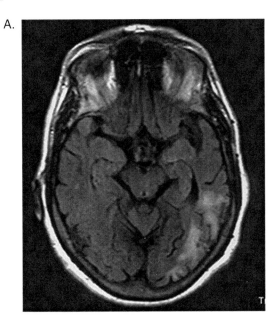

B.

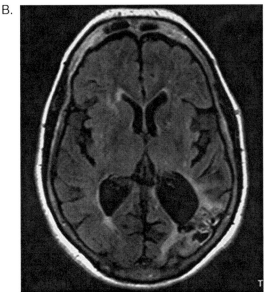

Figure 12.4 Visuoconstructive disorders in multiple infarct dementia. (A–D) 63-year-old woman with infarcts in the left hemisphere responsible for dementia. Mini Mental State Examination: 19/30. (E, F) Inability to copy the Mini Mental State Examination figure with oversimplification and omission of one component.

C.

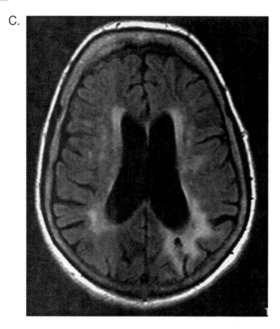

D.

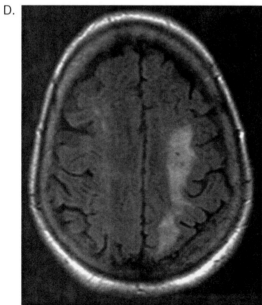

Figure 12.4 (*Cont.*)

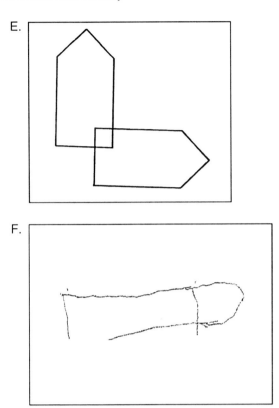

Figure 12.4 (*Cont.*)

Characteristics of strokes responsible for visuoconstructive disorders

A systematic study is required to determine the characteristics of stroke type and the territory of infarct inducing visuoconstructive disorders. Clinical practice indicates that infarcts in the middle cerebral artery induce visuoconstructive disorders, which may be observed even in infarcts limited to the inferior or deep branches. Drawing of complex figures may be impaired in large or bilateral infarcts in the anterior cerebral artery territory. In unilateral posterior cerebral artery infarct, we have frequently observed normal performance on drawing tests in patients without visual agnosia. A study suggests that cube drawing is impaired in patients with small infarcts, although sparing of visuo-constructive ability is expected in pure lacunar stroke (Fushimi *et al.*, 1996). Impaired performance on drawing of complex figures is frequent in complicated ruptured aneurysm of the anterior communicating artery. Finally, preliminary results suggest that visuoconstructive abilities are frequently spared in cerebral venous thrombosis.

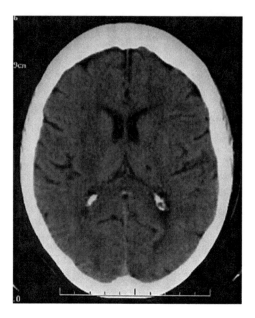

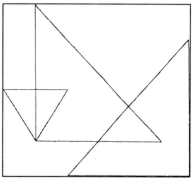

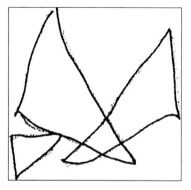

Figure 12.5 Visuoconstructive disorders in left thalamic infarct. (A) 73-year-old woman with a left thalamic infarct on CT-scan. Mini Mental State Examination: 27/30. (B,C) The copy of embedded triangles shows the global disorganization with errors in the spatial relations between triangles.

Key points Main types of stroke responsible for visuoconstructive disorders

Stroke type	Territory/characteristics
Infarct	Middle cerebral artery (inferior or deep branches)
	anterior cerebral artery: large infarct
	posterior cerebral artery: rare
Aneurysm	Anterior communicating artery

Assessment of visuoconstructive disorders in stroke

Assessment at the bedside uses free drawing and copying of simple drawings (square, triangle, daisy, star...). Figures of intermediate complexity, such as house, bicycle, face, cube, and clock, may be used, but their interpretation requires normative data (Kirk and Kertesz, 1989). One possibility is to use one version of the clock drawing test with a standardized scoring system. The study by Suhr *et al.* (1998) used six scoring systems (Sunderland *et al.*, 1989; Mendez *et al.*, 1992; Rouleau *et al.*, 1992; Ishiai *et al.*, 1993; Watson *et al.*, 1993; Freedman *et al.*, 1994) in stroke patients. They found a very good interrater reliability for five systems and a similar sensitivity of the global score to lesion sites (Suhr *et al.*, 1998). In addition, qualitative scoring (size, graphic difficulty, stimulus bound, conceptual difficulty, spatial planning, perseveration) (Rouleau *et al.*, 1992) provided a good interrater reliability (Suhr *et al.*, 1998). Standardized assessment of visuoconstructive deficit is usually based on the complex figure (Rey, 1959) or the block design subtest of the Wechsler Adult Intelligence Scale. The interpretation of performance requires control for perceptual and motor disorders. The contribution of low visual acuity, visual agnosia, simultagnosia, and Bálint's syndrome is estimated by the patient's ability to identify the figure to be copied and by comparing free drawing and copying of simple drawings. More complete testing is required in selected cases. Hemineglect contributes to drawing impairment and

Key points Neuropsychological assessment of visuoconstructive disorders

Clinical examination
Free and copy of simple drawings (square, triangle, daisy, star...)
Clock Drawing test (standardized scoring system)

Neuropsychological assessment
Complex figure
Block design subtest
And related disorders: hemineglect, visual agnosia, simultagnosia

has to be assessed separately using a specific procedure (see Chapter 9) especially with cancellation tests which do not require drawing. Motor, cerebellar, and extrapyramidal disorders are easily detected by clinical examination.

Prognosis and management

Key points Prognosis and management of visuoconstructive disorders

Marker of stroke severity
Frequent partial recovery
Rehabilitation in selected cases?

The observation of visuoconstructive disorders at the acute stage is a marker of stroke severity and is predictive of an overall poor prognosis (Andrews *et al.*, 1980; Friedman, 1991; Adunsky *et al.*, 2002). In surviving patients, recovery is frequently observed, although a persisting disorder was still observed at one year in about 20% of patients with right hemisphere stroke (Hier *et al.*, 1983). Rehabilitation has been proposed in selected cases, but, to our knowledge, no class I randomized trials have investigated the clinical benefit of this modality.

REFERENCES

Adunsky, A., Fleissig, Y., Levenkrohn, S., Arad, M. and Noy, S. (2002). Clock drawing task, mini-mental state examination and cognitive-functional independence measure: Relation to functional outcome of stroke patients. *Arch. Gerontol. Geriatr.*, **45**, 153–60.

Ajuriaguerra, J., Hécaen, H. and Anguelergues, R. (1960). Les apraxies: Variétés cliniques et latéralisation lésionnelle. *Rev. Neurol.*, **102**, 566–94.

Andrews, K., Brocklehurst, J. C., Richards, B. and Laycock, P. J. (1980). The prognostic value of picture drawings by stroke patients. *Rheumatol. Rehabil.*, **19**, 180–8.

Arena, R. and Gainotti, G. (1978). Constructional apraxia and visuoperceptive disabilities in relation to laterality of cerebral lesions. *Cortex*, **14**, 463–73.

Arrigoni, G. and De Renzi, E. (1964). Constructional apraxia and hemispheric locus of lesion. *Cortex*, **1**, 180–97.

Benton, A. L. (1967). Constructional apraxia and the minor hemisphere. *Confinia Neurologica*, **29**, 1–16.

(1968). Differential effects in frontal lobe disease. *Neuropsychologia*, **6**, 53–60.

Binder, L. M. (1982). Constructional strategies on complex figure drawings after unilateral brain damage. *J. Clin. Neuropsychol.*, **4**, 51–8.

De Renzi, E. and Faglioni, P. (1967). The relationship between visuospatial impairment and constructional apraxia. *Cortex*, **3**, 227–342.

Dérouesné, J., Seron, X. and Signoret, J. L. (1975). La rééducation de patients avec lésion frontale. *Rev. Neurol.*, **131**, 677–89.

Duensing, F. (1953). Raumagnostische und ideatorisch-apraktische storung des gestaltenden handelns. *Deutsch Zietschrift Nervenheilkd*, **170**, 72–94.

Engstad, T., Almkvist, O., Viitanen, M. and Arnesen, E. (2003). Impaired motor speed, visuospatial episodic memory and verbal fluency characterize cognition in long-term stroke survivors: The Tromso Study. *Neuroepidemiology*, **22**, 326–31.

Freedman, M., Leach, L., Kaplan, E., *et al.* (1994). *Clock Drawing: A Neuropsychological Analysis*, New York: Oxford University Press.

Friedman, P. J. (1991). Clock drawing in acute stroke. *Age Ageing*, **20**, 140–5.

Fushimi, H., Inoue, T., Yamada, Y., Udaka, F. and Kameyama, M. (1996). Asymptomatic cerebral small infarcts (lacunae), their risk factors and intellectual disturbances. *Diabetes*, **45** (Suppl. 3), S98–S100.

Gainotti, G. (1972). A quantitative study of the 'closing in' phenomenon symptom in children and in brain damaged patients. *Neuropsychologia*, **10**, 429–36.

(1985). Constructional apraxia. In J. A. M. Frederiks, ed., *Handbook of Clinical Neurology* Vol **1**. Amsterdam: Elsevier, pp. 491–506.

Gainotti, G., D'Erme, P. and Diodato, S. (1985). Are drawing errors differed in right-sided and left-sided constructional apraxics? *Ital. J. Neurol. Sci.*, **6**, 495–501.

Hécaen, H., Ajuriaguerra, J. and Massonet, J. (1951). *Les troubles visuoconstructifs par lésions pariéto-occipitales droites. Rôle des perturbations vestibulaires. Encéphale*. 122–79.

Hécaen, H. and Assal, G. (1970). A comparison of constructive deficits following right and left hemispherics lesions. *Neuropsychologia*, **8**, 289–303.

Hier, D. B., Mondlock, J. and Caplan, L. R. (1983). Recovery of behavioral abnormalities after right hemisphere stroke. *Neurology*, **33**, 345–50.

Hochstenbach, J., Mulder, T., Van Limbeek, J., Donders, R. and Schoonderwaldt, H. (1998). Cognitive decline following stroke: A comprehensive study of cognitive decline following stroke. *J. Clin. Exp. Neuropsychol.*, **20**, 503–17.

Hochstenbach, J. B., den Otter, R. and Mulder, T. W. (2003). Cognitive recovery after stroke: A 2-year follow-up. *Arch. Phys. Med. Rehabil.*, **84**, 1499–504.

Ishiai, S., Sugishita, M., Ichikawa, T., Gono, S. and Watabiki, S. (1993). Clock drawing test and unilateral spatial neglect. *Neurology*, **43**, 106–10.

Kirk, A. and Kertesz, A. (1989). Hemispheric contributions to drawing. *Neuropsychologia*, **27**, 881–6.

(1993). Subcortical contribution to drawing. *Brain Lang.*, **21**, 57–70.

Kleist, K. (1934). *Gehirnpathologie*, Leipzig: Barth.

Kreiter, K. T., Copeland, D., Bernardini, G. L., *et al.* (2002). Predictors of cognitive dysfunction after subarachnoid hemorrhage. *Stroke*, **33**, 200–8.

Lhermitte, F., Dérouesné, J. and Signoret, J. L. (1972). L'analyse neuropsychologique du syndrome frontal. *Rev. Neurol.*, **127**, 415–40.

Luria, A. R. and Tsvetkova, L. S. (1964). The programming of constructive activity in local brain injury. *Neuropsychologia*, **2**, 95—108.

Marshall, R. S., Lazar, R. M., Binder, J. R., *et al.* (1994). Intrahemispheric localization of drawing dysfunction. *Neuropsychologia*, **32**, 493—501.

Mayer, S. A., Kreiter, K. T., Copeland, D., *et al.* (2002). Global and domain-specific cognitive impairment and outcome after subarachnoid hemorrhage. *Neurology*, **59**, 1750—8.

Mendez, M., Ala, T. and Underwood, K. (1992). Development of scoring criteria for the clock drawing task in Alzheimer's disease. *J. Am. Geriatr. Soc.*, **40**, 1095—99.

Ogden, J. A., Mee, E. W. and Henning, M. (1993). A prospective study of impairment of cognition and memory and recovery after subarachnoid hemorrhage. *Neurosurgery*, **33**, 572—86.

Pillon, B. (1981). Troubles visuoconstructifs et méthodes de compensation: Résultats de 85 patients atteints de lésions cérébrales. *Neuropsychologia*, **19**, 375—83.

Rey, A. (1959). *Test de Copie d'une Figure Complexe*. Paris: Edition du Centre de Psychologie Appliquée.

Rosen, W. (1983). *The Rosen drawing Test*. New York: Veterans Administration Medical Center.

Rouleau, I., Salmon, D., Butters, N., Kennedy, C. and McGuife, K. (1992). Quantitative and qualitative analyses of clock drawings in Alzheimer's and Huntington's disease. *Brain Cogn.*, **18**, 70—87.

Sachdev, P. S., Brodaty, H., Valenzuela, M. J., *et al.* (2004). The neuropsychological profile of vascular cognitive impairment in stroke and TIA patients. *Neurology*, **62**, 912—19.

Shallice, T. (1989). *From Neuropsychology to Mental Structures*. Cambridge, UK: Cambridge University Press.

Suhr, J., Grace, J., Allen, J., Nadler, J. and McKenna, M. (1998). Quantitative and qualitative performance of stroke versus normal elderly on six clock drawing systems. *Arch. Clin. Neuropsychol.*, **13**, 495—502.

Sunderland, T., Hill, J. L. Mellow, A. M., *et al.* (1989). Clock drawing in Alzheimer's disease. A novel measure of dementia severity. *J. Am. Geriatr. Soc.*, **37**(8), 725—29.

Sunderland, A., Tinson, D. and Bradley, L. (1994). Differences in recovery from constructional apraxia after right and left hemisphere stroke? *J. Clin. Exp. Neuropsychol.*, **16**, 916—20.

Swindell, C. S., Holland, A. L., Fromm, D. and Greenhouse, J. B. (1988). Characteristics of recovery of drawing ability in left and right brain-damaged patients. *Brain Cogn.*, **7**, 16—30.

Tatemichi, T. K., Desmond, D. W., Stern, Y., *et al.* (1994). Cognitive impairment after stroke: Frequency, patterns, and relationship to functional abilities. *J. Neurol. Neurosurg. Psychiatry*, **57**, 202—7.

Warrington, E. K., James, M. and Kinsbourne, M. (1966). Drawing disability in relation to laterality of cerebral lesion. *Brain*, **89**, 53—82.

Watson, Y. I., Arfken, C. L. and Birge, S. J. (1993). Clock completion: An objective screening test for dementia. *J. Am. Geriatr. Soc.*, **41**, 1235—40.

13

Topographical disorientation

Bertille Périn and Olivier Godefroy

University Hospital, Amiens, France

General description of topographical disorientation

Topographical disorientation — the inability to find one's way in familiar or unfamiliar environments — remains poorly studied and is probably underestimated in stroke patients. However, recognition of this condition is usually easy and improves patient management.

This chapter deals with the selective loss of ability to find one's way in a familiar environment and to learn new paths. This disorder is generally known as "topographical disorientation," but terms such as "topographical agnosia" and "topographical amnesia" have also been used to refer to similar conditions. Topographical disorientation is defined by a relatively selective loss of ability to find one's way in a familiar environment in the absence of global amnesia, severe disorders of visual perception or confusion. Following initial case reports (Foerster, 1890; Jackson, 1932; Meyer, 1900), numerous cases have been reported and their diversity suggests the existence of several varieties of topographical disorientation. Several influential reviews of the literature and classifications have been proposed (e.g. Levine *et al.*, 1985; Farrell, 1996; Barrash, 1998; Aguirre and D'Esposito, 1999).

The presence of topographical disorientation is easily demonstrated in patients with difficulties finding their way in familiar places. The patient or caregiver may spontaneously report the difficulty, but clinical practice suggests that systematic interview significantly increases detection of the disorder. The disorder is especially striking in ambulatory patients. Difficulties in the familiar environment usually concern the hospital, home town (finding one's way to main public places, major buildings, familiar trips...) and in severe cases may even be observed in the patient's home. Difficulties may also impair the ability to learn new paths in a novel environment (hospital, unusual route...). Some patients spontaneously develop compensatory strategies: they use verbal indices such as room numbers, street names, station names and house numbers, or consult a map and verbal notes.

Two additional features may be observed in some patients and have been used to propose a classification of the disorder:

1. Although patients are able to report their final destination, their ability to describe or draw a familiar route may be spared or impaired (suggesting a deficit of spatial memory).

2. Some patients have a severe deficit in recognizing familiar places and buildings. Thus, they are unable to use these prominent environmental features for the purposes of orientation and this contributes to their difficulties. Most patients remain confined to the hospital or home and usually refuse to go out without a companion.

Topographical disorientation is frequently associated with hemianopia, prosopagnosia and central achromatopsia, but is not explained by these deficits, as shown by selective deficits with double dissociation (i.e. visual agnosia without topographical disorientation, and vice versa) (Levine *et al.*, 1985; Aguirre and D'Esposito, 1999). In the same vein, a deficit of visual–spatial memory may be observed in some patients, but does not account for all cases of topographical disorientation (Barrash, 1998; Aguirre and D'Esposito, 1999). Route finding difficulties secondary to severe hemineglect and Bálint's syndrome are usually not classified as topographical disorientation. Topographical disorientation should be distinguished from spatial disorientation, which impairs the orientation to place and is observed in other disorders. Finally, reduplicative paramnesia for places is a different disorder in which a patient repeatedly and consistently misidentifies a familiar place, sometimes including occupants, as a duplicate. Patients correctly identify their whereabouts (e.g. the room in the Amiens Neurology department), but think and maintain that they are (or this room is) also located in another place (e.g. their home in another city), which is a duplicate (sometimes described as an expansion) of the original one. Despite their ability to perceive the absurdity of this interpretation, they fail to reject it. Reduplicative paramnesia is not frequent — although observed in up to 8% of cases of focal damage in the study by Murai *et al.* (1997) — and is usually observed in right-sided or bilateral damage.

Topographical disorientation has been reported in different diseases, including stroke (Meyer, 1900; De Renzi, 1977b), dementia, traumatic brain injury, viral encephalitis (McCarthy *et al.*, 1996), paraneoplastic limbic encephalitis (Hirayama *et al.*, 2003), and tumor (Jackson, 1932). Temporal surgery may impair spatial memory, remembering and way-finding in the environment (Maguire *et al.*, 1996a). In focal pathology, the lesions more frequently concern the posterior cortex, and unilateral lesions are prominently located in the right hemisphere (Barrash, 1998). Most studies support the role of the right medial occipito-temporal (lingual gyrus) and the right medial temporal regions (especially the hippocampus and parahippocampal gyrus) (Maguire *et al.*, 1996b; Bohbot, 1998; Nunn *et al.*, 1999; Barrash *et al.*, 2000). The possible contribution of lesions of the left temporo-occipital lobe and inferior parietal lobe requires further studies (Barrash 1998; Aguirre and D'Esposito, 1999).

Several classifications of the disorder have been proposed according to the pattern of impairment and the presumed underlying deficit (Levine *et al.*, 1985; Farrell, 1996; Aguirre and D'Esposito, 1999). Two main neuropsychological mechanisms can underlie topographical disorientation.

1. A deficit of spatial memory is usually claimed to play a major role. The basic deficit is the inability to retrieve a representation of the map of the route, the specification of spatial relations between places and the use of this information to orient navigation (Meyer, 1900; De Renzi *et al.*, 1977a). This variety of topographical disorientation is frequently called "topographical amnesia."

2. Several studies have emphasized the failure to recognize familiar environments (buildings, landscapes), sometimes labeled "topographical or environmental or landmark agnosia" (Pallis, 1955; Whiteley and Warrington, 1978; Landis *et al.*, 1986). This deficit is frequently associated with prosopagnosia and is observed in lesions of the right parahippocampal region and anterior half of the lingual and fusiform gyri (Habib and Sirigu, 1987; Takahashi and Kawamura, 2002). However, the inability to recognize familiar environments is not a constant feature of topographical disorientation and its contribution to the patient's disability has been questioned by De Renzi (1977a), who observed a patient who did not improve in taking his bearings when the name of buildings was provided.

Aguirre and D'Esposito (1999) have proposed four categories:

1. Egocentric disorientation (deficit in representing location of objects with respect to self) is responsible for inaccurate route descriptions and usually associated with parietal lobe lesion.

2. Heading disorientation (deficit of orientation with respect to external environment) occurs when landmarks do not evoke any directional information.

3. Agnosia for landmarks is due to a deficit in recognizing landmarks associated with lesions of the lingual gyrus.

4. Anterograde disorientation occurs when patients are unable to navigate in new surroundings, to learn and follow new routes to specific destinations, associated with lesion of the parahippocampal region.

Key points Main characteristics of topographical disorientation

Topographical disorientation
Selective loss of ability to find one's way in a familiar environment
Inability to learn new paths
In the absence of global amnesia, severe disorders of visual perception or confusion
Associated in most patients with:
  –inability to use spatial information to orient the navigation
  –inability to retrieve a representation of the map of the route
  –failure to recognize familiar environment

Topographical disorientation and stroke

Although stroke is a frequent cause of topographical disorientation (De Renzi, 1977b), its prevalence has not been established to our knowledge.

A review of 41 well-documented cases reported during the last 20 years shows that the majority of strokes are due to infarcts (Table 13.1). Stroke is unilateral in most cases and located in the right occipito-temporal or medio-temporal regions. The arterial territory is rarely specified, but the description suggests the territory of the posterior cerebral artery in most cases (Landis *et al.*, 1986; Habib and Sirigu, 1987; Pai, 1997; Katayama *et al.*, 1999; Luzzi *et al.*, 2000; Ohra *et al.*, 2000; Lin and Pai, 2000; Takahashi and Kawamura, 2002; Mendez and Cherrier, 2003; Aoki *et al.*, 2003; Martinez-Fernandez *et al.*, 2003). Several patients suffer from stroke involving the region of the splenium, posterior cingulate cortex, and medial parietal lobe (including the cuneus area) (Cammalleri *et al.*, 1996; Suzuki *et al.*, 1998; Katayama *et al.*, 1999; Alsaadi *et al.*, 2000; Martinez-Fernandez *et al.*, 2003) and this appears to be the second most frequent site of the lesion. A few patients suffer from stroke restricted to a specific region (Table 13.1), such as the parahippocampal gyrus, occipital lobe, right parietal lobe, internal capsule (in one case documented by CT scan), or right thalamus. Most patients had right-sided lesions, a few cases had bilateral posterior lesions and a pure left lesion was found to be very rare in right-handed patients (Obi *et al.*, 1992; Sato *et al.*, 1998; Alsaadi *et al.*, 2000). Finally, pure topographical disorientation due to infarct in the inferior–posterior branch of the middle cerebral artery (responsible for inferior parietal infarct) was not observed in this review of the literature. These clinical–anatomical correlations suggest that another cause (especially Alzheimer's disease, another frequent cause of topographical disorientation in the elderly) should be suspected in patients with

Table 13.1. Stroke characteristics in recent cases of topographical disorientation

Study	n	Age	Imaging	Stroke type	Lesion location
Landis et al. (1986)	13	16–64	CT-scan	Infarct 12 Hematoma 1	8 R temporo-occipital 2 R parieto-occipital 2 R medial occipital (including 1 bilateral) 1 R medial parietal
Habib and Sirigu (1987)	4	26–60	CT-scan	Infarct	Territory of R PCA
Hublet and Demeurisse (1992)	1	72	CT-scan	Infarct	R internal capsule
Obi et al. (1992)	1	59	MRI	Infarct	L parieto-occipital and L splenium
Ishii et al. (1992)	1	80	MRI	Hematoma	Bilateral temporo-occipital
Cammalleri et al. (1996)	1	53	MRI	Angioma	R cingulate cortex
Pai (1997)	2	55–58	CT-scan	Infarct	Territory of R PCA
Suzuki et al. (1998)	1	70	MRI	Hematoma	R medial parietal (precuneus)
Sato et al. (1998)	1	67	MRI	Infarct	L temporo-occipital
Katayama et al. (1999)	1	82	MRI	Infarct	R splenium & posterior cingulate cortex
Luzzi et al. (2000)	1	75	CT-scan	Infarct	R parahippocampal gyrus
Alsaadi et al. (2000)	3	50–62	CT-scan: 2MRI: 1	Infarct	R splenium and cuneus Bilateral temporo-occipital (right prominence) L parieto-occipital and left splenium
Ohra et al. (2000)	1	70	MRI	Infarct	R occipital
Lin and Pai (2000)	1	55	MRI	Infarct	Territory of R PCA
Takahashi and Kawamura (2002)	4	69–73	MRI	Infarct	2 R temporo-occipital 2 R temporal
Yoshimura and Otsuki (2002)	1	73	MRI	Infarct	Territory of R anterior choroidal artery (thalamus and caudate tail)
Mendez and Cherrier (2003)	1	76	MRI	Infarct	R temporo-occipital
Aoki et al. (2003)	1	70	MRI	Infarct	R temporo-occipital
Martinez-Fernandez et al. (2003)	2	71–77	CT-scan	Infarct	Territory of R PCA

R: right; L: left; PCA: posterior cerebral artery

topographical disorientation and stroke in an unexpected site, especially when the territory of the right posterior cerebral artery is spared. Episodes of topographical disorientation attributed to epilepsy have been reported in one patient with an angioma in the right posterior cingulate cortex (Camalleri *et al.*, 1996).

Mitochondrial encephalomyopathy, lactic acidosis plus stroke-like episodes (MELAS) is responsible for stroke-like acute dysfunction and may induce topographical disorientation (Funakawa *et al.*, 1994). Transient topographical disorientation seems to be rarely due to transient ischemic attack (Stracciari *et al.*, 1994; Gil-Neciga *et al.*, 2002) and is probably due to a mechanism similar to that of transient global amnesia. These patients are usually older than 50 years and suffer from a short-lasting inability to find their way in a familiar environment, while they remain conscious and are able to recall what happened. Contrary to transient global amnesia, there is no lacunar amnesia and recall of the episode is preserved. Since such transient disorder may also be observed at the very early stage of Alzheimer's disease, a detailed examination is required.

Key points Main types of stroke responsible for topographical disorientation

Stroke type	Region/Territory
Infarct	Most cases: territory of the right posterior cerebral artery involving the following regions: –occipito-temporal –medio-temporal –medio-parietal, splenium and posterior cingulate gyrus Rare cases: parahippocampal gyrus, occipital lobe, right parietal lobe, internal capsule with a prominence of right sided lesions
Hematoma	occipito-temporal and medio-parietal regions

Assessment of topographical disorientation in stroke patients

Clinical examination

An excellent history taken from both the patient and the family is essential. It reveals (1) the patient's inability to find his/her way in familiar environments and the major difficulties learning new paths, contrasting with his/her previous abilities, (2) the contrast between difficulties in finding the way and the preserved ability to indicate the final destination, and (3) in some patients, the use of compensatory strategies such as the use of verbal tags (name of the street...).

When possible, clinical examination in a familiar place illustrates the patient's difficulties: inability to find the way back to his/her room, the possible use of room number or verbal tags, the frequent inability to give a verbal description (or to indicate on a map) the route to be followed. In addition, the examination may reveal the presence of hemianopia, visual agnosia (especially prosopagnosia), and excludes the presence of confusion, severe global memory deficit, and dementia.

Neuropsychological assessment

A general neuropsychological assessment is required and, in this situation, must more specifically examine episodic memory for verbal and visual material, visual–spatial exploration, visual identification (especially prosopagnosia and achromatopsia), language, and general intellectual efficiency.

The specific assessment of topographic orientation is based on familiar ways and landscapes, and consequently varies greatly from place to place and from one subject to another. Several tests have been proposed.

Short-term spatial memory is usually assessed by the Block-Tapping Task (Corsi, 1972). The subject is presented with nine cubes on a board in an irregular arrangement; the examiner taps in sequences of increasing length that the subject is required to reproduce. This test is usually performed as part of the general neuropsychological assessment and must be performed in patients with topographical disorientation. However, dissociations are frequently observed: a normal span may be observed in a disoriented patient, and vice versa.

Key points Neuropsychological assessment of topographical disorientation

---

Clinical examination

History: inability to find one's way in familiar environments and to learn new paths, preserved ability to indicate the final destination

possible use of compensatory strategies (use of verbal tags . . .), failure to recognize familiar environment

Examination when possible: orientation and displacement in familiar environment

Ability to describe or indicate in a map the route to follow

Neuropsychological assessment

Short term and episodic spatial memory

Identification of famous buildings and places

Semantic spatial knowledge

Perceptual disorders (agnosia especially prosopagnosia, visuospatial exploration and hemineglect)

General assessment: general intellectual efficiency, language, and verbal memory

---

The assessment of episodic memory should include examination of *visual–spatial memory*. Recall of the Rey Complex Figure (Rey, 1959) is frequently used, but does not specifically assess the spatial component. The Object Location Test requires the patient first to recall objects that have been presented in a specific location and, second, their spatial locations (Bohbot *et al.*, 1998; 2000). Several maze tests have been proposed with variable degrees of normative data, such as a "visually guided maze learning test" (which consists of 64 square buttons in 8 rows and columns and requires the subject to learn the correct path between the starting and ending points) (Milner, 1965; De Renzi, 1977a) and a "locomotor maze test" (where the subject is asked to find a way in a large room with landmarks taped on the walls and a map indicating the route) (Hecaen *et al.*, 1980). Recently computer-based tasks have been designed for research purposes (Barrash, 1994; McCarthy *et al.*, 1996).

The ability to identify famous buildings and places (and to describe them verbally) is usually required to assess "topographical agnosia." When famous places are located in a familiar environment, the subject is asked to describe the route from one place to another.

The use of a country map (requiring the placement of several important cities) is frequently used to examine *semantic spatial knowledge*. Its interpretation requires normative data. Impairment may be observed in numerous other conditions, and especially hemineglect, which induces omissions on one side reversed when the opposite north–south axis is used (see Chapter 7).

Outcome and management

Key points Management of topographical disorientation

Inability to learn new paths frequently persists
Disorientation for familiar environment may improve
Rehabilitation may be proposed in selected cases

The natural course of topographical disorientation has not been systematically studied to our knowledge. In most cases, this condition is detected in the rehabilitation center or after discharge home. When improvement is mentioned, persistence of difficulties in learning new paths (Habib and Sirigu, 1987; Barrash, 1998) appears to be frequent. This disorder is severely disabling and most patients refuse to leave home alone. Rehabilitation may be proposed in selected cases and must take into account the underlying mechanisms of topographical disorientation.

REFERENCES

Aguirre, G. K. and D'Esposito, M. (1999). Topographical disorientation: A synthesis and taxonomy. *Brain*, **122**, 1613–28.

Alsaadi, T., Binder, J. R., Lazar, R. M., Doorani, T. and Mohr, J. P. (2000). Pure topographic disorientation: A distinctive syndrome with varied localization. *Neurology*, **54**, 1864–6.

Aoki, K., Hiroki, M., Bando, M., Miyamoto, K. and Hirai, S. (2003). A case of agnosia for streets without visual memory disturbance. *Rinsho Shinkeigaku*, **43**, 335–40.

Barrash, J. (1994). Age-related decline in route learning ability. *Dev. Neuropsychol.*, **10**, 189–201.

(1998). A historical review of topographical disorientation and its neuroanatomical correlates. *J. Clin. Exp. Neuropsychol.*, **20**, 807–27.

Barrash, J., Damasio, H., Adolphs, R. and Tranel, D. (2000). The neuroanatomical correlates of route learning impairment. *Neuropsychologia*, **38**, 820–36.

Bohbot, V. D., Allen, J. J. and Nadel, L. (2000). Memory deficits characterized by patterns of lesions to the hippocampus and parahippocampal cortex. *Ann. N. Y. Acad. Sci.*, **911**, 355–68.

Bohbot, V. D., Kalina, M., Stepankova, K., *et al.* (1998). Spatial memory deficits in patients with lesions to the right hippocampus and to the right parahippocampal cortex. *Neuropsychologia*, **36**, 1217–38.

Cammalleri, R., Gangitano, M., D'Amelio, M., *et al.* (1996). Transient topographical amnesia and cingulate cortex damage: A case report. *Neuropsychologia*, **34**, 321–6.

Corsi, P. M. (1972). Human memory and the medial temporal region of the brain. *Dissertation Abstracts International*, **34**, 819B.

De Renzi, E., Faglioni, P. and Villa, P. (1977a). Topographical amnesia. *J. Neurol. Neurosurg. Psychiatry*, **40**, 498–505.

De Renzi, E., Faglioni, P. and Previdi, P. (1977b). Spatial memory and hemispheric locus of lesion. *Cortex*, **13**, 424–33.

Farrell, M. J. (1996). Topographical disorientation. *Neurocase*, **2**, 509–20.

Foerster, R. (1890). Ueber Rinden blindheit. *Albrecht v. Graefe Arch. Ophtalmol.*, **38**, 94–108.

Funakawa, I., Mukai, K., Terao, A., Kawashima, S. and Mori, T. (1994). A case of MELAS associated with prosopagnosia, topographical disorientation and PLED. *Rinsho Shinkeigaku*, **34**, 1052–4.

Gil-Neciga, E., Alberca, R., Boza, F., *et al.* (2002). Transient topographical disorientation. *Eur. Neurol.*, **48**, 191–9.

Habib, M. and Sirigu, A. (1987). Pure topographical disorientation: A definition and anatomical basis. *Cortex*, **23**, 73–85.

Hecaen, H., Tzortzis, C. and Rondot, P. (1980). Loss of topographical memory with learning deficits. *Cortex*, **16**, 525–42.

Hirayama, K., Taguchi, Y., Sato, M. and Tsukamoto, T. (2003). Limbic encephalitis presenting with topographical disorientation and amnesia. *J. Neurol. Neurosurg. Psychiatry*, **74**, 110–12.

Hublet, C. and Demeurisse, G. (1992). Pure topographical disorientation due to a deep-seated lesion with cortical remote effects. *Cortex*, **28**, 123–8.

Ishii, K., Kita, Y., Nagura, H., Bandoh, M. and Yamanouchi, H. (1992). A case report of cerebral achromatopsia with bilateral occipital lesion. *Rinsho Shinkeigaku*, **32**, 293–8.

Jackson, J. H. (1932). Case of large cerebral tumour with optic neuritis and with left hemiplegia and imperception. In J. H. Jackson, ed., *Selected Writings*. London: Taylor, pp. 146–52.

Katayama, K., Takahashi, N., Ogawara, K. and Hattori, T. (1999). Pure topographical disorientation due to right posterior cingulate lesion. *Cortex*, **35**, 279–82.

Landis, T., Cummings, J. L., Benson, D. F. and Palmer, E. P. (1986). Loss of topographic familiarity. An environmental agnosia. *Arch. Neurol.*, **43**, 132–6.

Levine, D. N., Warrash, J. and Farah, M. J. (1985). Two visual systems in mental imagery: Dissociation of the "what" and "where" in imagery disorders due to bilateral posterior cerebral lesions. *Neurology*, **35**, 1010–18.

Lin, C. C. and Pai, M. C. (2000). Transient topographical disorientation as a manifestation of cerebral ischaemic attack. *J. Formos. Med. Assoc.*, **99**, 653–5.

Luzzi, S., Pucci, E., Di Bella, P. and Piccirilli, M. (2000). Topographical disorientation consequent to amnesia of spatial location in a patient with right parahippocampal damage. *Cortex*, **36**, 427–34.

Maguire, E. A., Burke, T., Phillips, J. and Staunton, H. (1996a). Topographical disorientation following unilateral temporal lobe lesions in humans. *Neuropsychologia*, **34**, 993–1001.

Maguire, E. A., Frackowiak, R. S. and Frith, C. D. (1996b). Learning to find your way: A role for the human hippocampal formation. *Proc. R. Soc. Lond. B. Biol. Sci.*, **263**, 1745–50.

Martinez-Fernandez, E., Gil-Neciga, E., Boza-Garcia, F., Montes, E. and Donaire, A. (2003). Topographical disorientation associated with infarction in the territory of the right posterior cerebral artery. *Revista de Neurologica*, **36**, 224–6.

McCarthy, R. A., Evans, J. J. and Hodges, J. R. (1996). Topographic amnesia: Spatial memory disorder, perceptual dysfunction, or category specific semantic memory impairment? *J. Neurol. Neurosurg. Psychiatry*, **60**, 318–25.

Mendez, M. F. and Cherrier, M. M. (2003). Agnosia for scenes in topographagnosia. *Neuropsychologia*, **41**, 1387–95.

Meyer, O. (1900). Ein-und doppelseitige homonyme Hemianopsie mit Orientierungstoerungen. *Monatschr. Psychiatr. Neurol.*, **8**, 40–56.

Milner, B. (1965). Visually-guided maze learning in man: Effects of bilateral hippocampal, bilateral frontal and unilateral cerebral lesions. *Neuropsychologia*, **3**, 317–38.

Murai, T., Toichi, M., Sengoku, A., Miyoshi, K., Morimune, S. (1997). Reduplicative paramnesia in patients with focal brain damage. *Neuropsychiatry Neuropsychol. Behav. Neurol.*, **10**(3), 190–6.

Nunn, J. A., Graydon, F. J., Polkey, C. E. and Morris, R. G. (1999). Differential spatial memory impairment after right temporal lobectomy demonstrated using temporal titration. *Brain*, **122**(Pt 1), 47–59.

Obi, T., Bando, M., Takeda, K. and Sakuta, M. (1992). A case of topographical disturbance following a left medial parieto-occipital lobe infarction. *Rinsho Shinkeigaku*, **32**, 426–9.

Ohra, S., Otsuki, M., Omura, E., *et al.* (2000). A case of agnosia for streets and houses unaccompanied by prosopagnosia of familiar faces due to the right occipital lobe infarction. *Rinsho Shinkeigaku*, **40**, 891–5.

Pai, M. C. (1997). Topographic disorientation: Two cases. *J. Formos. Med. Assoc.*, **96**, 660–3.

Pallis, C. A. (1955). Impaired identification of locus and places with agnosia for colours. *J. Neurol. Neurosurg. Psychiatry*, **18**, 218–24.

Rey, A. (1959). *Test de copie d'une figure complexe.* Editions du centre de psychologie appliquée.

Sato, K., Sakajiri, K., Komai, K. and Takamori, M. (1998). A patient with amnesic syndrome with defective route finding due to left posterior cerebral artery territory infarction. *No To Shinkei*, **50**, 69–73.

Stracciari, A., Lorusso, S. and Pazzaglia, P. (1994). Transient topographical amnesia. *J. Neurol. Neurosurg. Psychiatry*, **57**, 1423–5.

Suzuki, K., Yamadori, A., Hayakawa, Y. and Fujii, T. (1998). Pure topographical disorientation related to dysfunction of the viewpoint dependent visual system. *Cortex*, **34**, 589–99.

Takahashi, N. and Kawamura, M. (2002). Pure topographical disorientation – the anatomical basis of landmark agnosia. *Cortex*, **38**, 717–25.

Whiteley, A. M. and Warrington, E. K. (1978). Selective impairment of topographical memory: A single case study. *J. Neurol. Neurosurg. Psychiatry*, **41**, 575–8.

Yoshimura, N. and Otsuki, M. (2002). A case of topographic disorientation without right occipital lesion. *No To Shinkei*, **54**, 601–4.

14

Cortical blindness

Alain Vighetto and Pierre Krolak-Salmon

Hôpital neurologique Pierre Wertheimer, Lyon and Université Claude Bernard Lyon I

Introduction

Cortical blindness refers to a total loss of vision caused by a bilateral lesion or dysfunction of the occipital lobe. It represents a subset of cerebral blindness, a more general term which indicates blindness from any damage to both visual pathways posterior to the lateral geniculate bodies. Cortical blindness results typically from direct insult to both the primary visual areas lying in the calcarine cortex. As the responsible lesion does not usually limit to the cortex, but also encompasses the posterior part of the optic radiations and variably the extrastriate visual areas, both de-afferentation and de-efferentation of the primary visual cortex may also contribute to the visual dysfunction that is observed at the acute and at the recovered stages as well. Ischemic strokes are the major cause of cortical blindness.

Description

Clinical symptoms

By definition, cortical blindness is defined by a bilateral and total loss of vision. Thus, affected subjects can no longer identify visual forms, colors, location, orientation or movement of objects, nor even differentiate light from dark. They are usually distressfully aware of their deficit. At the acute stage, however, degree of awareness is variable. Patients may not report spontaneously their problem or seem indifferent to it. A minority of patients may even deny any visual loss or attribute their faulty performance to external factors, such as unfitted eyeglasses or poor room illumination. This inappropriate behavior, called anosognosia for blindness, or Anton's syndrome (Symonds and Mackenzie, 1957), may add to the difficulty for the clinician in making the diagnosis in an emergency setting. Release hallucinations are present in over half of the cases during the initial period (Gloning et al., 1967). Hallucinations related to the acute occipital lobe lesion are usually elementary ones, described as spots of colors, streaks, or simple geometrical patterns (Kolmel, 1985; Fisher, 1986; Vaphiades et al., 1996).

Well-formed and complex hallucinations usually indicate extension of the lesion to the cortex of the temporal lobe, but can also be observed in occipital lobe lesion (Beniczky *et al.*, 2002).They usually start a few days after visual loss onset and may stop after days or persist over months (Lance, 1976). Patients may be reluctant to report them and they have to be specifically asked for. Both preservation of pupillary light reflexes and normal ocular fundi are characteristic findings that differentiate cortical blindness from more anterior causes of bilateral blindness. Onset and evolution profiles of cortical blindness depend on the etiology. Overwhelmingly, onset is acute, as a consequence of its most prevalent, vascular, cause. Vision loss is usually durable but it can also occur as a transient manifestation.

Incomplete or partly recovered forms of cortical blindness may be less rare than the complete form. Often, some crude light perception may remain, allowing detection of high luminance contrast, especially when flickering or moving stimuli are used. Other less severe cases present as degraded vision, with bilaterally reduced visual acuity, or as bilateral homonymous hemianopia, with spared acuity and central field of vision (Levin, 2005).

Residual vision

A proportion of patients having longlasting hemianopia or cortical blindness keep some visual abilities in their perimetrically blind areas. Such residual function refers to two related entities, that deal mainly with spatial attributes of vision and differ by the degree of awareness linked to this spared vision. The first entity, clinically derived, is called Riddoch's phenomenon. It designates a retained capacity to detect consciously moving but not stationary objects. Indeed, it is common clinical observation to find a degree of dissociation between detection of moving versus static objects during the recovering phase of cortical blindness. Such "stato-kinetic dissociation" can be shown while comparing Goldmann (kinetic) and automated (static) perimetry charts in patients with hemianopia or partly recovered cortical blindness, static perimetry being more pessimistic in terms of remnant visual field (Finkelstein and Johnson, 1989). In a few cases, proper use of optical flow generated while walking may render patients able to correctly ambulate and avoid obstacles despite (near) total blindness in the common sense (Mestre *et al.*, 1992). The second entity, laboratory derived, is called *blindsight*. Blindsight was initially showed in monkeys after removal of both occipital lobes and secondarily in patients with hemianopia or cortical blindness (Perenin *et al.*, 1980; Stoerig and Cowey, 1997; Danckert *et al.*, 2003; Weiskrantz, 2004). It refers to a non-conscious, implicit, behaviorally demonstrated vision, allowing patients to discriminate movement or detect orientation of contrast gratings, to orient their gaze or point manually to a visual target in a visual field that is supposedly blind. These preserved skills need to be revealed by forcing the patient to react to a visual event they are not aware of. Indeed, these two entities are probably the two ends of a unique spectrum, as degree of unawareness varies from patient to patient and from task to task. Residual vision, whether or not conscious, relates mainly to visual attributes that are processed by the magnocellular stream of the visual system. Since only a proportion of patients with cortical blindness demonstrate such residual vision, anatomical correlates have to be searched for. Actually, explanation for this phenomenon is still debated. Some advocate a degraded normal vision, due to incomplete damage to primary visual cortex, while most authors favor vision function that is provided by other parts of the visual system than the geniculostriate pathway. In the latter line, candidates are either subcortical structures, such as the superior colliculus and pulvinar, or extrastriate cortical structures, such as V5, which can be fed from direct thalamic inputs (both lateral geniculate bodies and pulvinar). The two explanations may well be complementary, depending on the cases. It can be speculated that gating between conscious and unconscious residual vision may relate to the relative amount of respectively cortical (especially V5) versus subcortical processing involved in a particular task condition (Sahraie *et al.*, 1997; Zeki and Ffytche, 1998).

The concept that some implicit visual processing can modulate our behavior despite apparent total blindness is of great theoretical interest. However, its clinical implications are limited. Blindsight cannot be demonstrated at the bedside. It is not clear whether blindsight contributes to ecological behavior in patients showing it, or can be manipulated for rehabilitation purpose, or is associated with a better visually related functional outcome.

Main causes

Most causes of cortical blindness relate to ischemic/hypoxic changes affecting the occipital lobes. Many other conditions may, however, be encountered (Table 14.1).

Cortical blindness of vascular origin

Clinical symptoms

Cortical blindness is a rare event, occurring in less than 5% of cases of posterior cerebral artery strokes (Brandt *et al.*, 2000). Blindness may occur suddenly in a normal seeing patient or as a two-stage deficit in a patient having previously homonymous hemianopia. In a series of 58 cases with unilateral occipital lobe infarction, it was found that 22% had a second stroke leading to cortical blindness over a mean period of 39.6 months (Bogousslavsky *et al.*, 1983). In such a case, it is not unusual that hemianopia secondary to the first posterior cerebral artery stroke

Table 14.1. Non exhaustive list of causes of cortical blindness

Embolic infarction in both posterior cerebral artery territories

Cardiac arrest

Severe hypotension

Carbon monoxide poisoning

Hypoxia

Bilateral occipital lobe hemorrhage (trauma, amyloid angiopathy)

Hypertensive encephalopathy (malignant hypertension, eclampsia, pheochromocytoma)

Other causes of posterior reversible leukoencephalopathy (ciclosporine or tacrolimus
    toxicity, iodine contrast agent)

Cerebral venous thrombosis

Subclavian vein catheterization

Post partum pulmonary embolus

Temporal arteritis

Wegener's granulomatosis

Sarcoidosis

Head trauma

Occipital lobe tumors

MELAS

Hypoglycemia

Uremia

Acute intermittent porphyria

Encephalitis/meningitis

Subacute sclerosing leukoencephalopathy

White matter diseases: Schilder's disease, adrenoleukodystrophy, metachromatic
    leukodystrophy, progressive multifocal leukoencephalopathy

Hydrocephalus, shunt dysfunction (in children)

Creutzfeldt-Jakob disease (Heidenhain's variant)

Migraine with aura

Occipital lobe epilepsy (ictal or post ictal blindness)

Congenital (hypoxemic-ischemic encephalopathy, periventricular leukomalacia,
    cortical dysplasia)

Sources: Liu *et al.*, 2001 and Levin *et al.*, 2005.

goes unrecognized until the second and contralateral stroke happens, leading then
to complete blindness. More rarely, it presents as transient episodes of bilateral
amaurosis, particularly in cases of postural hypotension after the introduction of
vigorous treatment against hypertension.

   Cortical blindness is isolated whenever the stroke is limited to the calcarine
artery territory. The other symptoms that may be associated to blindness are
related to the extension of the vascular lesion beyond the striate cortex, including

the temporal lobes, the thalami or the mesencephalon. Typically, involvement of the whole superficial territory of the posterior cerebral artery results in blindness associated with cognitive deficits, such as mental confusion or Korsakoff's-type amnestic disorder, agitated behavior, anomic or transcortical sensory aphasia. Involvement of the rostral midbrain leads to the "top of the basilar syndrome," in which blindness may be an additional sign to lethargy, vertical gaze deficits, ocular motor palsy, pupillary defects, or hemiplegia (Caplan, 1980).

Evolution

Prognosis for vision return is usually poor. However, spontaneous recovery of vision has been reported. From a total of 111 patients gathered from various studies in the literature, it was found that 73% showed recovery of vision, with considerable differences in terms of time course and extent of recovery (Zihl, 2000). In this series, complete recovery occurred in only 6% of cases. Recovery took place within 8–12 weeks, but was occasionally observed up to 2 years after injury. The pattern of recovery follows relatively definite stages. Light perception recovers first, allowing the patients to detect sudden illumination, especially when the luminance contrast is temporally modulated, through flickering or movement. This observation suggests that the magnocellular stream is implicated first during recovery. At this stage, patients may be able to grossly localize the incoming light in space, but are usually not able to indicate direction or speed of movement. Recovery of movement perception always precedes that of form and color perception, the only exception being exceptional cases of akinetopsia (Zeki, 1991). Then, patients can report vague perception of contours, while vision is described as foggy, and acuity is no more than counting fingers. When colors are perceived, they appear pale and hue discrimination is poor. Further improvement can lead to more or less successful recognition of objects, faces, and whereabouts. During the whole phase, hallucinations may be present, including palinopsia and polyopia. Recovery of vision usually occurs in the central field region. This may be related to the better compensation of the vascular supply of the occipital pole subserving central vision by the middle cerebral artery. Some patients may even recover 10/10 visual acuity, in spite of enduring visual deficit due to tubular field limited to the central 2 or 5 degrees, a condition termed "double homonymous hemianopia." Other patients can recover part of their peripheral field of vision. In terms of visual fields, numerous patterns of residual deficits can be found, depending on:

1. the more or less completeness of homonymous hemianopia
2. the presence of unilateral or bilateral homonymous deficit, as defined with respect to the vertical meridian
3. the symmetry of the deficit between the two sides.

Thus, main residual deficit include homonymous hemianopia or quadranta-nopia, altitudinal superior or inferior hemianopia, crossed quadrantanopia, central or paracentral homonymous scotomas, double hemianopia with macular sparing, temporal crescent sparing or involvement (Vighetto, 2004). Somewhat independently of the quality and quantity of the acuity and visual fields that recover, patients are often left with various kinds of visual agnosias, including apperceptive visual agnosia, alexia without agraphia, simultanagnosia, and Bálint's syndrome. In reference to age of onset, children are more likely to experience recovery from cortical blindness than adults.

Prognosis of vision recovery in cortical blindness is the poorest for ischemic strokes. The extent of recovery of vision has been found to be negatively correlated with time elapsed since stroke onset, history of diabetes or hypertension, age, associated cognitive deficits, and presence of bilateral lucencies on the initial CT scan (Aldrich *et al.*, 1987).

Strokes responsible for cortical blindness

Arterial supply of the primary visual cortex comes from the calcarine artery, a branch of the posterior cerebral artery, but the most posterior part of the occipital pole may also be supplied by a branch from the middle cerebral artery. Whenever such vascular compensation of the posterior pole is efficient, it may explain macular sparing observed after unilateral or bilateral posterior cerebral artery infarct. Ischemic infarcts resulting in cortical blindness are the consequence of occlusion of both calcarine arteries. Depending on the locus of the arterial occlusion, from the calcarine artery to the posterior cerebral artery trunk, the extent of the infarct may be confined respectively to the inner part of the occipital lobes resulting in pure cortical blindness, or may involve the internal and inferior temporal lobes, the thalamus or the mesencephalon, resulting in associated symptoms.

Most posterior cerebral artery trunk occlusions are caused by emboli, coming from the heart or from atherosclerotic artery-to-artery migration originating from the vertebral or basilar arteries (Chavez and Caplan, 2001). Fisher (1986) found in 95% of his 47 personal cases necropsy evidence of embolism. Bilateral infarcts that develop simultaneously usually result from embolism or extension of a thrombus in the distal basilar artery to the two posterior cerebral arteries. Those who develop consecutively have the same causes as found in unilateral infarcts, but are more likely to have additionally bilateral posterior cerebral artery atherosclerotic stenosis (Chavez and Caplan, 2001). Hemodynamic failure secondary to cardiac arrest or prolonged hypotension can result in cortical blindness from bilateral

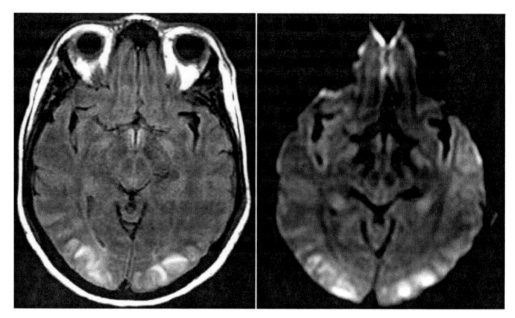

Figure 14.1 T2-weighted axial MRI showing bilateral occipital infarct as a consequence of eclampsia in a 24-year-old woman with cortical blindness.

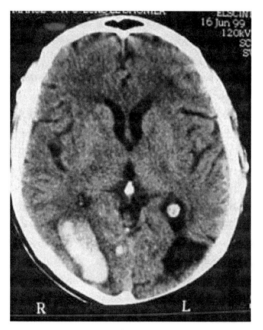

Figure 14.2 CT scan of a 78-year-old man showing cortical blindness as a consequence of amyloid angiopathy. A first left occipital ischemic event led to right hemianopia and blindness occurred after a second, left occipital, hemorrhagic stroke.

watershed infarction between posterior cerebral artery and carotid artery territories. Bilateral posterior cerebral artery infarct due to compression of the arteries onto the edge of the infratentorial tent may be observed after severe intracranial hypertension due to mass effect (Keane, 1980). Bilateral posterior infarcts have anecdotally been described in various vascular diseases, such as migraine (Moen *et al.*, 1988), dissection of either the distal basilar artery (Jay *et al.*, 2003) or the vertebral artery, temporal arteritis, and other angeitis. Carotid pathology may also rarely result in cortical blindness (Heeney and Koo, 1980). Among various causes of hemorrhagic strokes, arteriovenous malformations and amyloid angiopathy may present as cortical blindness (Yong *et al.*, 1992).

Bilateral infarcts of posterior cerebral artery territory have to be distinguished from metabolic–edematous leukoencephalopathy or capillary-leak syndrome resulting from severe increase of blood pressure in hypertensive encephalopathy.

Assessment

Clinical neuro-ophthalmological assessment

At the acute stage, exam is limited and informal testing can be done at the bedside. Observation is essential. Should the patient deny any trouble, their behavior betrays their blindness, as they demonstrate inability to avoid obstacles while walking, both to identify and reach for objects showed to them, and to orient gaze to visually presented objects. More formal testing includes light perception and automatic lid/eye movements triggered by visual stimuli. Patients should be tested for perception of bright light, presented in a static then moving condition. They have to be asked simple questions with binary responses (Is there a light in front of you? Is the light stationary or moving? Is the movement horizontal or vertical?) and tested several times to eliminate chance-level correct guesses. According to severity of visual deficit, the patient can then be described as having light perception versus no light perception, and in the former case as keeping (or not) movement detection, and movement direction detection. Automatic responses which are anticipated to be abolished in total cortical blindness are blink to visual threat or bright light exposure, and optokinetic nystagmus to moving scenes. It is very important to assess pupil reaction to light . Cortical blindness is associated with normal pupillary reaction to light, as the afferent pathways for the reflex diverge from the visual pathways at the level of the geniculate nucleus. In contrast to alleged total blindness, cortical blindness is the only organic condition that is tenable when pupils react normally to light. Perhaps the most difficult differential

Table 14.2. Main diagnostic clinical clues between different types of behavioral blindness

	Form recognition	Spatially oriented behavior	Gaze orientation	Optokinetic responses	Blink to threat	Pupils light reaction	Fundi
Cortical blindness	+	+	+	+	+	0	0
Aperceptive agnosia	+[*]	0	0	0	0	0	0
Bálint syndrome	0	+	+	+	+	0	0
Retrobulbar optic neuropathies	+	+	+	+	+	+	+[**]
Non organic blindness	+[***]	+[***]	+	0	0	0	0

+: deficit; 0: normal. *: patients do not recognize objects, but discriminate simple forms; **: fundi are normal initially, but atrophic changes occur in a few days; ***: dissociations are observed in behavior (i.e. better performance in "spontaneous" behavior than in examination setting)

diagnosis to be made at this stage is psychogenic blindness, in which pupils also react normally. Pupils may sometimes be poorly reactive in cortical blindness, when the brainstem is additionally involved. Oculomotor dysfunction is also present in such cases, comprising unilateral or bilateral fascicular third nerve palsy, nuclear third nerve palsy, vertical conjugate gaze palsy, skew deviation, torsional or vertical nystagmus (Vighetto, 2004). It is important for neurologists to assess ocular fundi. Both papillae should appear normal and this finding in conjunction with normal pupillary reactions rules out bilateral optic nerve dysfunction, such as ischemic anterior optic neuropathy or retrobulbar neuropathies. Should papilloedema be present in the context of acute cortical blindness, the diagnosis to be suspected is malignant hypertensive encephalopathy. Table 14.2 lists the main differential diagnosis.

Later on, in cases of longstanding blindness, patients can be tested for remnant visual mental imagery. Tests may include verbal descriptions of prototypical animals (tiger, squirrel), well-known places and routes, or hand drawings of common objects. Some patients can thus be shown to have lost their mental imagery, in totality or with specificity for spatial or object material (Goldenberg, 1992), while some others keep this ability (Goldenberg et al., 1995). In the same line, visual content of dreams may be lost.

More formal testing becomes possible as soon as recovery takes place. At the bedside, vision can be grossly evaluated through the maximum distance at which counting fingers is accurate (i.e. count fingers at 50 cm). Visual acuity measure is checked first with letters charts. Exam may be difficult and sensitivity of central retina may be underestimated, due to the small amount of useful visual fields, to attention and exploration disorders, to agnosic alexia, or simultanagnosia. Measure of visual acuity with luminance gratings, presented on charts or generated on a TV screen, is a most rewarding and precise method, but that is rarely used in practice. Visual fields recovery may be difficult to map during the initial stage. Goldmann perimetry is superior to automated perimetries for several reasons. It is easier to perform in a severely deficient patient, due to human interaction that allows tailoring of the testing procedure to patient ability, and to a better detection of moving stimuli as compared to static ones. Moreover, Goldmann is more prone to detect recovery in periphery beyond 45° of excentricity, one example being the monocular temporal crescent sparing. However, static perimetry is useful and should be done whenever vision and attention are sufficient. Campimetric deficits are usually larger when assessed with static as compared to kinetic perimetry, and they may relate more closely to the "real" visual loss experienced by the patients (Finkelstein and Johnson, 1989). Noticeably, such stato-kinetic dissociation is very common in retrogeniculate vision disorders, but has no territorial specificity, as it may also be found in pregeniculate visual deficits (Safran and Glaser, 1980). Color perception should be tested whenever acuity is over 3/10. Ishihara color plates are not appropriate, as they have been devised to detect congenital deficits and as they rely upon recognition of letters and figures. Using 15-hue saturated then desaturated tokens offers in our experience a good compromise between sensibility and duration of exam. Although the 100-hue Farnsworth—Maunsell test is more informative, it is a time-consuming test that can be done to further evaluate a case of suspected central dyschromatopsia. Apperceptive agnosia is a degraded vision, in which form vision, such as objects, persons, letters, as well as colors, is altered in contrast to spatial vision, such as grasping objects, following moving objects, avoiding obstacles. It is evaluated through different tests of elementary form vision (see Chapter 17). Visual fields show usually unilateral or bilateral deficits that predominate in the upper homonymous region. In Bálint's syndrome, patients may behave as if they were blind, but examination shows that form vision is spared and that deficit deals with spatial functions. Clinical evaluation of Bálint's syndrome may be difficult (see Chapter 15). Perimetry mapping is uneasy as performance may be variable due to fluctuations of spatial attention. Constricted visual fields or lower homonymous deficits are the most usual pattern. Optic ataxia shoud be tested in central vision, with free gaze, then in peripheral vision, using either hand. Eye movement disorders typically involve saccades and foveal pursuit directed to visual targets, while spontaneous as well as reflex eye movements are spared. Simultanagnosia may be evaluated by asking the patient to enumerate a number of line drawings on a sheet of paper, or to describe a visual scene, such as photography or more formally using Poppelreuter's superimposed figures.

EEG

Alpha rhythm recorded through the occipital electrodes when the patient closes their eyes is abolished by vision. In cortical blindness, there is no change of rhythms in the occipital regions when the patient either closes or opens their eyes (Aldrich *et al.*, 1987).

VEP

Visual evoked potentials (VEPs) do not seem helpful either to establish diagnosis or prognosis of cortical blindness. One case study showed normal VEP to light in a totally blind patient who was found at autopsy to have bilateral destruction of cortical visual areas (Spehlmann *et al.*, 1977). Other studies showed normal responses in both complete and incomplete cortical blindness (Celesia *et al.*, 1980; Hess *et al.*, 1982). In such cases, VEPs were thought to be generated through extrageniculate pathways. In another study, pattern and flash VEPs were found abnormal in 15 out of 19 patients with cortical blindness, but no correlation was found between potentials alterations and severity of visual loss or visual outcome (Aldrich *et al.*, 1987). So, in cases of "non-anterior" blindness, normality or presence of VEP responses does not rule out cortical blindness, and clinicians should avoid making a diagnosis of psychogenic disorder on this argument.

Management

Until recently, it was held that nothing worthwhile could be done to help these distressed patients. Actually, for many patients are still left without support. However, rehabilitation may be very helpful for these patients, for improving ambulation or reading. Its objectives should be realistic and tailored according to the patient's residual capacities and needs. Rehabilitation requires a multi-disciplinary approach with low-vision trained orthoptists, in conjunction with ergotherapists, neuropsychologists, and psychologists. In totally blind patients, rehabilitation techniques should rely upon development of non-visual vicariant strategies. In patients with partially recovered vision, three general rehabilitation strategies can be proposed, depending on the visual status, the motivation level of the patient, and the local experience and availability of methods. Aside from optical aids, the proposed methods rely upon either improving compensatory strategies, such as visual search strategies by oculomotor training (Kerkhoff *et al.*, 1994; Zihl, 1995) or attempting to enlarge the residual visual field through specific training (Kasten *et al.*, 1998; Julkunen *et al.*, 2003). Repetitive photic stimulation has also be advocated (Widdig *et al.*, 2003). Although the benefit of these techniques remains to be formally established, they seem to be ecologically beneficial (Pambakian *et al.*, 2005).

REFERENCES

Aldrich, M. S., Alessi, A. G., *et al.* (1987). Cortical blindness: Etiology, diagnosis, and prognosis. *Ann. Neurol.*, **21**(2), 149–58.

Beniczky, S., Keri, S., *et al.* (2002). Complex hallucinations following occipital lobe damage. *Eur. J. Neurol.*, **9**(2), 175–6.

Bogousslavsky, J., Regli, F., *et al.* (1983). Unilateral occipital infarction: Evaluation of the risks of developing bilateral loss of vision. *J. Neurol. Neurosurg. Psychiatry*, **46**(1), 78–80.

Brandt, T., Steinke, W., *et al.* (2000). Posterior cerebral artery territory infarcts: Clinical features, infarct topography, causes and outcome. Multicenter results and a review of the literature. *Cerebrovasc. Dis.*, **10**(3), 170–82.

Caplan, L. R. (1980). Top of the basilar syndrome. *Neurology*, **30**(1), 72–9.

Celesia, G. G., Archer, C. R., *et al.* (1980). Visual function of the extrageniculo-calcarine system in man: Relationship to cortical blindness. *Arch. Neurol.*, **37**(11), 704–6.

Chavez, C. J. and Caplan, L. (2001). Posterior cerebral artery syndromes. In *Stroke Syndromes*, ed. L. C. J. Bogousslavsky. Cambridge: Cambridge University Press, pp. 479–89.

Danckert, J., Revol, P., *et al.* (2003). Measuring unconscious actions in action-blindsight: Exploring the kinematics of pointing movements to targets in the blind field of two patients with cortical hemianopia. *Neuropsychologia*, **41**(8), 1068–81.

Finkelstein, J. I. and Johnson, L. N. (1989). Relative scotoma and statokinetic dissociation (Riddoch's phenomenon) from occipital lobe dysfunction. *Trans. Pa. Acad. Ophthalmol. Otolaryngol.*, **41**, 789–92.

Fisher, C. M. (1986). The posterior cerebral artery syndrome. *Can. J. Neurol. Sci.*, **13**(3), 232–9.

Gloning, I., Gloning, K., *et al.* (1967). On optic hallucinations. A study based on 241 patients with lesions of the occipital lobe and its surrounding regions verified by autopsy or surgery. *Wien Z Nervenheilkd Grenzgeb*, **25**(1), 1–19.

Goldenberg, G. (1992). Loss of visual imagery and loss of visual knowledge – a case study. *Neuropsychologia*, **30**(12), 1081–99.

Goldenberg, G., Mullbacher, W., *et al.* (1995). Imagery without perception – a case study of anosognosia for cortical blindness. *Neuropsychologia*, **33**(11), 1373–82.

Heeney, D. J. and Koo, A. H. (1980). Bilateral cortical blindness associated with carotid stenosis in a patient with a persistent trigeminal artery: Case report. *J. Neurosurg.*, **52**(5), 709–11.

Hess, C. W., Meienberg, O., et al. (1982). Visual evoked potentials in acute occipital blindness. Diagnostic and prognostic value. *J. Neurol.*, **227**(4), 193–200.

Jay, W. M., Shah, M. I., et al. (2003). Bilateral occipital-parietal hemorrhagic infarctions following chiropractic cervical manipulation. *Semin. Ophthalmol.*, **18**(4), 205–9.

Julkunen, L., Tenovuo, O., et al. (2003). Rehabilitation of chronic post-stroke visual field defect with computer-assisted training: A clinical and neurophysiological study. *Restor. Neurol. Neurosci.*, **21**(1–2), 19–28.

Kasten, E., Wust, S., et al. (1998). Computer-based training for the treatment of partial blindness. *Nat. Med.*, **4**(9), 1083–7.

Keane, J. R. (1980). Blindness following tentorial herniation. *Ann. Neurol.*, **8**(2), 186–90.

Kerkhoff, G., Munssinger, U., et al. (1994). Neurovisual rehabilitation in cerebral blindness. *Arch. Neurol.*, **51**(5), 474–81.

Kolmel, H. W. (1985). Complex visual hallucinations in the hemianopic field. *J. Neurol. Neurosurg. Psychiatry*, **48**(1), 29–38.

Lance, J. W. (1976). Simple formed hallucinations confined to the area of a specific visual field defect. *Brain*, **99**(4), 719–34.

Levin, L. A. (2005). Topical diagnosis of chiasmal and retrochiasmal disorders. *Walsh and Hoyt's Clinical Neuro-ophthalmology*, 6th edition, ed. N. R. Miller, N. J. Newman, V. Biousse and J. B. Kerrison. Philadelphia: Lippincott Williams & Wilkins, pp. 503–73.

Liu, G. T., Volpe, N. J. and Galetta, S. L. (2001). *Neuro-ophthalmology: Diagnosis and Management.* Philadelphia: W. B. Saunders Company.

Mestre, D. R., Brouchon, M., et al. (1992). Perception of optical flow in cortical blindness: A case report. *Neuropsychologia*, **30**(9), 783–95.

Moen, M., Levine, S. R., et al. (1988). Bilateral posterior cerebral artery strokes in a young migraine sufferer. *Stroke*, **19**(4), 525–8.

Pambakian, A., Currie, J., et al. (2005). Rehabilitation strategies for patients with homonymous visual field defects. *J. Neuroophthalmol.*, **25**(2), 136–42.

Perenin, M. T., Ruel, J., et al. (1980). Residual visual capacities in a case of cortical blindness. *Cortex*, **16**(4), 605–12.

Safran, A. B. and Glaser, J. S. (1980). Statokinetic dissociation in lesions of the anterior visual pathways. A reappraisal of the Riddoch phenomenon. *Arch. Ophthalmol.*, **98**(2), 291–5.

Sahraie, A., Weiskrantz, L., et al. (1997). Pattern of neuronal activity associated with conscious and unconscious processing of visual signals. *Proc. Natl. Acad. Sci. USA*, **94**(17), 9406–11.

Spehlmann, R., Gross, R. A., et al. (1977). Visual evoked potentials and postmortem findings in a case of cortical blindness. *Ann. Neurol.*, **2**(6), 531–4.

Stoerig, P. and Cowey, A. (1997). Blindsight in man and monkey. *Brain*, **120**(Pt 3), 535–59.

Symonds, C. and Mackenzie, I. (1957). Bilateral loss of vision from cerebral infarction. *Brain*, **80**(4), 415–55.

Vaphiades, M. S., Celesia, G. G., et al. (1996). Positive spontaneous visual phenomena limited to the hemianopic field in lesions of central visual pathways. *Neurology*, **47**(2), 408–17.

Vighetto, A. (2004). Accidents vasculaires cérébraux du territoire vertébro-basilaire. *Neuro-ophtalmologie*, ed. A. B. Safran, A. Vighetto, T. Landis and E. Cabanis. Paris: Masson 477–85.

Weiskrantz, L. (2004). Roots of blindsight. *Prog. Brain Res.*, **144**, 229–41.

Widdig, W., Pleger, B., *et al.* (2003). Repetitive visual stimulation: A neuropsychological approach to the treatment of cortical blindness. *NeuroRehabilitation*, **18**(3), 227–37.

Yong, W. H., Robert, M. E., *et al.* (1992). Cerebral hemorrhage with biopsy-proved amyloid angiopathy. *Arch. Neurol.*, **49**(1), 51–8.

Zeki, S. (1991). Cerebral akinetopsia (visual motion blindness). A review. *Brain*, **114**(Pt 2), 811–24.

Zeki, S. and Ffytche, D. H. (1998). The Riddoch syndrome: Insights into the neurobiology of conscious vision. *Brain*, **121**(Pt 1), 25–45.

Zihl, J. (1995). Visual scanning behavior in patients with homonymous hemianopia. *Neuropsychologia*, **33**(3), 287–303.

(2000). *Rehabilitation of Visual Disorders After Brain Injury*. In *Neuropsychological Rehabilitation: A Modular Handbook*. Hove: Psychology Press

15

Bálint's syndrome

Alain Vighetto and Pierre Krolak-Salmon

Hôpital neurologique Pierre Wertheimer, Lyon and Université Claude Bernard Lyon I

Introduction

Bálint's syndrome is a clinical entity which combines variously a set of complex spatial behavior disorders following bilateral damage to the occipital–parietal junction. The core syndrome is a triad, namely optic ataxia, gaze apraxia, and simultanagosia, to which visual–spatial perception deficits can be associated. Both diversity of terminology used in literature and bias in clinical descriptions, which often reflect a particular opinion of the authors on underlying mechanisms, add to the difficulty in describing and comprehending this rare and devastating syndrome. As the components are not elementary symptoms, and as they are not necessarily present in each case, indicating they do not rely upon a single brain mechanism, validity of the complex as a syndrome has been questioned (Rizzo and Vecera, 2002). Despite these flaws, Bálint's syndrome can be identified at the bedside examination and it allows robust anticipation of lesion localization.

Historically, Bálint provided in 1909 a thorough clinical and postmortem description of a patient who exhibited hitherto undescribed symptoms, he named *Seelenlähmung des "Schauens," optische Ataxie, raümliche Störung der Aufmerksamkeit*, usually translated as psychic paralysis of gaze, optic ataxia, and spatial disorder of attention. He related these symptoms to a bilateral area of ischemic suffering in the posterior parietal and anterior occipital regions, including the angular gyrus and underlying white matter on both sides. In Bálint's view, psychic paralysis of gaze was a consequence of attention impairment and not of eye movement disorder per se; meanwhile optic ataxia was explained in terms of disconnection between visual and motor centers. Independently, Holmes (1918) reported a series of six patients with penetrating missile wounds of the brain, under the heading of "visual disorientation," stressing oculomotor disturbances and spatial misperception, without individualizing optic ataxia. It is not clear whether Bálint's and Holmes' descriptions are truly different or merely reflect different focus on a range of symptoms (Husain and Stein, 1988). Hecaen first coined the term "Bálint's syndrome" (Hecaen and De Ajuriaguerra, 1954).

De Renzi suggested associating Bálint and Holmes to acknowledge the complementary contribution of the two authors and to encompass the whole spectrum of symptoms (De Renzi, 1989). Interestingly, these two seminal papers had been preceded by two recently rediscovered contributions (Badal, 1888; Inouye, 1904). Among minor forms of Bálint's syndrome, those resulting from unilateral lesion mainly result in impaired visually guided manual reaching, a symptom ascribed to general visual disorientation, in Holmes' line (Riddoch, 1935, Brain, 1941), or as optic ataxia – a specific disorder – following Bálint's view (Garcin *et al.*, 1967; Perenin and Vighetto, 1988).

Bálint's syndrome is not only a rare neurological curiosity. It is gaining new interest from progress in vision neurosciences as it provides some insight into the functional roles assigned to the neuronal populations of the occipital–parietal region. These functions include spatial perception, gating, and directing spatial attention, as well as spatial coding of eye and hand movements in the immediate extrapersonal space. In particular, a number of papers have focused on isolated optic ataxia, as a human model for studying visuomotor transformations processed in the dorsal visual stream.

General presentation of Bálint's syndrome

Complete Bálint's syndrome

Patients with full-blown syndrome are severely impaired. Their behavior is at first suggestive of blindness. Hence, their movements are hesitant and awkward, their gaze is mostly kept immobile, sometimes in the wrong direction with respect to the ongoing action, and patients are unable, for example, to pick up food from a tray or to walk on their own. However, examination shows definitely that they can see. They demonstrate surprising ability to recognize objects, even of tiny size, although they may require time to spot them, especially when several items are present. Further examination indicates their visual deficit is selective for visual–spatial material. They are no longer able to reach for objects under visual guidance, to direct gaze to visual location of objects, to find their way in familiar surroundings, to estimate size, orientation, or distance of objects. Patients are aware of their deficits, but usually they have much difficulty in conceptualizing them. Analysis of each component of the syndrome may be rendered difficult by fluctuation of performance and possible interdependency between certain symptoms, such as reciprocal interactions between optic ataxia, simultanagnosia, and visual–spatial disorders, or between gaze apraxia and simultanagnosia (Guard *et al.*, 1984). Moreover, these symptoms have to be disentangled from consequences of primary sensory deficits, especially visual field defects, which are often associated.

Optic Ataxia

Optic ataxia refers to inaccuracy in reaching and grasping visually presented objects, and more generally in exploring manually peri-personal visual space, that cannot be explained in terms of elementary visual, proprioceptive, or motor deficit. According to Bálint's view, optic ataxia is secondary to an inability to use visual information to guide movements, in the same way as tabetic ataxia results from loss of proprioceptive information. Alternative names have been proposed, such as visuomotor ataxia (Rondot *et al.*, 1977), or visuomotor apraxia (Classen *et al.*, 1995), but the original term has persisted. Optic ataxia enlightens a dissociation in brain function such that visual−spatial attributes of a particular object are still processed in terms of conscious experience and verbal description but are no longer implemented to calibrate movement of the limb. Several spatiotemporal abnormalities of visual guidance of hand movement can be described from clinical observation and kinematic recordings (Jakobson *et al.*, 1991; Jeannerod *et al.*, 1994). The whole movement is both delayed and slowed. The trajectory of hand movement is grossly impaired in terms of direction and amplitude, while the hand is held largely open, the posture grip being inadequate with respect to the form and orientation of the target object. Movement usually fails to reach the goal, although corrections may be possible with groping movements until a contact eventually elicits grasping.

Optic ataxia may be present in central vision but it always predominated in the peripheral field. Typically, optic ataxia is observed for the two hands in the whole field of vision, but it can also be present only in one homonymous or in both peripheral fields, or it may be limited to one hand (such as in Bálint's case). Limitation of optic ataxia to the peripheral field implies that the symptom has specifically to be looked for in these cases, as deficit is not apparent when prehension is performed in the natural condition of foveal vision. Limitation of optic ataxia to one hand demonstrates that the symptom is independent from any visual−spatial deficit and results from visuomotor incoordination, provided that proprioception is intact. Patients often exhibit striking decoupling of eye−hand coordination, in such a way that the eyes are not aligned to the place the hand is reaching to. Some harbor abnormal eye−hand recoupling, resulting in attraction of hand movement towards the place the patient's eyes are foveating, a phenomenon called "magnetic misreaching" (Carey *et al.*, 1997; Jackson *et al.*, 2005). Deficiency of visuomotor coordination observed in optic ataxia interferes with several daily activities, such as drawing, writing, eating, and filling a glass. For example, patients may be unable to draw a line between two points or to pick up a piece of food with a fork. Difficulty in navigating around and avoiding obstacles are related to the same dysfunction (Schindler *et al.*, 2004). Beyond limb movements, whole-body movements may also be impaired, resulting in difficulty for these patients in properly orienting their body with respect to the chair they intend to sit in, or to the bed they want to get in (Kase *et al.*, 1977). Optic ataxia may not be the sole cause of such impressive disorder, and both axial apraxia and visual—spatial misperception may also be contributive factors.

In contrast with movements directed to visual targets, those directed to body parts are accurate. Patients can point precisely with a finger to the body parts that are touched by the examiner, indicating that somesthetic—motor coordination is spared. Finally, although optic ataxia is described as a specific visuomotor transformation deficit, it may also be demonstrated for non-visually guided movements. Thus, reaching without vision of the hand may be even more impaired than reaching under visual feedback, and some patients may show in addition auditory ataxia (Guard *et al.*, 1984). Performance may vary according to the hand, the sensory or cross-sensory modality, but also the action space related to the body (Valenza *et al.*, 2004). These observations indicate that optic ataxia may be understood as a dysfunction of supramodal sensorimotor transformation control of movements in the immediate peri-personal space.

Gaze apraxia

Eye movement disorders have been variously labeled "psychic paralysis of gaze," "oculomotor disorders" (Holmes, 1918), or ocular motor apraxia (Cogan and Adams, 1953). These nebulous terms reflect the difficulty in assigning ocular motor deficits to a well-defined dysfunction as well as spectrum of eye movement problems observed from case to case. As no single term is satisfactory, we will use here the label *gaze apraxia* to indicate that deficit refers to eye movements in space (gaze), and that deficit of saccade function may be dissociated according to cognitive context (apraxia). Gaze apraxia should not be confounded with "oculomotor apraxia," a developmental syndrome of horizontal saccades deficit in children.

Gaze apraxia is characterized by severe abnormalities of generation of eye movements in response to visual targets in space, in the absence of ocular motor palsy, ascertained by full reflexive eye movements. The more constant observation in these patients is poverty of eye movements that may culminate in a condition often referred to as "spasm of fixation," or "visual grasp reflex." Patients stare open-eyed, with the gaze being locked to the place they are fixating, and they may be able to disrupt such sticky fixation only after a blink. In more severe cases, patients are not able to initiate intentional saccades, in response to a visual stimulus or to verbal command. Only occurrence of some automatic saccades to novel stimuli, such as unexpected sound or sudden touch to their own body, and sparing of REM during sleep, may distinguish this condition from saccadic paralysis (Michel *et al.*, 1963; Pierrot-Deseilligny *et al.*, 1988). Usually patients keep moving their eyes "spontaneously" or on verbal command, while they are impaired in performing visually guided saccades. The more attention and complex visual processing the eye movement requires, the less it is likely to be performed. In this line, visual search behavior is particularly vulnerable. Hence, when the patient is asked to move their eyes to a target suddenly appearing in the peripheral field, they may generate no movement, or initiate wandering eye movement, that results in erratic displacement of eyes in space, ending with incidental acquisition of the target. Even at this point the target may be lost due to lability of perception and instability of fixation, and a new search pattern has to be activated. Saccadic behavior is abnormal in a rich (natural) environment array, which requires continuous selection between concurrent stimuli, but it may be normal in a simplified context, when for example the task is to direct eyes to a peripheral LED in the dark (Guard *et al.*, 1984). Beside saccades, other visually guided eye movements are impaired, such as smooth foveal pursuit and optokinetic responses. Convergence onto a visual target is altered, and blink to visual threat is usually abolished. In addition to ocular movements abnormalities, some patients have lost spontaneous blinking (Watson and Rapcsak, 1989). Eye movement recordings usually show several abnormalities, such as prolonged latency, fragmentation, and hypometria of saccades, fixation drift and absence of smooth pursuit (Michel *et al.*, 1963; Girotti *et al.*, 1982). The pattern of oculomotor scanning is highly abnormal during scene exploration (Zihl, 2000). Both accuracy of fixation and saccadic localization are impaired, and spatiotemporal organization of eye displacements does not fit with the spatial configuration of the scene to be analyzed (Tyler, 1968).

Taking into account the facts that eye movement deficit is enhanced whenever attentional demand is high, and that a gradient of declining deficit exists between visually guided, pure intentional, and reflexive movements, one can formulate that gaze apraxia is the product of both visual and attention processing deficits in eye movements.

Simultanagnosia

"Spatial disorder of attention" (Bálint, 1909), "restriction/shrinkage of attention field" (Michel and Henaff, 2004), "bilateral neglect syndrome," or "disorder of simultaneous perception" (Luria, 1959) are equivalent terms to designate a complex symptom that can be viewed as a limitation of visual–spatial attention resources.

Patients do not seem to perceive visual targets located away from a small area, which is usually the area of foveation. They exhibit a reduction of "useful field of vision," operationally defined as the field of space that can be attended to while keeping central fixation (Rizzo and Vecera, 2002). This can be tested by asking patients either to direct their eyes or their hand to, or to name, an object presented extrafoveally. Evaluation using a motor response may be affected by concurrent optic ataxia and gaze apraxia, while verbal response more directly probes conscious/attentive perception. Generally, responses are more likely to be given after verbal encouragement, a finding that indicates that the deficit is not a consequence of a reduction of the visual fields but of attention scanning for non-central events. Shrinkage of the attention field reduces detection of multiple objects and may render patients able to perceive just one item at a time. Bálint's patient was not able to perceive the light of a match while focusing on a cigarette until he felt a burning pain. This limited capacity of attentive vision for only one object at a time does not depend upon the size of the object. This is another distinction from a visual field deficit. In addition, single object attention is reduced, as perception may be reported as "vanishing" and the patient may even have difficulty in binding several attributes of one object, such as color and form (Friedman-Hill et al., 1995). Using Posner's paradigm, it was shown that patients exhibit a defect in shifting spatial attention (Verfaellie et al., 1990), or in dis-engaging attention from fixated objects (Rizzo and Vecera, 2002), a difficulty which may be central for the visual grasp reflex to occur. As a general consequence, patients fail to perceive at any time the totality of the items forming a visual scene. Description or copying of complex figures is laborious and slow, patients focusing serially on details, apprehending portions of the pictures with a piecemeal approach, but failing to switch attention from local details to global structures. Similarly, performance for counting objects is altered. Patients explore working space in a disorganized fashion and may focus several times on the same object, their behavior betraying impairment of short-term memory for spatial location of items already explored. Alexia is often prominent, with difficulties in assembling words in a text, while letters and isolated words are usually well identified. In all these tasks, the severe perceptual deficit linked to attention capacity limitation increases when visual environment is complex and when stimuli are presented for a brief period. Although blinking in these patients is often reduced, some patients learn unconsciously to close their eyes either to enhance perception of a vanishing object being fixated, or conversely to break fixation from one object so they can look at another one (Gottlieb et al., 1991). Finally, this attention-related deficit may be limited to a part of the spatial field, resulting in hemispatial neglect (Bálint, 1909), or in altitudinal neglect (Rapcsak et al., 1988).

Spatial attention disorders may have impact on the other components of Bálint's syndrome, and for some authors constitute the central core of the syndrome (Rizzo and Vecera, 2002). Although eye movement patterns have been recorded as normal in some cases of simultanagnosia (Rizzo and Hurtig, 1987), spatial attention disorders are likely to participate in oculomotor deficits by altering visual exploratory behavior, by increasing latency of visually guided saccades, and by facilitating spasms of fixation. They play a role also in hand misreaching, by increasing visual misperception of the target, which may "vanish" whenever the hand is approaching the goal (Perenin and Vighetto, 1988). Finally, they play a key role in several visual–perceptual deficits, by affecting judgment of relative position and distances of objects, reading, and apprehension of complex pictures.

Associated deficits

Visual–spatial perception disorders can variously be found, depending on the case, and on the manner in which both the examination is performed and the results are interpreted. In most severe cases, patients have lost cardinal orientation in space, resulting in an inability to distinguish the right from the left side (or up from down) in egocentric space, or an inability to discriminate whether a given object is orientated to the right or to the left (orientation agnosia). Other aspects include difficulty in judging absolute distance, in estimating positions of objects relative to the subject, in depth perception and stereopsis, in visual motion perception and structure from motion perception, in perception of egomotion, and in directional heading (De Renzi, 1989; Rizzo and Vecera, 2002).

Additional symptoms depend on the extension of the lesion in the parietal lobes and in the adjacent occipital and temporal regions. They include anomic or transcortical sensory aphasia, pure agraphia, alexia without agraphia or with agraphia, Gerstmann's syndrome, hemispatial neglect, constructional apraxia, dressing apraxia, or apperceptive agnosia. Visual fields are typically full. However, Goldmann's perimetry may show slight constriction of peripheral isopters and fluctuations of measurements, as a consequence of peripheral attention deficit. Due to lesion extension in the optic radiations in the parietal lobe, patients often have homonymous hemianopia, unilateral or bilateral lower homonymous quadrantanopia.

Minor forms of Bálint's syndrome

These cases comprise those having the whole spectrum of symptoms, but in attenuated form (Hecaen and De Ajuriaguerra, 1954), and those showing only a limited range of symptoms. The latter cases have both theoretical and practical importance, as they indicate that each symptom can be isolated or predominant. A bilateral lesion may result in (almost) isolated simultanagnosia, in isolated optic ataxia (Damasio and Benton, 1979) or in associated optic ataxia and simultan-agnosia, without gaze apraxia (Michel and Henaff, 2004). On the other hand, a unilateral lesion of the posterior parietal region results in near-isolated optic ataxia (Garcin *et al.*, 1967; Castaigne *et al.*, 1975; Auerbach and Alexander, 1981; Ferro, 1984; Perenin and Vighetto, 1988).

Optic ataxia from a unilateral lesion resembles that after a bilateral lesion. However, visuomotor deficit is observed only in the peripheral visual field, as it is corrected with foveation (Vighetto and Perenin, 1981). In addition, the symptom is lateralized, mainly affecting both the hand and the visual field contralateral to the lesion. Such a lateralization of optic ataxia rules out an explanation in terms of motor, sensory, or visual deficit. In the involved hemifield, it can be demonstrated that optic ataxia can occur independently from perceptual disorder of spatial position or orientation discrimination. This offers a dissociation in brain function between visual spatial representations that are used respectively for perceiving and for generating action (Goodale and Milner, 1992). The pattern of visuomotor deficit may differ according to the site (Rondot *et al.*, 1977) and the side of the lesion (Perenin and Vighetto, 1988). Optic ataxia resulting from a right-sided lesion tends to involve the two hands in the left visual hemifield, while a left-sided lesion is more prone to affect the right hand in either visual field. The contrast between such "field effect" and "hand effect" may reflect some aspect of hemisphere specialization in motor control.

Movement analysis indicates that the two segmental components of the upper limb are altered in optic ataxia. These are (1) the reaching movement towards the spatial location of the target, which involves proximal musculature, and (2) the grasping movement, formed by the anticipated shaping of the hand and fingers to fit conformational features of the target, which involves distal musculature (Jeannerod *et al.*, 1994). These two components that implicate different limb parts and that are fed with different visual inputs from the target, define two visuomotor parallel channels processing goal-directed limb movement. Alteration of the former leads to spatial errors in hand transportation, while alteration of the latter results in mis-orientation and mis-shaping of the hand (Perenin and Vighetto, 1988). There are a few cases showing dissociation between the two visuomotor components (Binkofski *et al.*, 1998). Additionally, a related form of optic ataxia has been described after a unilateral parietal lesion, manifesting as impaired reaching for an object seen through a mirror (Binkofski *et al.*, 1999).

Finally, two psychophysical studies in patients with optic ataxia have provided new insight into some visuomotor operations performed in the parietal lobe. In the first one, it was shown that patients having recovered from optic ataxia in central vision are not able to adjust movement if the target location is unexpectedly changed upon movement initiation (Pisella *et al.*, 2000). This observation strongly indicates that optic ataxia more likely results from a deficit of real-time automatic trajectory adjustment than from a deficit of initial motor planning (Roy *et al.*, 2004). In the second one, it has been shown that hand reaching accuracy much improves whenever a delay is introduced between target presentation and movement onset, suggesting that optic ataxia is a specific impairment of fast visuomotor control rather than global impairment of goal-directed actions, and that an alternate visuomotor route activated in a different behavioral context is able to partly compensate for its deficit (Rossetti *et al.*, 2003; 2005).

Location of lesions and functional correlations

Bálint's syndrome usually results from large and more or less symmetrical lesions involving the posterior parietal region, including extensively the superior parietal lobule, as well as part of the inferior parietal lobule and the superior part of the occipital lobe. Depending on the causes, cortex of Brodmann's areas 7, 39 and 19, as well as underlying white matter, are involved. Extension of lesions is, however, quite variable. This is particularly true when Balint's syndrome results from infarction in the watershed areas. In such cases, lesions can extend anteriorly to the frontal lobes or posteriorly to the occipital lobes. Functionally, a lesion in the posterior parietal cortex also disconnects its cortical and subcortical targets, namely several areas in the premotor/prefrontal cortex and deep layers of the superior colliculus. Diversity in clinical expression of each component of the syndrome reflects variability of lesion extension and functional disconnection. There is no minimal lesion sufficient for producing the whole syndrome and it is likely that anatomical correlation for each component is relatively independent. Simultanagnosia may follow bilateral lesion of the superior aspect of the occipital lobes and the superior parietal lobule (Rizzo and Hurtig, 1987). This region is part of a cortical network for visual–spatial attention, that also includes the dorsolateral prefrontal cortex (Astafiev *et al.*, 2003; Woldorff *et al.*, 2004). This network may contribute to attentive vision for recognition of multiple objects, by selecting objects of interest, enhancing pertinent sensory information, maintaining a representation of information for a brief period of time in the working memory system for spatial location, disengaging attention, and shifting from one object to another one in a different location (Rizzo and Vecera, 2002). The core lesion for optic ataxia after a unilateral lesion was found to lie in the intraparietal sulcus and adjacent superior parietal lobule (Perenin and Vighetto, 1988). Recently, its location was refined to the nearby parietal–occipital junction (Karnath and Perenin, 2005). A recent fMRI study showed consistently that humans performing a visually guided pointing movement activate a fronto-parietal cortical network, including two specific areas for visuomotor control forming the "parietal reach region," namely the medial part of the intraparietal sulcus and the parietal–occipital junction, the former being activated whether pointing is performed in foveal or in peripheral vision, the latter being specifically activated in pointing in peripheral vision (Prado *et al.*, 2005). Deficit in visually guided saccades may be the consequence of a lesion in the "parietal eye field," a region in the superior parietal lobule and the intraparietal sulcus that may include several areas identified by fMRI studies (Müri *et al.*, 1996; Schluppeck *et al.*, 2005). However, extension of the lesions to the frontal lobe, encroaching the "frontal eye field," may explain additional loss of intentional, self-generated, saccades (Michel *et al.*, 1963; Pierrot-Deseilligny *et al.*, 1988).

Natural actions such as directing gaze or a hand towards a visual target, grasping and manipulating an object, require the brain to compute in parallel a complex set of coordinated motor commands for each segmental effector, based on multiple sensory information coming from both the extrapersonal and the body spaces. In short, the target has to be selected, its visual coordinates need to be transformed into different body-centered spaces, hand trajectory and final position has to be programmed, command has to be transcribed in a spatiotemporal pattern of muscle activation and inhibition, and ongoing movement has to be monitored and adjusted through sensory feedback and motor efferent copy (Rizzo and Vecera, 2002). The posterior parietal cortex is fed with visual inputs from the dorsal stream and processes spatial information, using different routes for spatial perception and action organization (Rizzolatti and Matelli, 2003). For the latter, it plays a particular role in building short-lived spatial representations that are directly used by the motor system (Goodale and Milner, 1992; Rossetti, 1998). It also combines visual with other sensory inputs, and it has direct projections onto cortical and subcortical motor areas. These anatomical properties give the posterior parietal cortex a central role for a supramodal fusion of updated information relating the body to objects in the surrounding world and for computation of spatial characteristics of visual objects to generate goal-directed movements. At the posterior parietal cortex level, visually guided movement is organized into discrete parallel visuomotor modules, recruiting different motor outputs (eye, arm, hand) and different spatial representations of visual information, with reference to eye, head, or body reference frames. These modules project to specific premotor cortex targets, defining a parietal–frontal cortical network of parallel circuits for generation of visually guided movements (Battaglia-Mayer *et al.*, 2003). Activity of individual neurons during a given task (as studied from electrophysiological recordings in monkey), or activity of a limited neuron set (as studied from functional MRI in humans), demonstrates several properties in the posterior parietal cortex of area 7, parietooccipital junction, and intraparietal sulcus that are relevant to the roles assigned to this part of the brain. Neuron populations are organized in discrete areas, defined by different response characteristics, consistent with functional parcellation. Most respond to visual information, which is implemented in retinal, as well as head and body-centered coordinates, often in combination with somesthetic inputs, and their activity is strongly enhanced by attention to the cognitively relevant visual stimulus.

Some populations respond to concomitant hand reaching, manipulation, saccade, or combined eye–hand movement (Andersen, 1997; Colby and Goldberg, 1999; Battaglia-Mayer *et al.*, 2000; Crawford *et al.*, 2004). Thus, neurons from the medial part of the intraparietal sulcus (area MIP) are activated during reaching to a visual target, as well as neurons in area V6A, a probable monkey equivalent to the human parieto-occipital junction (Colby and Goldberg, 1999; Galletti *et al.*, 2003), while neurons from the anterior part of the intraparietal sulcus (area AIP) are recruited during object manipulation (Binkofski *et al.*, 1998). Neurons in the lateral part of the intraparietal sulcus (area LIP) discharge in relation to visually guided saccades or to saliency of visual events, and they may contribute to spatial constancy by anticipating perceptual consequences of displacing gaze (Duhamel *et al.*, 1992; Heide *et al.*, 1995; Bellebaum *et al.*, 2005). However, the way these multiple representations shift from one to the other, depending on the particular spatial task and the required movement (Valenza *et al.*, 2004), and the way visuomotor signals converge for coordinated movements, remain largely unknown.

Differential diagnosis

Thorough examination of the patient should eliminate the erroneous diagnosis of blindness, visual object agnosia, or psychogenic disorder. However, diagnosis of individual components and of the whole syndrome may remain difficult, especially when elementary motor, sensory, and visual deficits coexist. This is the case when Bálint's syndrome shows up after recovery from cortical blindness, at a stage when patients keep degraded low-level vision, with visual field defect and apperceptive agnosia, caused by occipital lesions. Association of hemispatial neglect with contralateral hemianopia can mimic simultanagnosia (Rizzo and Vecera, 2002).

Causes of Bálint's syndrome

There are numerous diseases leading to Bálint's syndrome (Table 15.1). Traumatic brain lesions have been historically described after war injuries (Inouye, 1904; Holmes, 1918), but currently result from traffic accidents in patients having had severe ischemic/anoxic or hemorrhagic suffering in the posterior part of the hemispheres. Vascular origin is frequent, and has yielded most clinico-anatomical correlation studies, due to relatively discrete topography of lesions and to a number of cases who came to autopsy (Bálint, 1909; Kase *et al.*, 1977; Pierrot-Deseilligny *et al.*, 1986). The most frequent cause is probably cortical degeneration. Thus, Bálint's syndrome may develop in 30% of patients with Alzheimer's disease (Mendez *et al.*, 1990), and up to 82% of cases with posterior cortical atrophy of Benson's type (Tang-Wai *et al.*, 2004).

Table 15.1. Main causes of Bálint's syndrome

Infarction
Eclampsia
Hemorrhage
Amyloid angiopathy
Hypertensive encephalopathy
Tumors ("butterfly" parietal malignant glioma, bilateral metastases)
Degenerative cortical lesions (Alzheimer's disease, posterior cortical atrophy, cortico-basal
    degeneration, diffuse Lewy bodies disease)
Infection (Creutzfeldt-Jakob's disease, progressive multifocal leukoencephalopathy,
    HIV encephalitis)
Inflammatory diseases (Balo's concentric sclerosis)
Adrenoleukodystrophy
Drug toxicity (methotrexate)
Traumatic brain injury
Cerebral anoxia
Carbon monoxide intoxication

Bálint's syndrome in stroke

Bálint's syndrome resulting from stroke is usually of acute onset. It may be apparent from the beginning, or it appears secondarily after regression of cortical blindness, hemiparesis, or hypoesthesia. Rarely, symptoms follow a unilateral stroke in a patient having previously had a contralateral event.

Ischemic Bálint's syndrome is often related to watershed infarcts in the vertebrobasilar territory. In these cases, Bálint's syndrome is often heralded by transient cortical blindness. In most cases with bilateral lesions, infarcts are simultaneous and result from acute hemodynamic failure, consecutive to cardiac surgery or severe hypotension (Montero *et al.*, 1982; Hijdra and Meerwaldt, 1984). Other mechanisms include vasospastic angiopathy (Pisella *et al.*, 2000). In these hemodynamic crises, the upper occipital and parieto-occipital region appears to be the most vulnerable to ischemia, but the lateral aspect of the lower occipital lobe may also be involved (Figure 15.1). Less usually, the same vascular context leads to Bálint's syndrome after bilateral infarcts in the carotid artery territory. Severe stenosis or thrombosis of the carotid arteries is often present and infarcts result from occlusion of the posterior parietal branches of the middle cerebral artery or from a watershed infarct that may occasionally extend beyond the posterior parietal region to the sagittal border-zone between middle cerebral and anterior cerebral arteries (Michel *et al.*, 1963; Pierrot-Deseilligny *et al.*, 1988). Bilateral infarcts that occur usually successively may result from an embolic cardiac source

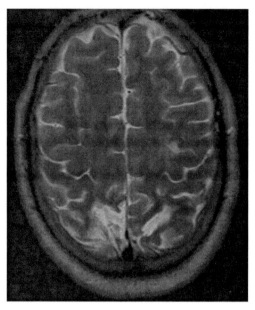

Figure 15.1A MRI with axial T2 sequence showing asymmetrical posterior parietal lesion (Brodmann's area 7) in a patient with Bálint's syndrome after watershed infarct in the territory of the posterior cerebral artery.

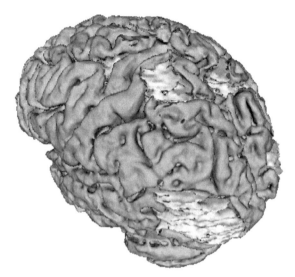

Figure 15.1B 3D reconstruction of the lesions in the same patient. Lesions involve both the medial part of the posterior parietal cortex (upper lesion) and the lateral part of the occipital cortex (lower lesion). For a color version of this figure please see www.cambridge.org/9780521106955.

(Pierrot-Deseilligny *et al.*, 1986). Unilateral infarct cases are observed after occlusion of the posterior parietal branch of the middle cerebral artery, or the parietal branch of the posterior cerebral artery. Amyloid angiopathy is probably a growing cause of vascular Bálint's syndrome that is still underdiagnosed. Symptoms result more frequently from sequential than from simultaneous lesions, and imagery shows evidence of bilateral hematomas in the superior parietal region or of combined hematoma on one side and infarct on the other side (Inoue *et al.*, 1988).

Assessment

Diagnosis of Bálint's syndrome is often difficult because of complexity of symptoms that can hardly be analyzed at the bedside. Actually, the syndrome is underdiagnosed and often missed. Diagnosis of isolated optic ataxia may also be missed, but for a different reason, as the symptom is usually covert and only identified through specific search.

Assessment needs first evaluation of elementary motor and sensory functions, such as strength and coordination, touch sense and kinesthesia, as well as "low-level" vision. Bedside examination of vision indicates only that objects or colors are recognized, provided they are presented centrally and time is allowed for evaluation, and that visual fields are full in confrontation testing. Formal testing is necessary. Visual acuity is usually normal, but the ophthalmologist should be aware of simultanagnosia and gaze apraxia, which may jeopardize reading the letter strings. Visual fields are typically full, but they may show homonymous deficits, such as lower quadrantanopia or paracentral scotoma, or exhibit constriction of peripheral isopters on Goldmann's perimetry, as a consequence of fluctuating spatial attention.

Visual–spatial functions may be evaluated by many informal tests. Interpretation of results should take into account the function being tested and more crucially spatial attention that is required to perform each test. Globally, the more attention resources the test recruits, the more it is likely to be altered. Tests include judgment of the relative distance of two objects from the patient (which one is the nearest?), of the absolute distance of an object from the patient, of relative placement of two objects previously identified by the patient (which one is above? on your right side?), of orientation of a single object (vertical? tilted? on which side?), of relative size between two objects, or movement of an object. Paper and pencil tests include discrimination of a dot location respective to a series of lines or to a geometrical form, discrimination between lines of different length or different orientation, finding the exit from a maze, and the copying of simple drawings (Michel and Henaff, 2004). More formal tests evaluate orientation discrimination (Benton's Judgment of Line Orientation), stereopsis (Titmus' test or random-dot anaglyph tests), motion perception (using a variety of computer tasks assessing elementary perception of moving dots, or higher level motion processing, such as identification of motion-defined shapes or biological motion), and global and local processing (Navon's test).

Optic ataxia is easily suggested when the patient fails to grasp an object they can still recognize and usually look at. Inaccuracy of upper limb movements aimed at visually presented (and identifiable) objects at reaching distance contrasts with accuracy of movements to somesthetic targets, such as to the contralateral thumb. A requisite condition for optic ataxia to be acknowledged is that misreaching should not be explained on the basis of elementary sensory or motor deficit, and that the visual field should be spared in the area tested for visuomotor deficit. In many cases, especially after unilateral lesion, optic ataxia has to be searched for in the peripheral vision, as misreaching is no longer present in the natural condition when the patient can direct their eyes to the target. Here, evaluation needs a systematic way of examination. The patient should be seated with the head and the eyes kept still, and the examiner should be placed behind, in order to avoid giving visual cues other than the target position. The patient is asked to perform a fast and accurate movement to grasp the object the examiner is presenting rapidly in the peripheral field. Each hand is successively tested in the two peripheral fields (with respect to both retina and body coordinate frames), allowing comparisons in terms of spatial errors between the different hand–field combinations. Due to these stringent conditions, numerous cases of optic ataxia are probably missed during standard testing in stroke units. Optic ataxia may be tested not only for evaluation of arm misreaching, but also for hand mis-shaping. This can be systematically approached with analysis of orientation errors of hand movements passing through an oriented slit, using the same general procedure as the one used for manual reaching (Perenin and Vighetto, 1988). Finally, optic ataxia may also be evaluated during paper and pencil tasks, as it impairs for example connecting a set of dots, copying, drawing, and writing.

Gaze apraxia has to be evaluated clinically. Indeed, eye movement recordings can rarely be done easily and, although they provide quantitative information, they do not add much to diagnosis of this complex symptom. A first step, particularly in the most severe cases when patients keep fixed gaze, is to rule out peripheral or central gaze palsies. This is achieved through demonstration of sparing of the vestibulo-ocular reflex and observation of spontaneous saccades. Optokinetic nystagmus may be abolished when tested with the rotatory drum, which elicits mostly foveal pursuit, but it is expected to be preserved when tested using full-field pattern stimulation. Saccade behavior is abnormal in terms of initiation delay and spatial accuracy. Analysis may be difficult, but it is best achieved through systematic evaluation of the different types of cognitive saccades. Non-visually guided intentional saccades (i.e. verbal command of looking to the side) are more easily elicited than visually or non-visually driven automatic saccades (i.e. looking at a novel object or sound appearing in the periphery, or at a part of their body being touched), which are in turn more easily triggered than visual attentive saccades (looking at the place of a particular object in the array, being present or after its removal). Deficit of attentive saccades may informally be tested by asking the patient to direct their gaze alternately between two different objects placed laterally, or by observing spontaneous behavior while searching for an object among distractors or exploring a complex picture. According to severity, deficit ranges from wandering eye and head displacements in space to only delayed target acquisition with saccadic hypometria. Other classes of visually guided eye movements are grossly impaired, such as foveal smooth pursuit and convergence to visual stimulus, which can easily be evaluated at bedside examination. Blink to visual threat may also be abolished.

Visual attention deficits are probably the more difficult to analyze as they cannot be easily disentangled at the bedside from visual field, spatial perception, and oculomotor deficits. As a general rule, they result in impaired (perceptive and motor) performance as far as attention resources are needed, and in reduced speed of processing. Conscious perception is limited to objects presented in the central field of vision, while a peripherally located object goes ignored, both verbally and behaviorally, unless strong encouragement is provided to the patient and time is allocated to the observer for the task. Moreover, reduction of central attention resources results in an inability to perceive more than one object at the same time. Less severe deficit results in "extinction" of one (the more peripheral) of two objects, while each of them presented in isolation is perceived. Simultanagnosia can be evaluated clinically by asking the patient to describe verbally a complex picture, such as the Cookie Theft Picture, or to count objects displayed in front of them or drawn on a sheet of paper. Typically, the picture is analyzed only through a succession of details, picked up randomly in terms of spatial location. Counting objects is affected in proportion to the number of items and complexity of the visual scene. Attention spatial span can be grossly evaluated by the number of simultaneous items that can be identified when presented for a limited number of seconds. This can be approached more precisely with computer-generated Treisman's tasks, that contrast automatic perception (pop-out vision) and attentive perception (visual search). Only the latter is altered, as shown by difficulties in detecting a target among an increasing set of distractors, by a decreased number of targets that can be counted when presented for a limited period, or by form recognition impairment under crowding conditions (Rizzo and Vecera, 2002; Michel and Henaff, 2004). Some attempts have been made to measure attention resolution across the spatial field, leading to representation of an attentional visual field (Michel and Henaff, 2004). Other computer tasks using Posner's paradigm may demonstrate predominant difficulties in disengaging attention (Michel and Henaff, 2004). Paper and pencil tests checking abilities to cross-out or to bisect lines displayed on a sheet of paper may reveal additional hemispatial neglect. Finally, reading is usually severely compromised at the single word or at the text level. Simultanagnosia may alter concomitant perception of the whole string of letters forming a word, or successive visual processing of words during text reading.

Prognosis and management

In patients with unilateral lesions harboring optic ataxia, functional consequence is modest, as visual–spatial functions are mostly spared and reaching is normal when performed in natural, central fixation. In contrast, the consequences of full Bálint's syndrome are devastating. Functional prognosis is poor as a result of diffusion of lesions that usually precludes significant recovery. However, spontaneous recovery can occur, after a delay ranging from weeks to years (Allison *et al.*, 1969; Montero *et al.*, 1982; Pisella *et al.*, 2000). Even in these cases, recovery is partial, leaving impaired simultaneous perception and reading difficulties (Allison *et al.*, 1969). Improvement of optic ataxia normalizes reaching accuracy in the foveal condition, but leaves the movement inaccurate in peripheral vision (Pisella *et al.*, 2000). Rehabilitation strategies are largely empirical and individually tailored, based on thorough clinical analysis of impaired and spared functions, especially in terms of patient's "lower" and "higher" visual spatial abilities (Al-Khawaja and Haboubi, 2001). An adaptative strategy uses preserved skills to compensate for problems and it aims at altering the patient's environment to lessen his or her disabilities. The remedial strategy is based upon training of perceptual and visuomotor defective functions in order to get generalization across all activities of daily living. Exercises usually include eye movement fixation, saccades, and pursuit of visual targets with the initial help of additional auditory or proprioceptive cues, manual reaching and pointing, as well as perception of a growing number of simultaneously presented objects. Evaluation of treatment procedures is to be developed. Reports of beneficial retraining are scarce and mostly limited to single cases (Al-Khawaja and Haboubi, 2001; Kerkhoff, 2001; Perez *et al.*, 1996; Rosselli *et al.*, 2001). Visual exploration and fixation has partly improved after systematic training of oculomotor functions in three patients with Bálint's syndrome (Zihl, 2000). This improvement seems transferable to daily activities, as these patients have gained better ability in finding their way in familiar surroundings. These data should encourage the development of rehabilitation programs.

Acknowledgment

The authors thank F. Cotton and L. Pijella for providing the MRI data.

REFERENCES

Al-Khawaja, I. and Haboubi, N. H. (2001). Neurovisual rehabilitation in Balint's syndrome. *J. Neurol. Neurosurg. Psychiatry*, **70**(3), 416.

Allison, R. S., Hurwitz, L. J., *et al.* (1969). A follow-up study of a patient with Balint's syndrome. *Neuropsychologia*, **7**, 319−33.

Andersen, R. A. (1997). Multimodal integration for the representation of space in the posterior parietal cortex. *Phil. Trans. R. Soc. Lond.*, **352**, 1421−8.

Astafiev, S. Y., Shulman, G. I., *et al.* (2003). Functional organisation of human parietal and frontal cortex for attending, looking and pointing. *J. Neurosci.*, **23**, 4689−99.

Auerbach, S. H. and Alexander, M. P. (1981). Pure agraphia and unilateral optic ataxia associated with a left superior parietal lobule lesion. *J. Neurol. Neurosurg. Psychiatry*, **44**(5), 430−2.

Badal, J. (1888). Contribution à l'étude des cécités psychiques: Alexie, agraphie, hémianopsie inférieure, trouble du sens de l'espace. *Arch. Ophthalmol.*, **140**, 97−117.

Bálint, R. (1909). Seelenlähmung des Schauens, optische Ataxie, räumliche Störung der Aufmerksamkeit. *Monatsschrift für Psychiatrie und Neurologie*, **25**, 51−81.

Battaglia-Mayer, A., Caminiti, R., *et al.* (2003). Multiple levels of representation of reaching in the parieto-frontal network. *Cereb. Cortex*, **13**, 1009−22.

Battaglia-Mayer, A., Ferraina, S., *et al.* (2000). Early coding of reaching in the parietooccipital cortex. *J. Neurophysiol.*, **83**, 2374−91.

Bellebaum, C., Hoffmann, K. P., and Daum, I. (2005). Post-saccadic updating of visual space in the posterior parietal cortex in humans. *Behav. Brain Res.*, **163**, 194−203.

Binkofski, F., Buccino, G., *et al.* (1999). Mirror agnosia and mirror ataxia constitute different parietal lobe disorders. *Ann. Neurol.*, **46**, 51−61.

Binkofski, F., Dohle, C., *et al.* (1998). Human anterior intraparietal area subserves prehension: a combined lesion and functional MRI activation study. *Neurology*, **50**(5), 1253−9.

Brain, R. (1941). Visual discrimination with special reference to lesions of the right hemisphere. *Brain*, **64**, 244−72.

Carey, D. P., Coleman, R. J., *et al.* (1997). Magnetic misreaching. *Cortex*, **33**(4), 639−52.

Castaigne, P., Rondot, P., *et al.* (1975). Ataxie optique localisée au côté gauche des deux hémichamps visuels homonymes. *Rev. Neurol. (Paris)*, **131**(1), 23−8.

Classen, J., Kunesch, E., *et al.* (1995). Subcortical origin of visuomotor apraxia. *Brain*, **118**, 1365−74.

Cogan, D. G. and Adams, R. D. (1953). A type of paralysis of conjugate gaze (ocular motor apraxia). *Arch. Ophthalmol.*, **50**(4), 434–42.

Colby, C. L. and Goldberg, M. E. (1999). Space and attention in parietal cortex. *Ann. Rev. Neurosci.*, **22**, 319–49.

Crawford, J. D., Medendorp, W. P., *et al.* (2004). Spatial transformations for eye-hand coordination. *J. Neurophysiol.*, **92**, 10–19.

Damasio, A. R. and Benton, A. L. (1979). Impairment of hand movements under visual guidance. *Neurology*, **29**, 170–4.

De Renzi, E. (1989). Balint-Holmes syndrome. In *Classic Cases in Neuropsychology*. Hove: Psychology Press, pp.123–43.

Duhamel, J. R., Colby, C. L., *et al.* (1992). The updating of the representation of visual space in parietal cortex by intended eye movements. *Science*, **255** (5040), 90–2.

Ferro, J. M. (1984). Transient inaccuracy in reaching caused by a posterior parietal lobe lesion. *J. Neurol. Neurosurg. Psychiatry*, **47**(9), 1016–19.

Friedman-Hill, S. R., Robertson, L. C., *et al.* (1995). Parietal contributions to visual feature binding: Evidence from a patient with bilateral lesions. *Science*, **269**(5225), 853–5.

Galletti, C., Kutz, D. F., *et al.* (2003). Role of the medial parieto-occipital cortex in the control of reaching and grasping movements. *Exp. Brain Res.*, **153**(2), 158–70. Epub 2003 Sep 27.

Garcin, R., Rondot, P., *et al.* (1967). Ataxie optique localisée aux deux hémichamps visuels homonymes gauches. *Rev. Neurol. (Paris)*, **116**(6), 707–14.

Girotti, F., Milanese, C., *et al.* (1982). Oculomotor disturbances in Balint's syndrome: Anatomoclinical findings and electrooculographic analysis in a case. *Cortex*, **18**(4), 603–14.

Goodale, M. A. and Milner, A. D. (1992). Separate visual pathways for perception and action. *Trends Neurosci.*, **15**, 20–5.

Gottlieb, D., Calvanio, R., *et al.* (1991). Reappearance of the visual percept after intentional blinking in a patient with Balint's syndrome. *J. Clin. Neuroophthalmol.*, **11**(1), 62–5.

Guard, O., Perenin, M. T., *et al.* (1984). Syndrome pariétal bilatéral ressemblant au syndrome de Balint. *Rev. Neurol.*, **140**(5), 358–67.

Hecaen, H. and De Ajuriaguerra, J. (1954). Balint's syndrome (psychic paralysis of visual fixation) and its minor forms. *Brain*, **77**(3), 373–400.

Heide, W., Blankenburg, M., *et al.* (1995). Cortical control of double-step saccades: Implications for spatial orientation. *Ann. Neurol.*, **38**, 739–48.

Holmes, G. (1918). Disturbances of visual orientation. *Brit. J. Ophthalmol.*, **2**, 449–68, 506–18.

Hijdra, A. and Meerwaldt, J. D. (1984). Balint's syndrome in a man with border-zone infarcts caused by atrial fibrillation. *Clin. Neurol. Neurosurg.*, **86**(1), 51–4.

Husain, M. and Stein, J. (1988). Rezso Balint and his most celebrated case. *Arch. Neurol.*, **45**(1), 89–93.

Inoue, A., Sato, K., *et al.* (1988). A case of multiple cerebral hemorrhage related to cerebral amyloid angiopathy. *No Shinkei Geka*, **16**(Suppl. 5), 544–9.

Inouye, T. (1904). Cited by Rizzo and Vecera (2002).

Jackson, S. R., Newport, R., *et al.* (2005). Where the eye looks, the hand follows; limb-dependent magnetic misreaching in optic ataxia. *Curr. Biol.*, **15**(1), 42–6.

Jakobson, L. S., Archibald, Y. M., *et al.* (1991). A kinematic analysis of reaching and grasping movements in a patient recovering from optic ataxia. *Neuropsychologia*, **29**(8), 803–9.

Jeannerod, M., Decety, J., *et al.* (1994). Impairment of grasping movements following bilateral posterior parietal lesion. *Neuropsychologia*, **32**, 369–80.

Karnath, H. O. and Perenin, M. T. (2005). Cortical control of visually guided reaching: Evidence from patients with optic ataxia. *Cereb. Cortex*, **15**(10), 1561–9.

Kase, C. S., Troncoso, J. F., *et al.* (1977). Global spatial disorientation. Clinico-pathologic correlations. *J. Neurol. Sci.*, **34**(2), 267–78.

Kerkhoff, G. (2000). Neurovisual rehabilitation: Recent developments and future directions. *J. Neurol. Neurosurg. Psychiatr.*, **68**, 691–706.

Kerkhoff, G. (2001). Neurovisual rehabilitation in Balint's syndrome: Reply. *J. Neurol. Neurosurg. Psychiat.*, **70**, 416.

Luria, A. R. (1959). Disorders of simultaneous perception in a case of occipito-parietal brain injury. *Brain*, **82**, 437–49.

Mendez, M. F., Tomsak, R. L. and Remler, B. (1990). Disorders of the visual system in Alzheimer's disease. *J. Clin. Neuroophthalmol.*, **10**, 62–9.

Michel, F. and Henaff, M. A. (2004). Seeing without the occipito-parietal cortex: Simultagnosia as a shrinkage of the attentional visual field. *Behav. Neurol.*, **15**(1-2), 3–13.

Michel, F., Jeannerod, M., *et al.* (1963). Un cas de désorientation visuelle dans les trois dimensions de l'espace (A propos du syndrome de Balint et du syndrome décrit par G Holmes). *Rev. Neurol. (Paris)*, **108**, 983–4.

Montero, J., Pena, J., *et al.* (1982). Balint's syndrome. Report of four cases with watershed parieto-occipital lesions from vertebrobasilar ischemia or systemic hypotension. *Acta Neurol. Belg.*, **82**(5), 270–80.

Müri, R. M., Iba-Zizen, M. T., *et al.* (1996). Location of the human posterior eye field with functional magnetic resonance imaging. *J. Neurol. Neurosurg. Psychiat.*, **60**, 445–48.

Perenin, M. T. and Vighetto, A. (1988). Optic ataxia: A specific disruption in visuomotor mechanisms. I. Different aspects of the deficit in reaching for objects. *Brain*, **111**(Pt 3), 643–74.

Perez, F. M., Tunkel, R. S., *et al.* (1996). Balint's syndrome arising from bilateral posterior cortical atrophy or infarction: Rehabilitation strategies and their limitation. *Disabil. Rehabil.*, **18**(6), 300–4.

Pierrot-Deseilligny, C., Gautier, J. C., *et al.* (1988). Acquired ocular motor apraxia due to bilateral frontoparietal infarcts. *Ann. Neurol.*, **23**(2), 199–202.

Pierrot-Deseilligny, C., Gray, F., *et al.* (1986). Infarcts of both inferior parietal lobules with impairment of visually guided eye movements, peripheral visual inattention and optic ataxia. *Brain*, **109**, 81–97.

Pisella, L., Grea, H., *et al.* (2000). An 'automatic pilot' for the hand in human posterior parietal cortex: Toward reinterpreting optic ataxia. *Nat. Neurosci.*, **3**(7), 729–36.

Prado, J., Clavagnier, S., *et al.* (2005). Two cortical systems for reaching in central and peripheral vision. *Neuron*, **48**, 849–58.

Rapcsak, S. Z., Cimino, C. R., *et al.* (1988). Altitudinal neglect. *Neurology*, **38**(2), 277–81.

Riddoch, G. (1935). Visual disorientation in homonymous half-fields. *Brain*, **58**, 376–82.

Rizzo, M. and Hurtig, R. (1987). Looking but not seeing: Attention, perception, and eye movements in simultanagnosia. *Neurology*, **37**, 1642–8.

Rizzo, M. and Vecera, S. P. (2002). Psychoanatomical substrates of Balint's syndrome. *J. Neurol. Neurosurg. Psychiatry*, **72**(2), 162–78.

Rizzolatti, G. and Matelli, M. (2003). Two different streams form the dorsal visual system: anatomy and functions. *Exp. Brain Res.*, **153**(2), 146–57.

Rondot, P., de Recondo, J., *et al.* (1977). Visuomotor ataxia. *Brain*, **100**(2), 355–76.

Rosselli, M., Ardila, A., *et al.* (2001). Rehabilitation of Balint's syndrome: A single case report. *Appl. Neuropsychol.*, **8**(4), 242–7.

Rossetti, Y. (1998). Implicit short-lived motor representations of space in brain damaged and healthy subjects. *Consciousness and Cognition*, **7**, 520–58.

Rossetti, Y., Pisella, L., *et al.* (2003). Optic ataxia revisited: Visually guided action versus immediate visuomotor control. *Exp. Brain Res.*, **153**(2), 171–9.

Rossetti, Y., Revol, P., *et al.* (2005). Visually guided reaching: Bilateral posterior parietal lesions cause a switch from fast visuomotor to slow cognitive control. *Neuropsychologia*, **43**(2), 162–77.

Roy, A. C., Stefanini, S., *et al.* (2004). Early movement impairments in a patient recovering from optic ataxia. *Neuropsychologia*, **42**(7), 847–54.

Schindler, I., Rice, N. J., *et al.* (2004). Automatic avoidance of obstacles is a dorsal stream function: Evidence from optic ataxia. *Nat. Neurosci.*, **7**(7), 779–84.

Schluppeck, D., Glimcher, P. and Heeger, D. J. (2005). Topographic organization for delayed saccades in human posterior parietal cortex. *J. Neurophysiol.*, **94**, 1372–84.

Tang-Wai, D. F., Graff-Radford, N. R., *et al.* (2004). Clinical, genetic, and neuropathologic characteristics of posterior cortical atrophy. *Neurology*, **63**(7), 1168–74.

Tyler, H. R. (1968). Abnormalities of perception with defective eye movements (Balint's syndrome). *Cortex*, **4**, 154–71.

Valenza, N., Murray, M. M., *et al.* (2004). The space of senses: Impaired crossmodal interactions in a patient with Balint syndrome after bilateral parietal damage. *Neuropsychologia*, **42**(13), 1737–48.

Verfaellie, M., Rapcsak, S. Z., *et al.* (1990). Impaired shifting of attention in Balint's syndrome. *Brain Cogn.*, **12**(2), 195–204.

Vighetto, A. and Perenin, M. T. (1981). Ataxie optique: Analyse des réponses oculaires et manuelles lors du pointage vers des cibles visuelles. *Rev. Neurol.*, **137**(5), 357–72.

Watson, R. T. and Rapcsak, S. Z. (1989). Loss of spontaneous blinking in a patient with Balint's syndrome. *Arch. Neurol.*, **46**(5), 567–70.

Woldorff, M. G., Hazlitt, C. J., *et al.* (2004). Functional parcellation of attentional control region of the brain. *J. Cogn. Neurosci.*, **16**, 149–65.

Zihl, J. (2000). Rehabilitation of visual disorders after brain injury. In *Neuropsychological Rehabilitation: A Modular Handbook*. Hove: Psychology Press Ltd.

16

Prosopagnosia

Eugene Mayer[1] and Bruno Rossion[2]

[1]University Hospital of Geneva, Switzerland
[2]University of Louvain, Belgium

General presentation of the disorder

Prosopagnosia is classically defined as an inability to recognize faces of people known to the patient on the basis of visual perception, despite the absence of low-level visual impairments, or cognitive alterations such as mental confusion or amnesia, with a preserved ability to recognize people through other cues: voice or other visual traits such as gait, size, clothes, or even facial features (moustache, scar, blemish) or accessories (ear-rings, eyeglasses). Prosopagnosics also have access to semantic knowledge concerning people.

According to Grüsser and Landis (1991), this condition seems to have been first described by Wigan (1844), in a book in which he expressed his views on the interaction of the two cerebral hemispheres. Wigan stated (pp. 128–9):

A gentleman of middle age, or a little past that period, lamented to me his utter inability to remember faces. He would converse with a person for an hour, but after an interval of a day could not recognise him again. Even friends, with whom he had been engaged in business transactions, he was unconscious of ever having seen (. . .) it was not till he heard the voice, that he could recognise men with whom he had constant intercourse (. . .) When I inquire more fully into the matter, I found that there was no defect in vision, except that his eyes were weak, and that any long continued employment of them gave him pain (. . .). He was quite determined to conceal it, if possible, and it was impossible to convince him that it did not depend solely on the eyes.

Early descriptions of prosopagnosia were also provided by Quaglino and Borelli (1867; a patient with right hemisphere stroke), Charcot (1883), Wilbrand (1887; 1892; stroke with bilateral posterior lesions). Frequently, prosopagnosia was found to be associated with other deficits such as achromatopsia and topographical disorientation (Quaglino and Borelli, 1867; Wilbrand, 1887; 1892), or even color and object agnosia (Charcot, 1883). A number of similar observations were published in the next 60 years (see Grüsser and Landis, 1991, for an historical review). Nevertheless, disturbance in face recognition was considered to be part of a complex visual agnosic disorder until the paper of Hoff and Pötzl (1937).

These authors considered for the first time the inability to identify familiar faces as a specific form of visual agnosia. Ten years later, Bodamer (1947) isolated the failure to recognize familiar persons on the basis of facial appearance from other disorder of visual perception and coined the term *prosopagnosia*.

Patients with prosopagnosia are generally able to make fine visual discriminations. For example, they are able to read. They can also categorize a visual stimulus as a face. But prevented from using the voice, clothes, gait, or specific attributes such as glasses, ear-rings, or moustaches, they cannot identify a familiar person, and even themselves in some cases. For example, Charcot's patient (1883) mistook his own mirror image for a stranger and apologized for blocking the way. Years ago, we filmed a woman who was prosopagnosic and we projected her own image to her on-line, without sound. We asked her to describe what she saw. She told us: "I see a woman, . . . she is speaking, . . . she is wearing a scarf." Asked about the identity of this woman, the patient responded "it could be one of my neighbours." This patient denied having any specific problem with face recognition even if she admitted to not being a physionomist. Nevertheless, absence of awareness of the disorder is not the rule. Other patients sometimes report that they do not recognize familiar people until they talk and base their visual recognition on clothes or hairstyle for instance.

The simplest and still the best way to determine clinically whether a patient is prosopagnosic or not is to confront him or her with several persons, of the same sex and age, uniformly dressed, among which one is familiar. Ideally, the hair should be masked with a cap. The persons should remain completely silent and move as little as possible, without smiling. In this condition, a prosopagnosic will not recognize the familiar person. If this familiar person is immediately identified when she begins to speak, the diagnosis is made. Even though low-level visual impairments are likely to be present due to the extension of the lesions to early visual areas, the deficit must not be *explainable* by alterations of lower-level visual impairments, hence the importance of detailed assessment of the patient's neuropsychological profile (see later).

A number of reviews of the anatomical basis and functional aspects of prosopagnosia and other face disorders have been published over the years (e.g. Barton, 2003; Behrmann and Moscovitch, 2001; Goldsmith and Liu, 2001; Grüsser and Landis, 1991). In line with the objectives of this volume, we have intended to provide a distinct account of this spectacular deficit, first by focusing on the assessment and rehabilitation of prosopagnosia, and second to highlight certain aspects of the deficit that are recent and/or relatively unknown. In the next section, the relationship between the localization of the lesions causing prosopagnosia and the neural basis of face processing in the normal brain will be discussed. Then we discuss recent findings illustrating how prosopagnosic patients can still process faces to some extent, something that may be critical to define for any attempt at rehabilitation of this deficit.

Key points Main characteristics of prosopagnosia

Inability to recognize familiar person on the basis of visual perception, despite the absence of low level visual impairments or cognitive alterations

Relative sparing of person recognition through other cues (essentially voice, but also gait, size, clothes, or facial features or accessories)

Frequently associated with left hemianopia, achromatopsia, and topographical disorientation

Due to right or bilateral lesion in the inferomedial part of the temporo-occipital region (fusiform and lingual gyri)

Etiology and lesion localization

Prosopagnosia is extremely rare. For example, Zihl and Von Cramon (1986) did not find any pure prosopagnosics in a series of 258 patients suffering from posterior brain lesions of different origins (closed head injury, encephalitis, tumors, surgical lesions for epilepsy, hemorrhages, and cerebral infarcts). If prosopagnosia is considered as one symptom among other visual and neuropsychological defects, the frequency is higher – for example 6% in the study of Hécaen and Angelergues (1962; 1963) concerning 382 patients with posterior cerebral lesions of different origins. Prosopagnosia of vascular origin is due to posterior cerebral artery infarcts (PCAIs). This latter disease represents 5–11% of all strokes in the general population (Brandt *et al.*, 2000). Among PCAI, prosopagnosia can be present in pure cortical infarct (4%), cortical and deep infarct (4%), and bilateral infarcts (7%) (Kumral *et al.*, 2004). If unilateral, the infarct must be on the right side in order to produce prosopagnosia (Cals *et al.*, 2002; De Renzi *et al.*, 1994; Grüsser and Landis, 1991; Milandre *et al.*, 1994; Uttner *et al.*, 2002; Wada and Yamamoto, 2001). Other etiologies include a carbon monoxide poisoning, temporal lobectomy, encephalitis, neoplasm, right temporal lobe atrophy, trauma, Parkinson's disease, and Alzheimer's disease. The debate about the localization of lesions has for long been restricted to the question of whether a right hemisphere lesion was sufficient and/or necessary, or not, to cause the deficit (e.g. see Damasio *et al.*, 1982; Ettlin *et al.*, 1992; Michel *et al.*, 1989). It is now widely admitted that a lesion of the right hemisphere is *necessary* to cause prosopagnosia, even though one case has been described with a lesion apparently restricted to the left hemisphere (see Mattson *et al.*, 2000). The fact that there is only a single case of prosopagnosia following a left hemisphere lesion is remarkable, given the contribution of the left hemisphere during normal face processing, as evidenced by lateralized visual field studies (e.g. Hillger and Koenig, 1991), and more recently by neuroimaging (e.g. Sergent *et al.*, 1992; Kanwisher *et al.*, 1997) and event-related potential (e.g. Rossion *et al.*, 2003b) studies. Face processes performed in the left hemisphere thus appear to complement a massively right localized function, and may not be critical for this function. Alternatively, a lesion in the left occipitotemporal cortex may cause only subtle face processing deficits that are usually not detected by conventional neuropsychological tests, perhaps because left unilateral brain-damaged patients present other, more spectacular, symptoms (e.g. alexia; see Farah, 1990).

However, the notion that a single right hemisphere lesion is *sufficient* to cause prosopagnosia, or whether a bilateral lesion was always necessary, has proved more difficult to resolve. This question originated from the analysis of visual field defects in prosopagnosic patients (Hécaen and Angelergues, 1962; Meadows, 1974). The presence of a left visual field defect, in particular a left superior quadrantanopia, is the most common low-level visual defect observed in cases of prosopagnosia, but there are also prosopagnosic patients that have exclusive right visual field defects (Bouvier and Engel, 2006; Meadows, 1974; Goldsmith and Liu, 2001). In any case, a left visual field defect associated more often with prosopagnosia cannot be used as a reliable criterion to support the view that a right hemisphere lesion is sufficient to cause the deficit, since cases of prosopagnosia would not present visual field defects if posterior cerebral lesions spare the optic radiations and striate cortex (Damasio *et al.*, 1982).

With the advent of structural imaging (CT scans, and then MRI; see Damasio and Damasio, 1989), it was clearly established that a right hemisphere lesion can be sufficient to cause prosopagnosia and several such cases have been reported (three cases in Barton *et al.*, 2002; Landis *et al.*, 1988; Marotta *et al.*, 2001: case 2; Sergent and Signoret, 1992: cases 1 & 2; Sergent and Villemure, 1989; Uttner *et al.*, 2002; Wada and Yamamoto, 2001), most of them following right posterior cerebral artery infarct. Furthermore, functional neuroimaging examination (positron emission tomography, PET; or functional magnetic resonance imaging, fMRI) performed in some of these cases indicated a normal metabolism in the left hemisphere (see Sergent and Signoret, 1992).

The lesions causing prosopagnosia are generally located in the inferomedial part of the temporo-occipital area, in the fusiform gyrus, the lingual gyrus, and the posterior part of the parahippocampic gyrus (Damasio *et al.*, 1982; Grüsser and Landis, 1991). Within this large cortical territory, PET and mainly fMRI studies conducted on the normal brain have identified at least two small (a few mm^3) areas responding preferentially to faces, as compared to other object categories, or scrambled face stimuli. These areas are localized in the inferior occipital gyrus (IOG) and in the lateral part of the middle fusiform gyrus (MFG), (e.g. Kanwisher *et al.*, 1997; Rossion *et al.*, 2000; 2003a; Sergent *et al.*, 1992; for a review see Haxby *et al.*, 2000). They can be localized in individual subjects with a certain amount of interindividual variability in location, sensitivity, and size (Rossion *et al.*, 2003a). The area in the right midfusiform gyrus that responds most strongly to face stimuli has been termed by some the "fusiform face area" (FFA) (Kanwisher *et al.*, 1997). However, isolated lesions in the vicinity of the right midfusiform that do not include the occipital cortex are rare because the blood supply comes from both the posterior and middle cerebral arteries thereby protecting it from ischemic damage. In contrast, there are more cases of prosopagnosia with a lesion encompassing the right IOG and sparing the right MFG (Bouvier and Engel, 2006; Figure 16.1). A recent analysis of the lesions causing prosopagnosia has shown that the area of maximal lesion overlap concerns a small territory in the right IOG, exactly where a preferential response to faces is observed in the normal brain (Bouvier and Engel, 2006). From these observations, it can be concluded that a lesion of the right IOG is sufficient to cause prosopagnosia, but it is yet unclear whether an isolated lesion of the right MFG can also, in itself, cause a massive face impairment as found in prosopagnosia (see the discussions in Rossion *et al.*, 2003a; Schiltz *et al.*, 2006).

Finally, given that the face processing system is bilateral and widely distributed (Haxby *et al.*, 2000), with a number of key regions in the right hemisphere, it is not

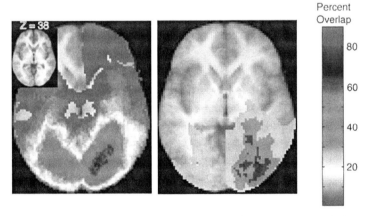

Figure 16.1 (Left) Lesion overlap of prosopagnosia cases. The prosopagnosia lesion overlap contains lesions from all cases with prosopagnosia regardless of achromatopsia diagnosis (*n* = 52). The inserts show the Talairach Z-coordinate at the average axial slice location. (Right) Lesion overlap of prosopagnosia cases with single disorder. The prosopagnosia lesion overlap (right) contains lesions from cases of prosopagnosia and intact color processing (*n* = 8). The scale bar indicates 1 cm. Figures taken from Bouvier, S. E. & Engel, S. A. (2005), with permission. For a color version of this figure please see www.cambridge.org/9780521106955.

strictly necessary to have a lesion in either of these two areas for prosopagnosia to occur. For instance, cases of prosopagnosia with more anterior lesions in the right temporal lobe due to closed head injury (Bukach *et al.*, 2006) or progressive right cortical atrophy (e.g. Evans *et al.*, 1995; Joubert *et al.*, 2003) may show a clear prosopagnosic deficit. Regions in the right inferotemporal lobe (i.e. Brodmann area 20) are rarely reported in fMRI studies of normal subjects due to magnetic susceptibility artifacts in the temporal lobe, but PET studies indicate that they play a role in the discrimination of familiar and unfamiliar faces and recollection of semantic information from faces (e.g. Leveroni *et al.* 2000; Rossion *et al.*, 2001).

Key points Strokes responsible for the disorder

Stroke type	Territory/characteristics
Arterial Infarct	posterior cerebral artery: right or bilateral
Hemorrhage	infero-medial part of the temporo-occipital area

Associated deficits and functional aspects of prosopagnosia

Associated deficits

As discussed previously, most prosopagnosic patients have a visual field defect, especially in the left upper quadrant (Bouvier and Engel, 2006; Goldsmith and Liu, 2001; Grüsser and Landis, 1991). As for low-level vision, impairments can be found in luminance discrimination, spatial resolution, curvature, line orientation or contrast at low spatial frequencies, but these deficits are rare and are unlikely to contribute to the prosopagnosic deficit (Barton *et al.*, 2004). Contrast sensitivity at higher frequencies may be more frequent (Barton *et al.*, 2004; Caldara *et al.*, 2005; Rizzo *et al.*, 1986) and directly related to the ability to extract fine-grained information about facial identity. One of the most frequent associations with prosopagnosia is achromatopsia — about 60% overlap in the meta-analysis of Bouvier and Engel (2006) — a deficit in color perception often associated with unilateral or bilateral lesions in the temporo-occipital junction, in the anterior part of the fusiform and lingual gyri (Zeki, 1990).

Another deficit frequently associated with prosopagnosia is topographical disorientation (see also Chapter 13). Two types of topographical disorientation are usually described (Landis, 2004). One of them concerns an impairment of vectorial orientation (troubles in angle and distance processing). The other is bound to a loss of environmental familiarity and difficulties in using landmarks. This latter pathology was described in association with a lesion circumscribed in the posterior part of the parahippocampal gyrus and the anterior part of the lingual gyrus of the right hemisphere (Habib and Sirigu, 1987).

Larger lesions in bilateral posterior regions can produce, in addition to prosopagnosia, shape and object agnosia, or even pure alexia (Farah, 1990). If prosopagnosia can be found without any deficit in word recognition, especially following unilateral right hemisphere damage, prosopagnosics have usually clear associated deficits in object recognition (e.g. Clarke *et al.*, 1997; Gauthier *et al.*, 1999). A few cases have been presented as having a deficit restricted to faces (e.g. De Renzi, 1986; Henke *et al.*, 1998; Whitley and Warrington, 1977), but they have been criticized on methodological grounds (e.g. Sergent and Signoret, 1992) because their apparent normal performance at object recognition could be explained by more general perceptual deficits and/or the possibility that a face recognition task is simply more difficult than an object recognition task (Gauthier *et al.*, 1999). Even when the difficulty of face and non-face object discrimination is equated for normal controls and the same tasks are then used to assess the performance of a prosopagnosic patient, differential speed response between faces and non-face objects are usually not considered (e.g. Farah *et al.*, 1995), whereas response time measures may reveal concurrent object recognition difficulties in prosopagnosic patients (Gauthier *et al.*, 1999; Laeng and Caviness, 2001). Yet, certain brain-damaged prosopagnosic patients, such as the patient PS described in later sections, may show a deficit restricted to the category of faces even when response times are considered (Rossion *et al.*, 2003a; Schiltz *et al.*, 2005).

When there are clear impairments at object recognition, the deficits may concern object categories for which the patient had developed a visual expertise at recognizing prior to the lesion (e.g. flowers or cars; Clarke *et al.*, 1997). For instance, Assal *et al.* (1984) described a farmer who in addition to his prosopagnosia could not recognize his cows anymore. In some cases, however, the deficit can spare the category of expertise, such as cars (Sergent and Signoret, 1992: case RM) or sheep faces (McNeil and Warrington, 1993). Finally, an extremely rare associated deficit is metamorphopsia, or the perception of a deformation of faces, first described by Bodamer (1947: case 3). In such cases, the deficit can also extend to familiar objects. For instance, Seron *et al.* (1995) described the case of a patient who suffered transient metamorphopsia following a small right occipitotemporal hemorrhage, in the area of the middle fusiform gyrus, and who, in addition to his prosopagnosia, perceived faces and objects such as cars as spatially distorted.

Subtypes of prosopagnosic deficits or functional aspects of prosopagnosia

It has been proposed that there may be several subtypes of prosopagnosia (de Renzi *et al.*, 1991; Damasio *et al.*, 1990). Two broad categories are apperceptive

and associative prosopagnosia (de Renzi *et al.*, 1991). In apperceptive prosopagnosia, the chief deficit is held to be impairment in generating an adequate percept
of the face, such that it cannot be matched to stored representations of previously
seen faces. In associative prosopagnosia, the process of generating the percept is
intact but the percept cannot be matched to store representations, either because
of disconnection from, or destruction of, the facial memory stores. However,
Farah (1990) and other authors (Davidoff and Landis, 1990) have cast doubts on
the existence of pure associative visual (prosop)agnosia, claiming that when tested
in detail, all visual agnosic patients, including prosopagnosics, show deficits at the
perceptual level. For instance, a few prosopagnosics have been reported to perform
in the normal range in face matching tasks on unfamiliar faces like the Benton face
recognition test (Benton *et al.*, 1983), but appear to take excessive time to do so
(e.g. Bukach *et al.*, 2006; Delvenne *et al.*, 2004; Davidoff and Landis, 1990).
All prosopagnosic patients may thus present perceptual deficits at the root of their
face impairment, even when the lesion spares the right visual cortex and concern
the anterior temporal lobe only (e.g. Joubert *et al.*, 2003; Bukach *et al.*, 2006).
Yet, there is a large amount of interindividual variability between prosopagnosic
patients in terms of their perceptual deficits (e.g. Barton *et al.*, 2004; Sergent and
Signoret, 1992; Schweich and Bruyer, 1993), such that distinctions between
apperceptive and associative prosopagnosia are more a matter of degree of visual
impairment than of kind. Recent studies suggest that prosopagnosic patients
are impaired at extracting *configural* information on faces: the perception of the
relationships between the features (i.e. metric distances) rather than the features
(eyes, mouth, nose . . .) themselves would be impaired (Barton *et al.*, 2002; Joubert
et al., 2003) (Figure 16.2). Other studies have indicated a deficit at integrating the
facial features into holistic representations (Boutsen and Humphreys, 2003;
Sergent and Signoret, 1992; Sergent and Villemure, 1989; for a review clarifying the
different kinds of configural information, see Maurer *et al.*, 2002). This inability to
integrate facial features into a whole representation and to extract metric distances
between features is in line with the absence of a decrease of performance for faces
presented upside-down generally found in prosopagnosia (e.g. Boutsen and
Humphreys, 2003; Delvenne *et al.*, 2004; Marotta *et al.*, 2002): prosopagnosic
patients appear to process faces in a piecemeal, analytical manner. Very recently,
two independent studies showed that prosopagnosics may present a marked
deficit at extracting diagnostic information to recognize faces on the upper part of
the face, i.e. the eyes region (Bukach *et al.*, 2006; Caldara *et al.*, 2005). Caldara
and collaborators used a learning and response classification method to show that
their prosopagnosic patient PS rather used the mouth and the external features of
the face, whereas normal controls relied on the eyes and the internal features
in general (Figure 16.3). This specific loss of the ability to extract diagnostic

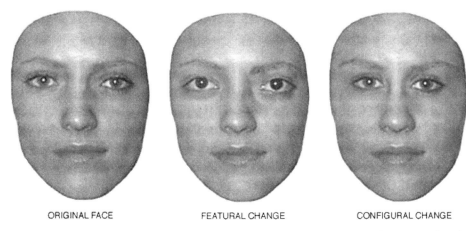

ORIGINAL FACE   FEATURAL CHANGE   CONFIGURAL CHANGE

Figure 16.2 Diagnostic information to discriminate and recognize individual faces can be *'featural'*, i.e. concern a modification in the shape and surface properties of a local feature such as the eyes, or *'configural'*, i.e. concern a modification in the relative properties (metric distances) of the features rather than the features themselves. There is evidence that prosopagnosic patients are particularly impaired at extracting configural differences between faces (e.g. Barton *et al.*, 2002).

Prosopagnosic patient   Normal controls

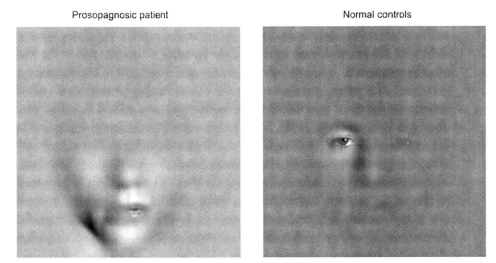

Figure 16.3 Areas of the face stimulus used by a brain-damaged prosopagnosic patient (PS) with deficit restricted to faces (see Rossion *et al.*, 2003a). PS used mainly the mouth area to recognize faces, as identified by a response classification method. In contrast, normal participants extract diagnostic information to recognize faces from the eyes on average, with a left visual field bias (Caldara *et al.*, 2005).

information from the eyes may be related to the impairment at processing configural information, which is heavily weighted in the upper part of the face (see Caldara *et al.*, 2005).

Finally, it is usually stated that prosopagnosics are able to tell apart men and women, estimate age from face, or categorize facial expression on faces (e.g. Bruyer *et al.*, 1983; Tranel *et al.*, 1988). However, these categorizations are usually easier than individual face recognition, and the patients may use external features such as the hair, or local cues (e.g. smile). When external cues such as the hair are masked, the prosopagnosic patient's performance is generally below normal range at these face judgments also (Sergent and Signoret, 1992).

Neuropsychological assessment

As stated in the introduction, it is relatively straightforward to define prosopagnosia in a brain-damaged patient, based on the behavior of the patient in a normal life situation. However, the question at stake is not simply to be able to classify the patient as being prosopagnosic, but to characterize the deficit (at which functional level it takes place) and define associated visual and memory impairments. Given the extension of the lesions, it is almost impossible to encounter a patient without any visual and/or memory deficits concerning non-face material. The question will be whether these deficits are directly related to (i.e. explain) the prosopagnosic deficit, or can be considered separately. For instance, achromatopsia – the loss of color perception – is most often (Bouvier and Engel, 2005), but not always associated with prosopagnosia, because the lesions causing prosopagnosia often encompass the visual area V4/V8 in the ventral pathway, critical for color processing in humans (Zeki, 1990). Even though color information may play a role in face recognition, it is not thought to be critical for the ability to discriminate and recognize faces. In any case, visual and mnesic impairments will have to be defined extensively, as they will help to determine the kind of tests that can be proposed to the patient to assess his/her face processing abilities. A patient with a visual short-term memory deficit cannot be tested in delayed face picture matching tasks for instance. Below, we provide a list of tests that could or should be used during the detailed assessment of prosopagnosia.

A first step should exclude a confusional state or a general intellectual impairment. The Wechsler Adult Intelligence Scale (WAIS III) is one of the best tools for this purpose. Furthermore, it allows the examiner to observe how the patient behaves on a wide array of tasks and can elicit cognitive dissociations (for example, better verbal than visual–spatial processing). The role of memory is crucial in the recognition of faces. In this optic, the Wechsler Memory Scale

(WMS III) evaluates verbal, visual, short- and long-term memory and, once more, can be useful in showing some specific impairment (for example, visual short-term memory deficit). The copy and recall of the Rey-Osterrieth figure (Spreen and Strauss, 1998) can give useful informations about visuo-constructive and/or visual memory impairments.

The evaluation of low-level visual capacities is made by a neuro-ophthalmologist. It generally comprises a test of visual acuity (Snellen or Monoyer's scale), an evaluation of contrast sensitivity (Ginsburg, 2003; Nadler *et al.*, 1990), a dynamic (Goldmann) or static (Octopus) visual field measure, an analysis of stereoptic vision (Buser and Imbert, 1987), color (Farnworth-Munsell; Ishihara) and movement perception (Cavanagh, 1992).

Some neuropsychological tests may also be useful in testing low-level visual capacities. For example, subtests two to five from the Birmingham Object Recognition Battery (BORB) (Riddoch and Humphreys, 1993) are suited to elicit pre-categorical visual processing impairments. These tests (matching tasks) are directed solely at the perception of basic properties of object forms — size, orientation, location, and length. Computerized versions of some tests of low-level vision (contrast sensitivity, spatial resolution, etc.) have been developed (Barton *et al.*, 2004). The "shape detection screening test" and the "incomplete letters test," two subtests from the Visual Object and Space Perception Battery (VOSP) (Warrington and James, 1991), as well as subtest six of the BORB ("the overlapping figure test"), can help to detect difficulties in figure/ground perception. More elaborated tests would involve determining whether three-dimensional figures are structurally possible or impossible (Farah, 1990; Delvenne *et al.*, 2004).

The next step is to test for the presence of a visual agnosia for non-face objects. Subtests seven and eight of the BORB point on difficulties in object recognition across different viewpoints. However, these may be achieved successfully through slow feature matching, even in visual agnosic patients (Delvenne *et al.*, 2004). A complete testing of normal object perception should include the simultaneous matching of novel (non-existent) objects and familiar objects presented in the same and in different viewpoints (Delvenne *et al.*, 2004; Rossion *et al.*, 2003b; Sergent and Signoret, 1992). At the associative level, tests nine to fourteen in BORB assess whether patients have the intact stored knowledge required to recognize and name visually presented objects. Another visual agnosia battery often used in the French community is the Montréal—Toulouse battery (Agniel *et al.*, 1992). Object naming can be tested with the Snodgrass and Vanderwart's (1980) set of line drawings, for which norms have been collected in several languages, and which are also available in gray scale and colorized versions (Rossion and Pourtois, 2004). As indicated in the previous section, accuracy measures are not sufficient to exclude a deficit in object recognition since prosopagnosic patients may achieve normal performance at object recognition when given unlimited time to respond (Farah, 1990). Response time measures may reveal concurrent object recognition difficulties in prosopagnosic patients (Delvenne *et al.*, 2004; Gauthier *et al.*, 1999; Laeng and Caviness, 2001). Since brain-damaged patients can be generally slowed down (Benton, 1986), it may be important to assess phasic reaction times (RT), or other baseline measures of RT. Alternatively, the performance of the patient can be compared to brain damaged controls without visual deficits.

Concerning face processing, the most popular test is the Benton face recognition test (Benton *et al.*, 1983), which is particularly well adapted to the detection of perceptual impairments. It requires matching unfamiliar faces that do not contain external face features, across changes of viewpoint and lighting. This test is highly diagnostic of prosopagnosia. Some authors have criticized this test because in rare cases the prosopagnosic patients can perform in the normal range, or because it would be possible to match faces on local features such as eyebrows (Duchaine and Weidenfeld, 2003). However, these criticisms are unjustified: when such strategies are used, RT measures will complement the accuracy scores and reveal that prosopagnosic patients take unusually long times to respond (e.g. Bukach *et al.*, 2006; Delvenne *et al.*, 2004). The recognition memory test (Warrington, 1984) evaluates non-verbal recognition memory with a facial recognition (old/new) test. A shorter version of this test is obtainable in the Camden Memory Battery (Warrington, 1996). The patient can also be tested with face photographs of personally familiar or famous people, but such tests should be developed on an individual basis. Other face processing functions such as gender categorization, facial expression, and age assessment can be performed with face stimuli without external cues (hair, earrings, etc.) again considering both accuracy rates and RT measures.

Key points Assessment of prosopagnosia

Tests aimed at assessing other cognitive or visual deficits:
– Wechsler adult intelligence scale (WAIS III)
– Wechsler memory scale (WMS III)
– Birmingham object recognition battery (BORB)
– Visual object and space perception battery (VOSP)
Tests aimed at evaluating facial perception and recognition:
– Benton face recognition test, with measure of accuracy and response times
– Warrington recognition memory test

Prognosis and management of the disorder

Prosopagnosia due to vascular disease is always associated with posterior cerebral artery territory infarcts (PCAIs). In the course of PCAI, death is rare, varying from 0% (Brandt *et al.*, 2000), to 3% (Yamamoto *et al.*, 1999), 5% (Pessin *et al.*, 1987), and 7% (Kumral *et al.*, 2004; Milandre *et al.*, 1994). Mortality and major disability were found to be strongly associated with cardioembolism and athero-sclerotic large-artery disease of the vertebrobasilar artery and PCA (Brandt *et al.*, 2000; Kumral *et al.*, 2004). Outcome is usually good (Brandt *et al.*, 2000). As discussed before, prosopagnosia is due to lesions in the inferomedial part of the temporo-occipital area, and the outcome of prosopagnosia depends on the size of infarction in these regions. Cognitive rehabilitation of prosopagnosia is rarely described. In fact we found only four publications on this subject (Beyn and Knyazeva, 1962; Glowic and Violon, 1981; Ellis and Young, 1988; Polster and Rapcsak, 1996). For the two first studies, the therapy methodology is poorly described. On the contrary, descriptions of Ellis and Young (1988) concerning the training of a young girl in face recognition are well-detailed (mostly face matching tasks), but the conclusions are dramatic. After more than two years of daily training, no improvement was observed. The authors concluded that any attempt at improving face recognition was vain, and that the patient should be trained to recognize persons by the mean of others cues such as the voice. Polster and Rapcsak (1996) tried to teach new faces to their prosopagnosic patient RJ. They concluded that semantic cuing (such as asking to associate the photograph of a face with a story concerning the person or with personality traits of this person) was more efficient than structural cuing (for example to determine the salient traits of a face). Nevertheless, the improvement was restricted to a specific viewpoint of the photograph and no generalization to other presentation of the photography could be made. Consequently, the techniques used to improve learning of new faces were inefficient in daily life, where faces are always seen from different viewpoints. We tried to improve face recognition in the patient PS, a state nursery school teacher who suffers from a particularly pure and severe prosopagnosia (Caldara *et al.*, 2005; Mayer *et al.*, 1999; Rossion *et al.*, 2003a; Schiltz *et al.*, 2005). For example, this patient did not recognize her daughter or her husband out of context when they kept silent. The revalidation strategy was based on the patient's spontaneous descriptions of known persons. We noted that the patient face's descriptions were based on the hair (length, color, presence of a fringe) and the global form of the face (round, lengthened, oval) as well as on visually derived semantic representations ("she looks Portuguese"). She never described the eyes, the nose, or the mouth. We made the hypothesis that the patient presented a deficit in the processing of the internal features of faces, as confirmed later (Caldara *et al.*, 2005). The processing of internal features, in particular the eyes, is essential to recognize familiar faces (Ellis *et al.*, 1979), and increases with face familiarity (O'Donnell and Bruce, 2001). Therefore we chose to train PS in the processing of internal traits. Rehabilitation was four months long with two sessions per week. First we established with the patient a list of terms related to faces features (for example, almond eyes, turned-up nose, shaggy eyebrows). Then we trained PS to analyze the internal features of faces (the nose, the mouth, eyes and eyebrows). Three types of face with increasing difficulty were presented: (1) personality caricature, (2) unknown faces of adults, and (3) unknown faces of children. Two tasks were proposed: first, PS had to sort face pictures by means of a given criterion (for example, the length of the mouth); then PS had to describe the internal features of face photographs. Finally, the last sessions were devoted to establishing a description in a card index of the prominent features of all the children in PS' class. PS had to fill those cards herself. Then, the descriptions were presented to the therapist, and sometimes modified after discussion. The card had to be learned by heart by PS, who should have been able to give one·or more prominent features when a child's name was given.

Two measures were employed in order to evaluate the rehabilitation efficacy:

1. The first consisted in testing the effective improvement of PS in the recognition of her class children from certain features (internal versus external) by comparing her scores to those of a colleague.

2. The second was a questionnaire based on subjective changes in the manner of processing faces (for more details see Mayer *et al.*, 1999).

Results showed that the improvement of PS was significantly better in the recognition of faces composed of internal features than in recognition of faces composed of external features. Moreover, the questionnaire showed a subjective improvement in the item concerning the identification of children with a hat, which indicate that PS was less impaired than before when she could not use the hair for identification. Among the cues spontaneously used for child identification, we noticed the apparition of the mouth and the eyes, even if the hair and the face outline remained the main cues used by PS. The consequences of PS' improvement in analyzing faces were important: before training, she could not go outside the school alone with her pupils; after training, she felt sufficiently secure to stay alone outside with the pupils. New training strategies may be developed based on the findings that PS, as well as other prosopagnosics, can use the mouth area to recognize faces, but is markedly impaired at the level of the eyes (Caldara *et al.*, 2005).

In conclusion, rehabilitation does not treat prosopagnosia — that is, it does not restore the possibility of recovering the familiarity of a known face. Nevertheless, it can diminish the consequences of such deficits in everyday life.

Key points Management and treatment

Spontaneous recovery: unusual

Revalidation:

– in selected patients

– strategy adapted to the deficit (internal features . . .)

– decrease the consequences of prosopagnosia in everyday life

This aim corresponds to the recent approach of neuropsychological rehabilitation, as described by Barbara Wilson for example:

The main purposes of neuropsychological rehabilitation are to enable people with disabilities to achieve their optimum level of well being, to reduce the impact of their problems on everyday life and to help them return to their most appropriate environments. (Wilson, 2003, p. 1)

REFERENCES

Agniel, A., Joanette, Y., Doyon, B. and Duchein, C. (1992). *Protocole Montréal-Toulouse, Évaluation des Gnosies Visuelles et Auditives.* Isbergues: L'ortho édition.

Assal, G., Favre, C. and Anderes, J. (1984). Nonrecognition of familiar animals by a farmer: Zooagnosia or prosopagnosia for animals. *Rev. Neurol.*, **140**, 580–4.

Barton, J. (2003). Disorders of face perception and recognition. *Neurol. Clin.*, **21**(2), 521–48.

Barton, J.J., Cherkasova, M.V., Press, D.Z., Intriligator, J.M. and O'Connor, M. (2004). Perceptual functions in prosopagnosia. *Perception*, **33**(8), 939–56.

Barton, J.J., Press, D.Z., Keenan, J.P. and O'Connor, M. (2002). Lesions of the fusiform face area impair perception of facial configuration in prosopagnosia. *Neurology*, **58**, 71–8.

Behrmann, M. and Moscovitch, M. (2001). Face recognition: Evidence from intact and impaired performance. In *Handbook of Neuropsychology*, Vol. 4, ed. F. Boller and J. Grafman Amsterdam: Elsevier, pp. 181–206.

Benton, A.L. (1986). Reaction time and brain disease: Some reflections. *Cortex*, **22**, 129–40.

Benton, A.L., Sivan, A.B., Hamsher, K., Varney, N.R. and Spreen, O. (1983). *Contributions to Neuropsychological Assessment: A Clinical Manual.* New York: Oxford University Press.

Beyn, E.S. and Knyazeva, G.R. (1962). The problem of prosopagnosia. *J. Neurol. Neurosurg. Psychiatry*, **25**, 154–8.

Bodamer, J. (1947). Die Prosop-Agnosie (Die Agnosie des Physiognomieerkennens). *Arch. Psychiatr. Nervenkr.*, **179**, 6–54. English translation by Ellis, H.D. and Florence, M. (1990). *Cogn. Neuropsychol.*, **7**, 81–105.

Boutsen, L. and Humphreys, G.W. (2003). The effect of inversion on the encoding of normal and "thatcherized" faces. *Q. J. Exp. Psychol.*, **56**(6), 955–75.

Bouvier, S. E. and Engel, S. A. (2006). Behavioral deficits and cortical damage loci in cerebral achromatopsia. *Cerebral Cortex*, **16**, 183–91.

Brandt, T., Steinke, W., Thie, A., Pessin, M. S. and Caplan, L. R. (2000). Posterior cerebral artery territory infarcts: Clinical features, infarct topography, causes and outcome. Multicenter results and a review of the literature. *Cerebrovasc. Dis.*, **10**, 172–82.

Bruyer, R., Laterre, C., Seron, X., *et al.* (1983). A case of prosopagnosia with some preserved covert remembrance of familiar faces. *Brain Cogn.*, **2**, 257–84.

Bukach, C. M., Bub, D. M., Gauthier, I. and Tarr, M. J. (2006). Perceptual expertise effects are not all or none: Local perceptual expertise for faces in a case of prosopagnosia. *J. Cogn. Neurosci.*, **18**, 48–63.

Buser, P. and Imbert, M. (1987). *Vision*. Paris: Hermann.

Caldara, R., Schyns, P., Mayer, E., *et al.* (2005). Does prosopagnosia take the eyes out from faces? Evidence for a defect in the use of diagnostic facial information in a brain-damaged patient. *J. Cogn. Neurosci.*, **17**, 1652–66.

Cals, N., Devuyst, G., Afsar, N., Karapanayiotides, T. and Bogousslavsky, J. (2002). Pure superficial posterior cerebral artery territory infarction in the Lausanne stroke registry. *J. Neurol.*, **249**, 855–61.

Cavanagh, P. (1992). Attention-based motion perception. *Science*, **257**, 1563–5.

Charcot, J. M. (1883). Un cas de suppression brusque et isolée de la vision mentale des signes et des objets (formes et couleurs). *Progr. Med.*, **11**, 568–71.

Clarke, S., Lindemann, A., Maeder, P., Borruat, F. X. and Assal, G. (1997). Face recognition and postero-inferior hemispheric lesions. *Neuropsychologia*, **35**, 1555–63.

Damasio, H. and Damasio, A. R. (1989). *Lesion Analysis in Neuropsychology*. New York: Oxford University Press.

Damasio, A. R., Damasio, H. and Van Hoesen, G. W. (1982). Prosopagnosia: Anatomic basis and behavioural mechanisms. *Neurology*, **32**, 331–41.

Damasio, A. R., Tranel, D. and Damasio, H. (1990). Face agnosia and the neural substrates of memory. *Ann. Rev. Neurosci.*, **13**, 89–109.

Davidoff, J. and Landis, T. (1990). Recognition of unfamiliar faces in prosopagnosia. *Neuropsychologia*, **28**(11), 1143–61.

De Renzi, E. (1986). Current issues on prosopagnosia. In *Aspects of Face Processing*, ed. H. D. Ellis, M. A. Jeeves, F. G. Newcombe and A. Young. Dordrecht: Martinus Nijhoff, pp. 243–52.

De Renzi, E., Faglioni, P., Grossi, D. and Nichelli, P. (1991). Apperceptive and associative forms of prosopagnosia. *Cortex*, **27**, 213–21.

De Renzi, E., Perani, D., Carlesimo, G. A., Silveri, M. C. and Fazio, F. (1994). Prosopagnosia can be associated with damage confined to the right hemisphere – an MRI and PET study and a review of the literature. *Neuropsychologia*, **8**, 893–902.

Delvenne, J. F., Seron, X., Coyette, F. and Rossion, B. (2004). Do perceptual deficits always co-occur with visual (prosop)agnosia? Evidence from neuropsychological investigation in a single-case study. *Neuropsychologia*, **42**, 597–612.

Duchaine, B. and Weidenfeld, A. (2003). An evaluation of two commonly used tests of unfamiliar face recognition. *Neuropsychologia*, **41**, 713–20.

Ellis, H. D., Shepherd, J. W. and Davies, G. M. (1979). Identification of familiar and unfamiliar faces from internal and external features: Some implications for theories of face recognition. *Perception*, **8**, 431–9.

Ellis, H. D. and Young, A. W. (1988). Training in face-processing skills for a child with acquired prosopagnosia. *Develop. Neuropsychol.*, **4**, 283–94.

Ettlin, T. M., Beckson, M., Benson, D. F., *et al.* (1992). Prosopagnosia: A bihemispheric disorder. *Cortex*, **28**, 129–34.

Evans, J. J., Heggs, A. J., Antoun, N. and Hodges, J. R. (1995). Progressive prosopagnosia with associated selective right temporal lobe atrophy: A new syndrome? *Brain*, **118**, 1–13.

Farah, M. J. (1990). *Visual Agnosia*. Cambridge: MIT Press.

Farah, M., Levinson, K. L. and Klein, K. L. (1995). Face perception and within-category discrimination in prosopagnosia. *Neuropsychologia*, **33**, 661–74.

Gauthier, I., Behrmann, M. and Tarr, M. J. (1999). Is prosopagnosia a general deficit in subordinate-level categorization? *J. Cogn. Neurosci.*, **11**, 349–70.

Ginsburg, A. P. (2003). Contrast sensitivity and functional vision. *Int. Ophthalmol. Clin.*, **43**, 5–15.

Glowic, C. and Violon, A. (1981). Un cas de prosopagnosie régressive. *Acta Neurol. Belgica.*, **81**, 86–97.

Goldsmith, Z. G. and Liu, G. T. (2001). Facial recognition and prosopagnosia: Past and present concepts. *Neuro-Ophthal.*, **25**, 177–92.

Grüsser, O. J. and Landis, T. (1991). Faces lost: Prosopagnosia. In *Visual Agnosias and Other Disturbances of Visual Perception and Cognition: Vision and Visual Dysfunction*, Vol. 12, Amsterdam: MacMillan, pp. 259–86.

Habib, M. and Sirigu, A. (1987). Pure topographical disorientation: A definition and anatomical basis. *Cortex*, **23**, 73–85.

Haxby, J. V., Hoffman, E. A. and Gobbini, M. I. (2000). The distributed human neural system for face perception. *Trends Cogn. Sci.*, **4**, 223–33.

Hécaen, H. and Angelergues, R. (1962). Agnosia for faces (prosopagnosia). *Arch. Neurol.*, **7**, 92–100.

(1963). *La Cécité Psychique*, Paris: Masson.

Henke, K., Schweinberger, S. R., Grigo, A., Klos, T. and Sommer, W. (1998). Specificity of face recognition: Recognition of exemplars of non-face objects in prosopagnosia. *Cortex*, **34**, 289–96.

Hillger, L. A. and Koenig, O. (1991). Separable mechanisms in face processing: Evidence from hemispheric specialization. *J. Cogn. Neurosci.*, **3**, 42–58.

Hoff, H. and Pötzl, O. (1937). Über eine optisch-agnostische Störung des "Physiognomie-Gedächtnisses". *Z. Ges. Neurol. Psychiat.*, **159**, 367–95.

Joubert, S., Felician, O., Barbeau, E., *et al.* (2003). Impaired configurational processing in a case of progressive prosopagnosia associated with predominant right temporal lobe atrophy. *Brain*, **126**, 2537–50.

Kanwisher, N., McDermott, J. and Chun, M. (1997). The fusiform face area: A module in human extrastriate cortex specialized for face perception. *J. Neurosci.*, **1711**, 4302–11.

Kumral, E., Bayulkem, G., Ataç, C. and Alper, Y. (2004). Spectrum of superficial posterior cerebral artery territory infarcts: Clinical and outcome correlates. *Eur. Neurol.*, **11**, 237–46.

Laeng, B. and Caviness, V. S. (2001). Prosopagnosia as a deficit in encoding curved surface. *J. Cogn. Neurosci.*, **13**, 556–76.

Landis, T. (2004). Désorientation topographique. In *Neuro-ophtalmologie*, ed. A. B. Safran, A. Vighetto, T. Landis and E. A. Cabanis. Paris: Masson, pp. 130–4.

Landis, T., Regard, M., Bliestle, A. and Kleihues, P. (1988). Prosopagnosia and agnosia for non-canonical views: An autopsied case. *Brain*, **111**, 1287–97.

Leveroni, C. L., Seidenberg, M., Mayer, A. R., *et al.* (2000). Neural systems underlying the recognition of familiar and newly learned faces. *J. Neurosci.*, **20**, 878–86.

Marotta, J. J., Genovese, C. R. and Behrmann, M. (2001). A functional MRI study of face recognition in patients with prosopagnosia. *Neuroreport*, **13**, 1581–7.

Marotta, J. J., McKeeff, T. J. and Behrmann, M. (2002). The effects of rotation and inversion on face processing in prosopagnosia. *Cogn. Neuropsychol.*, **19**, 31–47.

Mattson, A. J., Levin, H. S. and Grafman, J. (2000). A case of prosopagnosia following moderate closed head injury with left hemisphere focal lesion. *Cortex*, **36**, 125–37.

Maurer, D., Le Grand, R. and Mondloch, C. J. (2002). The many faces of configural processing. *Trends Cogn. Sci.*, **6**, 255–60.

Mayer, E., Fistarol, P. and Valenza, N. (1999). Prise en charge neuropsychologique d'une patiente prosopagnosique. In *La Rééducation en Neuropsychologie: Études de Cas*, ed. P. Azouvi, D. Perrier and M. Van der Linden. Marseille: Solal.

McNeil, J. E. and Warrington, E. K. (1993). Prosopagnosia: A face specific disorder. *Q. J. Exp. Psychol.*, **46A**, 1–10.

Meadows, J. C. (1974). The anatomical basis of prosopagnosia. *J. Neurol. Neurosurg. Psychiatry*, **37**, 489–501.

Michel, F., Poncet, M. and Signoret, J. L. (1989). Les lésions responsables de la prosopagnosie sont-elles toujours bilatérales? *Rev. Neurol.*, **145**, 764–70.

Milandre, L., Brosset, C., Botti, G. and Khalil, R. (1994). Etude de 82 infarctus du territoire des artères cérébrales postérieures. *Rev. Neurol.*, **150**, 133–41.

Nadler, M. P., Miller, D. and Nadler, D. J. (1990). *Glare and Contrast Sensitivity for Clinicians*, New York: Springer-Verlag.

O'Donnell, C. and Bruce, V. (2001). Familiarisation with faces selectively enhances sensitivity to changes made to the eyes. *Perception*, **30**, 755–64.

Pessin, M. S., Lathi, E. S., Cohen, M. B., *et al.* (1987). Clinical features and mechanism of occipital infarction. *Ann. Neurol.*, **21**, 290–9.

Polster, M. R. and Rapcsak, S. Z. (1996). Representations in learning new faces: Evidence from prosopagnosia. *J. Int. Neuropsych. Soc.*, **2**, 240–8.

Quaglino, A. and Borelli, G. (1867). Emiplegia sinistra con amaurosi – guarigione – perdita totale della percezione dei colori e della memoria della configurazione degli oggetti. *Giornale d'Oftalmologia Italiano*, **10**, 106–17.

Riddoch, M. J. and Humphreys, G. W. (1993). Birmingham object recognition battery. Hillsdale: Lawrence Erlbaum Associates.

Rizzo, M., Corbett, J. J., Thompson, H. S. and Damasio, A. R. (1986). Spatial contrast sensitivity in facial recognition. *Neurology*, **36**, 1254–6.

Rossion, B., Caldara, R., Seghier, M., *et al.* (2003a). A network of occipito-temporal face-sensitive areas besides the right middle fusiform gyrus is necessary for normal face processing. *Brain*, **126**, 2381–95.

Rossion, B., de Gelder, B., Dricot, L., *et al.* (2000). Hemispheric asymmetries for whole-based and parts-based face processing in the human fusiform gyrus. *J. Cogn. Neurosci.*, **12**, 793–802.

Rossion, B., Joyce, C., Cottrell, G. W. and Tarr, M. J. (2003b). Early lateralization and orientation tuning for face, word and object processing in the visual cortex. *Neuroimage*, **20**, 1609–24.

Rossion, B. and Pourtois, G. (2004). Revisiting Snodgrass and Vanderwart's object pictorial set: The role of surface detail in basic-level object recognition. *Perception*, **33**(2), 217–36.

Rossion, B., Schiltz, C., Robaye, L., Pirenne, D. and Crommelinck, M. (2001). How does the brain discriminate familiar and unfamiliar faces: A PET study of face categorical perception. *J. Cogn. Neurosci.*, **13**, 1019–34.

Schiltz, C., Sorger, B., Caldara, R., *et al.* (2006). Anomalous response to facial identity in the right middle fusiform gyrus underlies impaired face identification in acquired prosopagnosia. *Cerebral Cortex*, **16**, 574–86.

Schweich, M. and Bruyer, R. (1993). Heterogeneity in the cognitive manifestations of prosopagnosia: The study of a group of single cases. *Cogn. Neuropsych.*, **10**, 529–47.

Sergent, J., Otha, S. and MacDonald, B. (1992). Functional neuroanatomy of face and object processing. A positron emission tomography study. *Brain*, **115**, 15–36.

Sergent, J. and Signoret, J. L. (1992). Varieties of functional deficits in prosopagnosia. *Cerebral Cortex*, **2**, 375–88.

Sergent, J. and Villemure, J. G. (1989). Prosopagnosia in a right hemispherectomized patient. *Brain*, **112**, 975–95.

Seron, X., Mataigne, F., Coyette, F., *et al.* (1995). Etude d'un cas de métamorphopsie limitée aux visages et à certains objets familiers. *Rev. Neurol.*, **151**, 691–8.

Snodgrass, J. G. and Vanderwart, M. (1980). A standardized set of 260 pictures: Norms for name agreement, image agreement, familiarity, and visual complexity. *J. Exp. Psycho. [Learn. Mem. Cogn.]*, **6**, 174–215.

Spreen, O. and Strauss, E. (1998). *A Compendium of Neuropsychological Tests*, 2nd edn. New York, Oxford: Oxford University Press.

Tranel, D., Damasio, A. R. and Damasio, H. (1988). Intact recognition of facial expression, gender, and age in patients with impaired recognition of face identity. *Neurology*, **38**, 690–6.

Uttner, I., Bliem, H. and Danek, A. (2002). Prosopagnosia after unilateral right cerebral infarction. *J. Neurol.*, **249**, 933–5.

Wada, Y. and Yamamoto, T. (2001). Selective impairment of facial recognition due to a haematoma to the right fusiform and lateral occipital region. *J. Neurol. Neurosurg. Psychiatry*, **71**, 254–7.

Warrington, E. K. (1984). *Recognition Memory Test*. Windsor: NFER-Nelson.

(1996). *The Camden Memory Tests: Manual*. Hove: Psychology Press.

Warrington, E. K. and James, M. (1991). *The Visual Object and Space Perception Battery.* Bury St Edmunds: Thames Valley Test Company.

Whitely, A. M. and Warrington, E. K. (1977). Prosopagnosia: A clinical, psychological, and anatomical study of three patients. *J. Neurol. Neurosurg. Psychiatry,* **40**, 395−403.

Wigan, A. L. (1844). *A New View of Insanity: The Duality of the Mind.* London: Longman.

Wilbrand, H. (1887). *Die Seelenblindheit als Herderscheinung und ihre Beziehungen zur homonymen Hemianopsie.* Wiesbaden: J. F. Bergmann.

(1892). Ein Fall von Seelenblindheit und Hemianopsie mit Sectionsbefund. *Dtsch. Z. Nervenheilk.,* **2**, 361−87.

Wilson, B. (2003). The theory and practice of neuropsychological rehabilitation: An overview. In *Neuropsychological Rehabilitation,* ed. B. Wilson. Lisse: Swets & Zeitlinger.

Yamamoto, Y., Georgiadis, A. L., Chang, H. M. and Caplan, L. R. (1999). Posterior cerebral artery territory infarcts in the New England Medical Center Posterior Circulation Registry. *Arch. Neurol.,* **56**, 824−32.

Zeki, S. M. (1990). A century of cerebral achromatopsia. *Brain,* **113**, 1721−77.

Zihl, J. and Cramon, D. von (1986). *Zerebrale Sehstörungen.* Kohlhammer: Stuttgart.

17

Object and color agnosia

Georg Goldenbergh

Krankenhaus München-Bogenhausen, Germany

The visual agnosias

For seeing persons vision is the major source of object recognition. Although agnosia can affect recognition by other sensory channels (see Chapter 18) the majority of research and clinical interest in object agnosia concerns visual agnosia, which is also the topic of this chapter.

The term *agnosia* characterizes absent recognition in spite of preserved perception. Clinical diagnosis of visual agnosia is based on a model of visual recognition which was developed at the turning from the nineteenth to the twentieth century (Liepmann, 1908; Lissauer, 1890) but still serves as the starting point for cognitive analyses of visual recognition (Humphreys and Riddoch, 1987; Marr, 1982). This model distinguishes two stages leading from visual perception to recognition. At the "apperceptive" stage, elements of primary visual perceptions, like contours, brightness, texture, and color, are integrated into a coherent structural representation of the object. At the following "associative" stage, the structural representation gains access to semantic memory where knowledge about non-visual properties of the object is stored. Activation of knowledge about the object is equivalent to recognition and a necessary prerequisite for retrieving its name. Agnosia is classified as apperceptive or associative according to which of these stages is affected. Although modern neurophysiology casts doubts on the clean distinction between subsequent stages of visual recognition, the syndromes of "apperceptive agnosia" and "associative agnosia" have proven to correspond to salient and distinguishable clinical syndromes.

A further root of modern concepts of visual agnosia was the proposal that visual representations of objects may become disconnected from mental representations of their names, resulting in a selective disturbance of naming from vision, termed "optic aphasia" (Freund, 1889). This syndrome has also proven to correspond with clinical reality but is probably identical with one form of associative agnosia (see later).

Another tradition classifies agnosias according to the class of entities affected. Writing, colors, and faces have peculiarities which distinguish their disturbed recognition from object agnosia. Failure to recognize letters and words (alexia) and failure to recognize faces (prosopagnosia) are discussed elsewhere in this book, but this chapter will discuss disorders of color recognition in addition to object agnosia.

Object agnosia

The leading symptom of visual object agnosia is misnaming of visually presented objects contrasting with intact or at least much better retrieval of names in other situations. The differential diagnosis between agnosia and "elementary" visual perceptual disorders like visual field defects with insufficient visual exploration or diminution of visual acuity and contrast sensitivity may sometimes be difficult. The suspicion of "higher order" impairment is corroborated by dissociations between failure of recognition and preservation and other visually guided actions which put equal demands on visual exploration, visual fields, acuity, and contrast sensitivity. Both the kind of dissociations observed and the relationship between naming errors and properties of the visually presented object differ between the different variants of object agnosia.

Apperceptive agnosia

The patients' attempts at visual object naming reveal that they perceive single visual features but cannot combine them to a coherent image of the object. Depending on which features are perceived, two variants of apperceptive agnosia can be distinguished: patients with *form agnosia* perceive surface properties like brightness, color, or lustre, as well as movements, but no coherent contours. Patients with *integrative agnosia* perceive single contours but are not able to integrate them to a coherent structure of the whole object.

Form agnosia

This most severe form of visual agnosia is rare. It develops in recovery from initially complete cortical blindness (Adler, 1944; Benson and Greenberg, 1969; Gloning *et al.*, 1962; Goldenberg, 2002b; Landis *et al.*, 1982; Milner *et al.*, 1991). Patients cannot perceive coherent contours. When lines are curved or interrupted they loose their trace. Recognition of line drawings is virtually impossible, but perception of surface structure and color may eventually lead to recognition of real objects and photographs (Steeves *et al.*, 2004).

Severely disturbed perception of static forms may contrast with much better perception of the shape of movements. Letters or simple forms may be recognized when the movements of writing or drawing are observed (Benson and Greenberg, 1969; Goldenberg, 2002b; Landis *et al.*, 1982). Possibly the continuous movement unifies the parts of the shape and distinguishes the coherent shape from the background. A report of a patient who could fully compensate a severe form agnosia by exploratory movements of head or fingers, however, did not withstand a critical re-evaluation (Goldenberg, 2002a; Goldstein and Gelb, 1918).

Visual features like the orientation or length of contours which are inaccessible to conscious perception can be employed for visuomotor coordination. There is a report of a patient who performed at chance level when asked to indicate the orientation of a slit with a piece of cardboard held in her hand but who could insert the cardboard into the slit swiftly and accurately (Milner *et al.*, 1991). She was unable to indicate with her fingers the width of an object but could grasp that object with a perfectly adapted precision grip (Goodale *et al.*, 1994). Exploitation of visual information for visuomotor coordination was bound to actual grasping. When the patient was asked to demonstrate the grasp immediately after seeing the object or closely besides the visible object, the adaptation of grip width to the width of the object collapsed.

Integrative agnosia

Integrative agnosia may develop in recovery from agnosia (Adler, 1950) or may be a primary symptom of brain damage. It is more frequent than form agnosia and is sometimes referred to as "apperceptive agnosia" without further qualification.

Patients recognize single contours but cannot integrate local and global shapes to a coherent object. Their naming errors typically display visual similarity to either the global shape (e.g. clarinet: "telescope"; iron: "automobile") or single details (e.g. Swiss cheese: "dice") of the presented object. After description of several details they may eventually arrive at correctly guessing the object.

Real objects are more likely to be recognized than pictures. For pictures, success depends on the technique of pictorial representation: silhouettes and schematic line drawings are easier to recognize than line drawings rich in details, and colored images easier than monochrome ones. Unusual views of objects and line drawings representing complex three-dimensional structures are particularly difficult (Turnbull *et al.*, 2004).

Associative agnosia

In associative agnosia the integration of visual percepts to a coherent structural representation of the object is intact but fails to activate object-related knowledge in semantic memory. Consequently the object is not recognized and cannot be correctly named. Naming errors frequently show a semantic relationship to the target but need not be visually similar (e.g. airplane − "locomotive";

banana — "apple tree"). When patients attempt to name series of pictures, items from the same semantic field may continue to be produced in response to subsequent semantically unrelated pictures (Goldenberg and Karlbauer, 1998; Lhermitte and Beauvois, 1973; Poeck, 1984).

The relationship between naming errors and non-visual properties of visually presented objects proves that perceptual integration was sufficient to evoke in semantic memory some knowledge about the seen object. The source of errors is the selection of the correct entry in semantic memory and its distinction from other objects of the same semantic field. There are two possible causes for this failure: access from visual perception to semantic memory may be disconnected, or semantic memory may be impoverished. These two causes correspond to clinically and anatomically distinct variants of associative agnosia.

Associative agnosia from disconnection

Misnaming of visually presented objects contrasts with correct naming of the same objects when they are perceived by other sensory modalities, as for example by tactile exploration, by characteristic sounds, or by verbal definitions. Even for misnamed visually presented objects patients can frequently select the correct name when it is presented together with distracters which may include their own errors. Patients perform non-verbal tasks requiring access to semantic memory, like sorting objects according to categories, better than naming (though not faultless), and some patients are able to pantomime the use of visually presented tools in spite of misnaming them (Schnider *et al.*, 1994). A consistently observed peculiarity is better visual naming of actions than objects (Gainotti, 2004; Goldenberg and Karlbauer, 1998; Teixeira-Ferreira *et al.*, 1997).

This clinical constellation has been termed "associative agnosia" (Lissauer, 1890), "semantic access agnosia" (Riddoch and Humphreys, 1987), "optic aphasia" (Freund, 1889; Lhermitte and Beauvois, 1973), and "modality-specific misnaming" (De Renzi and Saetti, 1997; Goldenberg and Karlbauer, 1998). The divergence of names reflects divergent views on the pathogenesis of the syndrome. There is unanimity that it is due to disconnection but controversy as to where the flow of information from visual perception to semantic memory and language is interrupted. The competing theories emphasize different aspects of the clinical syndrome.

The designation "optic aphasia" emphasizes that the leading symptom is verbal misnaming, contrasting with better performance on tests tapping access to semantic memory non-verbally. Consequently disconnection is assumed to interrupt access from semantic memory to the lexicon. However, as semantic memory is generally believed to be a common stock of knowledge where information from all sensory modalities converges, it is difficult to conceive of a mechanism that hinders output from semantic memory to lexical retrieval only for information stemming from one sensory channel, vision.

The interpretation as "associative agnosia" or "semantic access agnosia" emphasizes that performance on non-verbal probes of access to semantic memory may be less error-prone than naming but is not perfect. Particularly when correct performance requires fine-grained distinctions within a semantic class, patients regularly come into difficulties. As naming does afford such fine-grained distinctions between an object and other objects of the same semantic class, misnaming is the most conspicuous manifestation of an incomplete disconnection between visual perception and semantics. However, if specification of the object in semantic memory is insufficient, patients should be unable to recognize the correct name when it is spoken to them, but they regularly are much better or even perfect on matching the heard name with the seen picture.

Apparently the interactions between consecutive stages of visual recognition and naming cannot satisfactorily be accounted for by a strictly sequential order of independent stages of visual, semantic, and linguistic processing. Connectionist models assuming neuronal interactions crossing the boundaries of consecutive stages are better able to account for the dynamics of recognition and naming than the traditional modular models (Goldenberg and Karlbauer, 1998; Plaut and Shallice, 1993; Sitton *et al.*, 2001).

Associative agnosia from loss of semantic knowledge

Associative agnosia can be one symptom of a widespread degradation of semantic memory. Because patients have lost their knowledge of objects, naming does not improve when objects are presented through other sensory modalities than vision or by verbal definitions, and patients do not recognize the correct name when it is spoken to them. Misnaming reflects the gradual degradation of semantic memory. Frequently the superordinate category is preserved, but all exemplars are given the name of one of its instances (e.g. all animals are designated as "cat" or "dog") or replaced by the designation of the category ("an animal").

Degradation of semantic memory can occur in diffuse brain damage which also encroaches upon the cortical areas responsible for perceptual integration. This may lead to a combination of apperceptive and associative agnosia where the frequency of semantic errors increases with increasing visual complexity of the stimulus (Done and Hajilou, 2004).

Achromatopsia and color agnosia

Similarly to the distinction between apperceptive and associative agnosia, disturbed recognition of colors can take two forms according to whether perceptual processing or access to knowledge is compromised. Defective perceptual processing is termed "achromatopsia," whereas the term "color agnosia" designates impaired recognition and naming of colors in spite of preserved perception.

Achromatopsia

Patients with achromatopsia complain that colors appear washed out and pale, or that they see the whole world only in shades of grey (Damasio *et al.*, 1980; Meadows, 1974; Zeki, 1990). Perception of shades of blue and green is usually affected most severely, whereas perception of red may be better preserved.

Similarly to the use of form information for visuomotor coordination in form agnosia, the visual system of patients with achromatopsia can exploit color information for other purposes than conscious perception of color. Patients can trace contours produced by boundaries between isoluminant but differentially colored areas although they do not perceive the difference between the colors (Cowey and Stoerig, 1991; Meadows, 1974), thus manifesting intact use of consciously inaccessible color information for the delimitation of contours.

Color agnosia

Patients with color agnosia do not notice any change of their color experience, but when asked to name colors they produce wrong color names. This visual misnaming contrasts with correct use of the same color names when they are required in a purely verbal context, as for example when patients are asked for the colors of hope, love, or grief, or for the ("red–green") coalition governing Germany at the beginning of the twenty-first century (Goldenberg, 1992; Lhermitte and Beauvois, 1973).

Key points Main characteristics of object and color visual agnosias

Visual agnosia: absent identification of visual stimuli in spite of preserved perception
1. Classified according to the class of entities affected:
– letters and words: alexia
– faces: prosopagnosia
– colors: central achromatopsia and color agnosia
– object: object agnosia
2. Classified according to the impaired stages:
– "apperceptive" stage: elements of primary perceptions (contours, brightness, texture, and color) are integrated into a coherent structural representation of the object
– "associative" stage: structural representation gains access to semantic memory (storage of knowledge about general, visual, and non-visual, properties of the object).

Main causes of visual agnosia

Form agnosia has been observed exclusively after cerebral anoxia or intoxication, and never after stroke. Associative agnosia from loss of semantic knowledge is a typical symptom of degenerative dementia. It may also result from encephalitis, particularly herpes simplex encephalitis, or head trauma. If the origin is vascular at all, it is part of vascular dementia from multiple lacunar lesions and raises a suspicion of accompanying degenerative cortical pathology (Jellinger, 2002). Integrative agnosia and achromatopsia may have many causes, including degenerative dementia (mainly for integrative agnosia), cerebral anoxia, and head trauma, but can also result from stroke. The disconnection variant of associative agnosia and color agnosia are most frequently caused by stroke, although there are single cases with other etiologies.

Strokes responsible for visual agnosia

Visual agnosia is not reported frequently in stroke patients; it concerns mainly patients suffering from an infarct in the territory of the posterior cerebral arteries (PCA). The responsible regions are located anterior of the primary visual cortex in the fusiform and lingual gyrus. Because of the vascular anatomy of the PCA, infarctions of these areas frequently encroach upon the calcarine cortex and cause visual field defects. It may be difficult to disentangle the symptoms of agnosia from the sequel of visual field restriction. In a study of pure superficial PCA infarct, visual agnosia was reported in 9% of patients, proposopagnosia in 6%, and color anomia in 5% (Cals *et al.*, 2002). This contrasts with the high frequency of visual field defects observed in about 90% of patients (Cals *et al.*, 2002).

Bilateral lesions are necessary for causing integrative agnosia, but extension in the right hemisphere is frequently more marked than in the left. If the right-sided lesion is large, left hemineglect and insufficient visual exploration may further complicate the differential diagnosis between "elementary" and higher order perceptual disturbances. Complete achromatopsia also affords bilateral lesions but there are rare observations of hemi-achromatopsia following a unilateral lesion (Meadows, 1974)

The disconnection form of associative agnosia and color agnosia are symptoms of left PCA infarction. Lesions causing these syndromes destroy the left calcarine cortex and encroach upon the splenium corporis callosi. This anatomical constellation accords well with the interpretation of the syndromes as being caused by disconnection. Destruction of primary visual cortex and subsequent right hemianopia deprive the left hemisphere of direct input from vision, and the splenial lesion makes transmission of visual information from the "seeing" right to the "blind" left hemisphere incomplete and error prone. Arguably the symptoms reflect either the attempts of the left hemisphere to derive meaning from the degraded visual information or the attempts of the right hemisphere to fulfill functions which normally are a domain of left hemisphere competence.

Visual agnosia may be observed, albeit rarely, following an occipito-temporal hemorrhage. Finally, complex visual disturbances are classical consequences of cerebral venous thrombosis but persisting visual agnosia seems to be rare in this pathology.

Key points Main types of stroke associated with object and color agnosia

Stroke type	Territory/characteristics
Arterial Infarct	posterior cerebral artery
Hemorrhage	Occipito-temporal region

Clinical assessment

Clinical assessment aims at delimitating the modality-specific visual nature of impaired recognition and at determining the stage of visual or semantic processing that is disturbed. These analyses may transgress the facilities and competence of neurologists working in acute clinical care. Their starting point, however, is the qualitative analysis of errors made in the clinical examination of visual picture and object naming.

Error analysis

Basically, error analysis searches for communalities between the correct designation of the visual stimulus and the wrong name or the description given by the patient. Visual errors have visual similarity with the presented stimulus but need not belong to the same semantic class nor have any other semantic or associative relationship to it. By contrast, semantic errors belong to the same superordinate category or have other semantic and associative links to the target but need not share visual features with it.

Fine-grained analysis of visual errors can help to differentiate integrative agnosia from sequel of visual field restriction. Restriction of visual fields as sole cause of errors becomes less likely when some of the errors resemble the global shape of the visually presented object rather than only small details.

Non-visual object recognition

Recognition of objects from modalities other than seeing can be examined by letting the patient tactually explore the real object, by presenting characteristic sounds made by the object (e.g. barking, pouring water, sound of automobile engine) or by giving verbal definitions of the object (e.g. a four-legged animal which is man's loyal companion and barks). Impaired non-visual naming points to a general degradation of semantic memory.

Copying and drawing from memory

Copying of a line drawing is frequently used for assessing the apperceptive stage of object recognition. A correct copy in spite of absent recognition has been taken as evidence for intact perceptual processing, but a correct copy can be achieved by joining together single details and need not indicate successful integration of these details into a coherent structure. On the other hand, visuo-constructional disorders can severely impair copying without having an impact on recognition and naming of the copied object. Copying nonetheless does provide valuable insight into perceptual processing but needs to be evaluated with caution and expertise.

Drawing objects from memory affords retrieval from semantic memory of a mental image of the object's visual appearance. In the disconnection form of associative agnosia, intact drawing from memory of unrecognized objects impressively demonstrates the preservation of semantic knowledge. The reverse conclusion that deficient drawing testifies to loss of semantic memory as being the source of deficient visual recognition is less straightforward. Impoverished drawing from memory has been observed in patients who have no problems with visual recognition at all (Gainotti *et al.*, 1983; Goldenberg, 1992; Goldenberg *et al.*, 2003).

Matching tests

Matching tests are the most important instruments for delimitating the stage of visual and semantic processing that is disturbed. Patients are presented an array of pictures and asked to select the one matching a target picture.

Matching of identical pictures can be achieved by a piecemeal comparison of local shapes. Patients with form agnosia fail but those with integrative agnosia may succeed. Matching of different views of the same object or of different exemplars of one class of object (e.g. different hats or dogs) requires recognition of the coherent structure of the whole object and appreciation of its characteristic features. Patients with integrative agnosia fail but those with associative agnosia succeed. Finally, matching by non-visual properties or associations (e.g. deciding whether an ostrich or a hen match the picture of an egg in an egg-cup) affords access to semantic memory and hence gives rise to errors in associative agnosia.

A somewhat problematic variant of matching by non-visual properties is matching by superordinate category (e.g. sorting pictures depicting tools or animals), because the exemplars of a category tend to be visually similar. Success on this task hence does not suffice for proving intact access to semantic memory, and a discrepancy between successful matching and impaired naming of the same items does not necessarily indicate that the disorder affects naming rather than access to semantic memory (De Renzi and Saetti, 1997).

Perception and categorization of colors

Perceptual discrimination of color is probed by presenting pairs of color batches which are either completely the same or have equal lightness but differ slightly in hue, and asking the patients to judge whether or not they are the same. Alternatively they can be asked to sort an array of color batches in such a way as to maximize the similarity between adjacent batches.

Access from color perception to color knowledge is probed by sorting of colored tokens (e.g. small balls of colored wools) into basic color categories (red, orange, yellow, green, etc.). Normal persons sort the colors without hesitation. Patients with color agnosia commit errors and their correct sorts are worked out in a laborious way: they compare each new specimen to each heap and select the one where the perceptual distance is smallest. This strategy leads to error when perceptual distance comes in conflict with color category. For example, a light green is perceptually more similar to yellow than to a dark green.

Key points Assessment of object and color agnosia

Clinical examination
Identification of objects and images presented in visual and non-visual modality
Copying and drawing from memory
Relatively spared copying as compared to identification impairment suggests associative agnosia
Neuropsychological tests

Prognosis and management

Some patients can cope astonishingly well with their object recognition disorder in daily life (Sparr *et al.*, 1991; Wilson and Davidoff, 1993). One reason may be that object agnosia affects object recognition but neither grasping objects nor the avoidance of obstacles. Another reason may be that patients learn to exploit the dissociations between defective and preserved visual functions and develop compensatory strategies based on the preserved aspect of object recognition.

Key points Management and treatment of visual agnosia

Rehabilitation
Used in selected patients
Controlled trials required

Therapeutic interventions must be tailored to the specific deficits and resources of the individual patient. Therapist and patient cooperate in the search for strategies to circumvent the disturbed stage of visual processing. Once found, strategies have to be extensively practiced in order to be readily available in daily life. Another important aspect of therapy is to help the patient to understand the bizarre symptoms and to develop ways for explaining the condition to relatives, friends, and strangers. Agnosia may lead to socially embarrassing situations, and patients who do not know how to handle these situations may end up with social retreat. For example, prosopagnosic patients fail to recognize – and hence also to greet – friends when they meet them unexpectedly on the street. Patients with object agnosia may be regarded as preposterous when they ask for help from other persons – e.g. for selecting an item in the supermarket – and explain that they have a problem with seeing but are then observed to navigate obstacles and grasp for objects like a normally sighted person.

An aspect of the apperceptive variants of object and color agnosia that is hard to measure but may contribute substantially to the patients' suffering is loss or change of aesthetic experience. Even if patients learn to recognize objects or colors they do not recover the normal experience of seeing (Sacks, 1995).

REFERENCES

Adler, A. (1944). Disintegration and restoration of optic recognition in visual agnosia. Analysis of a case. *Arch. Neurol.*, **51**, 243–59.

(1950). Course and outcome of visual agnosia. *J. Nerv. Ment. Dis.*, **111**, 41–51.

Benson, D. F. and Greenberg, J. P. (1969). Visual form agnosia – a specific defect in visual discrimination. *Arch. Neurol.*, **20**, 82–9.

Cals, N., Devuyst, G., Afsar, N., Karapanayiotides, T., and Bogousslavsky, J. (2002). Pure superficial posterior cerebral artery territory infarction in The Lausanne Stroke Registry. *J. Neurol.*, **249**, 855–61.

Cowey, A. and Stoerig, P. (1991). The neurobiology of blindsight. *Trends Neurosci.*, **14**, 140–5.

Damasio, A. R., Yamada, T., Damasio, H., Corbett, J. and McKee, J. (1980). Central achromatopsia: Behavioral, anatomic, and physiologic aspects. *Neurology*, **30**, 1064–71.

De Renzi, E. and Saetti, M. C. (1997). Associative agnosia and optic aphasia: Qualitative or quantitative difference? *Cortex*, **33**, 115–30.

Done, D. J. and Hajilou, B. B. (2004). Loss of high-level perceptual knowledge of object structure in DAT. *Neuropsychologia*, **43**, 60−8.

Freund, C. S. (1889). Ueber optische Aphasie und Seelenblindheit. *Archiv für Psychiatrie und Nervenkrankheiten*, **20**, 276−97, 371−416.

Gainotti, G. (2004). A metanalysis of impaired and spared naming for different categories of knowledge in patients with a visuo-verbal disconnection. *Neuropsychologia*, **42**, 299−319.

Gainotti, G., Silveri, M. C., Villa, G. and Caltagirone, C. (1983). Drawing objects from memory in aphasia. *Brain*, **106**, 613−22.

Gloning, K., Hoff, H. and Tschabitscher, H. (1962). Die Rückbildung der kortikalen Blindheit. *Wiener Klinische Wochenschrift*, **74**, 406−7.

Goldenberg, G. (1992). Loss of visual imagery and loss of visual knowledge − a case study, *Neuropsychologia*, **30**, 1081−99.

(2002a). Goldstein and Gelb's case Schn. − a classic case in neuropsychology? In *Classic Cases in Neuropsychology, Vol.* 2, ed. C. Code *et al.* Hove: Psychology Press, pp. 281−99.

(2002b). *Neuropsychologie - Grundlagen, Klinik, Rehabilitation*, 3. Auflage Urban and Fischer, München.

Goldenberg, G., Hartmann, K. and Schlott, I. (2003). Defective pantomime of object use in left brain damage: Apraxia or asymbolia? *Neuropsychologia*, **41**, 1565−73.

Goldenberg, G. and Karlbauer, F. (1998). The more you know the less you can tell: Inhibitory effects of visuo-semantic activation on modality specific visual misnaming, *Cortex*, **34**, 471−92.

Goldstein, K. and Gelb, A. (1918). Psychologische Analysen hirnpathologischer Fälle auf Grund von Untersuchungen Hirnverletzter − I. Abhandlung. Zur Psychologie des optischen Wahrnehmungs- und Erkennungsvorganges. *Zeitschrift für die gesamte Neurologie und Psychiatrie*, **41**, 1−142.

Goodale, M. A., Jakobson, L. S., Milner, A. D., *et al.* (1994). The nature and limits of orientation and pattern processing supporting visuomotor control in a visual form agnosic. *J. Cogn. Neurosci.*, **6**, 46−56.

Humphreys, G. W. and Riddoch, M. J. (1987). The fractionation of visual agnosia. In *Visual Object Processing: A Cognitive Neuropsychological Approach*, ed. G. W. Humphreys and M. J. Riddoch. Hove London Hillsdale: Lawrence Erlbaum, pp. 281−306.

Jellinger, K. A. (2002). Alzheimer disease and cerebrovascular pathology: An update. *J. Neural Transm.*, **109**, 813−36.

Landis, T., Graves, R., Benson, D. F. and Hebben, N. (1982). Visual recognition through kinaesthetic mediation. *Psychol. Med.*, **12**, 515−31.

Lhermitte, F. and Beauvois, M. F. (1973). A visual-speech disconnection syndrome. Report of a case with optic aphasia, agnosic alexia and colour agnosia. *Brain*, **96**, 695−714.

Liepmann, H. (1908). Ueber die agnostischen Stoerungen, *Neurologisches Centralblatt*, **27**, 609−17, 664−75.

Lissauer, H. (1890). Ein Fall von Seelenblindheit nebst einem Beitrag zur Theorie derselben. *Archiv für Psychiatrie und Nervenkrankheiten*, **21**, 222−70.

Marr, D. (1982). *Vision: A Computational Investigation into the Human Representation and Processing of Visual Information*, San Francisco: W. H. Freeman and Co.

Meadows, J. C. (1974). Disturbed perception of colours associated with localized cerebral lesions. *Brain*, **97**, 615–32.

Milner, A. D., Perrett, D. I., Johnston, R. S., *et al.* (1991). Perception and action in 'visual form agnosia'. *Brain*, **114**, 405–28.

Plaut, D. C. and Shallice, T. (1993). Perseverative and semantic influences on visual object naming errors in optic aphasia: A connectionist account. *J. Cogn. Neurosci.*, **5**, 89–117.

Poeck, K. (1984). Neuropsychological demonstration of splenial interhemispheric disconnection in a case of 'optic anomia'. *Neuropsychologia*, **22**, 707–14.

Riddoch, M. J. and Humphreys, G. W. (1987). Visual object processing in optic aphasia: A case of semantic access agnosia. *Cogn. Neuropsychol.*, **4**, 131–85.

Sacks, O. (1995). The case of the colorblind painter. In *An Anthropologist on Mars*. New York: Vintage Books, pp. 3–41.

Schnider, A., Benson, D. F. and Scharre, D. W. (1994). Visual agnosia and optic aphasia: Are they anatomically distinct? *Cortex*, **30**, 445–58.

Sitton, M., Mozer, M. C. and Farah, M. J. (2001). Superadditive effects of multiple lesions in a connectionist architecture: Implications for the neuropsychology of optic aphasia. *Psychol. Rev.*, **107**, 709–34.

Sparr, S. A., Jay, M., Drislane, F. W. and Venna, N. (1991). A historical case of visual agnosia revisited after 40 years. *Brain*, **114**, 789–800.

Steeves, J. K. E., Humphrey, G. K., Culham, J. C., *et al.* (2004). Behavioral and neuroimaging evidence for a contribution of color and texture information to scene classification in a patient with visual form agnosia. *J. Cogn. Neurosci.*, **16**, 955–65.

Teixeira-Ferreira, C., Giusiano, B., Ceccaldi, M. and Poncet, M. (1997). Optic aphasia: Evidence of the contribution of different neural systems to object and action naming. *Cortex*, **33**, 499–514.

Turnbull, O. H., Driver, J. and McCarthy, R. (2004). 2D but not 3D: Pictorial-depth deficits in a case of visual agnosia. *Cortex*, **40**, 723–38.

Wilson, B. A. and Davidoff, J. (1993). Partial recovery from visual object agnosia: A 10 year follow-up study. *Cortex*, **29**, 529–42.

Zeki, S. (1990). A century of cerebral achromatopsia. *Brain*, **113**, 1721–77.

18

Auditory disorders related to strokes

Bernard Lechevalier,[1] Jany Lambert,[1,2] Sylvain Moreau,[3]
Hervé Platel,[2,4] and Fausto Viader,[1,2]

[1]Service de Neurologie, CHU de Caen
[2]Inserm E.0218
[3]Service d'ORL, CHU de Caen
[4]Université de Caen

Introduction

Following strokes, disorders of auditory perception produced by lesions located in the territory of the internal carotid artery or of the vertebrobasilar system can be observed. These disorders were gathered in several different clinical forms, now conventional: *auditory agnosia* is defined as the impossibility of recognizing environmental sounds, words, and music which the patient, however, is said to hear. *Pure word deafness* is the impossibility of understanding spoken language to repeat or to write under dictation in the absence of another sign of aphasia. *Cortical deafness* is defined as the feeling of being deaf contrasting with the integrity of the tonal audiogram. *Amusia* is auditory agnosia specific for music. These central disorders of auditory perception may result from lesions of either the right, left, or both cerebral hemispheres, usually involving parietotemporal cortical areas (Lechevalier *et al.*, 1999). The outcome may be favorable in some cases of cerebrovascular etiology. In reality, such clinical profiles are far from being so distinct. There are intermediate forms, for example: absolutely pure cases of word deafness (relating to only the sounds of language) are extremely rare. Moreover, evolutionary forms were published, initially observed as a form of cortical deafness, then like an auditory agnosia (Godefroy *et al.*, 1995). In spite of these irregularities it seems to us justified to maintain the individuality of these clinical entities, notably because of the acoustic characteristics of the three types of the sounds (musical, verbal sounds, and environmental sounds). Moreover, if all these kinds of sound are composed with a fundamental and harmonics, only musical sounds could have an invariance in time, even if they last only one-tenth of a second (approximate value of thirty-second note in a measurement at 4 times played at a tempo of 60, i.e. a black by second). Central deafness due to brainstem lesion and auditory hallucinations constitute complex other fields, attached to this chapter for convenience.

The study of these syndromes includes accurate knowledge of symptoms and signs that distinguish them from each other, the acoustic structure of various auditory stimuli, the methodology of audiometric testing and functional brain imaging. New insights have been brought about both by improved knowledge of systematic anatomy of the temporal cortex, and by recent neuroimaging studies. The prognosis of these disorders depends on their cause and lesion localizations.

Circumstances of diagnosis

Classic profile of strokes

After the initial phase, when the state of consciousness of the patient allows a brief exploration of the cognitive functions "at the bedside," some symptoms and signs can attract the attention in favor of a disorder of auditory perception. Sometimes two strokes occur, one in each cerebral hemisphere. These strokes follow one another after a variable interval of a few weeks to some months. The second stroke allows the auditory deficit to be highlighted. It is usually a bilateral temporal infarction. Generally, the attention is focused by the "auditory behavior of the patient": they seem to understand and answer questions badly or barely react to noises (auditory neglect). It is very rare that one can initially categorize and diagnose a perceptive disorder from one of the clinical signs previously presented, before a precise assessment is carried out by the speech therapist and the audiologist, which will be correlated with a rigorous cerebral imagery.

It is common that the diagnosis is wrongly directed towards a disorder of consciousness, a mild state of mental confusion, and even a pseudo-psychotic form. The patient seems distant, cannot fix their attention, they answer wrongly, and then a few days later (as for one of our patients) one is surprised to find them reading; one realizes that he carries out perfectly written instructions without complaining about hearing disorders, being apparently anosognosic! The diagnosis of aphasia is often evoked when the lesion is located in the left hemisphere, and it is not rare that aphasic and agnosic disorders cohabit. It will be worthwhile to distinguish *pure word deafness* and *word deafness* from an aphasic origin, returning within the background of the Wernicke aphasia; the diagnosis will be rectified by language assessment.

The hearing disorder can reveal stroke

It was thus observed in a 65-year-old choral director (Lechevalier, 2003) who during a repetition found that several of his chorus-singers sang wrong notes and that he had lost his ear for music. This symptom was isolated and revealed a right posterior temporal infarct due to occlusion of the internal carotid artery. The association with visual agnosia is an exceptional possibility (De la Sayette *et al.*, 1994).

The auditory syndrome can be delayed

The auditory syndrome can be delayed and preceded by the occurrence of various neurological symptoms, like disorders of the body representation. This was the case in a 26-year-old patient who suffered a right temporo-parietal infarction of embolic origin.

Transient hearing disorders

Transient hearing disorders, which could even be repeated several times, may rarely reveal transient ischemic attack, as shown by Sidtis and Feldmann (1990).

Major clinical syndromes according to cerebral lesion

Anatomical considerations

The auditory nerves conveying potentials from the cochlea leave the internal auditory meatus and arrive in the posterior cranial fossa — more precisely in the cerebellopontum angle formed by the pons and the cerebellum (Figure 18.1). They penetrate the side part of the cerebral trunk to the union of the medulla and the pons. The first neuron makes a synapse with the sensory cells and ends in the ventral and dorsal side of the cochlear nuclei. From these nuclei, the second neurons leave. The ventral fibers form the trapezoidal body (which plays a significant role in the localization of the sounds in space). Some fibers end in the olivary nucleus and others go up directly into the lateral lemniscus. The dorsal fibers delineate the acoustic bundles. The majority of these fibers cross the median line but some remain on the ipsilateral side. Olivary nuclei give rise to "top-down" fibers projected to the cochlea which end on the external hair cells on which they apply a modulating influence. The second neuron ends in the inferior colliculus, located in the mesencephalon, and projects directly or via an interneuron to the medial geniculate body, in close relation with the posterior thalamus. The acoustic radiations originate from the medial geniculate body, cross the very posterior part of the internal capsule, the temporal isthmus transversely, and end in the horizontal part of the superior temporal convolution (T1). The temporal convolution is divided into three areas with a tonotopic organization: in the center, the transverse gyrus of Heschl (A1), surrounded by the secondary auditory areas (A2), namely: behind, the caudomedial area (CM) also named planum temporale, and ahead, the rostral area (R). For Rauschecker (1997), the ventral

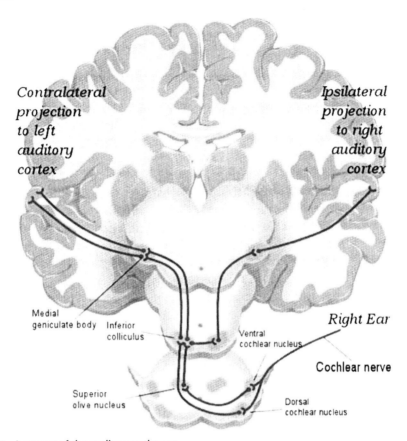

Figure 18.1   Anatomy of the auditory pathways.

part of the median geniculate body projects at the same time onto A1 and onto the rostral area with regard to pure sounds (without harmonics). Moreover, A1 is used as a relay for the CM. The dorsal part of the CGM projects onto the CM with regard to complex sounds and high frequencies (harmonics). For Mesulam, A1 would process at the same time the pitch of pure sounds which are also treated by the rostral area. The anterior part of T1 would process the phonetic aspects of the spoken language. The caudomedial area would specifically process complex sounds and music. Contrary to an old proposal, the visual and auditory areas would share similar functional organization (Rauschecker *et al.*, 1997) and especially a parallel organization of the modular type rather than a serial organization. The auditory system is organized according to tonotopy: a neuron that conveys signals from a given auditory frequency ends and is mainly connected with neurons conveying the same auditory frequency in brainstem relays and A1 and A2.

Table 18.1. Main characteristics of the disorders

	Cortical deafness	Pure word deafness	Auditory agnosia	Amusia
Tonal audiometry	+	+/−	−	−
Sound localization	+	−	−	+/−
Pitch perception	+	−	+/−	+
Rhythm perception	+	−	+/−	+
Rhythm production	+	−	+/−	+
Timbre perception	+	+/−	+/−	+
Environmental sound perception	+	−	+	+/−
Phoneme perception	+	+	+/−	−
Syllable perception	+	+	+/−	−
Voice perception	+	+	+/−	−
Word comprehension	+	+	−	−
Word production	+	+/−	−	−

+impaired; − usually preserved; +/− variable

For a summary of the main characteristics of disorders, see Table 18.1. Table 18.2 shows the anatomical locations of lesions.

Cortical deafness

For a long time, confusion existed in the terminology of the forms of auditory disorders, in particular between cortical deafness and auditory agnosia. François Michel (1980) characterized cortical deafness by bilateral abolition of the middle and late latencies of auditory potentials, testifying to bilateral lesions of the primary auditory cortices or Heschl's gyrus. The patient suffering a cortical deafness has the feeling of being deaf to all types of auditory stimuli. Nevertheless, the patient often says that they are *not* deaf, rather that they do not understand what is said to them. Curiously, such patients sometimes perceive a conversation with low voices (Mazzuchi *et al.*, 1982) or a very tiny noise like the rattling of keys (Mahoudeau *et al.*, 1958), or even music (Lechevalier *et al.*, 1984). It is possible that such perceptions are the result of the functionality of the median geniculate bodies or of the inferior colliculus, or of the integrity of some areas of the primary auditory cortices. Such phenomena are similar to those observed in cortical *blindness*, where the patient frequently states that they see whereas they do not avoid obstacles and cannot name what is presented visually to them. It is admitted that the degree of auditory neglect is proportionate to the intensity of cortical deafness. One of our personal observations (Lechevalier *et al.*, 1985) seems to

Table 18.2. Strokes usually responsible of the disorders

	Cortical deafness	Pure word deafness	Auditory agnosia	Amusia
Heschl gyrus	+ B	+/− L	+/− B	+/− R
Auditory cortex	+ B	+ L	+ B	+ R
Temporal pole	−	−	+/− B	+ B
Temporo-parietal junction	+/− B	+ L	+/− B	−
Broca's area	−	+/− L	+/− B	−
Prefrontal regions	−	−	−	+/− R
Parietal regions	−	+/− L	−	+/− R
Occipital regions	−	−	−	−

+ lesions often observed in this regions; − not or rarely observed; +/− sometimes observed; B, bilateral; L, left hemisphere dominant; R, right hemisphere dominant

contradict this assertion. In cortical deafness, the vocal audiogram is always "failed" whereas pure tone audiometry can be more or less preserved. In fact, we could note that the results were extremely inconsistent from one examination to another. Detection of pure sounds could be due to the preserved functionality of the median geniculate bodies. An objective cochleovestibular assessment shows no deterioration of the middle and internal ears and spared conduction in the auditory pathways of the brainstem. Conversely, middle and late latencies of auditory evoked potentials are abolished. Lesions responsible for cortical deafness are frequently bilateral temporal infarctions; bilateral hemorrhagic cortical–subcortical lesions involving the temporal cortex, temporal isthmus, and the posterior arm of the internal capsule are rarely observed (Godefroy *et al.*, 1995). Other causes exist (Lechevalier *et al.*, 1984).

We use the term *subcortical deafness* to indicate a state clinically identical to cortical deafness, due to lesions in subcortical areas of the brain. One could call it the syndrome of "Le Gros-Clark and Russell" who first described this possibility in 1938. The ischemic lesions involve the two external capsules and go down sufficiently low to interrupt acoustic radiations. Unilateral cortical deafness, or deafness of a unique cerebral hemisphere, represents the syndrome of "hemianacousia," described by Michel and collaborators in 1980. It is characterized by abolition of cortical auditory evoked potentials on one side accompanied by extinction on the dichotic listening test of the contralateral ear. This syndrome is seen less frequently than unilateral auditory agnosia (Pasquier *et al.*, 1991).

Pure word deafness

The term *pure word deafness* (PWD) was coined by Kussmaul (1884). Another term sometimes used is "verbal auditory agnosia." Lichtheim (1885) defined this syndrome as the failure to understand, repeat, and write from dictation verbal sounds in the context of the preservation of other linguistic processing (speaking abilities or writing, reading aloud, reading comprehension). The auditory dysfunction is highly specific. It affects speech perception but leaves relatively intact non-verbal auditory information such as environmental sounds or music.

Patients with PWD are always aware of their auditory speech problem: "I hear but I don't understand ... it's like noise ... vanishing words ... it sounds like a foreign language ... people speak too quickly." Cues such as lip-reading or contextual and pragmatic information are helpful but insufficient to compensate for the impairment of auditory verbal comprehension.

PWD must be differentiated from others central auditory syndromes: auditory agnosia, phonoagnosia which corresponds to the inability to recognize familiar voices, or amusia (see later). PWD in its pure form is quite rare. It provides with auditory agnosia evidence for a neuropsychological double dissociation between recognition of speech and of non-speech sounds. However, in a review, Buchman *et al.* (1986) concluded that most of patients diagnosed with PWD suffered from mild additional auditory processing impairment (auditory agnosia).

Neuropsychological tests are useful in characterizing PWD. *Linguistic assessment* using classical aphasia batteries (PALPA: e.g. Kay *et al.*, 1992) reveals impaired performance in all tasks which require verbal auditory perception. Repetition and writing under dictation are particularly difficult. Patients cannot give any response or make errors such as substitution with a word phonologically close to the target. More severe problems for sentences and non-words are noted. Verbal auditory comprehension is altered but patients may at times benefit from multiple choices in oral word to picture matching. Providing the patient with the context (e.g. topic of a conversation) improves comprehension. The effect of lip-reading has not been clearly demonstrated to be a facilitating factor. A striking disparity is noted between the alteration of verbal comprehension and the capacity to identify environmental sounds (i.e. animal cries, meaningful sounds). The remaining linguistic tasks show relatively intact performances (oral or written confrontation naming, verbal fluency, reading aloud, and written comprehension). Patients claim they experience increased difficulty with conversation between several individuals or in following speech in the presence of noise (Lambert, 1997).

Assessment of *phonemic perception* is useful to characterize the level of the underlying deficit. All studies have revealed dramatic phonetic or phonological deficits in tasks of discrimination and identification of syllables (Denes and Semenza, 1975; Saffran *et al.*, 1976; Auerbach *et al.*, 1982; Miceli, 1982; Tanaka *et al.*, 1987; Yaqub *et al.*, 1988; Kazui *et al.*, 1990; Praamstra *et al.*, 1991; Godefroy *et al.*, 1995; Wang *et al.*, 2000). Consonant perception is more affected than vowel perception. The impairment is more acute for phonemes which differ by one phonetic feature (voiced/unvoiced or place of articulation) than by two or more phonetic features. According to cognitive models of auditory comprehension (e.g. Ellis *et al.*, 1994), PWD results from damage at the level of the auditory analysis system whose function is to identify speech sounds in the speech wave. This impairment prevents normal processing of further stages: the auditory input lexicon whose role is to identify strings of phonemes as familiar words, and the semantic system which is involved in the extraction of a word's meaning. Damage localized to the auditory input lexicon is called "word-form deafness." Disruption between the auditory input lexicon and the semantic system leads to a pattern of "word-meaning deafness." When semantic representations themselves are degraded in the semantic system, a general semantic impairment is observed which affects comprehension whatever the input modality (auditory and written language).

Psychoacoustical analyses have shown that pure tone audiometry is normal or near normal and the mild pure tone hearing loss cannot explain the verbal auditory deficit. Ability to perceive static pitch, timbre, and loudness, and even sound localization is relatively adequate. Conversely, deficit in the temporal processing of speech has been noted. For example, Albert and Bear (1974) found that comprehension improved if the speech rate was reduced to one-third of the normal rate. It has also been mentioned for non-linguistic acoustic signals (Albert and Bear, 1974; Saffran *et al.*, 1976; Auerbach *et al.*, 1982): click-fusion tasks show a deficit in detection of rapid dynamic variations. Patients fused two clicks sounded at an interval of 15 ms or even 300 ms, while normal subjects are able to distinguish two clicks at 1–3 ms. Deficit in temporal auditory acuity has been emphasized to explain the speech perception disorder. Understanding language requires the ability to process temporal variations in the acoustic signal of speech which is characterized by rapid changes in fundamental frequency, intensity, and spectral properties. While vowels offer steady-state acoustic information, identification of consonants (especially stop consonants) depends on temporal changes such as transients that are click-like sounds, and rapid spectral changes between consonant and vowel called "formant transitions," with durations of a few milliseconds and around tens of milliseconds respectively. Thus the relative preservation of vowel identification as compared to consonant–vowel and consonant–vowel–consonant syllables suggests that the inability to process short dynamic patterns in speech signals is an important factor in PWD

(Phillips and Farmer, 1990; Wang *et al.*, 2000). A compromised cerebral time resolution mechanism is supposed to affect speech perception more than identification of environmental sounds whose acoustic characteristics do not imply such rapid acoustic variations.

The existence of two PWD subtypes has been proposed by Auerbach *et al.* 1982:
1. a "pre-phonemic" apperceptive disorder linked to an auditory temporal acuity disorder consecutive to bilateral temporal lobe lesions, and
2. a phonemic form associated with left unilateral lesion independent of auditory temporal resolution which is attributed to an impairment of phonemic discrimination.

Auditory agnosia

The border between pure word deafness and auditory agnosia is unclear because identification disorders of non-verbal sounds may be encountered in pure word deafness. We propose to call auditory agnosia a deficit of recognition of environmental sounds and/or music (amusia) and/or voice (phonoagnosia). When speech comprehension is also disturbed, one may prefer the label "pure word deafness," indicating that this terminology relates only exceptionally to a deficit limited to verbal sounds. The auditory agnosia can initially be complete, with all sounds (verbal and non-verbal) being confounded. The patient says that they hear, but they cannot distinguish anything. Auditory neglect is frequently associated, as shown by the lack of reaction of the subject to auditory stimuli. On the other hand, the appreciation of pitch and intensities of stimuli can be paradoxically preserved whereas the perception of musical rhythms or the lengths of sounds are disturbed. Because of the prevalent ischemic etiology, the disorder usually improves rapidly, with a course which frequently follows three stages: complete auditory agnosia, then agnosia limited to the non-verbal noises, and finally amusia. In some cases, the verbal message is well understood but the voice seems deformed and strange. One can call "emotional auditory agnosia" neutral perception, without prosody, of all voices. Lesions concern either temporal lobes or less frequently the right one only. They are generally asymmetrical cortical infarctions of the first temporal convolution and/or the white substance, injuring more or less the gyrus of Heschl. Subcortical strokes have been reported involving either of the external capsules extending into acoustic radiations, or the internal geniculate bodies. Contrary to cortical deafness, the auditory cortical (late latency) potentials are normal or moderately faded. A case of right unilateral auditory agnosia produced by a left lenticular hemorrhage was reported by Pasquier *et al.* (1991), and interpreted as a defect of activation of the ipsilateral cortex because of a diminution in the right temporoparietal cerebral blood flow.

Amusia

Disorders of music perception following cerebral damage can be divided into two categories:

1. multimode perceptive disorders affecting more or less selectively musical sounds, but with verbal and environmental sound difficulties
2. a pure amusia, where music perception only is affected.

Musical perception is not a uniform competence in the general population. Some patients will have had musical training, others not. Studies estimate that 5–10% of individuals in the general population are completely unable to distinguish the pitches of two notes of music or to memorize the smallest musical tune (Peretz, 2001). Musical competence can be evaluated by scales like the Wertheim and Botez classification (1959) which provides a classification into four categories. Although useful, its duration is long for clinical purpose, especially in stroke.

From a diagnostic point of view, there is an absence of standardized tools for investigation of musical competence. Old scales are still used, such as Seashore's test (1935), and the Montreal team developed a battery of musical evaluation (Ayotte et al., 2000). Without specific tools, clinical evaluation of the musical dimension is often neglected, although the occurrence of perceptive difficulties can often be revealed by a systematic exploration, even in the absence of an explicit complaint of the patient.

Musical abilities can be considered according to three dimensions: perception, representation, and expression (production). In conventional clinical assessment, only the perceptive dimension is really explored. It was believed for a long time that perceptive amusia (or auditory agnosia specific for music) was associated with right hemisphere lesions, because of some rare cases of musicians who, after a left sylvian infarction generating a Wernicke's aphasia, were able to carry on their composing careers (Luria et al., 1965; Basso and Capitani, 1985; Assal, 1973; Signoret et al., 1987). Some of these patients demonstrated "verbal" alexia but musical reading was spared. Modern studies suggest that this proposal is too simplistic: the left hemisphere would mediate the identification of familiar tunes, the perception of rhythms, as well as the elementary perception of pitch. On the other hand, the lesions responsible for the perception of timbre involve the right temporoparietal regions of the temporal lobe (Mazzuchi et al., 1982). It is the same for the failure of emotional perception and musical pleasure (Mazzoni et al., 1993; Lechevalier, 2003). Peretz (1990) opposes the global perception of melody (contour, which would be under the control of the right hemisphere) with the elementary perception of pitch (interval, which would depend on the left hemisphere).

Neuropsychological study of epileptic patients who have undergone a unilateral temporal cortectomy has contributed to our knowledge of the localization of musical functions (Liégeois-Chauvel *et al.*, 1998). A right temporal cortectomy disturbs melodic perception as well as the perception of pitch intervals, whereas a lobectomy on the left side does not disturb perception of the intervals. These results underline the key role of the superior temporal gyrus in discrimination of melodies. Cortectomy of the posterior part of T1, including the planum temporale, the side part of Heschl's gyrus and Brodmann's area 22, is more striking for the processing of pitch and variations of rhythm than cortectomy of the anterior part of T1. Disorders of the perception of rhythm and meter (recognition of a cadence of march or waltz) can be dissociated. The right and left anterior parts of T5 would be implicated in the processing of meter. The characteristics of epileptic lesions and the duration of the evaluation of these cases must be taken into account in any interpretation of these localizations.

Griffiths *et al.* (1997) report on a patient suffering from lesions of the median and posterior temporal areas, and the insula of the right hemisphere. The patient complained of not being able to appreciate music. A series of tests confirmed a deficit of musical perception without disturbance of the perception of noises, environmental sounds, and speech sounds. His ability to detect continuous changes of sound frequency was preserved. However, a disturbance in the analysis of rapid sequences of notes seemed to be the basis of his musical perception deficit. According to the authors, this observation shows that the occurrence of an amusia is not necessarily underlined by bilateral lesions. In addition, the patient presented a deficit in the perception of the movement of sounds. This observation is in agreement with PET studies suggesting the participation of associative areas of the primary auditory cortex in the perception of the movement of sounds. Neuroimaging studies overall support clinical data and, in addition, reveal that (1) rhythm perception activates area 44, and (2) detection of pitch changes relies on the left cuneus and precuneus. This latter localization is consistent with the hypothesis of a visual representation of the musical scale (Platel *et al.*, 1997). Lastly, some clinical observations as well as recent neuroimaging studies show the involvement of temporal areas (middle temporal gyrus on both sides) and prefrontal regions in long-term musical memory (Platel *et al.*, 2003).

Auditory neglect

Hemineglect (see Chapter 9) due to right parietal stroke is prominent in the visual modality and may also concern the auditory modality.

Clinical-anatomical correlations

Brodmann's areas 41 and 42 as well as the close language cortical regions (areas 22 and 21), corresponding to T1 and T2 respectively, are supplied by the middle cerebral artery. The posterior part of the internal capsule which includes acoustic radiations is supplied by the posterior communicating artery. At the mesencephalon level, the inferior colliculus is supplied by the quadrigeminal arteries, branches of the superior cerebellum arteries. The internal and median geniculate bodies belong to the epithalamus and are supplied by the thalamo-geniculate pedicle, deep territory of the posterior cerebral artery.

Cortical deafness is the consequence of bilateral destruction of the transverse gyrus of Heschl (primary auditory areas numbered BA 41). Right and left infarctions are seldom symmetrical in extent or in depth; they are often cortical–subcortical and can be different in age. We call "subcortical deafness" the clinical profile of cortical deafness due to bilateral ischemic (Le Gros–Clark and Russell, 1938) or hemorrhagic lesions (Godefroy et al., 1995) which interrupt acoustic radiations while sparing the auditory cortex. Auditory agnosia can be the consequence of bilateral lesions of the temporal lobes, variable in extent, excluding the gyrus of Heschl. A lesion of the first right temporal convolution in right-handed patients may initially produce auditory agnosia (including musical ability) which can be in the foreground, and then evolve to pure amusia. Impaired identification of a musical piece is always produced by a left hemisphere lesion.

Pure word deafness may be due to left or bilateral temporal lesions. They may be due to disconnection as described by Liepmann and Storch in 1902. A 67-year-old patient presented with three successive strokes. The first one was transient. Nine months later the second stroke led to an almost pure word deafness: the patient did not understand any word (that were perfectly heard), did not recognize melodies, and suffered from musical hallucinations. Five years later, a third stroke made him completely deaf for words and musical notes. Autopsy revealed a left-side hemorrhage located between the temporal isthmus in the bottom and outwards edges of the inferior internal capsule and the lenticular nuclei and inside "in the place where the fibers come from the left and right hemispheres (confirmed by the degeneration of the right tapetum) gather to the left temporal lobe." The authors suggest that this hemorrhage occurred at the same place as the first stroke. In the famous diagram "the small house of Lichtheim (1885)," pure word deafness is regarded as an interruption of the afferent subcortical pathway going to the center for auditory word "images." Poeppel refers to a sub-group of PWD caused by a left unilateral lesion of the temporal cortex. More frequent are cases of PWD from bilateral lesions of the posterior part of the posterior temporal cortex, excluding the gyrus of Heschl.

Hearing disorders due to brainstem lesions

Hearing disorders due to brainstem stroke are rare because of the bilateral projections of the central auditory pathways. However, a few studies have revealed (Cambier *et al.*, 1987) that pons stroke (infarction in the territory of the perforating arteries or paramedian hemorrhages) may cause deafness of varying severity which can be accompanied by a feeling of distortion of the sounds and by the impossibility of locating sounds in space. Audiometric analyses show the absence of cochlear disturbance with a normal impedance-metric and brainstem auditory evoked potentials, delayed latencies of I−V or I−III waves on one or both sides. Such central deafness is usually accompanied by other signs of brainstem lesions: hemianesthesia, paralysis of abducens and facial nerves, gaze disorders, cerebellar syndrome, gait disorders, and auditory hallucinations. MRI now makes it possible to locate with great precision even small lesions of the brainstem.

Auditory hallucinations

According to the usual definition, a hallucination is a perception without an object. Henry Ey distinguished between a *true hallucination*, when the patient is not aware of its abnormal nature, and *hallucinosis*, which is regarded as abnormal by the patient. The patient consents to the former but contests the latter, which they regard as pathological. Auditory hallucinations have multiple causes, including lesions of the inner ear and cochlear nerve, toxic encephalopathy, epilepsy, degenerative diseases (especially those leading to dementia), and psychosis. Stroke is a rare cause of auditory hallucinations.

Auditory hallucinations are observed in brainstem and temporal strokes. The phenomenon, called "peduncular hallucinosis" by Van Bogaert in 1927, had been described five years earlier by Jean Lhermitte. It concerned visual hallucinosis reported as "like an agitated spectacle, moving and colored which is held in silence, like a silent movie," and is observed in lesions of the peduncular cap. Patients described with accuracy the frequent and transient scenes they experienced. Cambier *et al.* (1987) published five purely auditory observations of hallucinosis: four were attributed to paramedian strokes of the pons (hemorrhagic in one case and ischemic in the others), and the fifth case to infarct of the dorsolateral mesencephalon, with abnormal wave V (brainstem auditory evoked potential) indicating a lesion in the area of the inferior colliculus (territory of the quadrigeminal artery). In these five cases, auditory hallucinations were similar: they were music tunes, classical or popular, with only one singer whom the patient identified with precision, or a choir, a whole orchestra, a military brass band, or opera. Conversations, "quarrels," and remarks about the patient were also observed to a lesser extent. Sometimes visual and auditory hallucinations follow one another. These hallucinations frequently occur in the evening, when the patients are inactive, and resemble "hypnagogic" hallucinations. Cambier and collaborators compare them to the first period of a dream.

Auditory hallucinations following temporal lesions are unusual and have different characteristics. Penfield and Perot (1963) had induced musical hallucinations by stimulation of right T1. In a review of cases of PWD, cortical deafness, and auditory agnosia (Lechevalier *et al.*, 1985), nine cases with hallucinations were detailed. They consisted of acoustic illusions, deformed and unpleasant sonorities, acouphenes, whistles, or elaborate hallucinations with musical or verbal content (Liepmann and Storch, 1902). For Ziegler's (1952) patient, the voices heard used several languages. Musical hallucinations are more frequent following right hemisphere lesions (Augustin *et al.*, 2001; Evers and Ellger, 2004).

Assessment of auditory disorders

Audiometry: Subjective tests
Standard pure tone audiometry

This technique detects the threshold of perception of pure tone. It is thus unsuited to testing the function of integration of sounds, i.e. the psycho-acoustic performance of an individual. Threshold is defined as the lowest intensity (measured in decibels) at which an individual can detect a pure tone or speech signal for more than 50% of the time. Standard tonal audiometry is usually within normal ranges in pure word deafness and auditory agnosia, although variable results may be observed in some patients. In cortical deafness, pure tone thresholds are generally disturbed.

Word discrimination test

This technique assesses the auditory comprehension of phonemes or words presented with various intensities. In central pathologies of hearing, this examination is always failed, but that is also the case in peripheral illness. Two features suggest a central disorder: the discrepancy between the word and tonal audiometry, and the inability to obtain a perfect identification of words or phonemes, whatever the intensity.

Specific audiometric tests
Dichotic listening test

The principle of this task is to present simultaneously different stimuli in each ear, but identical in intensity and duration. This test can be done with several kinds of stimuli (pure sounds, words, music) although routine use involves verbal stimuli. Subjects have to repeat (or identify) both stimuli. Such a procedure usually leads to a mild ear preference, and especially to a right ear preference for verbal stimuli in right-handed subjects — which is attributed to the prominence of crossed auditory pathway (right ear — left hemisphere). In unilateral brain damage, performance of the contralesional ear decreases dramatically and this contrasts with the normal performance during monaural presentation (i.e. stimuli presented separately in each ear), a phenomenon called "extinction." In addition, callosal lesions induce a left-ear extinction for verbal stimuli — attributed to the disruption of verbal sounds from the right temporal regions to the left hemisphere required for language processing.

The "hemianacousia" described by Michel is an association of the abolition of cortical evoked potentials on one side and extinction of the contralateral ear on the dichotic listening test.

Sequences of auditory signals

Subjects listen to two series of auditory signals, identical except for one signal. It is possible to vary the length or the frequency of the signal (long–long–short, long–short–long, or low–high–low, low–low–high). In bilateral temporal lesions, subjects cannot recognize the temporal sequence of two auditory stimuli. These tests are very sensitive in cases of cerebral lesion, but can also be disturbed in endocochlear deafness.

Audiometry: Objective tests

Oto-acoustic emissions (OAEs)

Kemp (1978) showed that the human ear is able to produce sounds (oto-acoustic emissions) in response to sound stimulation. The hair cells of the external Corti's organ are the origin of the emissions. They can be recorded by a probe placed in the external auditory canal. The source of the OAEs is thus upstream of the stage of transduction which transforms acoustic energy into nerve potential in the cochlear nerve. The occurrence of OAEs in deafness suggests an auditory neuropathy. Indeed it is sufficient to decrease the threshold to 30 dB (at 1 kHz) to make the OAEs disappear. This trivial fall could frequently coexist with a central pathology.

Evoked auditory potentials (EAPs)

Evoked auditory potentials use the same principles as electroencephalography. Recordings are made of early, middle, and late latency potentials in chronological order after the stimulus, representing the operation of increasingly central auditory pathways.

Brainstem EAPs (also known as early EAPs)

The response obtained proceeds 1–10 ms after the beginning of a short stimulation (click). These early EAPs are normal in deafness due to cortical–subcortical lesions.

EAPs of middle latency (or semi-early EAPs)

The response obtained proceeds 10–50 ms after the stimulus. Four waves (Na, Pa, Nb, Pb) can be identified according to the chronological order (a, b) and their positive (P) or negative (N) deflection. Pa seems to be generated by the thalamocortical ways, Pb by the core thalamic bodies, and Na comes from the cortical and subcortical regions. Analysis of these potentials consists primarily of looking for the presence or absence of the Na/Pa complex.

EAPs of late latency (or cortical EAPs)

The response obtained proceeds 50–250 ms after the beginning of the stimulus. The sequences of waves, alternately positive (P) and negative (N), are numbered in the order of appearance (N1, P1, N2, P2). Their nature is still debated, but it seems probable that N1–P1 and N2–P2 are associated with the primary auditory cortex.

Neuropsychological assessment

Investigations include verbal and non-verbal tasks.

Linguistic and speech perception tasks

All these verbal tasks are performed without lip-reading. Auditory input tasks (repetition, verbal comprehension, dictation) are compared to written input tasks with the same words (reading, written comprehension). The latter leads to normal scores in PWD. The most frequent comprehension tasks used are synonym judgments and word-to-picture matching including phonological distractors.

Within a cognitive approach, functionality of the different components of the auditory processing is assessed by identification and discrimination tasks using phonemes, music, environmental sounds, auditory lexical decision tasks, and semantic tasks.

Phonemic identification and discrimination tasks

The phonemic identification task requires subjects to name or to point to written vowels or syllables (consonant/vowel format). In the phonemic discrimination task, subjects hear a pair of vowels or syllables and have to judge whether they are identical or different. Consonants are always presented in a CV syllable with a constant vowel. Pairs of syllables using plosive (or fricative) consonants differ according to the phonemic proximity: several phonetic features (place of articulation, voice, manner: pa/za; place of articulation and voice: ka/ba) or a single phonetic feature (place of articulation: pa/ka, ba/ga; voice: pa/ba, sa/za).

Auditory lexical decision tasks
Subjects hear a list of words and non-words and have to decide whether an auditory stimulus is a word or not. The preservation of written lexical decision is useful in the diagnosis of PWD.

Evaluation of semantic access and of semantic processing
Subjects have to perform synonym/antonym judgments in auditory and written versions. Semantic association tasks such as "pyramids and palm trees" (Howard and Patterson, 1992) in different modalities of presentation (spoken word, written word, and picture) may also be useful. Only the auditory versions of these tasks are altered in PWD.

Non-speech sounds
Subjects have to identify animal cries (cat meowing), man-made and technical (car horn, hammer) or natural non-living sounds (thunder) or instruments (violin) played on a tape recorder. Identification is assessed by naming or pointing in a multiple choice of pictures or written names. The target is presented first with unrelated distractors and then with distractors drawn from the same category, or which present very close acoustic characteristics.

Receptive musical ability
This assesses several dimensions of sounds. *Intensity perception* is assessed by asking subjects to discriminate between two pure tones ("Which one is louder, the first or the second?") presented in each ear at 250, 1000 or 3000 Hz. *Tone (pitch) perception* is evaluated by asking subjects to determine whether a sequence of two tones of different intervals (1/2 step, whole step, second or third) is ascending or descending. *Rhythm perception* is assessed by asking subjects to determine whether two rhythm patterns of a pair are the same or different. *Rhythm production* assessment requires subjects to reproduce simple rhythm patterns. *Melody recognition* requires subjects to identify familiar songs. *Sound localization* is assessed by asking subjects to localize the azimuthal position of a brief click presented at one of several positions in a free field by pointing to its perceived position.

Prognosis and treatments

Clinical experience indicates that improvement of cerebral auditory perception is common in stroke patients. The first step in therapy of PWD is to inform patients and their relatives of the nature of the auditory disorder they have suffered — what is altered and what is preserved. The second step is to explain which aids they can benefit from, such as lip-reading, and the conditions in which they may be able to optimize auditory comprehension: conversation in a quiet room, and with one person at a time.

The aim of treatment is to restore the defective auditory analysis, or at least to improve auditory discrimination skills. The most frequent strategy used by speech therapists relies on stimulation throughout exercises of speech sound discrimination. The observations of Morris *et al.* (1996) represent a good example of this management, although their patients presented with several cognitive deficits. They proposed training for lip-reading, then various exercises of phonemic discrimination: phoneme-to-grapheme matching, auditory word-to-picture matching, auditory word-to-written-word matching, auditory word-to-picture judgment, and auditory word-to-written-word judgment, syllables (VC or CV) discrimination. Furthermore, practice followed a progression according to the phonemic contrast (several features, single feature) and to the hearing condition (natural voice + lip-reading, natural voice, registered voice on a tape-recorder). Computer-based auditory discrimination training can also be used (Audix system: Grawemeyer *et al.*, 2000). Management of auditory agnosia or amusia relies on the same general principles of therapy: stimulation, plus progressive training within a gradient of difficulty.

REFERENCES

Albert, M. L. and Bear, D. (1974). Time to understand. A case study of word deafness with reference to the role of time in auditory comprehension. *Brain*, **97**, 373–84.

Assal, G. (1973). Aphasie de Wernicke sans amusie chez un pianiste. *Rev. Neurol. (Paris)*, **129**, 251–5.

Auerbach, S. H., Allard, T., Naeser, M., Alexander, M. P. and Albert, M. L. (1982). Pure word deafness: Analysis of a case with bilateral lesions and a defect at the prephonemic level. *Brain*, **105**, 271–300.

Augustin, J., Guegan-Massardier, E., Levillain, D., *et al.* (2001). Musical hallucinosis following infarction of the right middle cerebral artery. *Rev. Neurol. (Paris)*, **157**, 289–92.

Ayotte, J., Peretz, I., Rousseau, I., Bart, C. and Bojanowski, M. (2000). Patterns of music associated with middle cerebral artery infarcts? *Brain*, **123**, 1926–38.

Basso, A. and Capitani, E. (1985). Spared musical abilities in a conductor with global aphasia and ideomotor apraxia. *J. Neurol. Neurosurg. Psychiatry*, **48**, 407–21.

Bogaert, van L. (1927). L'hallucinose pédonculaire. *Rev. Neurol. (Paris)*, **43**, 608–17.

Buchman, A., Garron, D. C., Trost-Cardamoze, J. E., Wichter, M. D. and Schwartz, M. (1986). Word deafness: One hundred years later. *J. Neurol. Neurosurg. Psychiatry*, **49**, 489–99.

Cambier, J., Decroix, J. P. and Masson, C. (1987). Auditory hallucinations in lesions of the brain stem. *Rev. Neurol. (Paris)*, **143**, 255–62.

De la Sayette, V., Dupuy, B., Eustache, F., *et al.* (1994). Multimodal or multisensorial agnosia? *Rev. Neurol. (Paris)*, **150**, 346–53.

Denes, G. and Semenza, C. (1975). Auditory modality-specific anomia: Evidence from a case of pure word deafness. *Cortex*, **11**, 401–11.

Ellis, A. W., Franklin, S. and Crerar, A. (1994). Cognitive neuropsychology and the remediation of disorders of spoken language. In M. S. Riddoch and G. W. Humphreys, eds., *Cognitive Neuropsychology and Cognitive Rehabilitation*. Hove: L. E. A. pp. 287–315.

Evers, S. and Ellger, T. (2004). The clinical spectrum of musical hallucinations. *J. Neurol. Sci.*, **227**, 55–65.

Godefroy, O., Leys, D., Furby, A., *et al.* (1995). Psychoacoustical deficits related to bilateral subcortical hemorrhages. A case with apperceptive auditory agnosia. *Cortex*, **31**, 149–59.

Grawemeyer, B., Cox, R. and Lum, C. (2000). AUDIX: A knowledge-based system for speech-therapy auditory discrimination exercises. *Stud. Health Informat.*, **77**, 568–72.

Griffiths, T. D., Rees, A., Witton, C., *et al.* (1997). Spatial and temporal auditory processing deficit following right hemisphere infarction. A psychophysical study. *Brain*, **120**, 785–94.

Howard, D. and Patterson, K. (1992). *The Pyramids and Palm Trees Test: A Test of Semantic Access from Words and Pictures*. Bury, St Edmunds: Thames Valley test Co.

Kay, J., Lesser, R. and Coltheart, M. (1992). *The Psycholinguistic Assessment of Language Processing in Aphasia*. Hove: Lawrence Erlbaum.

Kazui, S., Naritomi, H., Sawada, T., Inoue, N. and Okuda, J. (1990). Subcortical auditory agnosia. *Brain Lang.*, **38**, 476–87.

Kemp, D. T. (1978). Stimulated acoustic emissions from within the human auditory system. *J. Acoust. Soc. Am.*, **64**, 1386–91.

Kussmaull, A. (1884). Disturbances of speech. In *Cyclopedia of the Practice of Medicine*, ed. H. Von Ziemssen. New York: William Wood, **14**, 581–875. Les troubles de la parole (trad. française: Rueff A.) – Baillière et fils, Paris.

Lambert, J. (1997). Troubles de la perception du langage parlé: Approche cognitive et orientations thérapeutiques, In *Perception Auditive et Compréhension du Langage. Etat Initial, État Stable et Pathologie*, ed. J. Lambert and J. L. Nespoulous. Marseille: Solal, pp. 151–66.

Le Gros Clark, W. E. and Russell, W. R. (1938). Cortical deafness without aphasia. *Brain*, **61**, 375–83.

Lechevalier, B. (2003). *Le Cerveau de Mozart*, vol. **1**, Paris: Odile Jacod.

Lechevalier, B., Eustache, F. and Rossa, Y. (1985). *Les Troubles de la Perception de la Musique d'Origine Neurologique*, Paris: Masson.

Lechevalier, B., Lambert, J., Eustache, F. and Platel, H. (1999). Agnosies auditives et syndromes voisins: Etude clinique, cognitive et psychopathologique. *Encycl. Méd. Chir.* Paris: Elsevier, Neurologie, 17021 B[20], 9p.

Lechevalier, B., Rossa, Y., Eustache, F., *et al.* (1984). Un cas de surdité corticale épargnant en partie la musique. *Rev. Neurol. (Paris)*, **3**, 190–201.

Lichtheim, L. (1885). On aphasia. *Brain*, **7**, 433–84.

Liégeois-Chauvel, C., Peretz, I., Babaï, M., Laguitton, V. and Chauvel, P. (1998). Contribution of different cortical areas in the temporal lobes to music processing. *Brain*, **121**, 1853–67.

Liepmann, H. and Storch, E. (1902). Der mikroskopische gehirnbefund be idem fall Gorstelle. *Monatssch. Psychiatr. Neurol.*, **11**, 115–20.

Luria, A. R., Tsvetkova, L. and Futer, J. (1965). Aphasia in a composer. *J. Neurol. Sci.*, **2**, 288–92.

Mahoudeau, D., Lemoyne, J., Foncin, J. F. and Dubrisay, J. (1958). Considérations sur l'agnosie auditive (A propos d'un cas anatomoclinique). *Rev. Neurol.*, **99**, 454–71.

Mazzoni, M., Moretti, P., Pardossi, L., Vista, M. and Muratorio, A. (1993). A case of music imperception. *J. Neurol. Neurosurg. Psychiatry*, **56**, 322.

Mazzuchi, A., Marchini, C., Budai, R. and Parma, M. (1982). A case of receptive amusia with prominent timbre perception defect. *J. Neurol. Neurosurg. Psychiatry*, **45**, 644–7.

Miceli, G. (1982). The processing of speech sounds in a patient with cortical auditory disorder. *Neuropsychologia*, **20**, 5–20.

Michel, F. (1993). L'hémianacousie, un symptôme aussi fréquent que méconnu. *Rev. Neuropsychol.*, **3**, 365–75.

Morris, J., Franklin, S., Ellis, A., Turner, E. and Bayley, P. J. (1996). Remediating a speech perception deficit in an aphasic patient. *Aphasiology*, **10**, 137–58.

Pasquier, F., Leys, D., Steinling, M., *et al.* (1991). Agnosie auditive unilatérale droite consécutive à une hémorragie lenticulaire gauche. *Rev. Neurol.*, **147**, 129–37.

Peretz, I. (1990). Processing of local and global musical information by unilateral brain-damaged patients. *Brain*, **113**, 1185–205.

(2001) Brain specialization for music: New evidence from congenital amusia. In R. J. Zatorre and I. Peretz, eds., *The Biological Foundations of Music, Ann. N. Y. Acad. Sci.*, **930**, 153–65.

Phillips, D. P. and Farmer, M. E. (1990). Acquired word deafness, and the temporal grain of sound representation in the primary auditory cortex. *Behav. Brain Res.*, **40**, 85–94.

Penfield, W. and Perot, P. (1963). The brain's record of auditory and visual experience. A final summary and discussion. *Brain*, **86**, 595–696.

Platel, H., Baron, J. C., Desgranges, B., Bernard, F. and Eustache, F. (2003). Semantic and episodic memory of music are subserved by distinct neural networks. *NeuroImage*, **20**, 244–56.

Platel, H., Price, C., Baron, J. C., *et al.* (1997). The structural components of music perception: A functional anatomical study. *Brain*, **120**, 229–43.

Praamstra, P., Hagoost, P., Maassen, B. and Crul, T. (1991). Word deafness and auditory cortical function. *Brain*, **114**, 1197–225.

Rauschecker, J. P., Tian, B., Pons, J. and Mishkin, M. (1997). Serial and parallel processing in rhesus monkey auditory cortex. *J. Comp. Neurol.*, **382**, 89–103.

Saffran, E. M., Marin, O. S. and Yeni-Komshian, G. H. (1976). An analysis of speech perception in word deafness. *Brain Lang.*, **3**, 209–28.

Seashore, C. E. (1935). Measurement of musical talent, University of Iowa, *Studies in the Psychology of Music, Vol. 2*.

Sidtis, J. J. and Feldmann, E. (1990). Transient ischemic attacks presenting with a loss of pitch perception. *Cortex*, **26**, 469–71.

Signoret, J. L., Van Eeckout Ph., Poncet, M. and Castaigne, P. (1987). Aphasie sans amusie chez un organiste aveugle. *Rev. Neurol.*, **143**, 172–81.

Tanaka, Y., Yamadori, A. and Mori, E. (1987). Pure word deafness following bilateral lesions. A psychological analysis. *Brain*, **110**, 381–403.

Wang, E., Peach, R., Xu, P., Schneck, M. and Manry, C. (2000). Perception of dynamic acoustic patterns by an individual with unilateral verbal auditory agnosia. *Brain Lang.*, **73**, 442–55.

Wertheim, N. and Botez, M. I. (1959). Plan d'investigation des fonctions musicales. *L'Encéphale*, **48**, 246–55.

Yaqub, B., Gascon, G., Alnosha, M. and Whitaker, H. (1988). Pure word deafness (acquired verbal auditory agnosia) in an arabic speaking patient, *Brain*, **111**, 457–66.

Ziegler, D. K. (1952). Word deafness and Wernicke aphasia. *Arch. Neurol. Psychiatry*, **67**, 323–31.

19

Dysexecutive syndromes

Olivier Godefroy[1] and Donald Stuss[2,3]

[1]University Hospital, Amiens, France
[2]Rotman Research Institute, Baycrest
[3]University of Toronto

Introduction

Executive functions and response rapidity are frequently impaired in stroke patients and they represent a core deficit of post-stroke disability. The determinants of these deficits include several factors, the most classical of which is the site of the lesion. "Executive functions and deficits" encompass a large number of processes and impairments, and this terminology has been used with various meanings. Most frequently, executive functions refer to more central functions that control other abilities, and are most detectable in non-routine situations such as novel, conflicting, or complex tasks. The terminology "executive functions" (and dysexecutive syndrome) is now frequently preferred to "frontal functions" (and frontal syndrome) (although perhaps best instantiated in these anatomical areas) because these functions may also be impaired by non-frontal lesions. Disorders commonly considered to be "executive" in origin include a large number of behavioral changes and cognitive deficits. In addition, there is a huge overlap with some attentional processes such as selective, divided, and sustained attention (hence the term "supervisory attentional system") and these aspects are included in this review. Several reviews have covered this rapidly evolving field (Roberts *et al.*, 1996; Stuss and Alexander 2000; Godefroy, 2003). This review reports recent approaches to the dysexecutive syndrome from a clinical perspective. Several classes of executive disorders have been described and they can be roughly divided into behavioral and cognitive domains (Eslinger and Damasio, 1985; Bechara *et al.*, 1998). Such a distinction is compatible with the two major functional/anatomical dissociations within the frontal lobes (Sanides and Sas, 1970; Pandya and Yeterian, 1996; Stuss and Levine, 2002):

1. dorsolateral prefrontal regions evolving from the hippocampal–archicortical trend, primarily involved in *spatial and conceptual reasoning* processes.

2. ventral prefrontal cortex, part of the paleocortical trend emerging from the caudal orbitofrontal (olfactory) cortex, involved more in *emotional* processing (Nauta, 1971), including the acquisition and reversal of stimulus−reward associations (Mishkin, 1964; Rolls *et al.*, 1996; Fuster, 1997a; Rolls, 2000).

We will review these two aspects separately, and suggest that for clinical purposes it may be reasonable to even consider subclassifications within these two broad domains. The term "cognitive executive deficit" will refer to deficits of executive processes, such as planning, monitoring, and shifting as demonstrated on neuropsychological tests.

General presentation of the dysexecutive syndrome

The behavioral dysexecutive syndrome

The early description of clinical consequences of frontal damage has documented a large variety of behavioral disturbances such as abulia, apathy, aspontaneity, akinetic mutism, pseudodepressive state, lack of drive, poor motivation, inattention, indifference, euphoric state, distractibility, impulsivity, disinhibition, irritability, restlessness, moria, pseudopsychopathic state, anosognosia, indifference, confabulation, and perseveration (Rylander, 1939; Hécaen and de Ajuriaguerra, 1956; Fisher, 1983; Stuss and Benson, 1986). This area is still evolving and, for example, imitation and utilization behavior (Lhermitte *et al.*, 1986), loss of psychic autoactivation (Laplane *et al.*, 1981), and athymhormia (Habib and Poncet 1988) have been reported more recently. Some terms refer to similar clinical conditions (e.g. apathy, abulia, aspontaneity, and pseudodepressive state are used interchangeably) and have been identified by different approaches of behavior focusing on alteration of emotion, social interaction, or cognition (Stuss and Benson, 1986). From a clinical point of view, the recognition of behavioral disturbances is very important because it suggests or allows the diagnosis of dysexecutive syndrome and has major consequences for the patient's autonomy.

In order to simplify clinical assessment, a French cooperative group (Godefroy *et al.*, 2004) has proposed a list of the main behavioral changes, which distinguishes between highly suggestive and supportive disorders (Table 19.1). This proposal is based on a review of the literature and ongoing studies validating the specificity and frequency of behavioral changes. According to this approach, *global hypoactivity* consists of severe and otherwise unexplained reduction in self-triggered activities (walking, communication, eating, grooming...) and those triggered by the environment (orienting reaction, difficulty in initiating and sustaining various activities including tests). It is associated with abulia (defined by a reduction of movement and speech, slowed reactions, difficulty

Table 19.1. Main behavioral disorders suggestive of the dysexecutive syndrome

Highly suggestive
Global hypoactivity with abulia $\pm$ apathy $\pm$ aspontaneity
Global hyperactivity with distractibility–impulsivity $\pm$ disinhibition
Perseveration and stereotyped behavior
Syndrome of environmental dependency (manipulation, imitation, and utilization behavior)
Other supportive features
Disturbances of emotion and social behavior
Anosognosia, self awareness
Confabulation and reduplicative paramnesia
Disorders of sexual behavior, hyperorality and control of micturition

in sustaining activities) (Fisher, 1983), and/or apathy (defined by reduced motivation, loss of initiation, loss of interest, flat emotion and affect) (Marin, 1990; Robert *et al.*, 2002), and/or aspontaneity (defined by a severe reduction of self-triggered activities reversed by heteroactivation). *Global hyperactivity* concerns self-triggered activities (hyperkinetic state with restlessness, unceasing walking or talking, hyperphagia, and hyperorality) and reactions to the environment, such as distractibility–impulsivity (defined by inappropriate orientation and reaction to irrelevant information). Disinhibition is characterized by socially inappropriate behavior. *Perseverations* are suggestive of executive deficit when they consist of inappropriate maintenance or recurrence of the same set of actions ("stuck in set perseverations") and are observed in different domains. Although perseverations are a well-known behavioral sign of dysexecutive syndrome, their characterization requires neuropsychological assessment. Stereotypic behavior is characterized by the inappropriate repetition of a fixed sequence of actions. *The environmental dependency* syndrome includes abnormal prehension, manipulation, utilization of objects and imitation (Lhermitte *et al.*, 1986). Although this syndrome is usually demonstrated during clinical examination, caregivers may report "capture" of the patient's behavior by the environment (e.g. unmotivated manipulation of objects...). *Disturbances of emotion* refer to flat emotion (emotional blunting), as well as emotional lability, inability to perceive or represent the emotional content of a situation or another person's point of view (i.e. loss of empathy) (Stuss *et al.*, 2001c). This also includes loss and inability to appreciate humor that requires self-reflection (appreciation of slapstick humor may be intact) (Shammi and Stuss, 1999). *Impairment of social behavior* includes disturbances of interpersonal skills, adoption of a behavior which neglects the constraint of a given situation, and a deficit in acting in his/her self-interest with unfavorable decision-making (Stuss, 1991). This results in various behavioral changes ranging from tactlessness, irrelevant considerations or actions, to criminal acts.

Behavioral changes are more frequent in patients with frontal lesions in the medial and ventral regions. They may also be observed with a lower intensity in lesions of the caudate nucleus, thalamus, and centrum semiovale (Caplan *et al.*, 1990; Pedrazzi *et al.*, 1990; Godefroy *et al.*, 1992). The type of behavioral disorder depends on the site of the lesion (Stuss and Benson, 1986; Sarazin *et al.*, 2003) with clinical—anatomical correlations that require replications (for methodological considerations, see for example Godefroy *et al.*, 1998). Apathy has been found to depend on right medial lesions (Brodmann's area 10), and stereotypy is due to right orbitofrontal lesions (Brodmann's areas 11, 12, 13, and 14) (Sarazin *et al.*, 2003). Following attempts to increase the specificity of both cognitive and behavioral changes, various classes of apathy have been proposed as a means of operationally narrowing the broad characteristics within the label of apathy (Stuss *et al.*, 2000b). Apathy may be due either to a deficit of energization of behavior which depends on anterior cingulate/superior medial frontal, or to emotional disturbances which depends on ventral/orbitofrontal region (Stuss *et al.*, 2000b; 2005).

Dysexecutive behavioral disorders are due to different underlying deficits, which are still under study. First, some behavioral disorders are directly related to a cognitive deficit. Perseverations may reflect a deficit of set shifting (Milner, 1963), and distractibility a deficit of selective attention (Godefroy *et al.*, 1996) (see later). The environmental dependency syndrome would be due to a deficit of cognitive control, which results in capture of the behavior by environmental cues (Lhermitte *et al.*, 1986; Shallice *et al.*, 1989). Second, other behavioral changes may reflect disorders in the processing of emotional and social information and this would account for the preservation of routine test performance in some patients with severe behavioral disturbances. In these cases, because of the role of the ventral/medial frontal regions in reward processing, there are behavioral self-regulation problems in situations where cognitive analysis, habit, or environmental cues are not sufficient to determine the most adapted response (Harlow, 1868; Eslinger and Damasio, 1985). According to the somatic marker hypothesis (Damasio *et al.*, 1991; Bechara *et al.*, 1996), decision-making is a process that depends on emotion. Lesions of the ventromedial frontal cortex preclude the ability to use somatic (i.e. emotional) signals that are necessary to guide decisions in the advantageous direction. Patients with ventromedial damage fail to advantageously choose on a specific gambling test and this is correlated with their inability to acquire anticipatory skin conductance responses that are used as an index of somatic state (Bechara *et al.*, 1996). Such impairment might account for the disorders of social conduct and irrational behavior of frontal damaged patients. In the same vein, the ability to use and manipulate information relative to the social domain (such as determining the degree of intimacy between two persons depicted in the videotaped scene) was found to be impaired in frontal damage (Mah *et al.*, 2004) and this promising approach requires further studies.

The impairment of metacognitive abilities, especially "theory of mind," is likely to contribute to behavioral changes. Metacognitive abilities are the awareness of one's own mental states and beliefs, the relationships between these and external events and also the mental state of other people (Frith, 1989; Stuss *et al.*, 2001c). The "theory of mind" is conceived as an awareness of the likely content of other people's minds (Premack and Woodruff, 1978). The mental state attribution underlies the ability to understand and predict other people's behavior. A few studies have shown that frontal damage impairs tasks requiring inference of other people's experience, belief, or intention and the ability to recognize a "faux pas" (Stone *et al.*, 1998; Rowe *et al.*, 2001; Stuss *et al.*, 2001c). There is some suggestion in the literature that the theory of mind and humor may be related more to the polar frontal regions, where emotion and cognition might be integrated (Shammi and Stuss, 1999; Stuss and Alexander, 1999; 2000). The frontal poles (possibly more particularly on the right), are most recently evolved, and appear to bridge behavioral/self-regulatory and executive cognitive functions, because of their unique position to integrate the higher-level cognitive, executive cognitive functions, and emotional or drive-related inputs (Burgess *et al.*, 2005; Stuss and Alexander, 2000).

The cognitive dysexecutive syndrome

The development of neuropsychology has documented numerous cognitive deficits observed on specific tasks. Luria (1966) has suggested that behind the clinical diversity of frontal syndrome, patients were more specifically impaired in situations that require goal formulation, planning, carrying out goal-directed plans, and verification. This approach has been very influential and implicitly assumes that the unity of frontal functions lies in the domain of control functions operating in non-routine situations. Neuropsychological studies of disorders of executive functions have suggested that there is not a unique system controlling all aspects of behavior and cognition, but rather multiple executive processes that could be selectively impaired (Shallice and Burgess, 1996; Godefroy *et al.*, 1999). This accounts for the clinical variability of executive disorders and implies that a single neuropsychological test cannot resume the assessment of executive deficit. The exploration of executive deficit is still ongoing and the present review will

Table 19.2. Main cognitive disorders suggestive of the dysexecutive syndrome

Highly suggestive
Response initiation; response suppression and focused attention
Rule deduction; maintenance and shifting of set
Problem-solving and planning
Information generation

Supportive deficits and developing areas
Tasks coordination and divided attention
Sustained attention and alertness
Working memory deficit: delayed-response task, random generation, updating memory
Strategic mnemonic processes
Use of somatic markers
"Theory of mind"

focus on studies of executive processes closely connected with the assessment of stroke patients. Several theories have proposed an account of the dysexecutive syndrome, such as the model of working memory (Baddeley, 1986; Goldman-Rakic, 1987; Fuster, 1997b) and Shallice's model (Norman and Shallice, 1980; Shallice, 1982) (for a review, see Roberts *et al.*, 1996). From a clinical perspective, the present section will adopt a descriptive approach and reviews the main executive processes that are impaired in stroke patients.

A large number of executive disorders has been suggested from the study of patients and, to simplify routine assessment, a French cooperative group (Godefroy *et al.*, 2004) has proposed a list of the main deficits of executive processes, which distinguishes between highly suggestive and supportive disorders (Table 19.2).

Response initiation and suppression

These deficits are frequently observed during clinical examination when the patient is slow to answer or initiate action and when they are unable to suppress an automatic response. Neuropsychological studies have shown that frontal lesions can cause deficits in both response initiation (assessed by part A of the Trail Making test or by the naming and reading subtests of the Stroop test) and response suppression (assessed by Go/No-go, crossed tapping or Stroop tests) (Luria, 1966; Perret, 1974; Drewe, 1975). Both deficits may coexist and appear to be derived from opposite disorders. The deficit of response initiation would result from an underlying disorder of fast activation of routine response (Stuss *et al.*, 2001a; 2001b; Godefroy *et al.*, 2002). The deficit of response suppression would result from an underlying disorder of inhibition of fast, prepotent response; i.e. the inappropriate use of routine schemas (Burgess and Shallice, 1996a; Godefroy *et al.*, 1996). In addition, the persistent use of inappropriate routine schemas could be secondary to the decreased use of strategy (Burgess and Shallice, 1996a). From an attentional perspective,[1] the deficit of response suppression is interpreted in terms of disorders of selective attention (Posner and Petersen, 1990).

Rule deduction, maintenance and shifting of set, planning and problem-solving

These deficits are considered when patients are unable to cope with a simple problem, use inappropriate rules or make perseverations, especially if they repeatedly use the same rules. These deficits are well known in patients with frontal damage and are frequently assessed using the Wisconsin Card Sorting test. This test requires the patient to sort cards according to rules that have to be generated (color, shape, number) and used according to the examiner's feedback. It has been found to be more frequently impaired in frontal damage (Milner, 1963); it may also be impaired in patients with non-frontal lesions (Anderson *et al.*, 1991), but less so if potential problems in visual search and comprehension are not present (Stuss *et al.*, 2000a). Problem-solving tests such as card sorting, Tower of London (Shallice, 1982) or Six Elements tests (Shallice and Burgess, 1991) involve several executive processes including the generation and deduction of rules, the maintenance and shifting of rules, the ability to use cues to regulate behavior, and the ability to generate and use a strategy (Milner, 1963; Messerli *et al.*, 1979; Owen *et al.*, 1990; Delis *et al.*, 1992; Burgess and Shallice, 1996b; Levine *et al.*, 1998). Since these tests engage multiple and coordinated executive processes, impaired performance cannot be attributed to the deficit of a single process. Rule deduction may be assessed more specifically using some tests such as the Messerli test (Messerli *et al.*, 1979) and the Brixton

---

[1] Recent studies of attention disorders have been deeply influenced by the approach of Posner and Petersen (1990). According to this approach, attention is subdivided in different operations depending on specific networks: orienting to sensory stimuli, maintaining the alert state and executive functions. The network for covert orienting of visual signals involves parietal, thalamic, and mesencephalic regions. The alerting network is involved in maintaining readiness to react and would be supported by the right frontal and parietal lobes and locus coeruleus. The executive-control network is related to the "control of goal-directed behavior, error detection, conflict resolution and inhibition of automatic responses;" it includes frontal midline structures and part of the basal ganglia (Berger and Posner, 2000). We use this approach and add the division of attention, i.e., the ability to perform two tasks, either simultaneously or sequentially, which is not explicitly detailed in the Posner and Petersen review (1990). Thus we review the disorders of sustained attention (and its relation with the deficit of action initiation), selectivity (which is mentioned with the deficit of response suppression), and divided attention (which may be roughly assimilated to the ability to coordinate two tasks).

test (Burgess *et al.*, 1996). Perseverations are observed in a large variety of tests including simple sequencing task tests that require the patient to reproduce simple manual sequences (such as fist—palm—edge). These tests are sensitive (Truelle *et al.*, 1995) but not specific (Jason, 1985) to frontal damage. From a more general point of view, perseverative errors are one particular kind of impairment of action ordering in the correct temporal sequence which has been observed in various tasks (Sirigu *et al.*, 1995).

Deficit of information generation

The impairment on tests of verbal fluency was shown early in neuropsychological studies (Benton, 1968; Ramier and Hécaen, 1970). Briefly, these tests require the patient to produce a large number of words belonging to a category (e.g. animals or words beginning by the letter F) indicated by the examiner in a short time period (usually 1 or 2 minutes). Such a task requires access to lexical information and development of a strategy designed to retrieve the maximum number of words. The use of a strategy mainly depends on integrity of the prefrontal cortex (Stuss *et al.*, 1998).

Divided attention and task coordination

Stroke patients frequently complain of difficulty in performing two tasks simultaneously, suggesting a deficit of divided attention (Martin *et al.*, 2002). Few studies have formally assessed divided attention in patients with focal brain damage. These studies use a dual-task paradigm, which requires the patient to first perform both tasks (e.g., recall of digit series and visuomotor tracking) separately and then perform both tasks simultaneously. The decreased performance observed when both tasks are performed simultaneously is used to assess divided attention. Two studies showed a deficit in patients with frontal lesions (Cowey and Green, 1996; Leclercq *et al.*, 2000) and two studies showed a similar deficit in a subgroup of frontal damaged patients with either lesions including the medial region (Roussel-Pieronne *et al.*, in press), or neurobehavioral changes (Baddeley *et al.*, 1997). Two other studies used a sequential dual-task paradigm (e.g. Umilta *et al.*, 1992), which requires two simple tasks (such as a binary choice task and a recognition task) to be performed separately and then sequentially. Both studies showed that stroke patients with frontal damage are slower to respond in the dual-task condition (Godefroy *et al.*, 1999; Stablum *et al.*, 2000).

These studies indicate that deficits of divided attention and task coordination are observed in a subgroup of frontal damaged patients, especially with medial frontal lesions.

Working memory

Working memory is a system required for temporary storage and cognitive manipulation of information and is discussed in Chapter 21. According to Baddeley's model (Baddeley, 1986), working memory depends on a central system (the central executive) and on slave modality-specific systems that are responsible for the temporary storage of information. Severe impairment of storage capacity, assessed using forward digit span, has been mainly observed in parieto-insular lesions (Shallice and Vallar, 1990). The delayed-response tests, extensively studied in animals (Jacobsen, 1936), are impaired in humans with frontal lesions (D'Esposito and Postle, 1999), but they are rarely used in clinical practice. Some central executive functions have been found to be impaired in frontal damage such as task coordination and response suppression. Other processes are thought to depend on the central executive, such as random generation (Baddeley, 1966; Wiegersma *et al.*, 1990), memory ordering, and updating (Morris and Jones, 1990). The use of these tests in routine evaluation still requires further validation studies.

Sustained attention

Excessive fatigability and inability to maintain ongoing activity are frequently observed in frontal damaged patients. Although this may suggest a deficit of sustained attention, formal assessment has revealed controversial results, as some studies failed to show any deficit (Godefroy *et al.*, 1994), while others showed a deficit in patients with frontal damage (Wilkins *et al.*, 1987; Rueckert and Grafman, 1996) and posterior damage (Rueckert and Grafman, 1998). This issue remains largely unresolved because some studies used tests that failed to measure the temporal decline of performance (Wilkins *et al.*, 1987), with a poor sensitivity (Godefroy *et al.*, 1994), or assessed patients with mixed pathologies including traumatic lesions (Rueckert and Grafman, 1996). A study assessing the ability to sustain alertness (Posner and Petersen, 1990) during a simple detection test showed a disorder in frontal damaged patients (Godefroy *et al.*, 2002). The inability to repeatedly trigger a fast and simple response may underlie the deficit of initiation of action, but this requires further validation studies.

Strategic memory processes

A deficit of episodic memory is frequently observed in stroke patients and is discussed in Chapter 20. Word list learning tasks are used to distinguish between basic associative processes of cue–engram interaction (hippocampus/temporal lobes) and strategic encoding and retrieval process (frontal lobes) (Luria, 1966; Winocur and Moscovitch, 1990; Alexander *et al.*, 2003). The distinction is nicely summarized in the phrase that the frontal lobes "work with memory." In frontal damaged patients, several studies have suggested that disorders of episodic memory are due to impairment of strategic memory processes that are involved in active retrieval and selection of information. These deficits account for the high frequency of impairment of free recall and false recognition (Jetter *et al.*, 1986; Janowsky *et al.*, 1989; Incisa Della Rocchetta and Milner, 1993; Stuss *et al.*, 1994). Such a pattern of performance has been found to be specific to frontal damage (Pillon *et al.*, 1993) and it contributes to the diagnosis of dysexecutive syndrome (O. Godefroy, unpublished study).

A deficit of executive functions would also contribute to the presence of confabulations (Baddeley and Wilson, 1988; Dalla Barba, 1993; Burgess and Shallice, 1996c), especially when the selection of retrieved information according to contextual cues is impaired (Schnider and Ptak, 1999; Schnider *et al.*, 2000).

Response slowing

Response slowing is frequently reported in frontal damage and a recent re-examination has shown that it was the best predictor of frontal stroke, compared to posterior damage (Leskela *et al.*, 1999). The origin of response slowing on many of the measures remains undetermined and is presumably due to multiple factors: subtle perceptual, motor, and cognitive deficits may be responsible as well as attentional deficits. The presence of subtle impairment in dexterity of the ipsilateral hand (Desrosiers *et al.*, 1996; Sunderland *et al.*, 1999) and motor slowing of the affected hand (Cramer *et al.*, 1997) have been observed in stroke patients. Series of stroke patients subjected to reaction time measures have shown that response slowing was present on very simple tasks without additional lengthening with increased task complexity (e.g. Godefroy *et al.*, 1996). Such a pattern suggests the role of an attentional deficit and motor slowing (Godefroy *et al.*, 2002). There is some evidence of lesion specificity in relation to slowing. The majority of patients who were slow on simple and complex RT tasks had superior medial pathology, the region associated with activation, and in more severe lesions, with clinical syndromes such as abulia (Stuss *et al.*, 2002; Stuss *et al.*, 2005; Alexander *et al.*, 2005). Perhaps most surprisingly, many patients with other executive disorders had no significant slowing, again reflecting our proposal of increasing specificity in executive disorder assessment. According to Stuss *et al.* (2002), response slowing in patients with superior medial frontal damage is related to a deficit of an activation regulating function. Activation plays a key role in self-regulation. It is likely that much of the slowing seen in different frontal patients reflects this disorder of activation. Severe impairment results in global hypoactivity with apathy–abulia. Activation regulating functions deserve further specific study.

Key points Main characteristics of executive dysfunction

Executive functions: control functions especially involved in non-routine situations
Dysfunctions: induced various associations of behavioral and cognitive disorders including:
  behavioral changes: abulia, apathy, aspontaneity, loss of "psychic autoactivation,"
  distractibility, impulsivity, disinhibition, perseveration, stereotypic behavior,
  anosognosia, disturbances of emotion and social behavior, confabulations
  cognitive disorders: rule deduction, suppression of overlearned responses and selective
  attention, maintenance and shifting of set, information generation, divided attention
  and tasks coordination, planning and problem solving, response initiation –
  maintaining an alert state and sustained attention, strategic mnemonic processes

---

Executive disorders and stroke

Prevalence and determinants of the dysexecutive syndrome

Disorders of executive functions are frequently observed in stroke, regardless of its mechanism, as shown by several series of consecutive patients. These studies have generally been performed several months post-stroke in consecutive patients able to complete the battery of tests. These studies differ according to the time of assessment, patient selection (ischemic, hemorrhagic, postaneurysmal, or mixed causes of stroke), exclusion of demented patients, the battery of tests, and the criterion of deficit (a difference of 1 or 1.5 standard deviations from the mean value observed in controls; percentile 10 or 5). These methodological differences contribute to discrepancies in the prevalence of executive deficit. However, they provide convergent results supporting the high frequency of executive and attentional disorders in stroke.

Published studies provide a consistent picture of the high frequency of executive deficit across various types of stroke with about 20% of patients suffering from a deficit of rule deduction, abstract reasoning or set shifting, and with about 40% of patients suffering from response slowing, possibly secondary to attention disorder. In addition, these studies indicate that these impairments, although demonstrated on neuropsychological tests, are associated with disability in instrumental activities of daily living. To our knowledge, a systematic formal assessment of behavioral changes has not been performed. However, the Lausanne Emotion in Acute Stroke Study showed that disinhibition (defined by inappropriate jokes or laughing, or disinhibition) and indifference (defined by apathy, neglect in self-care, or a tendency to stay isolated) were observed in 38% of patients examined within the first four days post-stroke (Ghika-Schmid *et al.*, 1999). This high frequency may be attributable to numerous factors, and especially to the patient's experience of an acute disease. Apart from the high frequency of response slowing, a dominant pattern of executive deficit does not emerge from a review of the literature. The pattern of executive deficit is likely to depend mainly on the site of the lesion.

Several factors account for the development of executive deficit. The stroke site is usually considered to be the main determinant. Infarcts involve the frontal lobe with a high frequency estimated between 20% and 25% (Bogousslavsky, 1994; Leskela *et al.*, 1999). In addition, patients with a posterior stroke may present a prior stroke involving the frontal region with a frequency as high as 30% (Leskela *et al.*, 1999). However, a high frequency of frontal stroke is unlikely to exclusively account for the high frequency of executive deficit in stroke. Several studies have shown that anterior *and* posterior strokes result in impaired performance on tests of executive functions (e.g. Leskela *et al.*, 1999). Subcortical stroke involving the fronto-subcortical circuits (i.e. caudate nucleus, pallidum, thalamus, anterior centrum semiovale, anterior limb and genu of the internal capsule) proposed by Alexander and co-workers (1986) may contribute to the development of executive deficit. Fronto-subcortical connections include five parallel but independent circuits defined by their distinct major reciprocal subcortical connections (Alexander *et al.*, 1986; 1990; Cummings, 1993; Saint-Cyr, 2003). The cognitive aspects of executive functions are mainly supported by the circuit from the dorsolateral frontal cortex, and the behavioral component by the lateral orbital and medial frontal/anterior cingulate circuits. According to this approach, damage anywhere in each circuit will produce similar deficits. Although this approach fits well with data from degenerative diseases, the real consequence of subcortical stroke involving fronto-subcortical circuits on executive functions remains to be firmly established (Leskela *et al.*, 1999). Stroke location is not the sole determinant of executive deficit: white matter abnormalities (Ishii *et al.*, 1986; Pohjasvaara *et al.*, 2000; Mungas *et al.*, 2001; O'Brien *et al.*, 2002; Tullberg *et al.*, 2004), medial temporal atrophy (Vataja *et al.*, 2003) and pre-stroke cognitive disorders (Hénon *et al.*, 1997) also contribute to post-stroke executive deficit.

The presence of executive dysfunction on neuropsychological tests is associated in many cases with a poor functional outcome, as shown by the close connection with difficulties in Instrumental Activities of Daily Living in ischemic stroke (Pohjasvaara *et al.*, 2002; Sachdev *et al.*, 2004). An important area of future research is the understanding of potentially more precise relationships between specific executive disorders and daily life.

The dysexecutive syndrome and stroke characteristics

Disorders of executive functions have been studied more extensively in certain varieties of stroke.

Cerebral infarct and hemorrhage

A high frequency of executive and attentional disorders has been observed in ischemic strokes (Tatemichi *et al.*, 1994; Pohjasvaara *et al.*, 2002; Ballard *et al.*, 2003; Sachdev *et al.*, 2004) and mixed ischemic—hemorrhagic strokes (Hochstenbach *et al.*, 1998; Rasquin *et al.*, 2004). On tests assessing abstract reasoning, a deficit was observed in 20—30% of patients. In time-constrained tests, the deficit was much more frequent, observed in 33—60% on verbal fluency and attentional tests (Tatemichi *et al.*, 1994; Hochstenbach *et al.*, 1998; Ballard *et al.*, 2003; Rasquin *et al.*, 2004). A study using a global score of executive functions summarizing performance on verbal fluency, Wisconsin, Stroop interference and Trail Making B tests has shown a deficit in 41% of patients (Pohjasvaara *et al.*, 2002). These impressive frequencies decrease on retesting performed 6 months to 4 years post-stroke, suggesting that the deficit improves in about 25—30% of patients (Rasquin *et al.*, 2002; Hochstenbach *et al.*, 2003). However, a deficit of executive functions, motor speed, and episodic memory is still frequently observed in studies concerning long-term stroke survivors (Engstad *et al.*, 2003). This indicates that a large percentage of patients still suffer from attentional and executive disorders in the long term.

Territorial infarct

Executive deficits have been studied in infarcts in the territory of the middle and anterior cerebral arteries and in the anterior thalamus.

Middle cerebral artery (MCA) infarct   An infarct can involve significant lateral frontal convexity areas, those regions most often associated with cognitive executive deficits. Infarcts restricted to the superior—anterior branch of the middle cerebral artery induce a relatively pure frontal lateral infarct (albeit usually extending into the anterior parietal area) and they have been favored in studies of executive deficits. The executive deficit is usually prominent on the cognitive domain and may be especially marked on tests assessing rule deduction, maintenance and shifting of rules (such as the Wisconsin Card Sorting test), information generation (such as verbal fluency test), and maintenance of information in working memory. Conversely, the behavioral dysexecutive syndrome is frequently moderate and can even be absent. Global hypoactivity with abulia—apathy is the most frequent disorder and must be distinguished from depression which is frequently observed in stroke (Starkstein *et al.*, 1988) and in dominant hemisphere infarct, from mild aphasia. Hyperactivity with very mild distractibility—impulsivity may also be observed. The dysexecutive syndrome is rarely pure, especially at the acute stage, and is frequently associated with aphasic, perceptual, and constructional disorders that must be taken into account in the interpretation of cognitive and behavioral deficits.

However, MCA infarcts are not often restricted to the frontal lobes: cortical infarcts frequently concern both the superior and inferior (supplying the lateral part of the parietal and temporal lobes) territories of the MCA leading to classical left or right hemisphere syndrome (see Chapter 32). Second, infarcts in the subcortical territory of the MCA (deep branches, also called lenticulo-striate arteries) usually involve the dorsolateral caudate, dorsolateral anterior limb of the internal capsule, putamen (with a typical comma shape) and centrum semiovale (Figure 19.1). As noted above, stroke of this region can also result in deficits similar to those seen after frontal damage. The frontal dorsolateral convexity can be spared, but damage to deep frontal white matter can affect the connections from prefrontal convexity to posterior cortical regions, the ipsilateral medial frontal lobe, and the contralateral frontal lobe. This accounts for the presence of mild executive deficits in lenticulo-striate infarct, which may be associated with aphasia in left-sided stroke. Behavioral changes are usually minor in pure unilateral infarct: global hypoactivity with abulia—apathy or hyperactivity with distractibility—impulsivity may be observed (Mendez *et al.*, 1989; Caplan *et al.*, 1990; Pedrazzi *et al.*, 1990; Godefroy *et al.*, 1992). Cognitive executive deficits are usually very mild in pure unilateral lenticulo-striate infarct and concern tests assessing response activation and suppression, information generation, and rule deduction (Weiller *et al.*, 1990; Godefroy *et al.*, 1992). Bilateral infarcts due to anoxia (which are usually larger than the territory of the lenticulo-striate artery) are the usual cause of a behavioral disorder called "loss of psychic autoactivation" by Laplane *et al.* (1981; see also Habib and Poncet, 1988). This disorder results in severe global hypoactivity with abulia—apathy (usually associated with "empty mind") which is reversed by heteroactivation (usually following instructions from the examiner or the care-giver). This disorder, frequently confused with depression, results in severe loss of autonomy. The severity of behavioral changes contrasts with the relatively mild intensity of cognitive deficit on tests of executive functions and episodic memory and the relative preservation of other cognitive domains, contrary to the usual pattern of anoxic encephalopathy. This disorder has also been reported in bithalamic infarct (Bogousslavsky *et al.*, 1991).

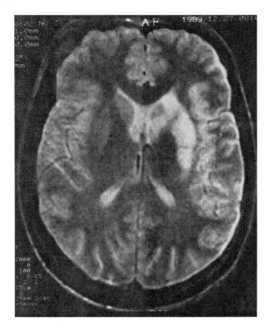

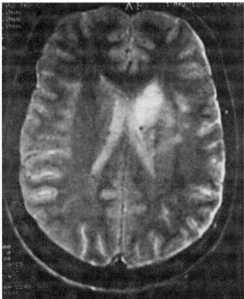

Figure 19.1 Lenticulostriate infarct (deep branch of the middle cerebral artery) with a typical comma shape. This right-handed 26-year-old woman (schooling: 11 years) was examined 6 months poststroke. Mini Mental State: 29/30. Transcortical motor aphasia of minor severity. Digit span: 4. Episodic memory, Trail Making test and Modified Card Sorting test: Normal. Minor behavioral changes (abulia).

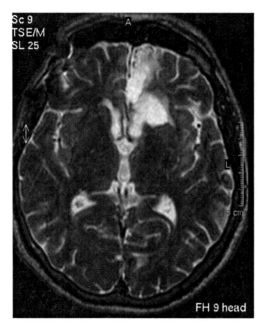

Figure 19.2 Anterior cerebral artery infarct in the superficial and deep (mediostriate arteries) territories. The lesion secondary to a ruptured anterior communicating artery aneurysm also involves the ventral striatum and basal forebrain. This right-handed 50-year-old patient (schooling: 6 years) was examined 2 years poststroke. Mini Mental State: 24/30. Digit span: 4. Response slowing on all tests. Stroop test: 21% errors (impaired) on the interference subtest. Modified Card Sorting test: 2 categories achieved with 21 errors (impaired). Episodic memory: Normal except for impaired free delayed recall.

Anterior cerebral artery (ACA) infarct This is a major, albeit rare, cause of the behavioral dysexecutive syndrome (Figure 19.2). Again, the extent of the damage is relevant, since ACA infarction can include the orbital cortex, frontal pole, anterior cingulate, and/or supplementary motor area. The lesions are bilateral when both ACAs arise from the same internal carotid artery. Involvement of the anterior corpus callosum may aggravate deficits caused by damage to the medial frontal cortex. Because ACA infarcts are rare, the pattern of dysexecutive syndrome remains poorly documented. In unilateral infarct, mild disorders of executive functions have been reported in case series usually associated with aphasia or hemineglect, and rarely with alien hand sign and diagonistic apraxia. Bilateral infarcts result frequently in akinetic mutism and, after the acute phase, the persistence of severe behavioral executive disorders is frequent and compromises autonomy (Bogousslavsky, 1994; Kumral *et al.*, 2002). Involvement of the deep territory of the ACA (especially the artery of Heubner) may damage the "limbic caudate" and thalamofrontal connections. Anterior communicating artery aneurysm (see later), a common cause of ACA infarction, may also affect the septal nuclei.

Anterior thalamic infarcts   In the territory of the tuberothalamic and paramedian arteries, infarcts are frequently claimed to cause executive deficits, although series of consecutive patients systematically assessed by neuropsychological tests remain rare (for reviews, see Bogousslavsky *et al.*, 1988; Van der Werf *et al.*, 2000; Schmahmann, 2003). The tuberothalamic artery (also called the thalamo-polar artery) arises from the posterior communicating artery. It is absent in nearly one-third of the normal population, in which case its territory is supplied by the paramedian artery (Percheron, 1976a; Bogousslavsky *et al.*, 1986). The paramedian artery (also called the thalamoperforating pedicle) arises from the proximal part of the posterior cerebral artery, close to arteries supplying the midbrain (paramedian mesencephalic pedicle) and this accounts for the frequent association with midbrain infarct (responsible for associated signs, especially vertical gaze palsy) (Percheron, 1976b). Each paramedian artery usually arises from the unilateral posterior cerebral artery, but they may also arise from a common trunk off one posterior cerebral artery. This accounts for the frequency of bilateral infarcts in the paramedian territory.

In anterior thalamic infarct, behavioral disorders are a classical component of the clinical picture at the acute phase. In unilateral lesions, they are usually of mild intensity and consist of global hypoactivity with abulia—apathy or less frequently impulsivity and disinhibition (Bogousslavsky *et al.*, 1986; Ghika-Schmid and Bogousslavsky, 2000; Van der Werf *et al.*, 2003). Perseveration and increased sensitivity to interference have also been observed, as well as disorders of temporal organization and coordination of actions (Ghika-Schmid and Bogousslavsky, 2000). In bilateral paramedian infarct, the picture is more severe with impaired consciousness at the acute phase and akinetic mutism. After the acute stage, mild behavioral disorders may persist. In patients with global hypoactivity, the possible role of hypersomnia has to be assessed, since it may contribute to difficulties in daily living, especially in bilateral paramedian infarcts.

Tests assessing executive functions may also be impaired in thalamic infarct. In the review by Van der Werf *et al.* (2000), about one-half of patients with anterior infarct and one-third of patients with infarct in the middle part of the thalamus had impaired executive functions. Impairment of executive functions and response speed was found to depend on several structures including the mediodorsal nucleus and internal medullary lamina (Van der Werf *et al.*, 2003). Executive disorders are usually associated with aphasia, or hemineglect and episodic memory deficit that must be taken into account when interpreting the tests. Follow-up examinations have shown that spectacular improvement is possible within a few months, even in patients with bilateral infarct (Krolak-Salmon et al., 2000). However, the persistence of mild behavioral changes, especially global hypoactivity with apathy or "loss of psychic autoactivation," is frequently reported (Bogousslavsky et al., 1991), as well as memory deficit. Outcome of cognitive executive deficit requires further studies. Persistent behavioral and cognitive disorders may be severe, especially in bilateral infarcts and they fit the criteria of so-called "thalamic dementia."

Lacunar infarcts

The presence of executive dysfunction is frequently claimed in patients with lacunar infarcts. This impairment was initially documented in a descriptive study of multiple lacunes (Wolfe et al., 1990). It has been supported by recent studies comparing subcortical ischemic vascular disease with either normal controls (Kramer et al., 2002) or other stroke types (Pohjasvaara et al., 2003). Although the presence of cognitive executive deficit in lacunes is well documented, its mechanism depends on several factors, as shown by recent studies. A first account highlights the prominence of lacunes in the basal ganglia and thalamus (Ishii et al., 1986), structures that are closely interconnected with the frontal lobes. Consistently, infarcts involving the fronto-subcortical loops (Alexander et al., 1986) (i.e. frontal cortex, caudate nucleus, pallidum, thalamus, genu and anterior limb of the internal capsule, and anterior centrum semiovale) were found to be more frequent in patients with executive dysfunction, a finding not subjected to multivariate analysis (Vataja et al., 2003). However, small vessel diseases, which are the usual cause of lacunes, are also associated with other cerebral abnormalities, such as white matter signal hyperintensities, reduced volume of cortical gray matter and medial temporal atrophy (Du et al., 2002). Studies performed in ischemic stroke (Vataja et al., 2003) and subcortical ischemic vascular disease (Mungas et al., 2001; Tullberg et al., 2004) showed that independent predictors of executive deficits were white matter lesions and cerebral atrophy but not lacunes (Mungas et al., 2001; Vataja et al., 2003; Tullberg et al., 2004). These results indicate that lacunes are a marker of pathology responsible for different lesions which contribute to executive deficit.

Subarachnoid hemorrhage

In subarachnoid hemorrhage, the frequency of executive deficit varies across studies: (1) on tests assessing abstract reasoning, a deficit was observed in 13–26%

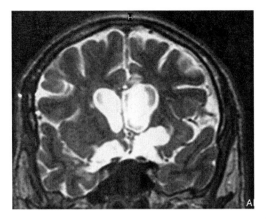

Figure 19.3 Frontobasal damage following rupture aneurysm of the anterior communicating artery. This right handed 42 year-old woman (schooling: 10 years) was examined 2 years following the treatment (clipping) of the ruptured aneurysm. She was not depressed and still complained from difficulties interfering with lifestyle (Rankin: 2) and quality of life. The MiniMental State was normal (29/30); significant impairment was observed on episodic memory (including recognition), copy of Rey Complex figure (18/36), whereas language assessment including verbal fluency was normal. Behavioral disorders were significant but restricted to a deficit of action initiation. Stroop and Trail Making tests were slowed and impairment was observed on the Modified Card Sorting test (5 categories achieved with 6 errors) and the dual task test.

of patients, and (2) on attentional tests, in 38–76% of patients (Ogden *et al.*, 1993; Kreiter *et al.*, 2002; Mayer *et al.*, 2002). Thus, a deficit in the domain of executive functions has been observed in 18–51% of patients (Ljunggren *et al.*, 1985; Hütter and Gilsbach 1993; Tidswell *et al.*, 1995; Mayer *et al.*, 2002; for a review, see Hütter, 2000). These deficits are observed in the postoperative period with intervals varying from 10 weeks to 2 years. The comparison between pre- and post-operative status in a small sample showed a significant albeit marginal decrease of performance, suggesting that treatment (mainly surgery) may contribute to cognitive deficit (Hillis *et al.*, 2000).

Executive deficits have been especially examined in patients with complicated rupture of an *anterior communicating artery aneurysm*. This pathology may induce lesions in frontal (especially in ventromedial and superior-medial regions), subcortical (ventral part of the head of the caudate nucleus and anterior limb of the internal capsule see Figure 19.2), basal forebrain (which includes septal nuclei) (see Figure 19.4) and anterior part of the corpus callosum regions. The disorder mainly concerns behavior, attention (especially selective attention as assessed by the Stroop task and divided attention as assessed by a dual-task

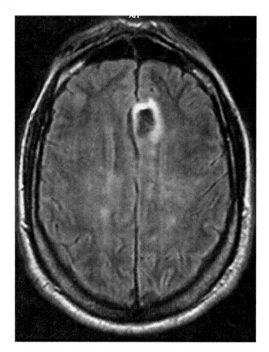

Figure 19.4 Spontaneous hemorrhage in the superior medial frontal region. This right-handed 43-year-old patient (schooling: 8 years) was examined 3 months poststroke. Progressive matrices: 20/47 (impaired). Digit span: 4. Rey Complex figure: copy: 19/36 (impaired). Response slowing on all tests. Stroop test: 85% errors (impaired) on the interference subtest. Modified Card Sorting test: 6 categories achieved with 20 errors (impaired). Episodic memory: impairment of free recall with normal recognition.

paradigm), and episodic memory with differing patterns (Jetter *et al.*, 1986; Stuss *et al.*, 1994; Wheeler *et al.*, 1995). Behavioral executive disorders include hypoactivity with abulia—apathy, hyperactivity with distractibility—disinhibition, perseveration and stereotypy, anosognosia, disturbances of emotion and social behavior, confabulation, and reduplicative paramnesia. These disorders may be observed in the same patient. A common situation is the observation of hypoactivity (even akinetic mutism) at the acute phase, followed by the progressive development of hyperactivity. Conversely the cognitive dysexecutive syndrome is usually mild except for the deficit of attention and response suppression; it may even be completely absent (pure behavioral dysexecutive syndrome). This stresses the need to formally assess behavioral changes in this pathology. Language, perceptual, and constructional abilities are usually spared. Although general intellectual abilities are frequently claimed to be spared, a mild decline on screening tests (such as the Mini Mental Status Examination) or batteries (such as the Wechsler Adult Intelligence Scale) is frequently observed in severely impaired patients (Rousseaux *et al.*, 1996).

Other Types of Stroke

In arteriovenous malformations, a few studies have shown the presence of attentional and executive deficits within the year post-surgery (Mahalick *et al.*, 1993) (Figure 19.4). In cerebral venous thrombosis, systematic assessment of cognitive deficits was performed in one study, which did not include attentional and memory assessment (De Bruijn *et al.*, 2000; Buccino *et al.*, 2003). A small unpublished study using a complete neuropsychological battery showed a similar pattern to that observed in arterial stroke with a high frequency of executive, attentional and memory deficits (J. M. Bugnicourt and O. Godefroy, personal communication). The authors also observed a few cases of severe and relatively isolated executive deficit in patients with frontal stroke due to superior sagittal sinus thrombosis.

Key points Main types of stroke associated to the dysexecutive syndrome

Stroke type	Territory/characteristics
Arterial infarct	Middle cerebral artery: deep and anterior branches
	Anterior cerebral artery
	Thalamus: Paramedian and tuberothalamic arteries
Ruptured aneurysm	Anterior communicating artery; pericallosal artery
Hemorrhage	Frontal, striatum and thalamus
Cerebral venous thrombosis	Superior sagittal sinus
Vascular dementia	Subcortical ischemic vascular disease

Assessment of executive disorders in stroke

Bedside neurobehavioral examination

A very important clinical tool is a thorough history. Evidence that there has been a major change in personality and behavior is essential. The basic neurological examination of patients with executive dysfunction, particularly when the pathology is not diffuse, is often normal. Nevertheless, careful assessment of motor function, including spontaneity of movement, can be revealing. Paresis and motor weakness are present if the damage involves the frontal motor regions, and may depend on the subcortical extent of the lesion; in many instances, the motor examination may be normal. Dorsolateral frontal damage may impair exploratory eye movements (frontal eye fields), but this is primarily intentional and not usually evident on routine testing of pursuit and saccadic eye movements. Certain reflexes may be present but are not necessarily diagnostic. A grasp reflex of varying severity, contralateral to supplementary motor area lesions, is frequent, although it may disappear with time. Sucking and rooting reflexes, inhibited after infancy, may re-emerge due to damage to frontal inhibition. Such frontal release signs (snout or glabellar) have been reported in up to 45% of non-demented stroke patients (Tatemichi *et al.*, 1993). Bilateral medial lesions, usually involving the supplementary motor area, can produce full akinetic mutism, reduced spontaneous movement, including speech. There are also lesser forms, such as hypokinesia—bradykinesia. Oppositional (increase in tone occurring in response to passive movement) and facilitatory (when the patient acts in the same direction as the passive movement) paratonia are well-known consequences of frontal damage, but have been especially observed in diffuse pathology (Beversdorf and Heilman, 1998). Careful analysis of language may reveal digressions, perseverations, stereotypy of speech, loss of prosody, and echolalia. These abnormalities may coexist with a transcortical motor aphasia (usually associated with global hypoactivity and aspontaneity), or with unceasing speech (usually associated with global hyperactivity).

Assessment of behavioral abnormalities includes analysis of orienting reaction, response rapidity, abulia, loss of spontaneity, restlessness, reactions to the environment, perseverations, stereotypic behavior and the presence of abnormal imitation or prehension, manipulation and utilization of objects. Sensory examination, including visual field testing, is usually normal, although there may be contralateral inattention resulting in reduced orienting and response to sensory or visual stimuli. For the rest of the bedside examination, clinical tools based on neuropsychological research may be useful, such as motor sequences (fist—palm—edge), crossed tapping ("tap once in response to a double tone and tap twice in response to a single tone") or Go/No-go ("tap once in response to a double tone and do not respond to a single tone"), word generation (verbal fluency), and word list learning. In most cases, neuropsychological examination is necessary to probe the details and specific characteristics of a potential dysexecutive disorder.

Neuropsychological assessment

There is no test that uniquely specifies executive disorder. All classical tests can be impaired due to even subtle impairments in language, memory, perception, attention, motivation, or effort. Nevertheless, several tests have a high specificity for frontal impairments when these posterior functions are intact. Moreover, recent research has helped to distinguish between various disorders. Our current knowledge of the dysexecutive syndrome allows us to assess the problems in a logical manner that was not feasible in the age when the disorder was viewed as unitary (considering the multiple advances in the past few years, it is highly likely that further refinement is possible). The ultimate rationale for this more targeted approach to the assessment of executive disorders is that it has the potential to guide management and treatment. An important corollary to this approach is that not all executive disorders will be seen after every stroke, and that lesion site is a relevant, albeit not the only, consideration. The following domains of assessment are proposed, following the classifications outlined above.

Behavioral dysexecutive disturbances

Several questionnaires are directed at identifying behavioral changes, and have had some success in various brain-damaged populations. The Behavioral Dyscontrol Scale (Grigsby et al., 1998), based on Luria's theory, includes tasks assessing both executive cognitive functions and self-regulatory behaviors. Personality changes can be assessed by the NeuroPsychiatric Inventory (Cummings et al., 1994) and the Frontal Lobe Personality Scale (Malloy and Richardson, 1994; Grace et al., 1999), which characterizes the various types of behavioral change described above. The Behavioral Assessment of the Dysexecutive Syndrome includes a questionnaire and six tests assessing executive functions (Wilson et al., 1996; 1998) and has been used in mixed pathologies (Burgess et al., 1998). A questionnaire developed by a French-speaking cooperative group based on diagnostic criteria of the behavioral syndrome is currently in the validation phase (Godefroy et al., 2004).

Executive cognitive functions

Executive cognitive functions (dorsolateral frontal circuitry) are those involved in the control and direction (activating, inhibiting, deduction, generation, maintenance and shifting of set, planning) of lower levels of automatic functions. Several measures are most frequently considered "cognitive executive," since they correspond to the above definition and are also generally not sensitive to orbitofrontal/ventral medial pathology (Stuss et al., 2001b; Stuss and Levine, 2002; Stuss et al., 2002). Commonly used tests are the Wisconsin Card Sorting Test, Trail Making Test Part B, Stroop test, and certain measures of verbal fluency tasks, but it is important to understand the limitations of these multi-factorial measures (Stuss et al., 2002; Stuss et al., 2001a,b; Troyer et al., 1998). Measures directed to isolate processes such as inhibition have more recently been devised and are in clinical usage (Burgess and Shallice, 1996a). The word list learning task can be used to demonstrate impairment of strategic encoding

Key points Assessment of executive dysfunction in stroke

Clinical examination
Clinical assessment of behavior
Grasp and sucking reflexes
Facilitatory and oppositional paratonia
Imitation and utilization behavior
Motor sequences (fist—palm—edge)
Crossed tapping or go/no-go
Word generation (verbal fluency)

Behavioral changes
Behavioral inventory: e.g., behavioral dyscontrol scale, neuropsychiatric inventory, frontal
lobe personality scale, behavioral assessment of the dysexecutive syndrome,
GREFEX inventory

Cognitive disorders
Verbal fluency, Stroop, trail making test, card sorting test
Episodic memory and strategic mnemonic processes

Optional and developing area
Divided attention: dual tasks test
Planning and problem solving: six element test, tower of London/Toronto
Reaction time tests (sustaining of attention)
Gambling task
Metacognitive processes

and retrieval processes (Luria, 1966; Winocur and Moscovitch, 1990; Alexander *et al.*, 2003). Dual-task tests are used to assess divided attention and task coordination. The role of the frontal lobes in working memory involves manipulation and control of information held on-line (Baddeley, 1986). The latest updates of the Wechsler Instruments have added new tasks stressing manipulation and control and even allow for a separate "working memory" composite score.

Optional and experimental assessments of executive dysfunction

Although behavioral questionnaires and previous tests are used routinely, they may fail to capture a selective or minor deficit. In addition, the domain is rapidly evolving and recent advances are likely to influence clinical assessment in the coming years. For these reasons, we mention additional tests here.

Several tasks have been devised to assess the difficulty encountered by patients with damage to the inferior medial frontal cortex to understand the *emotional consequences* of their behavior: gambling tasks (Bechara *et al.*, 1998; Rogers *et al.*, 1999), and naturalistic multiple subgoal tasks (Goel *et al.*, 1997; Burgess *et al.*, 1998; 2000; Levine *et al.*, 1995; 1997; 2000). These tasks remain experimental in nature, but are promising to provide quantitative measures of what is seen qualitatively. Tests evaluating the acquisition and reversal of *stimulus—reward associations* can be used, because of the role of the ventral prefrontal cortex in basic drives and rewards that help direct high-level decision-making (Fuster, 1997a; Rolls, 2000). It is possible to dissociate this affectively based reversal learning (interpreted as affective) from the impairment in attentional set-shifting more frequently associated with dorsolateral frontal lesions (Dias *et al.*, 1996; 1997). This finding further strengthens the distinction between cognitive and affective/emotional behavioral measures of executive disorder.

Mild disorders of *activation regulating function* are difficult to assess in clinical practice. Various tests can be used, including several bedside tests, to assess the capacity to rapidly generate and maintain actions or mental processes. Patients with damage to left or right medial (anterior cingulate and superior) frontal regions are slow in reaction time (RT) tasks (particularly if more demanding), are deficient in generating lists of words (particularly in the first 15 seconds), and have problems maintaining a selected target, such as in the Stroop interference test when the interference task is presented in a blocked format (Stuss *et al.*, 1998; 2001b; 2002). Reaction time tasks may be best, since they are more specific to activation deficit. Falling under the broad category of executive cognitive functions are *mechanisms of attention*, such as sustaining attention, monitoring information and variability in RT performance (Deutsch *et al.*, 1987; Wilkins *et al.*, 1987; Stuss *et al.*, 1989; Glosser and Goodglass, 1990; Godefroy *et al.*, 1996; Rueckert and Grafman, 1996; Robertson *et al.*, 1996; 1997; Godefroy *et al.*, 1999; Stuss *et al.*, 2005). Many of these findings have been revealed with experimental tests and are not in common clinical usage. Nevertheless, dissociations within frontal regions on different anterior attentional processes have been demonstrated, and will eventually be included in standard assessments (Stuss *et al.*, 2002; Stuss *et al.*, 2005).

The neuropsychological assessments of *metacognitive processes* are generally experimental, despite their importance. They include reactions to verbal and cartoon humor (Shammi and Stuss, 1999; Goel and Dolan, 2001), visual perspective taking tasks (Stone *et al.*, 1998; Stuss *et al.*, 2001c), and comparison of performance on remember—know memory tasks (Wheeler and Stuss, 2003). It is important to note that some individuals can solve these tasks on the basis of factual knowledge, not inference. Family reports often precisely describe the changes in behavior that have occurred: lack of empathy, unconcern, and inability to appreciate humor that requires self-reflection. In the absence of being able to use objective measures, an excellent history taken from both the patient and the family is the key.

Management and treatment

To our knowledge, class I randomized controlled trials addressing adequately the efficacy of pharmacological and rehabilitation treatment remain limited in the field of executive and attentional dysfunctions, especially in stroke (Lincoln *et al.*, 2000; Fleminger *et al.*, 2003; Forsyth and Jayamoni, 2003). The limited number of rehabilitation studies is due to the difficulty of establishing an operational definition of exactly which "executive disorders" need to be treated. Until the processes are specifically defined, specific rehabilitation procedures cannot be developed. Moreover, the relationship between the specific executive dysfunction and the impact on different aspects of daily life also remains to be determined. Nevertheless, the growing precision in the characterization of the severity and breadth of the disorder presents guidelines for prognosis and management. Three types of treatments have been utilized: pharmacological, cognitive, and compensatory.

Pharmacological treatment

Pharmacological intervention has been used in rare clinical trials for some behavioral disorders similar to those observed in dysexecutive syndrome. Most of them have been conducted in nonstroke patients, mainly suffering from closed head injury and dementia. Target disorders are either apathy–motivational deficit and akinetic mutism, or impulsivity–disinhibition–agitation. In apathy and motivational deficit, bromocriptine, amantadine and methylphenidate have been tried on the assumption that ascending monoamine pathways are damaged. Some studies concerning single cases, open trials (e.g. Powell *et al.*, 1996) and a double-blind placebo-controlled crossover trial (McDowell *et al.*, 1998) have reported significant behavioral improvement, sometimes maintained after bromocriptine withdrawal (Powell *et al.*, 1996). Benefit in everyday life activities remains to be examined. The same applies to methylphenidate (Forsyth and Jayamoni 2003). These promising results indicate the need for large randomized controlled trials. In patients with impulsivity, disinhibition, and agitation frequently due to traumatic brain injury, studies mainly based on open trials have reported the efficacy of beta-blockers (especially propranolol) (Shankle *et al.*, 1995), carbamazepine (Tariot *et al.*, 1998; Azouvi *et al.*, 1999; Tariot *et al.*, 1999), divalproate (Chatham Showalter and Kimmel, 2000), sertraline (Kant *et al.*, 1998), and clozapine (Michals *et al.*, 1993). However the Cochrane review (Fleminger *et al.*, 2003) highlights the need for better evaluations of drugs for these disorders.

Cognitive rehabilitation

Much effort has been directed to cognitive therapy attempting to improve executive dysfunction through drills or training of defective functions such as planning, sequencing, or problem-solving. A promising approach has been goal management therapy, specifically designed to address the problem of goal-directedness. The major objective of this therapy is to train individuals to stop and think before acting. Success in these cases may be assisted when the individual can use other abilities to help (self-talk — Stuss *et al.*, 1987). The rehabilitation of attentional disorders was found to improve measures of sustained attention and alertness (e.g. Stablum *et al.*, 2000), but with no evidence for significant improvement in everyday life activities according to the Cochrane review (Lincoln *et al.*, 2000).

Compensatory approach

In many cases, a compensatory approach is required. In a sense, this approach is directed to externalizing the support required for executive functioning, which in the frontal lobe literature has been called "becoming the frontal lobes" of the patient. The goals are to construct an environmental compensation that allows greater functional independence, limiting disability or handicap. There is no claim that executive dysfunction itself is treated. A similar but not identical approach has been used to address the problems in interpersonal relationships relative to problems in theory of mind. The first step is to ensure that the significant other (spouse, partner, sibling) is fully informed of the nature of the disorder.

Key points Management and treatment of executive dysfunction

Pharmacotherapy : possible interest in some patients but further trials required
apathy and akinetic mutism: bromocriptine, amantadine or methylphenidate
impulsivity, disinhibition and agitation: propanolol, carbamazepine,
divalproate, sertraline

Cognitive rehabilitation: further trials required
Goal management therapy
Rehabilitation of attentional disorders

Compensatory approach

REFERENCES

Alexander, G. E., Crutcher, M. D. and Delong, M. R. (1990). Basal ganglia-thalamocortical circuits: Parallel substrates for motor, oculomotor, 'prefrontal' and 'limbic' functions. *Prog. Brain Res.*, **85**, 119–46.

Alexander, G. E., DeLong, M. R. and Strick, P. L. (1986). Parallel organization of functionally segregated circuits linking basal ganglia and cortex. *Annu. Rev. Neurosci.*, **9**, 357–81.

Alexander, M. P., Stuss, D. T. and Fansabedian, N. (2003). California Verbal Learning Test: Performance by patients with focal frontal and non-frontal lesions. *Brain*, **126**, 1493–503.

Anderson, S. W., Damasio, H., Jones, R. D. and Tranel, D. (1991). Wisconsin Card Sorting Test performance as a measure of frontal lobe damage. *J. Clin. Exp. Neuropsychol.*, **13**, 909–22.

Azouvi, P., Jokic, C., Attal, N., *et al.* (1999). Carbamazepine in agitation and aggressive behaviour following severe closed-head injury: Results of an open trial. *Brain Inj.*, **13**, 797–804.

Alexander, M. P., Stuss, D. T., Shallice, T., Picton, T. W., and Gillingham, S. (2005). Impaired concentration due to frontal lobe damage from two distinct lesion sites. *Neurology*, **65**, 572–9.

Baddeley, A. D. (1966). The capacity for generating information by randomization. *Q. J. Exp. Psychol.*, **18**, 119–29.

(1986). *Working Memory*. New York: Oxford University Press.

Baddeley, A., Della Sala, S., Papagno, C. and Spinnler, H. (1997). Dual task performance in dysexecutive and non-dysexecutive patients with a frontal lesion. *Neuropsychology*, **11**, 187–94.

Baddeley, A. and Wilson, B. (1988). Frontal amnesia and the dysexecutive syndrome. *Brain Cogn.*, **7**, 212–30.

Ballard, C., Stephens, S., Kenny, R., *et al.* (2003). Profile of neuropsychological deficits in older stroke survivors without dementia. *Dement. Geriatr. Cogn. Disord.*, **16**, 52–6.

Bechara, A., Damasio, H., Tranel, D. and Anderson, S. W. (1998). Dissociation of working memory from decision making within the human prefrontal cortex. *J. Neurosci.*, **18**, 428–37.

Bechara, A., Tranel, D., Damasio, H. and Damasio, A. R. (1996). Failure to respond autonomically to anticipated future outcomes following damage to prefrontal cortex. *Cereb. Cortex*, **6**, 215–25.

Benton, A. L. (1968). Differential behavioral effects of frontal lobe disease. *Neuropsychologia*, **6**, 53–60.

Berger, A. and Posner, M. I. (2000). Pathologies of brain attentional networks. *Neuroscience Biobehav. Rev.*, **24**, 3–5.

Beversdorf, D. Q. and Heilman, K. M. (1998). Facilitory paratonia and frontal lobe functioning. *Neurology*, **51**, 968–71.

Bogousslavsky, J. (1994). Frontal stroke syndromes. *Eur. Neurol.*, **34**, 306–15.

Bogousslavsky, J., Regli, F. and Assal, G. (1986). The syndrome of unilateral tuberothalamic artery territory infarction. *Stroke*, **17**, 434–41.

Bogousslavsky, J., Regli, F., Delaloye, B., *et al.* (1991). Loss of psychic self-activation with bithalamic infarction: Neurobehavioural, CT, MRI and SPECT correlates. *Acta Neurol. Scand.*, **83**, 309–16.

Bogousslavsky, J., Regli, F. and Uske, A. (1988). Thalamic infarcts: Clinical syndromes, etiology, and prognosis. *Neurology*, **38**, 837–48.

Buccino, G., Scoditti, U., Patteri, I., Bertolino, C. and Mancia, D. (2003). Neurological and cognitive long-term outcome in patients with cerebral venous sinus thrombosis. *Acta Neurol. Scand.*, **107**, 330–5.

Burgess, P. W., Alderman, N., Evans, J. J., *et al.* (1996). Modified Six Element Test. In B. A. Wilson *et al.*, eds., *Behavioral Assessment of the Dysexecutive Syndrome*. Bury, St. Edmunds: Thames Valley Test Company.

Burgess, P. W., Alderman, N., Evans, J., Emslie, H. and Wilson, B. A. (1998). The ecological validity of tests of executive function. *J. Int. Neuropsychol. Soc.*, **4**, 547–58.

Burgess, P. W. and Shallice, T. (1996a). Response suppression, initiation and strategy use following frontal lobe lesions. *Neuropsychologia*, **34**, 263–73.

(1996b). Bizarre responses, rule deduction and frontal lobe lesions. *Cortex*, **32**, 241–61.

(1996c). Confabulation and the control of recollection. *Memory*, **4**, 359–411.

Burgess, P. W., Simons, J. S., Dumantheil, I., and Gilbert, S. J. (2005). The Gateway hypothesis of rostral prefrontal cortex (area 10) function. In J. Duncan, L. Phillips and P. McLeod, eds., *Speed, Control and Ageing: In Honour of Patrick Rabbitt.* Oxford: Oxford University Press, pp. 215–46.

Burgess, P. W., Veitch, E., de Lacy Costello, A. and Shallice, T. (2000). The cognitive and neuroanatomical correlates of multitasking. *Neuropsychologia*, **38**, 848–63.

Caplan, L. R., Schmahmann, J. D., Kase, C. S., *et al.* (1990). Caudate infarcts. *Arch. Neurol.*, **47**, 133–43.

Chatham Showalter, P. E. and Kimmel, D. N. (2000). Agitated symptom response to divalproex following acute brain injury. *J. Neuropsychiatry Clin. Neurosci.*, **12**, 395–7.

Cowey, C. M. and Green, S. (1996). The hippocampus: A working memory' structure? The effect of hippocampal sclerosis on working memory. *Memory*, **4**, 19–30.

Cramer, S. C., Nelles, G., Schaechter, J. D., Kaplan, J. D. and Finklestein, S. P. (1997). Computerized measurement of motor performance after stroke. *Stroke*, **28**, 2162–8.

Cummings, J. L. (1993). Frontal-subcortical circuits and human behavior. *Arch. Neurol.*, **50**, 873–80.

Cummings, J. L., Mega, M., Gray, K., *et al.* (1994). The Neuropsychiatric Inventory: Comprehensive assessment of psychopathology in dementia. *Neurology*, **44**, 2308–14.

de Bruijn, S. F., Budde, M., Teunisse, S., de Haan, R. J. and Stam, J. (2000). Long-term outcome of cognition and functional health after cerebral venous sinus thrombosis. *Neurology*, **25**, 1687–9.

D'Esposito, M. and Postle, B. R. (1999). The dependence of span and delayed-response performance on prefrontal cortex. *Neuropsychologia*, **37**, 1303–15.

Dalla Barba, G. (1993). Different patterns of confabulation. *Cortex*, **2**, 567–81.

Damasio, A. R., Tranel, D. and Damasio, H. (1991). Somatic markers and the guidance of behavior: Theory and preliminary testing. In H. S. Levin, H. M. Eisenberg and A. L. Benton, eds., *Frontal Lobe Function and Dysfunction*. Oxford: Oxford University Press, pp. 217–29.

Delis, D. C., Squire, L. R., Bihrle, A. and Massman, P. (1992). Componential analysis of problem-solving ability: Performance of patients with frontal lobe damage and amnesic patients on a new sorting test. *Neuropsychologia*, **30**, 683–97.

Desrosiers, J., Bourbonnais, D., Bravo, G., Roy, P. M. and Guay, M. (1996). Performance of the 'unaffected' upper extremity of elderly stroke patients. *Stroke*, **27**, 1564–70.

Deutsch, G., Papanicolaou, A. C., Bourbon, W. T. and Eisenberg, H. M. (1987). Cerebral blood flow evidence of right frontal activation in attention demanding tasks. *Int. J. Neurosci.*, **36**, 23–8.

Dias, R., Robins, T. W., and Roberts, A. C. (1996). Dissociation in prefrontal cortex of affective attentional shifts. *Nature*, **380**, 69–72.

Dias, R., Robins, T. W., and Roberts, A. C. (1997). Dissociable forms of inhibitory control within prefrontal cortex with an analog of the Wisconsin Card Sort Test: Restriction to novel situations and independence from 'on-line' processing. *J. Neurosci.*, **17**, 9285–97.

Drewe, E. A. (1975). Go No-Go learning after frontal lobe lesions in humans. *Cortex*, **11**, 8–16.

Du, A. T., Schuff, N., Laakso, M. P., *et al.* (2002). Effects of subcortical ischemic vascular dementia and AD on entorhinal cortex and hippocampus. *Neurology*, **58**, 1635–41.

Engstad, T., Almkvist, O., Viitanen, M. and Arnesen, E. (2003). Impaired motor speed, visuospatial episodic memory and verbal fluency characterize cognition in long-term stroke survivors: The Tromso Study. *Neuroepidemiology*, **22**, 326–31.

Eslinger, P. J. and Damasio, A. R. (1985). Severe disturbance of higher cognition following bilateral frontal lobe ablation: Patient EVR. *Neurology*, **35**, 1731–41.

Fisher, C. M. (1983). Abulia minor versus agitated behavior. *Clin. Neurosurg.*, **31**, 9–31.

Fleminger, S., Greenwood, R. J. and Oliver, D. L. (2003). Pharmacological management for agitation and aggression in people with acquired brain injury. *Cochrane Database Syst. Rev.*, **1**, CD003299.

Forsyth, R. and Jayamoni, B. (2003). Noradrenergic agonists for acute traumatic brain injury. *Cochrane Database Syst. Rev.*, **1**, CD003984.

Frith, U. (1989). A new look at language and communication in autism. *Br. J. Disord. Commun.*, **24**, 123–50.

Fuster, J. M. (1997a). Network memory. *Trends Neurosci.*, **20**, 451–9.

(1997b). *The Prefrontal Cortex: Anatomy, Physiology, and Neuropsychology of the Frontal Lobe.* New York: Lippincott-Raven.

Ghika-Schmid, F. and Bogousslavsky, J. (2000). The acute behavioral syndrome of anterior thalamic infarction: A prospective study of 12 cases. *Ann. Neurol.*, **48**, 220–7.

Ghika-Schmid, F., van Melle, G., Guex, P. and Bogousslavsky, J. (1999). Subjective experience and behavior in acute stroke: The Lausanne Emotion in Acute Stroke Study. *Neurology*, **52**, 22–8.

Glosser, G. and Goodglass, H. (1990). Disorders in executive control functions among aphasic and other brain-damaged patients. *J. Clin. Exp. Neuropsychol.*, **12**, 485–501.

Godefroy, O. (2003). Frontal syndromes and disorders of executive functions. *J. Neurol.*, **250**, 1–6.

Godefroy, O., Cabaret, M., Petit-Chenal, V., Pruvo, J.P. and Rousseaux, M. (1999). Control functions of the frontal lobes. Modularity of the central-supervisory system? *Cortex*, **35**, 1–20.

Godefroy, O., Cabaret, M. and Rousseaux, M. (1994). Vigilance and effects of fatigability, practice and motivation on simple reaction time tests in patients with lesion of the frontal lobe. *Neuropsychologia*, **32**, 983–90.

Godefroy, O., Duhamel, A., Leclerc, X., *et al.* (1998). Brain-behaviour relationships. Some models and related statistical procedures for the study of brain-damaged patients. *Brain*, **121**, 1545–56.

Godefroy, O. and GREFEX. (2004). Syndromes frontaux et dysexécutifs. *Rev. Neurol.*, **160**, 899–909.

Godefroy, O., Lhullier, C. and Rousseaux, M. (1996). Non-spatial attention disorders in patients with prefrontal or posterior brain damage. *Brain*, **119**, 191–202.

Godefroy, O., Lhullier-Lamy, C. and Rousseaux, M. (2002). SRT lengthening: Role of an alertness deficit in frontal damaged patients. *Neuropsychologia*, **40**, 2234–41.

Godefroy, O., Rousseaux, M., Leys, D., *et al.* (1992). Frontal lobe dysfunction in patients with unilateral lenticulo-striate infarcts. Prominent role of cortical lesion. *Arch. Neurol.*, **49**, 1285–89.

Goel, V. and Dolan, R.J. (2001). The functional anatomy of humor: Segregating cognitive and affective components. *Nat. Neurosci.*, **4**, 237–8.

Goel, V., Grafman, J., Tajik, J., Gana, S. and Danto, D. (1997). A study of the performance of patients with frontal lobe lesions in a financial planning task. *Brain*, **120**, 1805–22.

Goldman-Rakic, P.S. (1987). Circuitry of prefrontal cortex and regulation of behavior by representational memory. In F. Plum, ed., *Handbook of Physiology: The Nervous System V.* Berlin: Springer, pp. 373–417.

Grace, J., Stout, J.C. and Malloy, P.F. (1999). Assessment of frontal behavioral syndromes with the Frontal Lobe Personality Scale. *Assessment*, **6**, 269–84.

Grigsby, J., Kaye, K., Baxter, J., Shetterly, S.M. and Hamman, R.F. (1998). Executive cognitive abilities and functional status among community-dwelling older persons in the San Luis Valley Health and Aging Study. *J. Am. Geriatr. Soc.*, **46**, 590–6.

Habib, M. and Poncet, M. (1988). Perte de l'élan vital, de l'intérêt et de l'affectivité (syndrome athymhormique) au cours de lésions lacunaires des corps striés. *Rev. Neurol.*, **144**, 571–7.

Harlow, J.M. (1868). Recovery from the passage of an iron bar through the head. *Mass Med. Soc. Bost.*, **2**, 327–246.

Hécaen, H. and De Ajuriaguerra, J. (1956). *Troubles Mentaux au Cours des Tumeurs Intracraniennes.* Paris: Masson.

Hénon, H., Pasquier, F., Durieu, I., *et al.* (1997). Preexisting dementia in stroke patients. Baseline frequency, associated factors, and outcome. *Stroke*, **28**, 2429–36.

Hillis, A.E., Anderson, N., Sampath, P. and Rigamonti, D. (2000). Cognitive impairments after surgical repair of ruptured and unruptured aneurysms. *J. Neurol. Neurosurg. Psychiatry*, **69**, 608–15.

Hochstenbach, J., Mulder, T., Van Limbeek, J., Donders, R. and Schoonderwaldt, H. (1998). Cognitive decline following stroke: A comprehensive study of cognitive decline following stroke. *J. Clin. Exp. Neuropsychol.*, **20**, 503–17.

Hochstenbach, J. B., den Otter, R. and Mulder, T. W. (2003). Cognitive recovery after stroke: A 2-year follow-up. *Arch. Phys. Med. Rehabil.*, **84**, 1499–504.

Hütter, B. O. (2000). *Neuropsychological Sequelae of Subarachnoid Hemorrhage and its Treatment.* Wien: Springer-Verlag.

Hütter, B. O. and Gilsbach, J. M. (1993). Which neuropsychological deficits are hidden behind a good outcome (Glasgow=1) after aneurysmal subarachnoid hemorrhage? *Neurosurgery*, **33**, 999–1006.

Incisa Della Rocchetta, A. and Milner, B. (1993). Strategic search and retrieval inhibition: The role of frontal lobes. *Neuropsychologia*, **31**, 503–24.

Ishii, N., Nishihara, Y. and Imamura, T. (1986). Why do frontal lobe symptoms predominate in vascular dementia with lacunes? *Neurology*, **36**, 340–5.

Jacobsen, C. F. (1936). Studies of cerebral functions in the primates: I. The function of the frontal association areas in the monkeys. *Comp. Psychol. Monogr.*, **13**, 1–60.

Janowsky, J. S., Shimamura, A. P. and Squire, L. R. (1989). Source memory impairments in patients with frontal damage. *Neuropsychologia*, **27**, 1043–56.

Jason, G. W. (1985). Manual sequence learning after focal cortical lesions. *Neuropsychologia*, **23**(4), 483–96.

Jetter, W., Poser, U., Freeman, R. B. and Markowitsch, H. J. A. (1986). A verbal long term memory deficit in frontal lobe damaged patients. *Cortex*, **22**, 229–42.

Kant, R., Smith-Seemiller, L. and Zeiler, D. (1998). Treatment of aggression and irritability after head injury. *Brain Inj.*, **12**, 661–6.

Kramer, J. H., Reed, B. R., Mungas, D., Weiner, M. W. and Chui, H. C. (2002). Executive dysfunction in subcortical ischaemic vascular disease. *J. Neurol. Neurosurg. Psychiatry*, **72**, 217–20.

Kreiter, K. T., Copeland, D., Bernardini, G. L., *et al.* (2002). Predictors of cognitive dysfunction after subarachnoid hemorrhage. *Stroke*, **33**, 200–8.

Krolak-Salmon, P., Croisile, B., Houzard, C., *et al.* (2000). Total recovery after bilateral paramedian thalamic infarct. *Eur. Neurol.*, **44**, 216–18.

Kumral, E., Bayulkem, G., Evyapan, D. and Yunten, N. (2002). Spectrum of anterior cerebral artery territory infarction: Clinical and MRI findings. *Eur. J. Neurol.*, **9**, 615–24.

Laplane, D., Widlocher, D., Pillon, B., Baulac, M. and Binoux, F. (1981). Comportement compulsif d'allure obsessionnelle par nécrose circonscrite bilatérale pallido-striatale. *Rev. Neurol.*, **137**, 269–76.

Leclercq, M., Couillet, J., Azouvi, P., *et al.* (2000). Dual task performance after severe diffuse traumatic brain injury or vascular prefrontal damage. *J. Clin. Exp. Neuropsychol.*, **22**, 339–50.

Leskela, M., Hietanen, M., Kalska, H., *et al.* (1999). Executive functions and speed of mental processing in elderly patients with frontal or nonfrontal ischemic stroke. *Eur. J. Neurol.*, **6**, 653–61.

Levine, B., Dawson, D., Boutet, I., Schwartz, M. L. and Stuss, D. T. (2000). Assessment of strategic self-regulation in traumatic brain injury: Its relationship to injury severity and psychosocial outcome. *Neuropsychology*, **14**, 491−500.

Levine, B., Stuss, D. T. and Milberg, W. P. (1995). Concept generation: Validation of a test of executive functioning in a normal aging population. *J. Clin. Exp. Neuropsychol.*, **17**, 740−58. (1997). Effects of aging on conditional associative learning: Process analyses and comparison with focal frontal lesions. *Neuropsychology*, **11**, 367−81.

Levine, B., Stuss, D. T., Milberg, W. P., *et al.* (1998). The effects of focal and diffuse brain damage on strategy application: Evidence from focal lesions, traumatic brain injury and normal aging. *J. Int. Neuropsychol. Soc.*, **4**, 247−64.

Lhermitte, F., Pillon, B. and Serdaru, M. (1986). Human autonomy and the frontal lobes. Part I: Imitation and utilization behavior. *Ann. Neurol.*, **19**, 326−34.

Lincoln, N. B., Majid, M. J. and Weyman, N. (2000). Cognitive rehabilitation for attention deficits following stroke. *Cochrane Database Syst. Rev.*, **4**, CD002842.

Ljunggren, B., Sonesson, B., Säveland, H. and Brandt, L. (1985). Cognitive impairment and adjustment in patients without neurological deficits after aneurysmal SAH and early operation. *J. Neurosurg.*, **62**, 673−9.

Luria, A. R. (1966). *Higher Cortical Functions in Man.* New York: Basic Books Inc. Publishers.

Mah, L., Arnold, M. C. and Grafman, J. (2004). Impairment of social perception associated with lesions of the prefrontal cortex. *Am. J. Psychiatry*, **161**, 1247−55.

Mahalick, D. M., Ruff, R. M., Heary, R. F. and U, H. S. (1993). Preoperative versus postoperative neuropsychological sequelae of arteriovenous malformations. *Neurosurgery*, **33**, 563−70.

Malloy, P. F. and Richardson, E. D. (1994). Assessment of frontal lobe functions. *J. Neuropsychol. Clin. Neurosci.*, **6**, 399−410.

Marin, R. S. (1990). Differential diagnosis and classification of apathy. *Am. J. Psychiatry.*, **147**, 22−30.

Martin, C., Dellatolas, G., Viguier, D., Willadino-Braga, L. and Deloche, G. (2002). Subjective experience after stroke. *Appl. Neuropsychol.*, **9**, 148−58.

Mayer, S. A., Kreiter, K. T., Copeland, D., *et al.* (2002). Global and domain-specific cognitive impairment and outcome after subarachnoid hemorrhage. *Neurology*, **59**, 1750−8.

McDowell, S., Whyte, J. and D'Esposito, M. (1998). Differential effect of a dopaminergic agonist on prefrontal function in traumatic brain injury patients. *Brain*, **121**, 1155−64.

Mendez, M. F., Adams, N. L. and Lewandowski, K. S. (1989). Neurobehavioral changes associated with caudate lesions. *Neurology*, **39**, 349−54.

Messerli, P., Seron, X. and Tissot, R. (1979). Quelques aspects des troubles de la programmation dans le syndrome frontal. *Arch. Suisses Neurol., Neurochir. Psychiatrie*, **125**, 23−35.

Michals, M. L., Crismon, M. L., Roberts, S. and Childs, A. (1993). Clozapine response and adverse effects in nine brain-injured patients. *J. Clin. Psychopharmacol.*, **13**, 198−203.

Milner, B. (1963). Effects of different brain lesions on card sorting. *Arch. Neurol.*, **9**, 90−100.

Mishkin, M. (1964). Preservation of central sets after frontal lesions in monkeys. In J. M., Warren and K. Akert, eds., *The frontal granular cortex and behavior*. New York: McGraw Hill, pp. 219−41.

Morris, N. and Jones, D. M. (1990). Memory updating in working memory: The role of the central executive. *Br. J. Psychol.*, **81**, 111–21.

Mungas, D., Jagust, W. J., Reed, B. R., *et al.* (2001). MRI predictors of cognition in subcortical ischemic vascular disease and Alzheimer's disease. *Neurology*, **57**, 2229–35.

Nauta, W. J. (1971). The problem of the frontal lobe: A reinterpretation. *J. Psychiatr. Res.*, **8**, 167–87.

Norman, D. A. and Shallice, T. (1980). Attention to action: Willed and automatic control of behavior. Center for human information processing, Technical report N 99.

O'Brien, J. T., Wiseman, R., Burton, E. J., *et al.* (2002). Cognitive associations of subcortical white matter lesions in older people. *Ann. NY. Acad. Sci.*, **977**, 436–44.

Ogden, J. A., Mee, E. W. and Henning, M. (1993). A prospective study of impairment of cognition and memory and recovery after subarachnoid hemorrhage. *Neurosurgery*, **33**, 572–86.

Owen, A. M., Downes, J. J., Sahakian, B. J., Polkey, C. E. and Robbins, T. W. (1990). Planning and spatial working memory following frontal lobe lesions in man. *Neuropsychologia*, **28**, 1021–34.

Pandya, D. N. and Yeterian, E. H. (1996). Comparison of prefrontal architecture and connections. *Philos. Trans. R. Soc. Lond. B. Biol. Sci.*, **351**, 1423–32.

Pedrazzi, P., Bogousslavsky, J. and Regli, F. (1990). Hématome de la tête du noyau caudé. *Rev. Neurol.*, **146**, 726–38.

Percheron, G. (1976a). Les artères du thalamus humain, I: Artère et territoire thalamiques polaires de l'artère communicante postérieure. *Rev. Neurol.*, **132**, 297–307.

(1976b). Les artères du thalamus humain, II: Artères et territoire thalamiques paramédians de l'artère basilaire communicante. *Rev. Neurol.*, **132**, 309–24.

Perret, E. (1974). The left frontal lobe of man and the suppression of habitual responses in verbal categorical behaviour. *Neuropsychologia*, **12**, 323–40.

Pillon, B., Deweer, B., Agid, Y. and Dubois, B. (1993). Explicit memory in Alzheimer's, Huntington's, and Parkinson's diseases. *Arch. Neurol.*, **50**, 374–9.

Pohjasvaara, T., Leskela, M., Vataja, R., *et al.* (2002). Post-stroke depression, executive dysfunction and functional outcome. *Eur. J. Neurol.*, **9**, 269–75.

Pohjasvaara, T., Mantyla, R., Salonen, O., *et al.* (2000). How complex interactions of ischemic brain infarcts, white matter lesions, and atrophy relate to poststroke dementia. *Arch. Neurol.*, **57**, 1295–300.

Pohjasvaara, T., Mantyla, R., Ylikoski, R., Kaste, M. and Erkinjuntti, T. (2003). Clinical features of MRI-defined subcortical vascular disease. *Alzheimer Dis. Assoc. Disord.*, **17**, 236–42.

Posner, M. I. and Petersen, S. E. (1990). The attention system of the human brain. *Annu. Rev. Neurosci.*, **13**, 25–42.

Powell, J. H., al-Adawi, S., Morgan, J. and Greenwood, R. J. (1996). Motivational deficits after brain injury: Effects of bromocriptine in 11 patients. *J. Neurol. Neurosurg. Psychiatry*, **60**, 416–21.

Premack, D. and Woodruff, G. (1978). Does the chimpanzee have a theory of mind? *Behav. Brain Sci.*, **1**, 515–26.

Ramier, A. M. and Hécaen, H. (1970). Rôles respectifs des lésions frontales et de la latéralisation lésionnelle dans les déficits des fluences verbales. *Rev. Neurol.*, **123**, 17–22.

Rasquin, S. M., Lodder, J., Ponds, R. W., *et al.* (2004). Cognitive functioning after stroke: A one-year follow-up study. *Dement. Geriatr. Cogn. Disord.*, **18**, 138–44.

Rasquin, S. M., Verhey, F. R., Lousberg, R., Winkens, I. and Lodder, J. (2002). Vascular cognitive disorders: Memory, mental speed and cognitive flexibility after stroke. *J. Neurol. Sci.*, **203–4**, 115–19.

Robert, P. H., Clairet, S., Benoit, M., *et al.* (2002). The Apathy Inventory: Assessment of apathy and awareness in Alzheimer's disease, Parkinson's disease and mild cognitive impairment. *Int. J. Geriatr. Psychiatry*, **17**, 1099–105.

Roberts, A. C., Robbins, T. W. and Weiskrantz, L. (1996). Executive and cognitive functions of the prefrontal cortex. *Phil. Trans. R. Soc.*, **351B**, 1387–527.

Robertson, I. H., Manly, T., Andrade, J., Baddeley, B. T. and Yiend, J. (1997). 'Oops!': Performance correlates of everyday attentional failures in traumatic brain injured and normal subjects. *Neuropsychologia*, **35**, 747–58.

Robertson, I. H., Ward, T., Ridgeway, V. and Nimmo-Smith, I. (1996). The structure of normal human attention: The Test of Everyday Attention. *J. Int. Neuropsychol. Soc.*, **2**, 525–34.

Rogers, R. D., Owen, A. M., Middleton, H. C., *et al.* (1999). Choosing between small, likely rewards and large, unlikely rewards activates inferior and orbital prefrontal cortex. *J. Neurosci.*, **19**, 9029–38.

Rolls, E. T. (2000). Memory systems in the brain. *Annu. Rev. Psychol.*, **51**, 599–630.

Rolls, E. T., Critchley, H. D., Mason, R. and Wakeman, E. A. (1996). Orbitofrontal cortex neurons: Role in olfactory and visual association learning. *J. Neurophysiol.*, **75**, 1970–81.

Rousseaux, M., Godefroy, O., Cabaret, M., Benaim, C. and Pruvo, J. P. (1996). Analyse et évolution des déficits cognitifs après rupture d'un anéurysme de l'artère communicante anterieure. *Rev. Neurol.*, **152**, 678–87.

Roussel-Pieronne, M., Godefroy, O., Dujardin, K., *et al.* Perturbations de la mémoire de travail dans la pathologie cérébrale focale. *Rev. Neuropsychol.* (in press).

Rowe, A. D., Bullock, P. R., Polkey, C. E. and Morris, R. G. (2001). 'Theory of mind' impairments and their relationship to executive functioning following frontal lobe excisions. *Brain*, **124**, 600–16.

Rueckert, L. and Grafman, J. (1996). Sustained attention deficits in patients with right frontal lesions. *Neuropsychologia*, **34**, 953–63.
  (1998). Sustained attention deficits in patients with lesions of posterior cortex. *Neuropsychologia*, **36**, 653–60.

Rylander, G. (1939). Personality changes after operations on the frontal lobes. A clinical study of 32 cases. *Acta Psychiatr. Neurol. Scand.*, **Suppl 20**, 3–327.

Sachdev, P. S., Brodaty, H., Valenzuela, M. J., *et al.* (2004). The neuropsychological profile of vascular cognitive impairment in stroke and TIA patients. *Neurology*, **23**, 912–19.

Saint-Cyr, J. A. (2003). Frontal-striatal circuit functions: Context, sequence, and consequence. *J. Int. Neuropsychol. Soc.*, **9**, 103–27.

Sanides, F. and Sas, E. (1970). Persistence of horizontal cells of the Cajal foetal type and of the subpial granular layer in parts of the mammalian paleocortex. *Z. Mikrosk. Anat. Forsch.*, **82**, 570–88.

Sarazin, M., Michon, A., Pillon, B., *et al.* (2003). Metabolic correlates of behavioral and affective disturbances in frontal lobe pathologies. *J. Neurol.*, **250**, 827–33.

Schmahmann, J. D. (2003). Vascular syndromes of the thalamus. *Stroke*, **34**, 2264–78.

Schnider, A. and Ptak, R. (1999). Spontaneous confabulators fail to suppress currently irrelevant memory traces. *Nat. Neurosci.*, **2**, 677–81.

Schnider, A., Ptak, R., von Daniken, C. and Remonda, L. (2000). Recovery from spontaneous confabulations parallels recovery of temporal confusion in memory. *Neurology*, **55**, 74–83.

Shallice, T. (1982). Specific impairments of planning. *Phil. Trans. R. Soc. Lond.*, **B298**, 199–209.

Shallice, T. and Burgess, P. (1991). Deficits in strategy application after frontal lobe damage in man. *Brain*, **114**, 727–41.

(1996). The domain of supervisory processes and temporal organization of behaviour. *Phil. Trans. R. Soc. Lond.*, **B351**, 1405–12.

Shallice, T., Burgess, P. W., Schon, F. and Baxter, D. M. (1989). The origins of utilization behaviour. *Brain*, **112**, 1587–98.

Shallice, T. and Vallar, G. (1990). The impairment of auditory-verbal short term storage. In G. Vallar and T. Shallice, eds., *Neuropsychological Impairment of Short Term Memory*. Cambridge: Cambridge University Press, pp. 11–53.

Shammi, P. and Stuss, D. T. (1999). Humour appreciation: A role of the right frontal lobe. *Brain*, **122**, 657–66.

Shankle, W. R., Nielson, K. A. and Cotman, C. W. (1995). Low-dose propranolol reduces aggression and agitation resembling that associated with orbitofrontal dysfunction in elderly demented patients. *Alzheimer Dis. Assoc. Disord.*, **9**, 233–7.

Sirigu, A., Zalla, T., Pillon, B., *et al.* (1995). Selective impairments in managerial knowledge following prefrontal cortex damage. *Cortex*, **31**, 301–16.

Stablum, F., Umilta, C., Mogentale, C., Carlan, M. and Guerrini, C. (2000). Rehabilitation of executive deficits in closed head injury and anterior communicating artery aneurysm patients. *Psychol. Res.*, **63**, 265–78.

Starkstein, S. E., Robinson, R. G., Berthier, M. L. and Price, T. R. (1988). Depressive disorders following posterior circulation as compared with middle cerebral artery infarcts. *Brain*, **111**, 375–87.

Stone, V. E., Baron-Cohen, S. and Knight, R. T. (1998). Frontal lobe contributions to theory of mind. *J. Cogn. Neurosci.*, **10**, 640–56.

Stuss, D. T. (1991). Disturbances in self-awareness after frontal system damage. In G. Prigatano and D. Schacter, eds., *Awareness of Deficit After Brain Injury*. New York: Oxford University Press, pp. 63–83.

Stuss, D. T. and Alexander, M. P. (1999). Affectively burnt in: A proposed role of the right frontal lobe. In E. Tulving, ed., *Memory, Consciousness and the Brain: The Tallinn Conference*. Philadelphia: Psychology Press, pp. 215–27.

Stuss, D. T. and Alexander, M. P. (2000). Executive functions and the frontal lobes: A conceptual view. *Psychol. Res.*, **63**, 289–98.

Stuss, D. T., Alexander, M. P., Hamer, L., *et al.* (1998). The effects of focal anterior and posterior brain lesions on verbal fluency. *J. Int. Neuropsychol. Soc.*, **4**, 265–78.

Stuss, D. T., Alexander, M. P., Palumbo, C. L., *et al.* (1994). Organizational strategies of patients with unilateral or bilateral frontal lobe injury in word list learning tasks. *Neuropsychology*, **8**, 355–73.

Stuss, D. T., Alexander, M. P., Shallice, T., *et al.* (2005). Multiple frontal systems controlling response speed. *Neuropsychologia*, **43**, 396–417.

Stuss, D. T. and Benson, D. F. (1986). *The Frontal Lobes.* New York: Raven Press.

Stuss, D. T., Binns, M. A., Murphy, K. J. and Alexander, M. P. (2002). Dissociations within the anterior attentional system: Effects of task complexity and irrelevant information on reaction time speed and accuracy. *Neuropsychology*, **16**, 500–13.

Stuss, D. T., Bisschop, S. M., Alexander, M. P., *et al.* (2001a). The Trail Making Test: A study in focal lesion patients. *Psychol. Assess.*, **13**, 230–9.

Stuss, D. T., Delgado, M. and Guzman, D. A. (1987). Verbal regulation in the control of motor impersistence: A proposed rehabilitation procedure. *J. Neurol. Rehabil.*, **1**, 19–24.

Stuss, D. T., Floden, D., Alexander, M. P., Levine, B. and Katz, D. (2001b). Stroop performance in focal lesion patients: Dissociation of processes and frontal lobe lesion location. *Neuropsychologia*, **39**, 771–86.

Stuss, D. T., Gallup, G. G. and Alexander, M. P. (2001c). The frontal lobes are necessary for 'theory of mind'. *Brain*, **124**, 279–86.

Stuss, D. T. and Levine, B. (2002). Adult clinical neuropsychology: Lessons from studies of the frontal lobes. *Annu. Rev. of Psychol.*, **53**, 401–33.

Stuss, D. T., Levine, B., Alexander, M. P., *et al.* (2000a). Wisconsin Card Sorting Test performance in patients with focal frontal and posterior brain damage: Effects of lesion location and test structure on separable cognitive processes. *Neuropsychologia*, **38**, 388–402.

Stuss, D. T., Murphy, K. J., Binns, M. A. and Alexander, M. P. (2003). Staying on the job: The frontal lobes control individual performance variability. *Brain*, **126**, 2363–80.

Stuss, D. T., van Reekum, R. and Murphy, K. J. (2000b). Differentiation of states and causes of apathy. In J. Borod, ed., *The Neuropsychology of Emotion*. New York: Oxford University Press, pp. 340–63.

Stuss, D. T., Stethem, L. L., Hugenholtz, H., *et al.* (1989). Reaction time after head injury: Fatigue, divided and focused attention, and consistency of performance. *J. Neurol. Neurosurg. Psychiatry*, **52**, 742–8.

Sunderland, A., Bowers, M. P., Sluman, S. M., Wilcock, D. J. and Ardron, M. E. (1999). Impaired dexterity of the ipsilateral hand after stroke and the relationship to cognitive deficit. *Stroke*, **30**, 949–55.

Tariot, P. N., Erb, R., Podgorski, C. A., *et al.* (1998). Jan Efficacy and tolerability of carbamazepine for agitation and aggression in dementia. *Am. J. Psychiatry*, **155**, 54–61.

Tariot, P. N., Jakimovich, L. J., Erb, R., *et al.* (1999). Withdrawal from controlled carbamazepine therapy followed by further carbamazepine treatment in patients with dementia. *J. Clin. Psychiatry*, **60**, 684–9.

Tatemichi, T. K., Desmond, D. W., Paik, M., *et al.* (1993). Clinical determinants of dementia related to stroke. *Ann. Neurol.*, **33**, 568–75.

Tatemichi, T. K., Desmond, D. W., Stern, Y., et al. (1994). Cognitive impairement after stroke: Frequency, patterns, and relationship to functional abilities. *J. Neurol. Neurosurg. Psychiatry*, **57**, 202–7.

Tidswell, P., Dias, P. S., Sagar, H. J., Mayes, A. R. and Battersby, R. D. (1995). Cognitive outcome after aneurysm rupture: Relationship to aneurysm site and perioperative complications. *Neurology*, **45**, 875–82.

Troyer, A. K., Moscovitch, M., Winocur, G., Alexander, M. P. and Stuss, D. (1998). Clustering and switching on verbal fluency: The effects of focal frontal- and temporal-lobe lesions. *Neuropsychologia*, **36**, 499–504.

Truelle, J. L., Le Gall, D., Aubin, G., Derouesné, C. and Lezak, M. (1995). Movements disturbances following frontal lobe lesions: Qualitative analysis. *Neuropsychiatry Neuropsychol. Behav. Neurol.*, **8**, 14–19.

Tullberg, M., Fletcher, E., DeCarli, C., et al. (2004). White matter lesions impair frontal lobe function regardless of their location. *Neurology*, **63**, 246–53.

Umilta, C., Nicoletti, R., Simion, F., Tagliabue, M. E. and Bagnara, S. (1992). The cost of a strategy. *Eur. J. Cogn. Psychol.*, **4**, 21–40.

Van der Werf, Y. D., Scheltens, P., Lindeboom, J., et al. (2003). Deficits of memory, executive functioning and attention following infarction in the thalamus; A study of 22 cases with localised lesions. *Neuropsychologia*, **41**, 1330–44.

Van der Werf, Y. D., Witter, M. P., Uylings, H. B. and Jolles, J. (2000). Neuropsychology of infarctions in the thalamus: A review. *Neuropsychologia*, **38**, 613–627.

Vataja, R., Pohjasvaara, T., Mantyla, R., et al. (2003). MRI correlates of executive dysfunction in patients with ischaemic stroke. *Eur. J. Neurol.*, **10**, 625–31.

Weiller, C., Ringelstein, E. B., Reiche, W., Thron, A. and Buell, U. (1990). The large striato-capsular infarct. A clinical and pathophysiological entity. *Arch. Neurol.*, **47**, 1085–91.

Wheeler, M. A. and Stuss, D. T. (2003). Remembering and knowing in patients with frontal lobe injuries. *Cortex*, **39**, 827–46.

Wheeler, M. A. Stuss, D. T. and Tulving, E. (1995). Frontal lobe damage produces episodic memory impairment. *J. Internat. Neuropsychol. Soc.*, **1**, 525–36.

Wiegersma, S., Van der Scheer, E. and Human, R. (1990). Subjective ordering, short term memory and the frontal lobes. *Neuropsychologia*, **28**, 95–8.

Wilkins, A. J., Shallice, T. and McCarthy, R. (1987). Frontal lesions and sustained attention. *Neuropsychologia*, **25**, 359–65.

Wilson, B. A., Alderman, N., Burgess, P. W., Emslie, H., and Evans, J. J. (1996). *Behavioural Assessment of the Dysexecutive Syndrome*. Reading, England: Thames Valley Company.

Wilson, B. A., Evans, J. J., Emslie, H., Alderman, N. and Burgess, P. W. (1998). The development of an ecologically valid test for assessing patients with a dysexecutive syndrome. *Neuropsychol. Rehabil.*, **8**, 213–28.

Winocur, G. and Moscovitch, M. (1990). Hippocampal and prefrontal cortex contributions to learning and memory: Analysis of lesion and aging effects on maze learning in rats. *Behav. Neurosci.*, **104**, 544–51.

Wolfe, N., Linn, R., Babikian, V. L., et al. (1990). Frontal systems impairment following multiple lacunar infarcts. *Arch. Neurol.*, **47**, 129–32.

20

Disorders of episodic memory

Chun Lim and Michael P. Alexander

Beth Israel Deaconess Medical Center, Boston, MA

Introduction

Key points Main characteristics of disorders of episodic memory

---

Distinct forms of memory
Implicit memories:
- occur without specific knowledge or recollection of how they were learned
- include: classical conditioning, priming, motor skills, and mental procedures
Explicit memory:
- conscious recall of events, experiences, or information
- divided into *episodic memory* (recall of personal experiences) and *semantic memory* (body of facts, principles, and rules that make up our general knowledge of the world, consciously recalled without reference to a personal experience)

Disorders of episodic memory
- Induce memory complaint and/or forgetfulness
Differing patterns according to lesion location:
1. *true amnesia*: impaired recognition, little benefit from cues, and poor delayed recall
2. *disorder due to executive deficit* (especially due to some frontal damage): good items recognition (except for the possible presence of false recognition) and cued recall; impaired learning (as shown by a flat curve); little loss of items after delay
3. *modality effect according to lesion side* (especially in mediotemporal and thalamic lesions):
   left lesion: deficit of verbal memory (story recall, list learning) and some degree of visual memory (figures,
      designs)
   right lesion: configurational visual memory

Memory is not a unitary capacity — there are several distinct forms. *Implicit memories* are those that occur without specific knowledge or recollection of how they were learned and include diverse mental capacities: classical conditioning, priming, motor skills, and mental procedures. *Explicit memory* is the conscious recall of events, experiences, or information, and is further divided into episodic and semantic memory. *Episodic memory* is the recall of personal experiences. *Semantic memory* is the body of facts, principles, and rules that make up our general knowledge of the world, consciously recalled without reference to a personal experience. In everyday life these compartments of memory may operate simultaneously: moved by a piece of music while failing to recall the original experience (perceptual priming), your fingers may play out the rhythm (motor learning), triggering recollection of the name of composer (semantic knowledge) and a memory of a youthful piano lesson (episodic memory). Despite this interweaving of memories, this chapter will focus only on deficits in episodic memory caused by strokes.

Episodic memory

The neuroanatomical basis of episodic memory emerged from clinicopathological observations and from the effects of discrete experimental lesions in animals. In 1957, William Scoville removed both anterior medial temporal regions in patient HM in an attempt to treat his intractable epilepsy (Scoville and Milner, 1957). The surgery produced profound explicit memory loss, attributed to removal of the hippocampi, adjacent parahippocampal structures, and amygdala. Subsequent observations of patients with damage to medial temporal structures due to stroke (Victor *et al.*, 1961), paraneoplastic limbic encephalitis (Corsellis *et al.*, 1968), herpes simplex encephalitis (Cermak and O'Connor, 1983; Damasio *et al.*, 1985a), anoxia (Cummings *et al.*, 1984), and Alzheimer's Disease (Hyman *et al.*, 1984) confirmed that medial temporal regions are critical for memory.

It has been known for over 100 years that chronic alcoholics and other nutritionally deprived individuals could develop severe amnesia, but 70 years passed before investigators demonstrated that lesions of the dorsomedial nucleus of the thalamus (Victor *et al.*, 1971) and mammillary bodies (Mair *et al.*, 1979) were critical. Additional case reports and clinicopathological studies of patients with memory disorders confirmed the critical role of the diencephalon (Squire *et al.*, 1989) and also that of the septal nuclei (Whitehouse *et al.*, 1982; Damasio *et al.*, 1985b).

Anatomical studies in non-human primates and rodents (Nauta, 1961; Swanson and Cowan, 1975; 1977; Swanson, 1978; Zola-Morgan *et al.*, 1982; Rosene and Van Hoesen, 1987; De Olmos, 1990) have shown that these limbic structures form two related anatomical units. The first unit includes the hippocampal formation with projections to the septal region and the mammillary bodies of the hypothalamus (fornix), then from the mammillary bodies to the anterior nuclei of the thalamus (the mammillothalamic tract), followed by projections to the cingulate and retrosplenial cortices, and finally returning to the hippocampus (cingulum) — the so-called Papez circuit (Papez, 1995). The second unit involves the amygdala and projections to the septal nuclei and dorsomedial nucleus of the thalamus (ventral amygdalofugal pathway), and from the thalamus to the prefrontal cortex (thalamocortical projections). In animals these systems are complementary with lesions in any component or its pathways causing moderate amnesia, but damage to both systems causing profound amnesia (Mishkin, 1978). In humans significant episodic memory impairment appears to follow primarily damage to the first unit, although damage to the second unit can cause clinically significant amnesia.

In humans there is also a strong modality effect depending on the laterality of the injury. Whatever the cause, including stroke, damage to the left limbic structures produces impaired verbal memory (story recall, list learning, etc.) and some degree of visual memory (figures, designs, etc.). Damage to the right limbic structures produces impaired configurational visual memory and perhaps impaired spatial memory (visuospatial memory). Thus, without repeating the laterality effect for each stroke syndrome described below, these laterality effects can be assumed.

Lesions outside of the limbic systems can also cause deficits in memory. Damage to any perceptual or cognitive process can disrupt memory formation and recall dependent on that process. For example, a lesion in the language system that affects the lexicosemantic networks will interfere with the normal acquisition of novel verbal material. In addition, active learning and recall requires alertness, motivation, effort, perhaps a strategy, and inhibition of competing memories. Lesions that disrupt these processes will alter the strength and pattern of the memory engram and disrupt learning strategies or retrieval patterns. Clinically, this frequently presents as a deficiency in memory. Patients in confusional states, even when mild, have impaired attention and secondarily poor memory. Frontal lobe lesions may damage executive processes that modulate attention, effort, and inhibition.

Damage to any of these structures by stroke will result in memory deficits. It is the *location* of structural damage that determines memory impairment, not the etiology. Thus, both lobar hemorrhage in the left hippocampal region and infarction in the left PCA territory may produce identical memory loss; likewise anterior thalamic damage whether infarction from small vessel occlusive disease, vasculitis, basilar artery emboli, or hypertensive hemorrhages.

We will review the stroke syndromes that cause amnesia by damage to limbic structures, then the locations of strokes that impair the various processes, modality-specific and more generally strategic, that may impair learning and recall

Key points Summary of stroke subtypes causing memory disorders

Location/vascular territory	Anatomy	Memory deficits	Associated deficits
Infarct: PCA			
Left PCA	Hippocampus	Verbal memory	Visual field deficits
	Medial temporal lobe		Color agnosia
	Collateral isthmus		Alexia without agraphia
			Anomia
Right PCA	Hippocampus	Visuospatial memory	Visual field deficits
	Medial temporal lobe		Prosopagnosia
	Collateral isthmus		
Bilateral PCA	Hippocampus	Explicit memory	Cortical blindness
	Medial temporal lobe	Retrograde memory	Apperceptive agnosia
	Collateral isthmus		Associative agnosia
Infarct: anterior thalamus (polar artery)			
Left anterior thalamus	Anterior thalamus	Verbal memory	Executive dysfunction
	Mammillothalamic tract	Visuospatial memory	Mixed transcortical aphasia
	Internal medullary lamina		
Right anterior thalamus	Anterior thalamus	Visuospatial memory	Executive dysfunction
	Mammillothalamic tract		Visuoperceptual deficits
	Internal medullary lamina		
Infarct: Medial thalamic (paramedian thalamic artery)	Dorsomedial nucleus	Verbal memory	Hypersomnolence
	Centromedian nucleus	Visuospatial memory	Attentional deficits
	Internal medullary lamina	Retrograde amnesia	Ocular motility
Genu internal capsule (deep MCA or anterior choroidal artery)			
Left genu internal capsule	Anterior thalamic peduncle	Verbal memory	Frontal lobe system

Key point (Cont.)

Location/vascular territory	Anatomy	Memory deficits	Associated deficits
	Inferior thalamic peduncle		
Right genu internal capsule	Anterior thalamic peduncle	Visuospatial memory	Frontal lobe system
	Inferior thalamic peduncle		
Aneurysm of the ACoA: basal forebrain lesion	Septal nuclei	Verbal memory Visuospatial memory	Confabulation Executive impairment Anosognosia for amnesia

PCA: posterior cerebral artery; MCA: middle cerebral artery; ACoA: anterior communicating artery

without causing classical amnesia. Infarctions are constrained by vascular territory and hemorrhages are constrained by location and planes of dissection, and, thus, damage is rarely limited to regions solely subserving memory formation. Depending on the adjacent regions involved, strokes causing memory problems commonly co-occur with language, visuospatial, and executive deficits.

Many of the syndromes described below have been better characterized in patients who have suffered non-vascular injury such as surgical ablation and trauma. For the sake of faithfulness and brevity, the following discussion will be limited to the stroke literature.

Strokes causing amnesia

Medial temporal damage

Structures supplied by the posterior cerebral arteries (PCA) include the superior midbrain, portions of the posterior thalamus, the medial occipital lobes, and the medial and inferior portions of the temporal lobe, including the posterior hippocampus and the parahippocampal and occipitotemporal gyri. Bilateral PCA infarctions are caused by emboli that block the distal basilar artery bifurcation, by occlusive vascular disease of any cause of the rostral basilar artery, and, rarely, by cerebral herniation. Unilateral PCA lesions are usually caused by embolic infarctions. Hemorrhage involving this region is less frequent.

Bilateral PCA infarction involving the medial temporal lobe causes a profound deficit in explicit memory (Victor *et al.*, 1961). Similar to the deficits of patient HM, there is essentially total anterograde deficit and extensive retrograde amnesia extending over several years and involving both verbal (Victor *et al.*, 1961) and visuospatial memory (Ross, 1980a). Associated deficits (Caplan, 1980) depending upon exact lesion locations may include

1. a variety of visual field deficits, particularly in the superior quadrants, even cortical blindness
2. various visual processing disorders, such as alexia, anomia, agnosia, achromotopsia, or prosopagnosia
3. Balint's syndrome
4. agitated delirium.

Infarctions restricted to the left PCA territory appear to produce memory impairment as profound as bilateral lesions, at least in the acute phase, but the most lasting deficits are in verbal memory (Mohr *et al.*, 1971; Caplan and Hedley-Whyte, 1974; De Renzi *et al.*, 1987). The complete amnesic syndrome is usually transient (Geschwind and Fusillo, 1966) but may last as long as one year (Von Cramon *et al.*, 1988). Associated symptoms include right visual field defects, alexia without agraphia, anomia, and color agnosia (Damasio and Damasio, 1983; De Renzi *et al.*, 1987). Transient tactile memory loss has also been described (Ross, 1980b).

Right posterior cerebral artery territory infarcts produce impairments in visual memory and spatial memory. In addition to disturbed testing on figural and

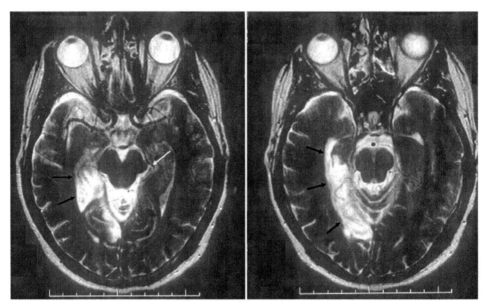

Figure 20.1 T2-weighted MRI images of a 62-year-old RH male who presented with acute onset left visual field defect, prosopagnosia, and visuospatial memory deficits. Images reveal a right PCA infarct (black arrows). White arrow points to the collateral sulcus, below which lies the collateral isthmus.

design tasks, clinically relevant memory deficits include difficulty learning to recognize new faces and impaired route learning (De Renzi *et al.*, 1987; Von Cramon *et al.*, 1988) and the inability to remember tactile objects placed in the contralateral hand (Ross, 1980b). Associated symptoms include left visual field defects and prosopagnosia.

The critical lesion for memory deficits after PCA infarctions is probably not the hippocampus but the afferent pathways to the entorhinal cortex and hippocampus that pass through a critical bottleneck deep to the parahippo-campal gyrus, the so-called collateral isthmus (Von Cramon *et al.*, 1988). This mechanism – damage to critical converging pathways – will recur in subsequent examples of stroke-related amnesia.

Thalamic lesions

The vascular supply to the thalamus is variable; thus the relationship between the area of infarction and the precise vessel involved can be quite variable, but lesions of the thalamus that result in memory disorders are in the anterior or medial regions. The most common cause of infarction in the thalamus is probably small vessel occlusive disease. The thalamus is also a common site of hypertensive hemorrhages.

Anterior thalamic infarctions are usually in the territory of the tuberothalamic artery or polar artery that typically arises from the posterior communicating artery. Infarcts in this territory will include the anterior nucleus, the mammil-lothalamic tract, and the internal medullary lamina (IML). The intralaminar region is another brain area where several critical pathways converge: the fornix descending to the mamillary bodies, the ascending mammillothalamic tracts and the ventral amygdalofugal pathways to dorsomedial thalamus. Anterior thalamic lesions of either hemisphere produce substantial executive dysfunction (Ghika-Schmid and Bogousslavsky, 2000), presumably due to damage to or disconnection of the thalamic–prefrontal systems, that impairs performance on all types of memory tests. Left-sided lesions also cause significant language impairment, at least anomia if not a mixed transcortical pattern of aphasia along with both verbal and visual memory deficits (Graff-Radford *et al.*, 1985). Right-sided lesions cause visuoperceptual deficits, including memory deficits (Graff-Radford *et al.*, 1985). Thus, with neither left nor right anterior thalamic lesions does amnesia appear in isolation. A recent study demonstrated some impairment of anterograde verbal memory after lesions of either anterior thalamic region although greater after left-sided lesions (Ghika-Schmid and Bogousslavsky, 2000). Recall was more impaired than recognition. The numerous intrusions, perseverations, and false recognitions produced by patients with lesions in either hemisphere illuminate the co-existing executive impairments in these patients.

Occlusion of the paramedian thalamic artery, also known as the interpeduncular profunda artery, typically the terminal small perforating artery of the basilar, can result in unilateral or bilateral infarctions. Thalamic damage is most prominent in the dorsomedial nucleus and the surrounding IML including the centromedian nucleus. In the acute phase these patients are usually hypersomnolent. As they improve there is continuing impairment in attention that produces deficits in all cognitive domains, including memory. Memory deficits include verbal and nonverbal and both anterograde and some retrograde memory (Katz *et al.*, 1987). There is no laterality effect on verbal or visual memory. With further improvement, there is continued reduction of sustained attention. These people are probably more accurately described as having an executive-dominant dementia than straightforward amnesia (Katz *et al.*, 1987) and significant impairments may be very persistent (Graff-Radford *et al.*, 1985; Von Cramon *et al.*, 1985; Gentilini *et al.*, 1987). Improvement is more likely with unilateral lesions.

Infarction of the inferior portion of the genu of the internal capsule in the territory of the perforating arteries arising from the internal carotid or from the anterior choroidal artery branches causes memory impairment, although again usually in the context of more pervasive deficits (Tatemichi *et al.*, 1992).

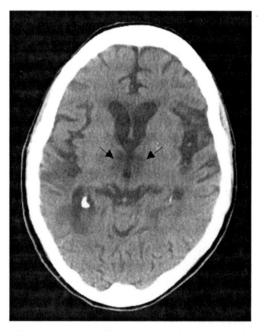

Figure 20.2 This is an 82-year-old RH woman who was found unresponsive by her husband. CT image on day 5 revealed bilateral medial thalamic infarcts (arrow).

This is also an example of critical converging pathways, in this case, the so-called "anterior thalamic peduncle" carrying the bi-directional connections of prefrontal structures and the thalamic nuclei. The clinical profile is similar to that of direct thalamic damage. Thus, typical features include fluctuating alertness, inattention, apathy, abulia, and psychomotor retardation – all consistent with a "frontal-lobe syndrome." As with the thalamic lesions, there is a modality–laterality effect with left-sided infarcts causing verbal memory loss and right-sided causing visuospatial memory impairment (Graff-Radford *et al.*, 1985). Limited long-term follow-up suggests that there is substantial recovery especially of the executive deficits (Madureira *et al.*, 1999).

Basal forebrain lesions

The only vascular etiology of basal forebrain lesions is rupture of an anterior communicating artery (ACoA) aneurysm. Extremely variable damage can arise from direct extension of hemorrhage, destruction or occlusion of the ACoA perforators, surgical isolation of the ACoA, or vasospasm in the proximal anterior cerebral arteries (ACAs) affecting the septal nuclei of the basal forebrain, the anterior hypothalamus, the medial forebrain bundle, the thalamofrontal connections, the ventral striatum, and the frontal cortex. The critical lesion for amnesia is probably in the septal nuclei that are the origin of the cholinergic pathways to the hippocampus, but there remains controversy about the specific role of the other regions in memory function.

Damage to the prefrontal cortex or to the anterior thalamic-prefrontal connections described above will cause considerable executive impairment. Associated signs may include hemiparesis, often worse in the leg, from ACA infarcts, lateralized grasp reflex, akinesia (unilateral or bilateral), and a period of mutism. Anterior hypothalamic injury can also cause a transient diabetes insipidus (Alexander and Freedman, 1984).

About 18% of survivors of ACoA rupture and surgery will have some cognitive deficit and severe amnesia is the most common (Lindqvist and Norlen, 1966; Takaku *et al.*, 1979), with most patients having complicated profiles of amnesia and executive impairment. Confabulation (discussed further below) is often much more prominent in these patients than after other causes of amnesia, attributed to the co-existing severe executive impairments that may blunt monitoring of responses and predispose to perseverative recollections (Damasio *et al.*, 1985a). Impaired recall of even very remote memories also appears more commonly in the "ACoA syndrome" (Gade and Mortensen, 1990). The mechanism of this retrograde amnesia is not known, nor is it universally observed (Alexander and Freedman, 1984), but it has been attributed to a failure to activate remote epochs of memory for a subsequent monitored fact checking (D'Esposito *et al.*, 1996).

More than with other causes of amnesia, patients with the "ACoA syndrome" are also likelier to be totally unaware of their deficits. This, in turn, causes substantial safety and behavioral problems. As amnesia alone does not cause lasting anosognosia for amnesia, the superimposition of executive impairments that blunt strategic analysis and monitoring has been blamed (Stuss *et al.*, 1978).

Confabulation is the recall of incorrect memories without intent to mislead. Some confabulations are simple, plausible filling in for failed recollection. If so, they are usually unelaborated and may change over repeated examinations. Other confabulations are intrusions of more detailed recollections from another similar epoch of experience: asked why he/she is hospitalized, the patient may relate an episode of hospitalization from years earlier. Others are more complex and variably implausible: asked why he/she is hospitalized, the patient may relate that he/she is making a sales call or serving meals. These are sometimes labeled "fantastical," and they may have the properties of fixed delusions (Stuss *et al.*, 1978). All patients with acute memory impairment may confabulate intermittently, perhaps responding to a sense that they should have the requested memory or because a related epoch comes to mind. As awareness of memory troubles increases, confabulation seems to be inhibited. The combination of

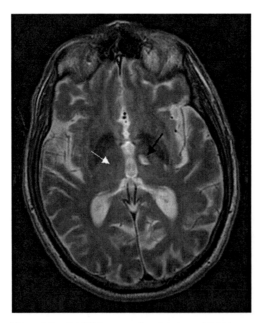

Figure 20.3 T2-weighted MRI image of a 75-year-old RH man who presented with acute onset of confusion, disorientation, right hemiparesis, and a mild aphasia with an infarct in the left anterior thalamus (black arrows). White arrow points to the intermedullary lamina.

Table 20.1. Summary of strokes affecting memory processing systems

Location/vascular territory	Processing system	Memory deficit
Left MCA	Lexical semantic system	Verbal memory
Left MCA	Parietal region — apraxia	Motor memory
Right MCA	Visuospatial	Visuospatial memory
Left frontal — lateral convexity	Executive	Verbal recall
Frontal — posterior medial	Executive	Verbal recall

memory loss and confusion or severe executive impairment appears to predispose to more elaborate and unlikely confabulations as well as to excessive false recognition (Verfaellie *et al.*, 2004). While not at all unique to patients with ACoA aneurysm rupture, these confabulations are quite common, and seem related to the severity of comorbid executive impairment in these patients (DeLuca and Cicerone, 1991).

Strokes affecting memory-processing systems

A summary of strokes affecting memory-processing systems is shown in Table 20.1.

Language-dominant hemispheric lesions

Atherosclerotic, embolic, or hemorrhagic strokes of sufficient size almost anywhere in the territories of the left middle cerebral artery, superficial or deep, cause aphasia. It is trivial to observe that patients with severe aphasia will not learn or "recall" verbal information. If they do not understand the material, they cannot learn it. If they are not able to recall or produce words in direct confrontation of language, they are not going to be able to demonstrate "recollection" in a delayed task of memory. It is not trivial, however, that even patients with very mild aphasia may be quite impaired at verbal learning. The impairment does not appear to be related directly to specific lesion locations or to traditional aphasia classifications. It is, however, closely related to deficits in specific linguistic systems (Risse *et al.*, 1984; Ween *et al.*, 1996). Patients with mild residual aphasia but persistent phonological impairments measured as phonemic paraphasias have normal verbal memory as usually tested with list learning and story recall, although they do have reduced working memory measured as forward and reverse digit span. Patients with mild residual aphasia but persistent lexical–semantic impairments measured as semantic paraphasias and low naming scores have normal working memory but impaired verbal memory. Patients with mild residual aphasia and both phonological and lexical–semantic impairments are impaired in both domains of memory. Mildly aphasic patients often complain that they have memory problems, but they are only reflecting sensitivity to word-finding problems or to reduced immediate verbal span. Their experiential memories, as long as specific verbal recall and lengthy immediate verbal span are not required, are quite normal.

Left hemisphere lesions and motor memory

Damage to the left parietal region, with or without accompanying aphasia, often produces apraxia (Liepmann and Mass, 1907). There is an enormous and conflicting literature about the proper nomenclature for apraxias, about the exact type of apraxia seen with parietal lesions, and about exactly where in the left parietal lobe lesions are most likely to cause apraxia (see Chapter 3). Attempting to avoid distraction by a semiological quarrel about apraxia itself, we propose that left parietal lesions cause disruption in the controlled production of learned movements, particularly critical in the preferred hand, in response to a stimulus (request, imitation, context, etc.) that normally produces the movement. In this sense, the parallel with the discussion above about aphasia should be obvious. If patients with apraxia cannot produce a learned movement when confronted with an evocative stimulus, the underlying system for organized control of movement is damaged. These patients also have difficulty learning a list of gestures (Rothi and Heilman, 1984) and acquiring a new motor skill (Heilman *et al.*, 1975). This is clinically significance in the setting of rehabilitation when therapists may try to teach new motor patterns to compensate for weakness. Repetition alone may be successful (implicit memory/motor skill) when explicit strategies fail.

Right hemisphere lesions and spatial memory

Right hemisphere lesions frequently cause disorders in visual spatial processing (Brain, 1941) and thus these patients will frequently have difficulty with learning and remembering spatial information. On occasions, patients with no overt visuospatial perceptive problems but with spatial memory deficits have been described following strokes.

De Renzi and colleagues have examined numerous right posterior hemisphere damaged patients, primarily vascular in origin. They found that patients with right hemisphere damage with a visual field deficit were impaired in learning and remembering spatial sequences (De Renzi *et al.*, 1977a; Cremonini *et al.*, 1980) and a visual maze task (De Renzi *et al.*, 1977b). These studies did not provide accurate neuroanatomical details; but, based on EEG data and physical examination (visual field deficits), the authors speculate that the retro-rolandic area is involved.

Strokes affecting strategic or executive systems

Patients with purely frontal lesions do not develop a classical amnesia, but they do develop a variety of memory impairments. The effects of frontal lesions on memory have been very extensively studied in non-human primates, in patients with a variety of frontal lesions, and in normal subjects with functional imaging. These studies have been extensively reviewed (Alexander and Stuss, 2000; Chayer and Freedman, 2001; Fletcher and Henson, 2001; Gaffan, 2002), and there is considerable, but not complete, convergence of evidence. Memory deficits are secondary to defects in one or more executive functions such as attention, working memory, strategy formulation, inhibition of competing recollections, and monitoring of ongoing mental activity (Moscovitch and Winocur, 1995). Exactly how these executive deficits impair memory is unclear.

Conclusions about the effects of human frontal lesions are further complicated by methodological obstacles. Rarely has lesion site been specified more precisely than right, left, or bilateral. Few studies have been restricted to patients with infarcts, and those studies often can inform only about the effects of a portion of the frontal lobe, usually the lateral convexity, being topographically restricted by vascular supply. Other etiologies are likewise restricted. Traumatic contusions are overwhelmingly polar and orbital, and patients may have more diffuse axonal injury. Resections to control epilepsy are biased towards premotor and superior medial regions, and patients may still be affected by seizures and medications. Tumor resections may leave behind infiltrating tumor (malignant gliomas) or may have had minimal cerebral effects (benign gliomas and meningiomas). Intracerebral hemorrhages probably offer the widest, unconstrained range of lesion sites, but they are relatively less common than the other etiologies.

A comprehensive view of the potential effects of frontal strokes on memory may require studies that include all etiologies or that incorporate all of the varied topographically restricted studies into a single analysis. Some general observations appear agreed upon. Frontal lesions may not disrupt learning a set of experimental stimuli, but they may impair memory for the order in which they occurred (Milner *et al.*, 1985) (temporal order), or to which stimulus set they belonged (Johnson *et al.*, 1993) (source memory). They may disrupt the capacity to judge whether the stimulus is actually being recognized or if it just seems familiar (Schnyer *et al.*, 2004). When recall of the stimuli is impaired, recognition may be normal (Stuss *et al.*, 1994). This distinction is often used in neuropsychology to distinguish a "true amnesia" where even recognition is impaired. When recognition is impaired, it may be much more likely because of mistaken endorsement of non-stimuli than in patients with "true amnesia" (Schnyer *et al.*, 2004), suggesting an over-reliance on familiarity and an under-reliance on monitoring. All of these features of impaired memory after frontal lesions have been referred to as "metamemory" (Moscovitch and Winocur, 1995).

Other than attribution of impaired recognition memory to right frontal damage, there have been few claims for specific regional frontal effects. For example, a group in Toronto demonstrated regional differences in recall, recognition, and error types and suggested that the practice of analyzing the effects of frontal lesions by amalgamating all lesion locations into a single "frontal" study group might be ineffective (Stuss *et al.*, 1994).

In a subsequent study, the same group demonstrated distinctive profiles of verbal memory impairment associated with lesions in different regions of the frontal lobes (Alexander *et al.*, 2003). All non-progressive etiologies were allowed: infarction, hemorrhage, traumatic contusions, and resection of benign intracerebral tumors, as the group was purposefully heterogeneous with stroke being the most common etiology. Performance was analyzed regionally using a standard list-learning task.

Patients with left lateral convexity lesions had impaired recall, and the impairment correlated with reduced verbal fluency and confrontation naming. Although the naming deficits were generally very mild, this presumably reflects the

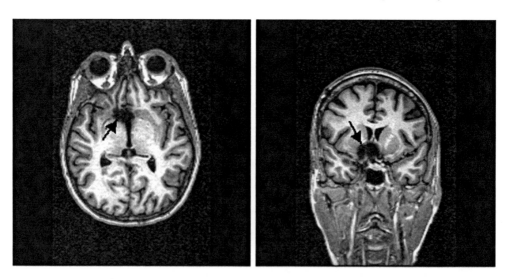

Figure 20.4 T1-weighted MRI images of a 58-year-old RH woman who is two years status post rupture of her anterior communicating artery aneurysm with lesion in the basal forebrain (R > L, arrows), extending into the septal nuclei (right figure).

same residual lexical–semantic impairment demonstrated in more overtly aphasic patients (see above). In addition, this group had poor recognition memory due to high false-positive endorsements of foils. Poor encoding secondary to mild semantic deficits appeared to leave them susceptible to bias – impaired setting of response criteria – with false-positive recognition resulting.

Patients with posterior, inferior medial lesions also had impaired recall. These patients had lesions that included the septal region. Their memory difficulties were presumably caused by the loss of cholinergic projections, and most of these patients actually had frontal damage secondary to ruptured ACoA aneurysms.

Patients with lesions limited to the right lateral, the right or left polar and the posterior, superior medial frontal regions had minimal deficits, but they did not utilize subjective organization as the normal controls did. That is, they did not consistently recall words paired together across sequential trials leading to inefficient acquisition of the entire list even if the final recall was normal.

Although etiologies were mixed, this study included a sufficient number of patients with lesions in all frontal regions that it serves as a preliminary template for the possible effects of frontal strokes – infarctions or hemorrhages – on memory.

Clinical assessment

The bedside assessment of the amnesic patient can be difficult. Patients should be alert, attentive, cooperative, motivated, and neither anxious nor depressed, and have intact perceptual processing systems or the assessment of memory is meaningless. Thus, clinical assessment of memory may, paradoxically, first involve assessment of possible comorbid deficits such as aphasia, alexia, visuoperceptual impairments, apraxia, and inattention. These cognitive deficits are more apparent than memory deficits and may complicate memory assessment, as discussed above. For patients who are initially lethargic or confused, it is best to wait until attention improves before reaching any definite conclusion about memory. Attention can be assessed with so-called mental control tasks: reciting the months of the year backwards, spelling words backwards or doing serial subtractions. Digit span forwards and backwards has the added benefit of determining the patient's list span, so subsequent memory tests such as serial list learning tasks can be modified accordingly, if necessary.

Once adequate attention, language, and perceptual functions have been demonstrated, memory can be evaluated. For some patients with low probability of memory deficits, the coherence and detail of the history provided by the patient may be sufficient testing. There is one verbal memory task that can be very informative along many dimensions: supraspan serial word list learning tasks, usually 9−10 words, from which the examiner can extract a learning curve, delayed recall, and a recognition score. Patients with executive deficits alone may have inefficient learning (a flat curve) or a tendency to repeat items within single presentations, but little loss of items after delay and good recognition. Patients with true amnesia may have variable, even good, learning curves, but poor recall and recognition. Utilizing a list-learning task of this sort can be awkward at the bedside and requires that the examiner be prepared with a list and a second list for recognition foils. A more universally practical bedside test of memory is telling the patient a coherent story with just three or four salient features, followed by a brief probe to be certain that the details have been noted, then probed again after a delay for uncued recall. Bedside tests, although useful, have a limited sensitivity.

Visual and spatial memory are rarely tested at the bedside because assessment is cumbersome. Copying and then, after a delay, reproducing abstract drawings is a reasonable assessment of visual memory. Observing the placement of a few objects in specific spatial relationships to each other and then, after delay, describing or drawing the relationship of the objects is a reasonable assessment of spatial memory.

Formal neuropsychological testing remains frequently warranted, especially in case of memory complaint (by the patient or informant), when bedside test is impaired or when the lesion concerns a region known to impair memory such as mediotemporal, thalamic, genu of the internal capsule, basal forebrain, and frontal regions. The standard neuropsychological tests of memory are valid, reliable, and standardized over a very wide age range. The tests can specify memory loss in all dimensions − short-term versus long-term, anterograde and retrograde, modality-specific, etc. − much better than casual bedside testing. Memory tests provide valuable information on the pattern of episodic memory deficit: true amnesia is characterized by poor recognition with poor benefit, if any, from cuing and greater loss of items on delayed recall. Conversely, executive deficits impair learning (as shown by a flat curve) and free recall whereas cued recall is typically good as recognition (except for the possible presence of false recognition); finally, there is little loss of items after delay. Severity of memory loss, severity and prognosis of medical/vascular condition, time since onset, comorbid neurological and medical diagnoses, age, and likely discharge setting are all factors that influence the decision to obtain neuropsychological testing. Clinicians should develop bedside tools that parallel standard neuropsychological tests but avoid using those tests so that they retain reliability in the contest of full testing. Clinicians should also recall that patients with attentional or executive impairments (e.g. frontal or thalamic strokes) and patients with mild language deficits may appear more memory impaired on standard tests than they actually are in real life.

Key point Assessment of episodic memory disorders in stroke

Deficit	Bedside testing	Neuropsychological tests
Possible associated deficits	aphasia, alexia, apraxia, visuoperceptual impairments, inattention	
Verbal memory	Supraspan word list	Rey auditory verbal learning
	Story recall	test
	Instruction recall	California verbal learning test
	Personal hospital history	Wechsler memory scale—revised
		Rivermead behavioral memory test
Visuospatial memory	Abstract drawing recall	Rey—Osterrieth complex figure
	Object location	Brief visual memory test—revised
Retrograde memory	Prior to hospitalized history	Autobiographical memory
	Autobiographical memory	interview

Prognosis

Some recovery can be anticipated after all strokes. The extent of recovery may be extremely variable, determined by size, location, and type of lesion and by age of the patient and comorbid medical and neurological factors. Neural systems with low redundancy and highly convergent pathways are at risk for limited recovery even with small lesions. The descending motor pathways for the hand and the geniculocalcarine visual pathways are the most obvious examples in the brain. As we noted above, however, the memory systems are also served by highly convergent systems — perforant pathway into hippocampus, collateral isthmus pathways into parahippocampal gyrus (and entorhinal cortex), intramedullary lamina with amygdala, hippocampal, and mamillary efferents all streaming close together, and anterior thalamic outflow. Even small critical lesions may produce permanent deficits in memory. Counterbalancing this anatomical risk of persistent deficits, event-based learning, and recollection is rarely modality specific, and unilateral lesions of the key structures usually will allow reasonable return of event learning and recollection.

Lesion in the basal forebrain are usually bilateral. In these patients, the combination of damage to the basal forebrain, striatum, and frontal lobes results in persistent, dense amnesia, while isolated basal forebrain damage is compatible with excellent recovery (Irle *et al.*, 1992). In addition, the retrograde amnesia improved in this group of ACoA aneurysm patients in parallel with recovery of executive functions (D'Esposito *et al.*, 1996). Better utilization of executive systems to check recollection, monitor possibilities, and utilize compensation may underlie improvement (Stablum *et al.*, 2000).

There are several physiological mechanisms of recovery. Acute-phase recovery is presumably due to resolution of edema, pressure effects, and sub-lethal ischemic injury, or even restitution of circulation. Later recovery must depend on more complex components of neural recovery and plasticity: resolution of diaschisis (Seitz *et al.*, 1999); regeneration of neural damaged elements such as regrowth of axons into damaged tracts (Lipton, 1989); possibly neurogenesis (Magavi *et al.*, 2000); and reorganization of undamaged brain to improve the function of a damaged region (Liepert *et al.*, 2000; Luft *et al.*, 2004). Reorganization may be local structural compensation, such as axonal sprouting (Carmichael, 2003) or dendritic reorganization (Kozlowski and Schallert, 1998), or it may be remote functional such as emergence of latent capacity in homologous, contralateral brain (Fisher, 1992). How any of these specifically evolve or even occur in recovery of memory after limbic lesions is not known. There is scant predictive information available beyond the lesion site and laterality factors noted above.

Management of disorders of episodic memory

There are two main approaches towards rehabilitation of stroke. One involves using adaptive strategies such as canes, orthotic devices, and cognitive and physical therapy. The second strategy involves attempts to enhance brain recovery.

Functional recovery can be modulated by the use of drugs such as neuroprotective agents (Park *et al.*, 1988) and growth factors (Kawamata *et al.*, 1998), but none has yet shown clinical efficacy. Norepinephrine (Goldstein, 1997) and amphetamine (Martinsson and Eksborg, 2004) have been shown to improve stroke outcome, possibly by influencing the physiological mechanisms of recovery discussed above. Recently, electrical stimulation has been used in an attempt to improve recovery. Direct cortical stimulation (Brown *et al.*, 2003) at the lesion site and transcranial magnetic stimulation (Oliveri *et al.*, 2001; Werhahn *et al.*, 2003; Naeser *et al.*, 2005) at the homologous contralateral hemisphere have improved recovery. These techniques are in their infancy and are limited to the motor, attentional, and language systems, so applicability to memory recovery is unknown.

Adaptive strategies for memory rehabilitation rely on cognitive remediation with two main approaches: retraining residual abilities and providing alternative resources to improve performance. Intense retraining of partially damaged neural systems has been successful for some limited aspects of motor recovery (constraint-induced hand therapy, bodyweight-supported treadmill gait therapy, etc.). Comparable treatments in cognitive and memory disorders have been less successful. Neither intensive training (Prigatano *et al.*, 1984; Godfrey and Knight, 1985), nor semantic elaboration (Wilson, 1982), nor visual imagery (Jones, 1974) has been effective in improving memory performance. More promising techniques such as "vanishing cues" (Glisky *et al.*, 1986), spacing of repetitions (Hillary *et al.*, 2003), errorless learning (Baddeley and Wilson, 1994), or combinations (Komatsu *et al.*, 2000), teach hyperspecific information. These techniques can be used for learning specific information or skills such as simple computer skills, but they do not result in a global improvement on memory performance.

Memory prostheses are an alternative resource that can be an effective compensation for defective memory. One long-term study demonstrated that patients were using memory aids and strategies to a greater extent during the follow-up evaluation than they had been during the rehabilitation period, suggesting considerable practical benefit (Harris and Sunderland, 1981). Notebooks, diaries, alarm watches, calendars, and posted signs containing useful information in critical areas around a person's living environment, or educating family members in cued supervision, can be useful (Evans *et al.*, 2003). Simple devices, such as pagers and voice organizers, can help a patient maintain a schedule or follow a medication regimen. They are simple to operate, require modest training, have demonstrated efficacy even in severely impaired individuals, and training effects may persist even after withdrawal of the device (Wilson *et al.*, 1997).

Key points Management and treatment of episodic memory dysfunction

---

Pharmacotherapy: possible interest in some patients but further trials required
Norepinephrine, amphetamine, or acetylcholinesterase inhibitor
Transcranial magnetic stimulation: possible interest in other disorders; trials required
Cognitive remediation:
intense re-training, semantic elaboration and visual imagery: poor efficacy
promising approaches: 'vanishing cues', spacing of repetitions, and errorless learning
Compensatory approach: practical benefit in most patients
notebooks, diaries, alarm watches, calendars, organization of living environment, and
    educating family members in cued supervision: useful
simple devices (pagers and voice organizers) to maintain a schedule or follow a medication
    regimen: efficacious even in severely amnesics
personal digital assistants and similar handheld pocket computers: only in selected patients
    with pure and mild to moderate amnesia

Recently, development of personal digital assistants and similar handheld pocket computers has the potential to help mildly amnestic patients, but the devices paradoxically require too much learning for the densely amnesic patient. In addition, many amnesics also have other problems — alexia (PCA strokes), poor motivation (thalamic and frontal strokes), etc. — that make them poor candidates for external aids.

Attempts to restore brain function directly are in their infancy and have no proven value in memory rehabilitation. Efforts to restore memory function through repetition and practice have only marginal value for isolated skills or tasks. Thus, current efforts should be directed towards compensating for memory impairments. External aids can be helpful, in mild to moderate amnestic patients, with the simpler to operate the better for patients. The latest group of external aids, the personal digital assistant devices, has the potential to be a valuable memory aid in this group of patients, provided that family members are willing to invest the time and training to properly learn to use these devices. The obvious amalgamation of memory rehabilitation is to use errorless learning techniques to teach amnestic patients how to reliably and properly use simple external memory aids.

REFERENCES

Alexander, M. P. and Freedman, M. (1984). Amnesia after anterior communicating artery aneurysm rupture. *Neurology*, **34**, 752–7.

Alexander, M. P. and Stuss, D. T. (2000). Disorders of frontal lobe functioning. *Sem. Neurol.*, **20**, 427–37.

Alexander, M. P., Stuss, D. T., *et al.* (2003). California Verbal Learning Test: Performance by patients with focal frontal and non-frontal lesions. *Brain*, **126**, 1493–503.

Baddeley, A. and Wilson, B. A. (1994). When implicit learning fails: Amnesia and the problem of error elimination. *Neuropsychologia*, **32**, 53–68.

Brain, W. R. (1941). Visual disorientation with special reference to lesions of the right cerebral hemisphere. *Brain*, **64**, 244–72.

Brown, J. A., Lutsep, H., *et al.* (2003). Motor cortex stimulation for enhancement of recovery after stroke: A case report. *Neurol. Res.*, **25**, 815–18.

Caplan, L. R. (1980). "Top of the basilar" syndrome. *Neurology*, **30**, 72–9.

Caplan, L. R. and Hedley-Whyte, T. (1974). Cuing and memory dysfunction in alexia without agraphia. *Brain*, **97**, 251–62.

Carmichael, S. T. (2003). Plasticity of cortical projections after stroke. *Neuroscientist*, **9**, 64–75.

Cermak, L. S. and O'Connor, M. (1983). The anterograde and retrograde retrieval ability of a patient with amnesia due to encephalitis. *Neuropsychologia*, **21**, 213–34.

Chayer, C. and Freedman, M. (2001). Frontal lobe functions. *Curr. Neurol. Neurosci. Rep.*, **1**, 547–52.

Corsellis, J. A., Goldberg, G. J., *et al.* (1968). "Limbic encephalitis" and its association with carcinoma. *Brain*, **91**, 481–96.

Cremonini, W., De Renzi, E., *et al.* (1980). Contrasting performance of right- and left-hemisphere patients on short-term and long-term sequential visual memory. *Neuropsychologia*, **18**, 9.

Cummings, J. L., Tomiyasu, U., *et al.* (1984). Amnesia with hippocampus lesions after cardiopulmonary arrest. *Neurology*, **34**, 679–81.

D'Esposito, M., Alexander, M. P., *et al.* (1996). Recovery of memory and executive function following anterior communicating artery aneurysm rupture. *J. Int. Neuropsychol. Soc.*, **2**, 565–70.

Damasio, A. R. and Damasio, H. (1983). The anatomic basis of pure alexia. *Neurology*, **33**, 1573–83.

Damasio, A. R., Eslinger, P. J., *et al.* (1985a). Multimodal amnesic syndrome following bilateral temporal and basal forebrain damage. *Arch. Neurol.*, **42**, 252–9.

Damasio, A. R., Graff-Radford, N. R., *et al.* (1985b). Amnesia following basal forebrain lesions. *Arch. Neurol.*, **42**, 263–71.

Deluca, J. and Cincerone, K. D. (1991). Confabulation following aneurysm of the anterior communicating artery. *Cortex*, **27**, 417–23.

De Olmos, J. S. (1990). Amygdala. In *The Human Nervous System*, ed. J. Paxinos. New York: Academic Press, Inc., pp. 583–710.

De Renzi, E., Faglioni, P., *et al.* (1977a). Spatial memory and hemispheric locus of lesion. *Cortex*, **13**, 424–33.

De Renzi, E., Faglioni, P., *et al.* (1977b). Topographical amnesia. *J. Neurol., Neurosurg. Psychiatry*, **40**, 498–505.

De Renzi, E., Zambolin, A., *et al.* (1987). The pattern of neuropsychological impairment associated with left posterior cerebral artery infarcts. *Brain*, **110**, 1099–116.

Evans, J. J., Wilson, B. A., *et al.* (2003). Who makes good use of memory aids? Results of a survey of people with acquired brain injury. *J. Int. Neuropsychol. Soc.*, **9**, 925–35.

Fisher, C. M. (1992). Concerning the mechanism of recovery in stroke hemiplegia. *Can. J. Neurol. Sci.*, **19**, 57–63.

Fletcher, P. C. and Henson, R. N. (2001). Frontal lobes and human memory: Insights from functional neuroimaging. *Brain*, **124**, 849–81.

Gade, A. and Mortensen, E. L. (1990). Temporal gradient in the remote memory impairment of amnesic patients with lesions in the basal forebrain. *Neuropsychologia*, **28**, 985–1001.

Gaffan, D. (2002). Against memory systems. *Philos. Trans. R. Soc. London.* [*Bio.*], **357**, 1111–21.

Gentilini, M., De Renzi, E., *et al.* (1987). Bilateral paramedian thalamic artery infarcts: Report of eight cases. *J. Neuro., Neurosurg. Psychiatry*, **50**, 900–9.

Geschwind, N. and Fusillo, M. (1966). Color-naming defects in association with alexia. *Arch. Neurol.*, **15**, 137–46.

Ghika-Schmid, F. and Bogousslavsky, J. (2000). The acute behavioral syndrome of anterior thalamic infarction: A prospective study of 12 cases. *Ann. Neurol.*, **48**, 220–7.

Glisky, E. L., Schacter, D. L., *et al.* (1986). Learning and retention of computer-related vocabulary in memory-impaired patients: Method of vanishing cues. *J. Clin. Exp. Neuropsychol.*, **8**, 292–312.

Godfrey, H. P. and Knight, R. G. (1985). Cognitive rehabilitation of memory functioning in amnesiac alcoholics. *J. Consult. Clin. Psychol.*, **53**, 555–7.

Goldstein, L. B. (1997). Influence of common drugs and related factors on stroke outcome. *Curr. Opin. Neurol.*, **10**, 52–7.

Graff-Radford, N. R., Damasio, H., *et al.* (1985). Nonhaemorrhagic thalamic infarction. *Brain*, **108**, 485–516.

Harris, J. E. and Sunderland, A. (1981). A brief survey of the management of memory disorders in rehabilitation units in Britain. *Int. Rehab. Med.*, **3**, 206–9.

Heilman, K. M., Schwartz, H. D., *et al.* (1975). Defective motor learning in ideomotor apraxia. *Neurology*, **25**, 1018–20.

Hillary, F. G., Schulthesis, M. T., *et al.* (2003). Spacing of repetitions improves learning and memory after moderate and servere TB1. *J. Clin. Exp. Neuropsychol.*, **25**, 49–58.

Hyman, B. T., Van Hoesen, G. W., *et al.* (1984). Alzheimer's disease: Cell-specific pathology isolates the hippocampal formation. *Science*, **225**, 1168–70.

Irle, E., Wowra, B., *et al.* (1992). Memory disturbances following anterior communicating artery rupture. *Ann. Neurol.*, **31**, 473–80.

Johnson, M. K., Hashtroudi, S., *et al.* (1993). Source monitoring. *Psychol. Bull.*, **114**, 3–28.

Jones, M. K. (1974). Imagery as a mnemonic aid after left temporal lobectomy: Contrast between material-specific and generalized memory disorders. *Neuropsychologia*, **12**, 21–30.

Katz, D. I., Alexander, M. P., *et al.* (1987). Dementia following strokes in the mesencephalon and diencephalon. *Arch. Neurol.*, **44**, 1127–33.

Kawamata, T., Ren, J., *et al.* (1998). Intracisternal osteogenic protein-1 enhances functional recovery following focal stroke. *Neuroreport*, **9**, 1441–5.

Komatsu, S., Mimura, M., *et al.* (2000). Errorless and effortful processes involved in learning of face-name associations by patients with alcoholic Korsakoff's syndrome. *Neuropsychol. Rehab.*, **10**, 113–32.

Kozlowski, D. A. and Schallert, T. (1998). Relationship between dendritic pruning and behavioral recovery following sensorimotor cortex lesions. *Behav. Brain Res.*, **97**, 89–98.

Liepert, J., Bauder, H., *et al.* (2000). Treatment-induced cortical reorganization after stroke in humans. *Stroke*, **31**, 1210–6.

Liepmann, H. and Mass, O. (1907). Ein Fall von linksseitiger Agraphie und Apraxie bei rechtsseitiger Lahmung. *J. Psychol. Neurol.*, **10**, 214–27.

Lindqvist, G. and Norlen, G. (1966). Korsakoff's syndrome after operation on ruptured aneurysm of the anterior communicating artery. *Acta Psychiatr. Scand.*, **42**, 24–34.

Lipton, S. A. (1989). Growth factors for neuronal survival and process regeneration. Implications in the mammalian central nervous system. *Arch. Neurol.*, **46**, 1241–8.

Luft, A. R., McCombe-Waller, S., *et al.* (2004). Repetitive bilateral arm training and motor cortex activation in chronic stroke: A randomized controlled trial. *JAMA*, **292**, 1853–61.

Madureira, S., Guerreiro, M., *et al.* (1999). A follow-up study of cognitive impairment due to inferior capsular genu infarction. *J. Neurol.*, **246**, 764–9.

Magavi, S. S., Leavitt, B. R., *et al.* (2000). Induction of neurogenesis in the neocortex of adult mice. *Nature*, **405**, 951–5.

Mair, W. G. P., Warrington, E. K., *et al.* (1979). Memory disorder in Korsakoff's psychosis: A neuropathological and neuropsychological investigation of two cases. *Brain*, **102**, 749–83.

Martinsson, L. and Eksborg, S. (2004). Drugs for stroke recovery: The example of amphetamines. *Drugs and Aging*, **21**, 67–79.

Milner, B., Petrides, M., *et al.* (1985). Frontal lobes and the temporal organization of memory. *Hum. Neurobiol.*, **4**, 137–42.

Mishkin, M. (1978). Memory in monkeys severely impaired by combined but not separate removal of the amygdala and hippocampus. *Nature*, **273**, 297–8.

Mohr, J. P., Leicester, J., *et al.* (1971). Right hemianopia with memory and color deficits in circumscribed left posterior cerebral artery territory infarction. *Neurology*, **21**, 1104–13.

Moscovitch, M. and Winocur, G. (1995). Frontal lobes, memory, and aging. *Ann. N. Y. Acad. Sci.*, **769**, 119–50.

Naeser, M. A., Martin, P. I., *et al.* (2005). Improved picture naming in chronic aphasia after TMS to part of right Broca's area: An open-protocol study. *Brain Lang.*, **93**, 95–105.

Nauta, W. J. (1961). Fibre degeneration following lesions of the amygdaloid complex in the monkey. *J. Anat.*, **95**, 515–31.

Oliveri, M., Bisiach, E., *et al.* (2001). rTMS of the unaffected hemisphere transiently reduces contralesional visuospatial hemineglect. *Neurology*, **57**, 1338–40.

Papez, J. W. (1995). A proposed mechanism of emotion. 1937. *J. Neuropsychiatry Clin. Neurosci.*, **7**, 103–12.

Park, C. K., Nehls, D. G., *et al.* (1988). The glutamate antagonist MK-801 reduces focal ischemic brain damage in the rat. *Ann. Neurol.*, **24**, 543–51.

Prigatano, G. P., Fordyce, D. J., *et al.* (1984). Neuropsychological rehabilitation after closed head injury in young adults. *J. Neurol., Neurosurg. Psychiatry*, **47**, 505–13.

Risse, G. L., Rubens, A. B., *et al.* (1984). Disturbances of long-term memory in aphasic patients. *Brain*, **107**, 605–17.

Rosene, D. L. and Van Hoesen, G. W. (1987). The hippocampal formation of the primate brain: A review of some comparative aspects of cytoarchitecture and connections. In *Cerebral Cortex*, ed. E. G. Jones and A. Peters. Plenum Publishing Corporation, pp. 345–456.

Ross, E. D. (1980a). Sensory-specific and fractional disorders of recent memory in man. I. Isolated loss of visual recent memory. *Arch. Neurol.*, **37**, 193–200.

(1980b). Sensory-specific and fractional disorders of recent memory in man. II. Unilateral loss of tactile recent memory. *Arch. Neurol.*, **37**, 267–72.

Rothi, L. J. and Heilman, K. M. (1984). Acquisition and retention of gestures by apraxic patients. *Brain Cogn.*, **3**, 426–37.

Schnyer, D. M., Verfaellie, M., *et al.* (2004). A role for right medial prefontal cortex in accurate feeling-of-knowing judgements: Evidence from patients with lesions to frontal cortex. *Neuropsychologia*, **42**, 957–66.

Scoville, W. B. and Milner, B. (1957). Loss of recent memory after bilateral hippocampal lesions. *J. Neurol., Neurosurg. Psychiatry*, **20**, 11–21.

Seitz, R. J., Azari, N. P., *et al.* (1999). The role of diaschisis in stroke recovery. *Stroke*, **30**, 1844–50.

Squire, L. R., Amaral, D. G., *et al.* (1989). Description of brain injury in the amnesic patient N.A. based on magnetic resonance imaging. *Exp. Neurol.*, **105**, 23–35.

Stablum, F., Umilta, C., *et al.* (2000). Rehabilitation of executive deficits in closed head injury and anterior communicating artery aneurysm patients. *Psychol. Res.*, **63**, 265–78.

Stuss, D. T., Alexander, M. P., *et al.* (1978). An extraordinary form of confabulation. *Neurology*, **28**, 1166–72.

Stuss, D. T., Alexander, M. P., *et al.* (1994). Organizational strategies of patients with unilateral or bilateral frontal lobe injury in word list learning tasks. *Neuropsychology*, **8**, 355–73.

Swanson, L. W. (1978). The anatomical organization of septo-hippocampal projections. In *Functions of the Septo-Hippocampal System*. Ciba Foundation Symposium, pp. 25–43.

Swanson, L. W. and Cowan, W. M. (1975). Hippocampo-hypothalamic connections: Origin in subicular cortex, not Ammon's horn. *Science*, **189**, 303–4.

(1977). An autoradiographic study of the organization of the efferent connections of the hippocampal formation in the rat. *J. Comp. Neurol.*, **172**, 49–84.

Takaku, A., Tanaka, S., *et al.* (1979). Postoperative complications in 1,000 cases of intracranial aneurysms. *Surg. Neurol.*, **12**, 137–44.

Tatemichi, T. K., Desmond, D. W., *et al.* (1992). Confusion and memory loss from capsular genu infarction: a thalamocortical disconnection syndrome? *Neurology*, **42**, 1966–79.

Verfaellie, M., Rapcsak, S. Z., *et al.* (2004). Elevated false recognition in patients with frontal lobe damage is neither a general nor a unitary phenomenon. *Neuropsychology*, **18**, 94–103.

Victor, M., Adams, R. D., *et al.* (1971). *The Wernicke-Korsakoff Syndrome*. Oxford, England, Blackwells.

Victor, M., Angevine, J. B., *et al.* (1961). Memory loss with lesions of hippocampal formation. *Arch. Neurol.*, **5**, 244–63.

Von Cramon, D. Y., Hebel, N., *et al.* (1985). A contribution to the anatomical basis of thalamic amnesia. *Brain*, **108**, 993–1008.

Von Cramon, D. Y., Hebel, N., *et al.* (1988). Verbal memory and learning in unilateral posterior cerebral infarction. *Brain*, **111**, 1061–77.

Ween, J. E., Verfaellie, M., *et al.* (1996). Verbal memory function in mild aphasia. *Neurology*, **47**, 795–801.

Werhahn, K. J., Conforto, A. B., *et al.* (2003). Contribution of the ipsilateral motor cortex to recovery after chronic stroke. *Ann. Neurol.*, **54**, 464–72.

Whitehouse, P. J., Price, D. L., *et al.* (1982). Alzheimer's disease and senile dementia: Loss of neurons in the basal forebrain. *Science*, **215**, 1237–9.

Wilson, B. (1982). Success and failure in memory training following a cerebral vascular accident. *Cortex*, **18**, 581–94.

Wilson, B. A., Evans, J. J., *et al.* (1997). Evaluation of NeuroPage: A new memory aid. *J. Neurol. Neurosurg. Psychiatry*, **63**, 113–15.

Zola-Morgan, S., Squire, L. R., *et al.* (1982). The neuroanatomy of amnesia: Amygdala-hippocampus versus temporal stem. *Science*, **218**, 1337–9.

21

Working memory dysfunctions in stroke patients

Martial Van der Linden,[1,2] Martine Poncelet,[2] and Steve Majerus[2,3]

[1]University of Geneva
[2]University of Liège
[3]Belgian National Fund of Scientific Research (FNRS)

Working memory and the Baddeley and Hitch multi-component model

Working memory refers to a system involved in the short-term maintenance and manipulation of information necessary for performing complex cognitive tasks. One of the most influential views of working memory has been put forth by Baddeley and Hitch (1974; see also Baddeley, 1986). The Baddeley and Hitch model comprises a modality-free controlling central executive that is aided by a number of subsidiary slave systems which ensure temporary maintenance of information. Two such systems have been more deeply explored: the phonological loop and the visuospatial sketchpad. The phonological loop system is specialized for processing acoustic and verbal material and is composed of two subsystems: a phonological store which can hold memory traces for a few seconds, and an articulatory rehearsal mechanism (analogous to subvocal speech) which permits memory traces to be refreshed. Neuropsychological and neuroimaging data (Baddeley, 2003) suggest that the phonological store and the articulatory rehearsal mechanism are associated with the left inferior parietal region (BA 40) and the left inferior frontal cortex (Broca's area)/premotor cortex (BA 6/44), respectively. The visuospatial sketchpad system is assumed to be involved in temporarily maintaining and manipulating visuospatial information. It may actually be composed of two distinct systems, one for maintaining visual representations, and another for spatial ones. A fractionation of the visuospatial sketchpad, analogous to that of the phonological loop, has also been proposed: a visual storage component and a more dynamic retrieval and rehearsal mechanism. Neuropsychological and neuroimaging studies (Baddeley, 2003) indicate that the visuospatial sketchpad may be principally represented within the right hemisphere (right inferior parietal cortex, BA 40; right premotor cortex, BA 6; right inferior frontal cortex, BA 47; and also the anterior extrastriate occipital cortex, BA 19). Recently, Baddeley (2000) has proposed a supplementary component, the episodic buffer. The episodic buffer represents a temporary storage system using a multimodal code, permitting integration of information from the subsidiary systems and from long-term memory. It has been suggested that the frontal lobes play an important role in the temporary retention of integrated information (Prabhakaran *et al.*, 2000), but it is likely that other regions are also involved. To our knowledge, no neuropsychological study has yet explored the episodic buffer by using a task specifically designed to measure its capacity.

The core of the working memory model is the central executive. The central executive is assumed to be an attentional control system responsible for strategy selection and for control and coordination of the various processes involved in short-term storage and more general processing. Numerous neuroimaging studies (Collette and Van der Linden, 2002) have examined the cerebral areas related to the central executive by using tasks that require the manipulation of information temporarily maintained in working memory (such as the alpha span task in which the participants are required to recall sequences of words not in serial order but according to the alphabetical order). These studies demonstrated the involvement of the dorsolateral prefrontal cortex (BA 9/46) but also of the parietal cortex. Baddeley (1986) has suggested that the supervisory attentional system (SAS) of the "attentional control of action" model proposed by Norman and Shallice (1980) might be an adequate approximation of the functions of the central executive system. Norman and Shallice assume the existence of two attentional control processes: the contention scheduling mechanism, which would be involved in making selections between conflicting routine actions, and the SAS which intervenes when the selection of routine actions is not sufficient (for instance, when coping with novel or dangerous situations). Additionally, the SAS is supposed to carry out a variety of processes that are relatively independent from each other. Accordingly, Miyake *et al.* (2000) recently found that three executive functions (shifting between mental sets or tasks, updating and monitoring of working memory contents, and inhibition of prepotent responses) are separable at a cognitive level, but are also moderately correlated with one another, thus indicating both unity and diversity of executive functions. In a recent neuroimaging study capitalizing on the framework proposed by Miyake *et al.*, we confirmed the unity and diversity of executive functions at a functional brain level (Collette *et al.*, 2005). Indeed, we observed that the three main executive functions identified by Miyake and co-workers (updating, shifting, and inhibition) activated common cerebral areas (the left superior parietal gyrus and the right intraparietal sulcus and, at a lower statistical threshold, the left middle and inferior frontal gyri). In addition to these common areas, each executive process also relied on specific sets of frontal and parietal areas.

Key points Main characteristics of working memory according to the Baddeley and Hitch model

> *Working memory*: short-term maintenance and manipulation of information; involved in simple (e.g. short-term maintenance of a phone number) and complex cognitive tasks (e.g. coordination of two simultaneous tasks)
> It includes:
> a modality-free controlling central executive (coordination of the various processes involved short-term storage)
> slave systems which ensure temporary maintenance of information:
> the phonological loop (verbal information) which is composed of a phonological store and articulatory rehearsal mechanism
> the visuospatial sketchpad (visuospatial information)

Impairment of the phonological loop

Assessment of the phonological loop

Phonological loop capacity is typically measured using verbal span tasks. In these tasks, the patient is asked to repeat back auditorily presented sequences of digits, letters, or words. The sequences are of increasing length and the memory span corresponds to the longest sequence length at which the sequence is correctly reproduced in, for example, 50% or 75% of trials. For a young healthy adult, the digit span is about seven digits (± 2). Word span is generally lower and depends on the length and lexical frequency of the words used. Another characteristic of performance in verbal span tasks is the phonological similarity effect, reflecting better recall of phonologically dissimilar sequences (e.g. *house, dog, car*) as opposed to phonologically similar sequences (e.g. *cat, map, ham*). The word-length effect represents better recall performance for lists of short words (e.g. *house, dog, ice*) relative to longer words (e.g. *locomotive, refrigerator, inauguration*). Based on Baddeley and Hitch's model, the word length and the phonological similarity effect are supposed to arise from two different sources. The phonological similarity effect is supposed to reflect the operation of the phonological store where phonological traces of the to-be-recalled information are stored, with more distinctive phonological traces leading to better recall performance (Baddeley, 1966). The word-length effect is the consequence of the articulatory rehearsal mechanism which depends on the speed of subvocal articulation and takes longer for long words than for short words, leading to more efficient refreshment of short words. It should be noted that the presence of phonological similarity and word-length effects can be variable even in healthy controls. Hence it is recommended to check for the consistency of the absence of these effects in short-term memory impaired patients, by taking at least 2−3 three different measures of these effects.

Phonological loop deficits in stroke patients

The precise prevalence of verbal short-term deficits in stroke patients has not been systematically studied to our knowledge. In most stroke patients, verbal short-term memory generally appears to be relatively spared when administering standardized (but often not very sensitive) neuropsychological test batteries. However, mild deficits are frequent in stroke patients presenting an infarct in the left middle cerebral artery territory, and they are often associated with other cognitive impairments such as aphasia and attentional problems (Bartha and Benke, 2003). In more rare cases of stroke patients, a selective phonological loop deficit has been observed. These patients typically present with reduced digit spans (1−4) and complain about difficulties following a conversation, summarizing the information of a phone call they just got, repeating telephone numbers, or doing mental arithmetic operations (e.g. Basso *et al.*, 1982; Silveri and Cappa, 2003). Otherwise, these patients present no other cognitive deficits: their visuospatial sketchpad is normal and they have preserved episodic long-term memory and general intellectual abilities. Language perception and production are also not significantly impaired. Nevertheless, it must be noted that the language tests used are not always very sensitive and thus the presence of subtle deficits at the level of perceptual and phonological processing cannot always be completely ruled out. This remark is very important as a number of these patients were aphasic immediately after the cerebral infarction, presenting most often with conduction aphasia, an aphasic syndrome characterized by severe difficulties in repeating even single words (e.g. patient PV: Basso *et al.*, 1982). Although the single word processing difficulties of these patients might recover, the presence of residual subtle impairments at the level of speech perception or planning cannot be completely ruled out and these might interact with the apparent selective phonological loop deficit that is later observed in these patients.

Most patients with phonological loop deficits present relatively normal phonological similarity effects but word-length effects are generally absent. However, phonological similarity effects are absent when the information is presented visually, contrary to healthy subjects, suggesting that the visually presented verbal information is not recoded in an auditory−phonological code. This pattern of performance is consistent with the interpretation that the patients avoid the use of their defective phonological store, despite having normal capacity to articulate, and try to use their preserved visual−spatial sketchpad capacities. More generally, it must be noted that the deficit in verbal span tasks is most severe for auditorily presented verbal information, with some patients showing normal performance when the word or digit lists are presented visually (Vallar and Papagno, 2002). A selective deficit in the articulatory rehearsal mechanism has been described by Belleville *et al.* (1992) in a stroke patient with a left temporoparietal lesion. Indeed, he showed a reduced verbal span, no word-length effect in both the visual and the auditory modalities, no phonological similarity effect in the visual modality, and, contrary to healthy subjects, no reduction of verbal span when subvocal rehearsal was prevented by requiring the patient to repeat an irrelevant sound. In addition, he presented a slowed articulation rate.

Another important characteristic of these patients is that they have severe difficulties in learning new phonological information, such as the vocabulary of a foreign language, suggesting that the phonological loop is involved in the acquisition of language. For example, PV, an Italian woman who presented severely reduced verbal spans after an infarction of the left parietal lobe, was unable to learn the Russian translation of familiar Italian words (Baddeley *et al.*, 1988). Sentence comprehension is also frequently affected in these patients (Van der Linden and Poncelet, 1998). Although short sentences are in general correctly understood, patients with phonological loop deficits have difficulties with long sentences where word order is important (e.g. *touch the large red square and the small green rectangle*) or that contain semantically reversible sentences (e.g. *the boy that the girl hit was my neighbor*).

In most stroke patients with a selective phonological loop deficit, the lesion involves the left parietal cortex, and, more specifically, the left supramarginal gyrus (Vallar and Papagno, 2002). However, a number of uncertainties remain with regard to the neuroanatomical substrate of the phonological loop. Indeed, many patients also presented lesions to the temporal lobes. For example, Takayama *et al.* (2004) presented a patient with selective verbal working memory deficits but apparently normal language processing who had a focal infarct of the posterior part of the left superior temporal gyrus. Thus both the superior temporal and the inferior parietal cortex seem to be involved in verbal working memory (see also Majerus *et al.*, 2003). The question that arises is whether these two regions play different roles during the temporary retention of verbal information. In verbal span tasks, two different types of information have to be retained: the items and their phonological and lexico-semantic characteristics as well as the order in which the items are presented. One possibility is that the parietal lobe is specifically involved in the retention of serial order information (Marshuetz *et al.*, 2000) and that the temporal region is related to item short-term storage (Majerus *et al.*, 2004). With respect to the stroke patients with a selective verbal working memory deficit, the issue of item and order recall has not yet been specifically investigated.

It is therefore impossible at present to determine whether the patients with selective lesions to the parietal cortex have more difficulties in retaining order than item information, and whether the reverse is true in patients with lesions limited to the posterior part of the superior temporal lobe.

A final theoretical issue pertains to an even more fine-grained distinction at the level of item representations themselves. Martin *et al.* (1994) reported two patients who showed different capacities for temporarily retaining phonological and lexico-semantic information. Patient EA was more impaired than patient AB on a task assessing short-term memory for phonological information (a rhyme probe task where the patient was asked to decide if a target stimulus rhymes with one of the words presented in a list just before the presentation of the target stimulus); while patient AB had greater difficulty on a task measuring short-term memory abilities for lexico-semantic information (a category probe task where the patient was asked to decide if a target stimulus belonged to the same category as one of the words presented in a list just before the presentation of the target stimulus). Patient EA had suffered from an infarct to the left superior temporal and inferior parietal cortex while patient AB had presented a left frontal hematoma. Other stroke patients with specific difficulties in the retention of lexico-semantic information have been described, involving the left prefrontal cortex, as well as the parietal and temporal cortex (patients ML and GR: Freedman and Martin, 2001). These lesion sites are too broad to provide a clear idea of what the cerebral substrates of these "semantic short-term storage abilities" might be. Nevertheless, these distinctions are important because they have implications with regard to the theoretical models of working memory and language processing. For example, Martin *et al.* (1994) showed that patients with phonological short-term storage deficits seem to have relatively preserved sentence comprehension but impaired sentence repetition abilities, while the reverse has been observed for patients with semantic short-term storage deficits.

Impairment of the visuospatial sketchpad

Spatial short-term memory is usually measured using the Corsi block tapping task which comprises an array of nine blocks. The examiner touches an (increasing) number of blocks following a pre-defined order; the subject then attempts to reproduce the sequence by touching the same blocks in the same order. In healthy persons, Corsi span is typically about two less than the digit span. Visual short-term memory is assessed by means of the pattern span task; here, the subject is shown for several seconds matrices of black and white cells, with half of the cells being black. After presentation of each target matrix, the subject is presented the same matrix, but containing this time only white cells; the patient has to indicate those cells that were black in the target matrix. The matrix size progressively increases, beginning with a 2×2 matrix.

The assessment of the visuospatial sketchpad in stroke patients has mainly been conducted by using the Corsi block tapping task. Kessels *et al.* (2000) applied the Corsi task to a group of healthy participants and a group of patients with cerebral lesions (mainly due to an ischemic stroke) and showed that the right hemisphere patients performed worse than the left hemisphere patients. Interestingly, Mayer *et al.* (2003) observed a significant correlation between performance on the Corsi task (forward and backward span) and written-digit calculation in patients with chronic single vascular brain lesions. On the other hand, performance on the digit span task (forward and backward) significantly correlated with oral calculation.

More recently, in two experiments, Malhotra *et al.* (2005) demonstrated that spatial working memory capacity is related to the neglect syndrome in neglect patients who suffered from a stroke that damaged regions within the right parietal lobe and insula. Spatial short-term storage was assessed using a vertical computerized variant of the Corsi task (experiment 1) and by another variant designed to provide a purer measure of spatial short-term storage, circumventing problems due to impaired memory for stimulus sequence or poor visuomotor control of manual responding (experiment 2). More specifically, the authors showed that as a group, right hemisphere patients with left neglect had impaired spatial working memory capacity. Moreover, poor performance on the second spatial storage task correlated with severity of left neglect on cancellation tasks. These results are consistent with the view that a deficit in keeping track of spatial locations (a spatial short-term storage deficit) interacts with a lateral spatial bias towards the right, to exacerbate neglect. In addition, the study by Malhotra and co-workers also suggested that some non-neglect patients may show a spatial short-term storage deficit if their lesions involve critical "spatial short-term memory" regions without inducing any lateral bias. Finally, other authors have also suggested that impairments in visuospatial working memory might contribute to representational aspects of neglect, and not only to perceptual neglect (e.g. Della Sala *et al.*, 2004).

Impairment of the central executive

At a very general level, the central executive can be measured by using tasks requiring not only storage and rehearsal (as do forward digit span and Corsi span tasks), but also the manipulation of the maintained information or the simultaneous processing of additional information. For example, backward digit and Corsi span tasks can be used; in these tasks, the patient is required either to repeat digit sequences (backward digit span) or to reproduce block sequences (Corsi span) in the reverse order. Other tasks interleave the presentation of to-be-remembered target stimuli, such as digits or words, with the presentation of a demanding, secondary processing task such as comprehending sentences or verifying equations. For example, the computation span task includes the presentation of series of cards on each of which an arithmetic problem is given. The second number in each arithmetic problem is framed and the solution is replaced by a question mark $(5 + \boxed{3} = ?; 6 - \boxed{5} = ?; 2 + \boxed{7} = ?)$. The patient is required to remember the framed digits in order while solving the problems. The number of arithmetic problems presented on each trial increases progressively from two to nine. At the end of each trial, the participant has to recall the series of framed digits. Similarly, the sentence span task requires reading (or hearing) and verifying whether a sentence is semantically or syntactically correct and then recalling the final word of each sentence (or an unrelated word). More specific tasks should be used to explore the specific functions (such as inhibition, updating, shifting) that are also attributed to the central executive system. However, the description of these tasks would considerably exceed the limits of the present chapter (see also Chapter 19).

Leskelä *et al.* (1999) found that elderly patients with a frontal infarct had lower performance in the backward digit span task, but not in the forward digit span task, relative to non-frontal patients and to control subjects. These data confirm that the frontal lobes contribute to central executive functioning. Central executive deficits (as assessed by working memory tasks requiring storage and processing, such as the sentence span task), along with normal performance on the digit or word span tasks, have also been observed in patients with isolated thalamic stroke (Dagenbach *et al.*, 2001) and in young patients with isolated infratentorial infarcts (Malm *et al.*, 1998), suggesting a role of the thalamus and the cerebellum in central executive functioning. Finally, Amberla *et al.* (2004) found that the backward digit span task is one of the most sensitive tests to differentiate pre- and post-stroke patients with CADASIL (cerebral autosomal dominant arteriopathy with subcortical infarcts and leukoencephalopathy). More generally, Vataja *et al.* (2003) showed that executive dysfunctions (as assessed by classical executive tasks such as the Stroop task, the Wisconsin Card Sorting Test, the verbal fluency test, or the Trail-Making Test) are frequent in patients with ischemic stroke and are related to brain infarcts and white matter lesions affecting the frontal–subcortical circuits or the pons (see Chapter 19). Finally, in a more analytical study, Ravizza and Ciranni (2002) showed that the ability to shift from one stimulus dimension to another (one of the executive functions identified by Miyake *et al.*, 2000) was impaired in stroke patients with prefrontal damage and that these shifting deficits did not appear to be the result of a reduced working memory capacity.

Key points Main types of stroke associated with working memory deficits

Stroke type	Territory/characteristics
Arterial Infarct	Middle cerebral artery: posterior/inferior and anterior/superior branches
	Thalamus

Key points Tasks commonly used to assess the components of the Baddeley and Hitch working memory model

Component of working memory	Method
Phonological loop	Forward digit span
	Word span
Phonological store	Phonological similarity effect
Articulatory rehearsal mechanisms	Word length effect
Visuospatial sketchpad:	
– spatial component	Corsi Block Tapping Test
– visual component	Pattern recall
Central executive	Backwards digit span
	Computation span
	Sentence span

Rehabilitation of working memory deficits

Rehabilitation of working memory deficits in stroke patients has been the focus of surprisingly few studies, despite the significant incidence of these impairments and their impact on other cognitive functions. Francis *et al.* (2003) focused on treating phonological loop impairment with related sentence comprehension deficits in a stroke patient showing some cerebral atrophy and an infarct of the left parietal lobe. The treatment consisted of repeating sentences of increasing length and syntactic complexity. Post-treatment assessment showed an increase in digit span and in the number of words recalled during sentence repetition. However, there was only limited generalization to sentence comprehension: although the patient could understand longer sentences and needed less repetition, significant deficits in sentence comprehension remained. The authors suggested that therapy improved the active central executive system rather than the passive phonological store.

In another recent study, we described an intervention which targeted limitations in passive storage capacity for phonological information more directly

Table 21.1. A selection of tests presented to BJ before and after therapy

	Initial assessment 1999	Pre-therapy 2001	Post-therapy 2003	Significance pre- vs. post-therapy
Digit span	3	3	5	Within normal limits after therapy
Word span	3	3	3	Unchanged after therapy
Proportion of words recalled	na	0.43	0.72	$\chi^2(1) = 27.14$, $p < 0.001$
Nonword span	< 2	< 2	3	Within normal limits after therapy
Proportion of nonwords recalled	0.00	0.00	0.38	$\chi^2(1) = 46.91$, $p < 0.001$
Rhyme judgment				
Words		1.00	0.99	n.s.
Nonwords		0.75	0.95	$\chi^2(1) = 15.69$, $p < 0.001$

(Majerus *et al.*, 2005). The treatment was administered to a patient (BJ) with selective and chronic phonological loop impairment due to a left perisylvian infarct. It consisted of single non-word delayed repetition for a large set of bisyllabic nonwords; the duration of the retention interval (during which the patient had to count backwards) was increased by two seconds each time the repetition performance for a given retention interval was successful. At post-therapy assessment (Table 21.1), a modest improvement was observed for digit and non-word span as well as significant increases for the number of non-words and words correctly repeated in word or non-word span tasks. Rhyme judgment for non-words also significantly improved. After treatment, the patient reported that her previous difficulties for sentence comprehension (which occurred when several people spoke at the same time) had decreased and she was again able to drive her car while speaking at the same time or listening to the radio. These results seem to be specific to the treatment program as performance in word and non-word span tasks had not changed in the years preceding the treatment, despite intensive speech-language therapy that targeted the patient's productive language difficulties she initially presented.

Key points Management and treatment of working memory dysfunction

---

Rehabilitation: further trials required
Successful treatment effects observed in some case studies for verbal short-term memory deficits

---

Finally, Malouin *et al.* (2004) demonstrated the contribution of working memory in physical rehabilitation after stroke. More specifically, they showed in 12 patients with residual motor impairment resulting from a first cerebrovascular accident that one session of physical practice combined with mental practice (recalling the kinesthetic sensations, visual images, and verbal descriptors associated with the proper motor strategy) resulted in an improvement in the loading of the affected leg during standing up and sitting down. The improvement of the motor skill was maintained one day after training. In addition, this learning effect was strongly related to working memory capacity especially in the visuo-spatial working memory domain. These data suggest that working memory deficits should be taken into account when selecting therapeutic approaches in physical rehabilitation.

Considering the critical nature of working memory to cognitive functioning and the diverse situations in which such a system seems to be important, it is to be hoped that in future more studies will be conducted in stroke patients to examine the relationships between working memory deficits and complex cognitive tasks in everyday life, and to explore the efficacy of specific rehabilitation strategies.

REFERENCES

Amberla, K., Wäljas, M., Tuominen, S., *et al.* (2004). Insidious cognitive decline in CADASIL. *Stroke*, **35**, 1598–602.

Baddeley, A. (1966). Short-term memory for word sequences as a function of acoustic, semantic and formal similarity. *Q. J. Exp. Psychol.*, **18**, 362–5.

(1986). *Working Memory*. Oxford: Clarendon Press.

(2000). The episodic buffer: A new component of working memory? *Trends Cogn. Sci.*, **4**, 417–23.

(2003). Working memory: Looking back and looking forward. *Nat. Rev. Neurosci.*, **4**, 829–39.

Baddeley, A. D. and Hitch, G. (1974). Working memory. In G. Bower, ed., *The Psychology of Learning and Motivation*, Vol. **8**, New York: Academic Press, pp. 47–90.

Baddeley, A. D., Papagno, C. and Vallar, G. (1988). When long-term learning depends on short-term storage. *J. Mem. Lang.*, **27**, 586–95.

Bartha, B. and Benke, T. (2003). Acute conduction aphasia: An analysis of 20 cases. *Brain Lang.*, **85**, 93–108.

Basso, A., Spinnler, H., Vallar, G. and Zanobio, M. E. (1982). Left hemisphere damage and selective impairment of auditory verbal short-term memory. A case study. *Neuropsychologia*, **20**, 263–74.

Belleville, S., Peretz, I. and Arguin, M. (1992). Contribution of articulatory rehearsal to short-term memory: Evidence from a case of selective disruption. *Brain Lang.*, **43**, 713–46.

Collette, F. and Van der Linden, M. (2002). Brain imaging of the central executive component of working memory. *Neurosci. Biobehav. Rev.*, **26**, 105–25.

Collette, F., Van der Linden, M., Laureys, S., *et al.* (2005). Exploring the unity and diversity of the neural substrates of executive functioning. *Human Brain Mapping*, **25**, 409–23.

Dagenbach, D., Kubat-Silman, A. K. and Absher, J. R. (2001). Human verbal working memory impairments associated with thalamic damage. *Int. J. Neurosci.*, **111**, 67–87.

Della Sala, S., Logie, R. H., Beschin, N. and Denis, M. (2004). Preserved visuo-spatial transformations in representational neglect. *Neuropsychologia*, **42**, 1358–64.

Francis, D. R., Clark, N. and Humphreys, G. W. (2003). The treatment of an auditory working memory deficit and the implications for sentence comprehension abilities in mild "receptive" aphasia. *Aphasiology*, **17**, 723–50.

Freedman, M. and Martin, R. C. (2001). Dissociable components of short-term memory and their relation to long-term learning. *Cogn. Neuropsychol.*, **18**, 193–226.

Kessels, R. P. C., Van Zandvoort, M. J. E., Postma, A., Kappelle, L. J. and De Haan, E. H. F. (2000). The Corsi block-tapping task: Standardization and normative data. *Appl. Neuropsychol.*, **7**, 252–8.

Leskelä, M., Hietanen, M., Kalska, H., *et al.* (1999). Executive functions and speed of mental processing in elderly patients with frontal or nonfrontal ischemic stroke. *Eur. J. Neurol.*, **6**, 653–61.

Majerus, S., Laureys, S., Collette, F., *et al.* (2003). Phonological STM networks after recovery of Landau-Kleffner syndrome. *Human Brain Mapping*, **19**, 133–44.

Majerus, S., Van der Kaa, M. A., Renard, C., Van der Linden, M. and Poncelet, M. (2005). Treating verbal short-term memory deficits by increasing the duration of temporary phonological representations: A case study. Brain Lang., **95**(1), 174–75.

Majerus, S., Van der Linden, M., Poncelet, M. and Metz-Lutz, M.-N. (2004). Can phonological and semantic STM be dissociated? Further evidence from Landau-Kleffner syndrome. *Cogn. Neuropsychol.*, **21**, 491–512.

Malhotra, P., Jäger, H. R., Parton, A., *et al.* (2005). Spatial working memory capacity in unilateral neglect. *Brain*, **128**, 424–35.

Malm, J., Kristensen, B., Karlsson, T., *et al.* (1998). Cognitive impairment in young adults with infratentorial infarcts. *Neurology*, **51**, 433–40.

Malouin, F., Belleville, S., Richards, C. L., Desrosiers, J. and Doyon, J. (2004). Working memory and mental practice outcomes after stroke. *Arch. Phys. Med. Rehabil.*, **85**, 177–83.

Marshuetz, C., Smith, E. E., Jonides, J., DeGutis, J. and Chenevert, T. L. (2000). Order information in working memory: FMRI evidence for parietal and prefrontal mechanisms. *J. Cogn. Neurosci.*, **12** (Suppl. 2), S130–S144.

Martin, R. C., Shelton, J. R. and Yaffee, L. S. (1994). Language processing and working memory: Neuropsychological evidence for separate phonological and semantic capacities. *J. Mem. Lang.*, **33**, 83–111.

Mayer, E., Reicherts, M., Deloche, G., *et al.* (2003). Number processing after stroke: Anatomoclinical correlations in oral and written codes. *J. Int. Neuropsychol. Soc.*, **9**, 899–912.

Miyake, A., Friedman N. P., Emerson, M. J., Witzki, A. H. and Howerter, A. (2000). The unity and diversity of executive functions and their contributions to complex "frontal lobe" tasks: A latent variable analysis. *Cogn. Psychol.*, **41**, 49–100.

Norman, D. A. and Shallice, T. (1980). Attention to action: Willed and automatic control of behavior. *Center for Human Information Processing (Technical report No.* 99). Reprinted in revised form in *Consciousness and Self-regulation. Advances in Research*, ed. R. J. Davidson, G. E. Schartz and Shapiro, (1986), Vol **4**, New York: Plenum Press, pp. 1–18.

Prabhakaran, V., Narayanan, K., Zhao, Z. and Gabrieli, J. D. E. (2000). Integration of diverse information in working memory within the frontal lobe. *Nature Neurosci.*, **3**, 85–90.

Ravizza, S. M. and Ciranni, M. A. (2002). Contributions of the prefrontal cortex and basal ganglia to set shifting. *J. Cogn. Neurosci.*, **14**, 472–83.

Silveri, M. A. and Cappa, A. (2003). Segregation of the neural correlates of language and phonological short-term memory. *Cortex*, **39**, 913–25.

Takayama, Y., Kinomoto, K. and Nakamura, K. (2004). Selective impairment of the auditory-verbal short-term memory due to a lesion of the superior temporal gyrus. *Eur. Neurol.*, **51**, 115–17.

Vallar G. and Papagno, C. (2002). Neuropsychological impairments of verbal short-term memory. In *Handbook of Memory Disorders, 2nd Edition*, ed. A. D. Baddeley, M. D. Kopelman and B. A. Wilson. John Wiley & Sons Ltd, pp. 249–70.

Van der Linden, M. and Poncelet, M. (1998). The role of working memory in language and communication disorders. In *Handbook of Neurolinguistics*, ed. B. Stemmer and H. A. Whitaker. Academic Press, pp. 289–300.

Vataja, R., Pohjasvaara, T., Mäntylä, R., *et al.* (2003). MRI correlates of executive dysfunction in patients with ischaemic stroke. *Eur. J. Neurol.*, **10**, 625–31.

22

Akinetic mutism and related disorders

Didier Leys and Hilde Henon

University Hospital of Lille, France

General characteristics of akinetic mutism

Neuropsychological deficits are of major importance in stroke patients: they are frequent, have a major diagnostic value as they may be the only clinical manifestation of stroke, require a specific management, and are a major determinant of residual disability. This chapter will focus on the main characteristics of akinetic mutism and related disorders, which are sometimes classified as "coma-like states."

Clinical description

The main characteristics of akinetic mutism and related disorders that may be misdiagnosed with akinetic mutism are summarized in the Key points table. All these conditions may occur after a coma of a variable length of time, and represent a favorable step between a comatose state and return to normality. The main difference between these conditions and coma is that sleep–wake cycles are present. This differentiation is important to determine the prognosis and to choose the most appropriate therapeutic strategy.

Akinetic mutism

Akinetic mutism is also called "abulia major," and was formerly called "coma vigile." Patients with akinetic mutism appear alert or at least wakeful, because their eyes are open and they have active gaze movements. They are mute and immobile, but they are able to follow the observer or moving objects with their eyes, to whisper a few monosyllables, and to have slow feeble voluntary movements under repetitive stimuli. The patients can answer questions, but otherwise never voluntarily start speaking. In extreme circumstances such as noxious stimuli, they can become agitated and even say appropriate words. This neuropsychological syndrome occurs despite the lack of obvious alteration of sensory motor functions. This syndrome results in impaired abilities in communicating and initiating motor activities. The speech disorder includes verbal inertia, hypophonia, perseveration, softened and at times slurred language

Key points Main clinical characteristics and neuropathological findings in patients
with akinetic mutism or related disorders

Clinical syndrome	Main clinical features	Lesion
Akinetic mutism (also called abulia major)	No cognitive function Sleep–wake cycles present Seems to be interested in environment No spontaneous movement Limited movements after noxious stimuli No major sensori-motor deficit	Bilateral basal medial frontal lobe
Locked-in syndrome	Alert and aware of the environment Quadriplegic Lower cranial nerve palsies Vertical gaze and blinking preserved Sleep–wake cycles present	Bilateral anterior pontine
Persistent vegetative state (also called "apallic syndrome")	No cognitive function Retained vegetative components Sleep–wake cycles present	Extensive cortical lesions or extensive subcortical lesions with relative preservation of the brainstem
Abulia (severe cases are classified as akinetic mutism)	Severe apathy Sleep–wake cycles present No ability to speak spontaneously No ability to move spontaneously Blunting of feelings, mentation, and behavior	Bilateral basal medial frontal lobe

(Nagaratnam *et al.*, 2004). The linguistic disturbances associated with akinetic mutism may consist of fluent, non-fluent, anomia and transcortical (motor, mixed) aphasias (Nagaratnam *et al.*, 2004), but they can usually hardly be diagnosed.

Two different types of akinetic mutism have been identified on the basis of the location of the cerebral lesion:

1. The fronto-diencephalic form is seen in patients with anterior cerebral artery territory infarcts and/or rupture of the anterior communicating artery aneurysms with vasospasm. Besides the classical neuropsychological deficits, patients may have urinary incontinence, normal wakefulness, grasping and generalized bifrontal slowing on electroencephalogram, with a lack of desynchronization after external stimuli.

2. The thalamic form of akinetic mutism is seen in patients with paramedian thalamic or thalamo-mesencephalic infarcts.

The clinical features of akinetic mutism are associated with vertical eye movement impairment and hypersomnia (Lhermitte *et al.*, 1963; Segarra, 1970).

Related disorders

Athymormia

A discrepancy may be present between hetero- and auto-activation, the patient having an almost normal behavior under external stimuli. This peculiar form of akinetic mutism has been reported as "athymormia," "loss of psychic self-activation" or "pure psychic akinesia" (Laplane *et al.*, 1984; Laplane, 1990; Bogousslavsky *et al.*, 1991).

Locked-in syndrome

The term "locked-in syndrome" was proposed in 1966 (Plum and Posner, 1980), but this condition was described one century before by Alexandre Dumas with the figure of M. Noirtier de Villefort, in his book *Le Comte de Monte-Cristo*, edited 1844–1845: "the Count was alert and oriented, but he could communicate only with his eyes" (Dumas, 1860).

Patients are alert and aware of their environment. They are quadriplegic and have lower cranial nerve palsies. They can communicate with vertical gaze movements and blinking. The patient cannot physically move any part of the body except the eyes, but is conscious and able to think. Vertical eye movements and eye blinking can be used to communicate and to operate environmental controls. A persistent trismus may occur (Krasnianski *et al.*, 2003), but the patient usually remains able to yawn. Yawning leads to a transient sedation of trismus (Krasnianski *et al.*, 2003).

Persistent vegetative state (formerly called apallic syndrome)

The term "apallic syndrome" used to describe a complete loss of higher functions with retention of brainstem functions, and implied the loss of the cortical gray matter (so-called pallium) or extensive white matter lesions that interrupts any cortical connection. This term is currently replaced by that of vegetative state. Arousal is present, but the ability to interact with the environment is not. Eye opening can be spontaneous or occur in response to stimulation. Patients are unable to speak or to obey, but spontaneous movements may occur. Systemic responses to pain exist, such as increased heart rate, increased respiration, posturing, or sweating. Sleep—wake cycles, respiratory functions, yawning, chewing, grimacing, and digestive functions are preserved (Giacino and Zasler, 1995). Patients have no awareness of the environment, but they have preserved sleep—wake cycles.

Abulia

Abulia is a term used to describe a less severe state than akinetic mutism (see also Chapter 20). Patients have a severe apathy. They have blunting of feelings, mentation, and behavior, leading to an inability to speak or to move spontaneously (Mesulam, 1986).

Differential diagnosis

Coma

The main differential diagnosis of akinetic mutism and related disorders is coma. Coma is defined as a state of unconsciousness from which the individual cannot be awakened, in which the individual responds minimally or not to stimuli, and initiates no voluntary activities. While in a deep coma, a patient may not move at all, even to painful stimuli, and may be unable to produce any voluntary actions or meaningful responses. They can show various levels of non-purposeful movements, and respond minimally or not at all to stimuli.

Anarthric tetraparesis

Anarthric tetraparesis is a differential diagnosis of akinetic mutism and of locked-in syndrome. The lesion is located in both internal capsules and results in tetraparesis with normal horizontal eye movements (Chia, 1984; De Smet *et al.*, 1990; Ferbert and Thron, 1992; Nicolai and Lazzarino, 1993).

Depression

Akinetic mutism is also sometimes misdiagnosed with depression (Nagaratnam *et al.*, 2004).

Non-fluent aphasia

Severe forms of Broca's, transcortical motor and global aphasias also induce a mutism. Severe transcortical motor aphasia is frequently due to large prefrontal lesions and usually associated with severe motor reduction, hence corresponding to the criteria of akinetic mutism. Conversely, spontaneous movements and attempts to communicate by gestures are usually observed in Broca's and global aphasias.

Causes and determinants

Akinetic mutism, abulia, abulia minor, and athymormia

The term "akinetic mutism" was introduced into the English language more than 60 years ago to describe the peculiar neuropsychological picture of a lady with an epidermoid cyst located in the third ventricle (Cairns *et al.*, 1941). This syndrome has also been reported in traumatic lesions, in carbon monoxide poisoning (Tengvar *et al.*, 2004), after surgery for hydrocephalus (Psarros *et al.*, 2003; Aidi *et al.*, 2000), and in astrocytoma infiltrating the fornices (Oberndorfer *et al.*, 2002). However, most cases of akinetic mutism have been reported in patients with anterior cerebral artery territory infarcts and/or rupture of an anterior communicating artery aneurysm with vaso-spasm: of eight patients with bilateral infarction in the anterior cerebral artery territory, seven were found to have akinetic mutism (Minagar and David, 1999). It has also been reported in paramedian thalamic or thalamo-mesencephalic infarcts.

Akinetic mutism is due to disruption of reticulo-thalamo-frontal and extra-thalamic reticulo-frontal afferent pathways (Figure 22.1). The main determinant is a lesion located in both cingulated gyri (cingulum), but such a lesion is usually not sufficient and should be associated with other lesions (Buge *et al.*, 1975; Plum and Posner, 1980). Akinetic mutism is regarded as a specific condition characterized by injury of the frontal neuronal systems which promote executive functions (Tengvar *et al.*, 2004). Akinetic mutism is a neurobehavioral condition that results when the dopaminergic pathways in the brain are damaged. The critical areas are the frontal (cingulate gyrus, supplementary motor area, and dorso-lateral border zone), basal ganglia (caudate, putamen), the mesence-phalon and thalamus (Nagaratnam *et al.*, 2004).

Stroke, akinetic mutism, and related disorders

Akinetic mutism, abulia, and athymormia

They have been reported in single case reports and short series of patients suffering from bilateral infarcts or hemorrhages in the basal ganglia, deep

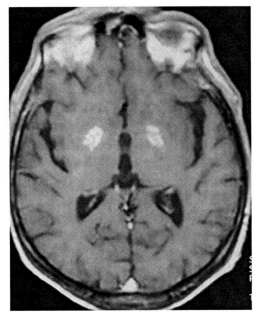

Figure 22.1   Patient with akinetic mutism after carbon monoxide poisoning (courtesy Prof. Pruvo).

Key points Main types of stroke associated with akinetic mutism

Stroke type	Territory/characteristics
Arterial infarct	thalamus: paramedian (bilateral)
	middle cerebral artery: deep
	branches (bilateral)
	anterior cerebral artery (bilateral)
Ruptured aneurysm	anterior communicating artery
	Pericallosal artery
Cerebral venous thrombosis	superior sagittal sinus

cerebral veins thrombosis (Laplane *et al.*, 1982; 1984; Richfield *et al.*, 1987; Habib and Poncet, 1988; Laplane, 1990; De Smet *et al.*, 1990; Baron, 1994; Bhatia and Marsden, 1994; Milandre *et al.*, 1995; Piccirilli *et al.*, 1995; Tatemichi *et al.*, 1995; Mega and Cohenour, 1997), thalamic infarcts (Lhermitte *et al.*, 1963; Bogousslavsky *et al.*, 1991), uni- or bilateral capsular genu infarcts

(Tatemichi *et al.*, 1993), midbrain infarcts or hemorrhages (Kemper and Romanul, 1967; Castaigne *et al.*, 1981; Hochman *et al.*, 1985), bilateral cingulate infarcts (Buge *et al.*, 1975; Laplane *et al.*, 1981; Habib and Poncet, 1988; Gugliotta *et al.*, 1989; Borggreve *et al.*, 1994), basal forebrain infarcts (Okawa *et al.*, 1980), or frontal strokes (Gautier *et al.*, 1983). Bilateral infarct in the anterior cerebral artery territory due to thrombosis is rare. Most cases are due to vasospasm following ruptured aneurysm of the anterior communicating artery and to a lesser extent of the pericallosal artery where a sudden akinetic mutism may even be the presenting picture. Akinetic mutism observed after repair of anterior communicating artery aneurysm is usually due to extensive bifrontal lesions (frequently associated with basal forebrain lesions). It usually improves but clinical practice suggests that it frequently indicates a poor cognitive outcome. Bilateral paramedian thalamic or thalamo-mesencephalic infarcts are another classical cause of akinetic mutism. It is usually observed following the improvement of the initial hypersomnia.

A lesser severity of abulia has been reported as "abulia minor" in bilateral caudate infarcts, and in polar thalamic infarcts (Fisher, 1983). Athymormia has been reported in patients with bilateral lesions located in the deep frontal white matter, or in the basal ganglia, especially the globus pallidus (Laplane *et al.*, 1984; Laplane, 1990; Bogousslavsky *et al.*, 1991). Most cases were due to anoxic encephalopathy.

Locked-in syndrome

The lesion is usually an infarct involving bilaterally the anterior part of the pons, and is the consequence of a basilar artery occlusion, bilateral occlusion of paramedian arteries and vertebral artery dissections (Rae-Grant *et al.*, 1989). Locked-in syndromes are almost always the consequence of infarcts located in both paramedian territories of the pons. It can also be due to bilateral midbrain infarcts (Karp and Hurtig, 1974; Patterson and Grabois, 1986). Transient forms have been reported after stellate ganglion block (Tuz *et al.*, 2003). Other causes have been reported, such as traumas or tumors (Inci and Ozgen, 2003).

Persistent vegetative state

Lesions are extensive cortical or subcortical lesions with preservation of the brainstem and they are usually not due to stroke. They can be encountered in severe head trauma, diffuse hypoxia, and various types of encephalopathies.

Management and outcome

Key points Management of akinetic mutism and locked-in syndrome

Akinetic mutism	Pharmacotherapy with dopaminergic agent: possible improvement in selected patients
Locked-in syndrome	Intensive and early rehabilitation

Akinetic mutism and abulia
It has been suggested that the clinical feature is the consequence of an impairment of the dopaminergic modulatory signals from the caudate nucleus to the frontal lobe. Dopaminergic agonists have been reported to be beneficial (Ross and Stewart, 1981; Aidi *et al.*, 2000; Alexander, 2001; Psarros *et al.*, 2003) but only in single case reports or small open series.

Locked-in syndrome
The relatives and staff caring for patients with a locked-in syndrome should be regularly reminded that the cognitive functions of the patient and awareness are strictly normal. Recovery is possible even after several months (McCusker *et al.*, 1982). Patients with initially stable locked-in syndromes can have prolonged survival, live in the community if there is enough support, and have some measure of quality of life (Doble *et al.*, 2003). Intensive and early rehabilitation, started within 1 month of the morbid event, improves the functional recovery and may reduce mortality (Casanova *et al.*, 2003)

Persistent vegetative state
The prognosis is very poor when the situation lasts more than 1 month (Childs *et al.*, 1993).

REFERENCES

Aidi, S., Elalaoui-Faris, M., Benabdeljlil, M., *et al.* (2000). Mutism akinétique et syndrome simulant une paralysie supranucléaire progressive après dérivation d'une hydrocéphalie obstructive. Efficacité d'un traitement par bromocriptine: Deux cas. *Rev. Neurol. (Paris)*, **156**, 380–3.

Alexander, M. P. (2001). Chronic akinetic mutism after mesencephalic-diencephalic infarction: Remediated with dopaminergic medications. *Neurorehabil. Neural Repair*, **15**, 151–6.

Baron, J. C. (1994). Conséquences des lésions des noyaux gris centraux sur l'activité métabolique cérébrale: Implications cliniques. *Rev. Neurol. (Paris)*, **150**, 599–604.

Bhatia, K. P. and Marsden, C. D. (1994). The behavioural and motor consequences of focal lesions of the basal ganglia in man. *Brain*, **117**, 859–76.

Bogousslavsky, J., Regli, F., Delaloye, B., *et al.* (1991). Loss of psychic self-activation with bithalamic infarction. Neurobehavioural, CT, MRI and SPECT correlates. *Acta Neurol. Scand.*, **83**, 309–16.

Borggreve, F., De Deyn, P. P., Marien, P., Cras, P. and Dierckx, R. A. (1994). Bilateral infarction in the anterior cerebral artery vascular territory due to an unusual anomaly of the circle of Willis. *Stroke*, **25**, 1279–81.

Buge, A., Escourolle, R., Rancurel, G. and Poisson, M. (1975). Mutisme akinetique et ramollissement bicingulaire. Trois cas anatomo-cliniques. *Rev. Neurol. (Paris)*, **131**, 121–31.

Cairns, H., Oldfield, R. C., Pennybacker, J. B. and Whitteridge, D. (1941). Akinetic mutism with an epidermoid cyst of the 3rd ventricle. *Brain*, **64**, 273–90.

Casanova, E., Lazzari, R. E., Lotta, S. and Mazzucchi, A. (2003). Locked-in syndrome: Improvement in the prognosis after an early intensive multidisciplinary rehabilitation. *Arch. Phys. Med. Rehabil.*, **84**, 862–7.

Castaigne, P., Lhermitte, F., Buge, A., *et al.* (1981). Paramedian thalamic and midbrain infarct: Clinical and neuropathological study. *Ann. Neurol.*, **10**, 127–48.

Chia, L. G. (1984). Locked-in state with bilateral internal capsule infarcts. *Neurology*, **34**, 1365–7.

Childs, N. L., Mercer, W. N. and Childs, H. W. (1993). Accuracy of diagnosis of persistent vegetative state. *Neurology*, **43**, 1465–7.

De Smet, Y., Rousseau, J. J. and Brucher, J. M. (1990). Infarctus putamino-capsulo-caudés bilatéraux, symmétriques et simultanés. *Rev. Neurol. (Paris)*, **146**, 415–19.

Doble, J. E., Haig, A. J., Anderson, C. and Katz, R. (2003). Impairment, activity, participation, life satisfaction, and survival in persons with locked-in syndrome for over a decade: Follow-up on a previously reported cohort. *J. Head Trauma Rehabil.*, **18**, 435–44.

Dumas, A. (1860). *Le Comte de Monte-Christo*. Paris: Calmann-Lévy. S.

Ferbert, A. and Thron, A. (1992). Bilateral anterior cerebral artery territory infarction in the differential diagnosis of basilar artery occlusion. *J. Neurol.*, **239**, 162–4.

Fisher, C. M. (1983). Honored guest presentation: Abulia minor vs. agitated behavior. *Clin. Neurosurg.*, **31**, 9–31.

Gautier, J. C., Awada, A. and Loron, P. A. (1983). A cerebrovascular accident with unusual features. *Stroke*, **14**, 808–10.

Giacino, J. and Zasler, N. (1995). Outcome after severe traumatic brain injury: Coma, the vegetative state, and the minimally responsive state. *J. Head Trauma Rehabil.*, **10**, 40–56.

Gugliotta, M. A., Silvestri, R., De Domenico, P., Galatioto, S. and Di Perri, R. (1989). Spontaneous bilateral anterior cerebral artery occlusion resulting in akinetic mutism. A case report. *Acta Neurol. (Napoli)*, **11**, 252–8.

Habib, M. and Poncet, M. (1988). Perte de vitalité, d'intérêt et des affects (syndrome athymormique) dans des lésions lacunaires du striatum. *Rev. Neurol. (Paris)*, **144**, 571–7.

Hochman, M. S., Sowers, J. J. and Bruce-Gregorios, J. (1985). Syndrome of the mesencephalic artery: Report of a case with CT and necropsy findings. *J. Neurol. Neurosurg. Psychiatry*, **48**, 1179–81.

Inci, S. and Ozgen, T. (2003). Locked-in syndrome due to metastatic pontomedullary tumor – case report. *Neurol. Med. Chir. (Tokyo)*, **43**, 497–500.

Karp, J. S., and Hurtig, H. I. (1974). "Locked-in" state with bilateral midbrain infarcts. *Arch. Neurol.*, **30**, 176–8.

Kemper, T. L., and Romanul, F. C. (1967). State resembling akinetic mutism in basilar artery occlusion. *Neurology*, **17**, 74–80.

Krasnianski, M., Gaul, C., Neudecker, S., *et al.* (2003). Yawning despite trismus in a patient with locked-in syndrome caused by a thrombosed megadolichobasilar artery. *Clin. Neurol. Neurosurg.*, **106**, 44–6.

Laplane, D. (1990). Perte d'auto-activation psychique. *Rev. Neurol. (Paris)*, **146**, 397–404.

Laplane, D., Baulac, M., Pillon, B. and Panayotopoulou-Achimastos, I. (1982). Perte d'autoactivation psychique. Activité compulsive obsessionnelle. Lésions lenticulaire bilatérale. *Rev. Neurol. (Paris)*, **138**, 137–41.

Laplane, D., Baulac, M., Widlocher, D. and Dubois, B. (1984). Pure psychic akinesia with bilateral lesions of basal ganglia. *J. Neurol. Neurosurg. Psychiatry*, **47**, 377–85.

Laplane, D., Degos, J. D., Baulac, M. and Gray, F. (1981). Bilateral infarction of the anterior cingulate gyri and of the fornices. Report of a case. *J. Neurol. Sci.*, **51**, 289–300.

Lhermitte, F., Gautier, J. C., Marteau, R. and Chain, F. (1963). Troubles de conscience et mutise akinétique. Etude anatomoclinique d'un ramollissement bilatéralparamédian des pédoncules cérébraux et du thalamus. *Rev. Neurol. (Paris)*, **109**, 115–31.

McCusker, E. A., Rudick, R. A., Honch, G. W. and Griggs, R. C. (1982). Recovery from the 'locked-in' syndrome. *Arch. Neurol.*, **39**, 145–7.

Mega, M. S. and Cohenour, R. C. (1997). Akinetic mutism: Disconnection of frontal-subcortical circuits. *Neuropsychiatry Neuropsychol. Behav. Neurol.* **10**, 254–9.

Mesulam, M. M. (1986). Frontal cortex and behavior. *Ann. Neurol.*, **19**, 320–5.

Milandre, L., Habib, M., Royere, M. L., Gouirand, R. and Khalil, R. (1995). Syndrome athymormique du à un infarctus striato-capsulaire. Maladie de Moya-Moya de l'adulte. *Rev. Neurol. (Paris)*, **151**, 383–7.

Minagar, A. and David, N. J. (1999). Bilateral infarction in the territory of the anterior cerebral arteries. *Neurology*, **52**, 886–8.

Nagaratnam, N., Nagaratnam, K., Ng, K. and Diu, P. (2004). Akinetic mutism following stroke. *J. Clin. Neurosci.*, **11**, 25–30.

Nicolai, A. and Lazzarino, L. G. (1993). Painful tonic spasms associated with subcortical infarction. *Acta Neurol. (Napoli)*, **15**, 87–91.

Oberndorfer, S., Urbanits, S., Lahrmann, H., *et al.* (2002). Akinetic mutism caused by bilateral infiltration of the fornix in a patient with astrocytoma. *Eur. J. Neurol.*, **9**, 311–13.

Okawa, M., Maeda, S., Nukui, H. and Kawafuchi, J. (1980). Psychiatric symptoms in ruptured anterior communicating aneurysms: Social prognosis. *Acta Psychiatr. Scand.*, **61**, 306–12.

Patterson, J. R. and Grabois, M. (1986). Locked-in syndrome: A review of 139 cases. *Stroke*, **17**, 758–64.

Piccirilli, M., Mazzi, P., Luccioli, R. and Sciarma, T. (1995). Selective bilateral lesion of the globus pallidus: Ten-year follow-up of memory impairment and frontal symptomatology. *Ital. J. Neurol. Sci.*, **16**, 635–40.

Plum, F. and Posner, J. B. (1980). *The Diagnosis of Stupor and Coma*. Philadelphia: Davis, 377.

Psarros, T., Zouros, A. and Coimbra, C. (2003). Bromocriptine-responsive akinetic mutism following endoscopy for ventricular neurocysticercosis. Case report and review of the literature. *J. Neurosurg.*, **99**, 397–401.

Rae-Grant, A. D., Lin, F., Yaeger, B. A., *et al.* (1989). Post traumatic extracranial vertebral artery dissection with locked-in syndrome: A case with MRI documentation and unusually favourable outcome. *J. Neurol. Neurosurg. Psychiatry*, **52**, 1191–3.

Richfield, E. K., Twyman, R. and Berent, S. (1987). Neurological syndrome following bilateral damage to the head of the caudate nuclei. *Ann. Neurol.*, **22**, 768–71.

Ross, E. D. and Stewart, R. M. (1981). Akinetic mutism from hypothalamic damage: Successful treatment with dopamine agonists. *Neurology*, **31**, 1435–9.

Segarra, J. M. (1970). Cerebral vascular disease and behavior. I. The syndrome of the mesencephalic artery (basilar artery bifurcation). *Arch. Neurol.*, **22**, 408–18.

Tatemichi, T. K., Desmond, D. W., Paik, M., *et al.* (1993). Clinical determinants of dementia related to stroke. *Ann. Neurol.*, **33**, 568–75.

Tatemichi, T. K., Desmond, D. W. and Prohovnik, I. (1995). Strategic infarcts in vascular dementia. A clinical and brain imaging experience. *Arzneimittelforschung*, **45**, 371–85.

Tengvar, C., Johansson, B. and Sorensen, J. (2004). Frontal lobe and cingulate cortical metabolic dysfunction in acquired akinetic mutism: A PET study of the interval form of carbon monoxide poisoning. *Brain Inj.*, **18**, 615–25.

Tuz, M., Erodlu, F., Dodru, H., Uygur, K. and Yavuz, L. (2003). Transient locked-in syndrome resulting from stellate ganglion block in the treatment of patients with sudden hearing loss. *Acta Anaesthesiol. Scand.*, **47**, 485–7.

23

Alterations of level of consciousness related to stroke

Marc D. Reichhart

Xigen Enterprises and CHUV, Lausanne, Switzerland

Introduction

Alteration of level of consciousness (ALC), which comprises deficient arousal, stupor, and rarely deep coma, is frequent at the acute stage of stroke. These conditions may cause fluctuating, fixed, or fast decrease of consciousness level, which in turn interferes with a detailed bedside neurological examination and neuropsychological assessment. Conversely, ALC constitutes a useful complementary sign both for the localization (syndrome) and cause (etiology) of cerebrovascular diseases (Adams, 1997). A typical example is the examination of a stuporous old patient with high blood pressure (220/120 mmHg), showing an ataxic hypesthetic hemiparesis with asterixis, bilateral Babinski signs, whereas neuro-ophthalmological evaluation of his (forced open) eyes reveals an upgaze palsy with downward gaze deviation: this stroke pattern suggests a contralateral large thalamic (syndrome) hemorrhage (etiology), as illustrated in Figure 23.1.

Patients who develop ALC, ranging from somnolence to stupor and coma, need immediate admission to the intensive care unit (ICU), particularly those without upper airways protection, absent gag reflex, and/or a Coma Glasgow Scale (CGS) below or equal to 6 (see later). Indeed, endotracheal intubation is mandatory in these cases before further CT-scan or MR imaging (MRI) studies, EEG and laboratory tests – i.e. hematocrit, electrolytes with quick capillary glucose, osmolality; renal, hepatic, arterial blood gases (pH, PCO_2, PO_2, HCO_3, HbCO, lactate), coagulations tests (aPTT, INR, platelets, smear, fibrinogen with fibrin degeneration products, D-dimer), blood and urine toxic screening, thyroid and hypophyse functions screening. In this context, spinal tap for CSF analysis (white and red cell count, protein, glucose, lactate, India ink stain, cryptococcal antigen, viral and eubacterial PCR) is usually performed after neuroimaging study (Howard and Hirsch, 1999; Ropper *et al.* 2004; Wijdicks, 2001; Wijdicks, 2000b).

As regards the evaluation of ALC, clinicians should first be certain that the patient suffers from acute CNS injury which induces stupor to coma states. The

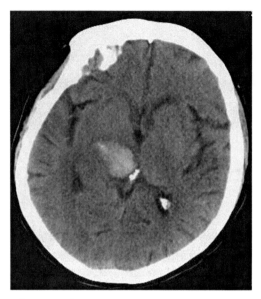

Figure 23.1 Admission plain CT-scan showing a right-sided thalamic hemorrhage extending toward the internal capsule.

second step is to search for basilar artery occlusion-associated coma, due to ventral pontine ischemia (see case 1, Figure 23.2), which is underestimated and needs prompt neuroimaging studies for thrombolytic therapy in order to avoid evolvement into a locked-in syndrome; and to rule out (1) acute inflammatory polyradiculoneuropathy (Landry–Guillain–Barré–Strohl syndrome), which in its most severe form can mimic a locked in syndrome or brain death, (2) botulism or tetanus, and only finally, (3) malingering.

Consciousness, arousal and mechanisms of ALC

Consciousness is the state of awareness of the self and the environment, and represents the primary cognitive level that integrates stimuli from the internal and external environments, whereas coma is its extreme opposite – the total absence of awareness despite applying external painful stimuli to the subject (Plum and Posner, 1980c). Two physiological aspects of conscious behavior have been recognized by Plum and Posner (1980c): arousal, which is closely linked to wakefulness or alertness, and its content which represents the sum of cognitive and affective mental function. This functional duality is essential in understanding the pathophysiology of ALC. However, the neuronal correlates of consciousness are

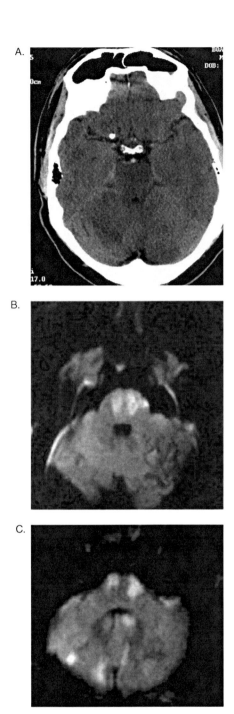

Figure 23.2 (A) Admission plain CT-scan showing pontine infarction with a dense basilar artery; (B–D) 24-hour post IA thrombolytic therapy DWI MR imaging confirmed bilateral ventropontine ischemic infarcts together with multiple and bilateral cerebellar infarcts (right-sided postero-inferior cerebellar artery territory infarct is also seen on CT scan), (E) Admission MRA-TOF shows complete occlusion of the basilar artery, with distal left vertebral artery (VA) occlusion and hypoplasic right VA.

D.

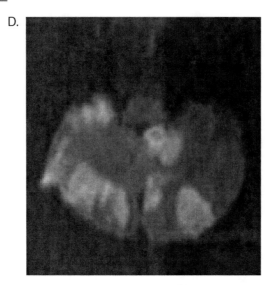

E.

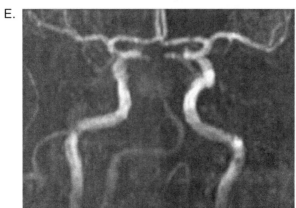

Figure 23.2   *(cont.)*

Clinical Case 1. (2001). A 45-year-old man developed a left thalamo-geniculate stroke of artery-to-artery secondary to a left vertebral artery dissection. One week later, while under oral anticoagulants with an INR of 1.8 (normal value, 1.2), he became suddenly comatose, with horizontal gaze palsy and ocular bobbing, tetraplegia with Babinski signs and prominent lower limbs shivering, muscles twitching, and polymyoclonus. Despite IA thrombolytic therapy, the patient evolved to locked-in syndrome.

still a matter of debate and research (Albright *et al.*, 2001; Crick *et al.*, 2004; John, 2002; Maia and Cleeremans, 2005; Searle, 2000; Sieb, 2004; Toates, 2006; Young and Pigott, 1999; Zeman, 2001).

The maintenance of consciousness (i.e. arousal) relies on interaction between the ascending reticular activating system (ARAS) and the cerebral hemisphere. The ARAS, first described in animal studies (Morison and Dempsey, 1942; Moruzzi and Magoun, 1949), constitutes the central core of the upper brainstem and diencephalon, that extends from the paramedian tegmentum of the dorsal upper pons (raphe nuclei) and midbrain (magnocellular medial nuclei) and lateral midbrain (parvocellular lateral nuclei) to the posterior hypothalamus and thalamus nuclei; i.e. intralaminar, ventral anterior and reticular (Brazis *et al.*, 1996; Plum and Posner, 1980c; Wijdicks, 2000b). The complexity of the suspected anatomy of the ARAS in humans must be regarded as a physiological entity, which comprises three main ascending pathways: one projects to the thalamic reticular nucleus and then to the cortex with complex thalamo-cortical and cortico-thalamic inputs, resonance and oscillations (for details, see Llinas and Ribary, 2001; Pinault, 2004); the second ascends through the hypothalamus to influence the basal forebrain and limbic system; the third includes serotoninergic neurons of the midbrain raphe, and noradrenergic neurons of the locus coeruleus, both projecting diffusely to the neocortex (Plum and Posner, 1980c). Cholinergic, noradrenergic, dopaminergic, serotoninergic, and histaminergic chemical complex subsystems resume the pharmacology of the ARAS (Zeman, 2001). The rostral brainstem and thalamus are implicated in the genesis of slow-wave and REM sleep, particularly cholinergic nuclei at the pontomesencephalic junction, the laterodorsal tegmentum and pediculopontine nuclei (Zeman, 2001). An excellent and comprehensive review on the ARAS has been summarized by Pappas and Carrion (1989). A schema of the ARAS is shown in Figure 23.3 (Parvizi and Damasio, 2001), and its pathways through the brainstem in Figure 23.4 (Pappas and Carrion, 1989) (for details, see Parvizi and Damasio, 2001; Parvizi and Damasio, 2003).

Between these two extreme states of normal and profound depressed consciousness, a continuum of the following *acute conditions* has been described (Howard and Hirsch, 1999; Plum and Posner, 1980c):

1. *Clouding of consciousness* is a state characterized by reduced wakefulness and awareness, which may alternate with irritability and hyperexcitability. Its hallmark is attention defect (Lipowsi, 1973). The subject is easily distracted, and stimuli may produce startles (myoclonic jerks), while sensorial perceptions (particularly visual ones) are misjudged. Although not disorientated, their thought processes are slow and unclear.

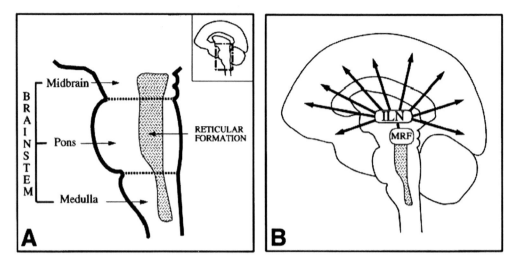

Figure 23.3 Schematic view of the ARAS. (A) The mesencephalic reticular formation (MRF) is the convergence and origin of the ARAS that activates the cortex via the intralaminar nuclei of the thalamus (ILN). (B) From Parvizi and Damasio (2001).

2. *Acute confusional state* represents a more severe impairment of consciousness with misinterpretation of stimuli, associated with time, place, or person disorientations, impairment of short-memory and mental state, and day-night reversal (see Chapter 24).

3. *Delirium* comprises disturbed consciousness with abnormal mental state, disorientation, misperception of stimuli, visual hallucinations, logorrhea, motor and psychic agitation (see Chapter 24).

4. *Obtundation* is characterized by mental blunting or torpidity. It is first an alteration of mental state, with mild to moderate reduction of alertness, and arousal is obtained slowly by responses to tactile or verbal stimuli. The patient shows poor interest in the environment, slow psychological responses to stimulation, and hypersomnia with drowsiness.

5. *Stupor* is a state of deep reduced wakefulness and awareness similar to sleep or behaviorally similar unresponsiveness. Arousal is obtained only after repeated and vigorous stimuli, with a typical waxing-waning lapsing return to initial unresponsive state as soon as repeated stimuli are stopped.

6. *Coma* is a state of continuous "eyes-closed" unconsciousness, in the absence of a sleep–wake cycle (Plum, 1991; Plum and Posner, 1980c; Zeman, 2001). It is a state of unresponsiveness in which the subject lies with eyes closed, showing neither understandable response to external stimuli nor inner need. The psychological aspects of coma have probably gradations in depth, which have been quantified by the universal and reliable CGS (Teasdale and

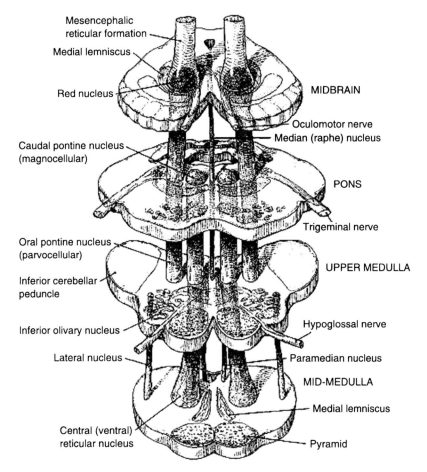

Mesencephalic
reticular formation

Medial lemniscus

Red nucleus

MIDBRAIN

Oculomotor nerve
Median (raphe) nucleus

Caudal pontine nucleus
(magnocellular)

PONS

Trigeminal nerve

Oral pontine nucleus
(parvocellular)

UPPER MEDULLA

Inferior cerebellar
peduncle

Inferior olivary nucleus

Hypoglossal nerve

Lateral nucleus

Paramedian nucleus

MID-MEDULLA

Medial lemniscus

Central (ventral)
reticular nucleus

Pyramid

Figure 23.4 Schematic view of the ARAS through the brainstem. From Pappas and Carrion (1989).

Jenett, 1974); i.e. sum of the best verbal, eyes opening, and motor responses to
noxious stimuli (see Table 23.1), ranging from 15 to 3, for normal
consciousness to deep coma, respectively. Recently, Wijdicks and colleagues
have validated a new coma score, i.e. the Full Outline of UnResponsiveness
(FOUR), developed since 1998 and more adapted for ICU-patients (Wijdicks
et al., 1998; 2005).

The following entities are states of subacute to chronic ALC:

1. *Hypersomnia* refers to excessive drowsiness, so-called sleep-like coma in the
   European literature, and is characterized by subacute progressive states
   of excessive but normal sleep in which the subject awakes when stimulated
   (Plum and Posner, 1980c).

Table 23.1. The Full Outline UnResponsiveness (FOUR) score and the Coma Glasgow Scale (CGS)

	FOUR score		CGS		
Eye response (eyelids)	Open or opened, tracking, or blinking to command	4	Eyes opening	4	Spontaneous
	Open but not tracking	3		3	To speech
	Closed but not open to loud voice	2		2	To pain
	Closed but open to pain	1		1	None
	Remains closed with pain	0	Best motor response (arm)	6	Obeying
Motor response	Thumbs-up, fist, or peace sign	4		5	Localizing pain
Withdrawal	Localizing to pain	3		4	Withdrawal
Abnormal flexing	Flexion response to pain	2		3	Abnormal flexing
Extensor response	Extension response to pain	1		2	Extensor response
None	No response to pain or generalized myoclonus status	0		1	None
Brainstem reflexes	Pupil and corneal reflexes present	4	Best verbal response	5	Oriented
Confused conversation	One pupil wide and fixed	3		4	Confused conversation
	Pupil or corneal reflexes absent	2		3	Inappropriate words
Incomprehensible words	Pupil and corneal reflexes absent	1		2	Incomprehensible words
None	Absent pupil, corneal, and cough reflex	0		1	None
Respiration	Not intubated, regular breathing pattern	4			
	Not intubated, Cheynes-Stokes breathing pattern	3			
	Not intubated, irregular breathing	2			
	Breaths above ventilator rate	1			
	Breaths are ventilator rate or apnea	0			

Source: FOUR – Wijdicks *et al.*, 2005; CGS – Teasdale and Jenett, 1974.

2. *Akinetic mutism* is characterized by silent, alert-appearing immobility, absence of response to pain, unresponsive to commands, questions, preserved alertness and wakefulness, double incontinence, preserved sleep—wake cycles, (see Chapter 22).

3. *Persistent vegetative state*, described by Jenett and Plum (1972), is a condition which follows coma due to severe diffuse brain injury (traumatic, anoxic—ischemic) with a return of wakefulness after 2—4 weeks (mean, 1 month). Subjects show apparent total lack of cognitive functions but they open eyes in response to verbal stimuli. Brainstem functions (chewing, swallowing, breathing, circulation control) and reflexes (pupillary, oculocephalic, corneal, gag) remain normal while sleep—wake cycles reappear; they may smile, shed tears, grunt, and scream spontaneously (Plum and Posner, 1980c; Wijdicks and Cranford, 2005; Zeman, 1997). Other similar states have been described as "the apallic syndrome" (Kretschmer, 1940), and "coma vigile" (Alajouanine, 1957). Neuropathologic studies of patients with persistent vegetative state following anoxic—ischemic injuries showed constantly damage of the forebrain, various cortical laminar necrosis which involved particularly the occipital and hippocampal areas, necrosis of the Ammon's horns and basal ganglia (including the thalamus), loss of Purkinje cells, and various infarctions of both hemispheres. The study of regional cerebral blood flow and glucose metabolism showed severe reduction of one-third to one-half (Ingvar *et al.*, 1978; Zeman, 1997). Electroencephalographic studies found various patterns ranging from isoelectric, alpha-like, delta, and theta activity (Ingvar *et al.*, 1978; Zeman, 1997). Recently, a subtype of persistent vegetative state with wakefulness and partial presence of awareness, suspected to carry a better outcome, has been defined as the minimally conscious state; their diagnosis criteria are summarized in Tables 23.2 and 23.3 (Giacino *et al.*, 2002; Multi-Society Task Force on PVS, 1994; Wijdicks and Cranford, 2005).

Locked-in syndrome, first described by Plum and Posner in 1966, is characterized by supranuclear motor deafferentation causing tetraplegia with lower cranial nerve palsies, giving a false appearance of permanent coma (Plum and Posner, 1980a; 1980c). Consciousness is intact but the subject cannot communicate by words or body movements. In some cases, the responsible lesion (ventral pons, see Figure 23.2) allows vertical eye movements or blinking to communicate their awareness of internal and external stimuli (Plum and Posner, 1980c). The first definition of locked-in syndrome was thus quadriplegia, lower cranial nerve palsies and mutism with preservation of consciousness, vertical gaze, and upper eyelids movements, but changed in 1986 to anarthria instead of mutism (Smith and Delargy, 2005). The first description of a locked-in syndrome is due to Alexandre Dumas' book *The Count of Monte Cristo*, and a famous French

Table 23.2. Criteria for the diagnosis of a persistent vegetative state (PVS), from the multi-society task force on PVS

1.	No evidence of awareness of themselves or their environment; they are incapable of interacting with others
2.	No evidence of sustained, reproducible, purposeful, or voluntary behavioral responses to visual, auditory, tactile, or noxious stimuli
3.	No evidence of language comprehension or expression
4.	Intermittent wakefulness manifested by the presence of sleep–wake cycles
5.	Sufficiently preserved hypothalamic and brainstem autonomic functions to survive if given medical and nursing care
6.	Bowel and bladder incontinence
7.	Variably preserved cranial nerve (pupillary, oculocephalic, corneal, vestibulo-ocular, and gag) and spinal reflexes

Source: Multi-Society Task Force on PVS, 1994.

Table 23.3. Criteria for a minimally conscious state (MCS)

To diagnose a MCS, limited but clearly discernible evidence of self- or environmental awareness must be demonstrated on a reproducible or sustained basis by 1 or more of the following behaviors:
1. follows simple commands
2. gestural or verbal yes/no responses (regardless of accuracy)
3. intelligible verbalization
4. purposeful behavior, including movements or affective behaviors that occur in contingent relationship to relevant environmental stimuli and are not due to reflexive activity. Some examples of qualifying purposeful behavior are:
5. appropriate smiling or crying in response to the linguistic or visual content of emotional but not neutral topics or stimuli
6. vocalizations or gestures that occur in direct responses to the linguistic content of questions
7. reaching for objects that demonstrates a clear relationship between object location of reach
8. touching or holding objects in a manner that accommodates the size and shape of the object
9. pursuit eye movement of sustained fixation that occurs in direct responses to moving or salient stimuli

Source: Giacino *et al.*, 2002.

journalist has written his own experience (Bauby, 1997), which has been later studied (Dudzinski, 2001), as a physician's poem relates the dramatic condition of a patient suffering from locked-in syndrome (Ginsberg, 2005).

Several mechanisms may account for ALC. Strokes which produce ALC comprise cerebral infarct and hemorrhage involving extensive areas of both hemispheres, either restricted regions: bilateral mesial frontal regions, paramedian diencephalon and upper brainstem (Brazis *et al.*, 1996; Plum and Posner, 1980c;

Wijdicks, 2000b). Unilateral large ischemic infarcts of the dominant hemisphere have been reputed to cause transient ALC (Plum and Posner, 1980c), but this has not been supported by more recent studies (cf. infra anterior circulation strokes). Vascular lesions involving the medulla oblongata (Wallenberg syndrome (latero-bulbar), Babinski-Nageotte syndrome (medio-bulbar), Déjerine syndrome (hemi-bulbar) and lower pons) may cause failure to drive respiration, vascular tone, and cardiac rhythm. Such failure may result in coma due to anoxia and hypercapnia (anoxic–ischemic diffuse encephalopathy) (Plum and Posner, 1980c; Wijdicks, 2000b). Furthermore, large expanding unilateral strokes, including those caused by CVT, may increase intra-cranial pressure (ICP) above 15 mmHg (17.5 cmH$_2$O) and this indirectly causes coma. Such mass effect may result in cerebral herniation; three main herniation syndromes have been described for supratentorial lesions (1–3 below), and one (4) for infratentorial lesions (Brazis et al., 1996; Plum and Posner, 1980a; 1980b; 1980c; Wijdicks, 2000b):

Lateral (uncal) herniation
The temporal uncus and hippocampal gyrus are pushed into the tentorium gap, producing an external compression of the third cranial nerve (fixed mydriasis) and of the posterior cerebral artery (ischemic/hemorrhagic occipital stroke) ipsilateral to stroke, whereas opposite compression of the cerebral peduncle against the (rigid) tentorium (Kernohan's notch) gives rise to hemiparesis ipsilateral to stroke, and secondary infarcts and hemorrhages (of Duret, see Figure 23.5) of the midbrain by tearing of paramedian basilar perforating arteries. At this stage, both pupils become in midsize fixed position (sympathic pathway lesions).

Central (transtentorial) downward herniation
Central (transtentorial) downward herniation has the classic central rostrocaudal deterioration syndrome, which comprises five stages: early and late diencephalic, midbrain–upper pons, lower pontine, and medullary. The early diencephalic stage is characterized by impaired attention and somnolence, normal respiration pattern interrupted by deep sighs, yawns, and pauses, tiny reactive pupils, roving eye movements (slow side to side) which are divergent in primary position, intact saccades and nystagmus on eliciting oculocephalic reflex (OCR) and caloric stimulation (oculo-vestibular reflex: OVR). Motor responses are adequate (noxious stimulation), and paratonia or "Gegenhalten" hypertonia with grasping and bilateral Babinski's signs are present. Late diencephalic stage produces true coma, Cheynes–Stokes respiration (crescendo/decrescendo hyperventilation with pauses), preserved OCR (opposite conjugate eyes deviation) and OVR (opposite nystagmus on cold water instillation in the ear), upward gaze paresis, small reactive pupils, with decorticate motor (upper limb flexion and

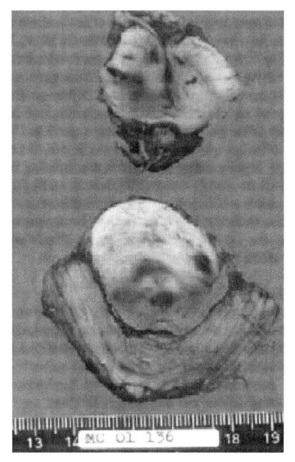

Figure 23.5 Macroscopic pictures of Duret's hemorrhages at the level of the midbrain (top) and pons (bottom). 72-year-old man with uncal herniation following left hemisphere ICH. MD Reichhart, Neurology Department; R.C. Janzer, Pathology Department, University of Lausanne.

lower limb extension) on noxious stimuli and bilateral extensor plantar responses. Both diencephalic stages may allow neurological recovery when promptly managed.

The hallmarks of the next midbrain−upper pons stage are: deeper coma with central hyperventilation (constant quick breathing); temperature oscillations with diabetes insipidus (hypothalamic dysfunction) or the cerebral salt wasting syndrome (personal observation); midsized, unequal, eccentric, and deformed fixed pupils (corectopia, Figure 23.6), restricted or absent OCR (particularly in vertical gaze) and OVR, disconjugate horizontal and vertical eyes movements, skew deviation (hypotropia contraversive to lateralized ponto-mesencephalic

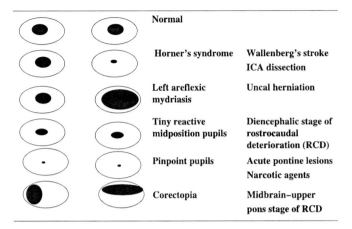

Figure 23.6   Synopsis of abnormal pupils pattern (MD Reichhart).

lesion); decerebrate posturing with rigidity (four-limb extension) and bilateral Babinski signs. The exitus is preceded by bilateral mydriasis due to anoxia with release of epinephrine. In the lower pontine stage, the respiration is quicker but shallower, and no eye movement can be elicited, the decerebrate rigidity decreases, while triple lower limb withdrawal in addition to plantar extensor responses may be seen after noxious stimuli. The medullary and agonal stage causes ataxic breathing, with gasps or deep sighs, followed by apnea, the blood pressure drops, and the pulse becomes irregular, slow, or fast.

As regards respiration patterns, contrary to ischemic syndromes of the lower pons or medulla, primary apneustic breathing per se is rarely present in the two latter caudal stages of central deterioration syndromes. Conversely, a specific central sleep apnea syndrome (Ondine's curse), with impaired respiration automatism mechanisms, has been reported in unilateral or bilateral medullary infarction (Bogousslavsky, 1990; Devereaux *et al.*, 1973; Levin and Margolis, 1977).

Cingulate herniation
Cingulate herniation is often paucisymptomatic but may prelude the aforementioned herniation. The cingulate gyrus is squeezed under the falx, and this produces contralateral and/or bilateral infarctions in the anterior cerebral artery manifested by frontal release signs, abulia, and contralateral or bilateral lower limb paresis.

Central (transtentorial) upward and downward herniation syndromes
These herniation syndromes are caused by infratentorial strokes – cerebellar infarction or hemorrhage. Such expansive lesions of the posterior fossa compress

the upper brainstem and cause upward transtentorial herniation, with either coma, hyperventilation, fixed pupils, and vertical ophthalmoplegia (dysfunction), or somnolence, pinpoint pupils (Figure 23.6), oculoparetic nystagmus on lateral gaze, truncal ataxia, depending whether such lesions impinge directly or secondarily on the midbrain tectum, or pontine tegmentum, respectively. Thus, two mechanisms of posterior fossa strokes may induce upper brainstem-associated ALC. Finally, the last downward herniation syndrome through the foramen magnum is characterized by secondary infarctions of the tonsils, medulla, and upper cervical spinal cord, with subsequent generalized anoxia (apnea) and circulatory failure (cardiopulmonary arrest). Noteworthy, the classical signs of increased ICP, so-called Kocher–Cushing signs, which include rising blood pressure and slowing of pulse rate, are frequently seen with infratentorial lesions. A synopsis of the aforementioned abnormal pupils is summarized in Figure 23.6.

Frequency and prognosis value of ALC

Strokes associated with ALC ranging from hypersomnia to coma have been reported in 17% of patients in the Lausanne Stroke Registry (Bogousslavsky et al., 1988b), and are due more often to intracranial hemorrhage (50%) than infarction (cardio-embolism, 12%). This was confirmed by other prospective series (Melo et al., 1992), which found coma at stroke onset more frequently in patients with intracranial hemorrhage (ICH) (72%), especially in deep hemorrhage (basal ganglia) followed by infarct (23%), and subarachnoid hemorrhage (5%). Coma related to ICH (CGS < 5) carried a short-term case fatality of 86%: the depth of coma (lowest CGS) was in turn correlated with radiological evidence of herniation in patients with ICH. Overall, specific predictors of death were a CGS below 5, anisocoria, abnormal flexion (decorticate) or no response to pain, and absent or only one brainstem reflex. A review of the literature found coma in 5–19% of patients with stroke, with a preponderance of ICH (38–56% of cases) (Bassetti, 2001; Bogousslavsky et al., 1988b; Melo et al., 1992). As regards the prognosis, the mortality is highest for patient with coma (80%), and decreases for those with stupor (60%), and somnolence (40%), respectively (Bassetti, 2001; Melo et al., 1992). Further studies confirmed that ALC quantified by the CGS was inversely correlated with poor outcome in acute ischemic stroke (Weir et al., 2003), and that a CGS < 10, requiring endotracheal intubation, together with absent pupillary light responses were strong predictors of poor prognosis for survival in patients with ischemic stroke and ICH (Bushnell et al., 1999).

Specific stroke syndromes associated with ALC

Posterior circulation strokes

As a general rule, lesions disrupting the rostral part of the ARAS — i.e. infarctions involving the thalamus surrounding the third ventricle and adjacent gray matter, the mesencephalic tegmentum, the periaqueductal gray matter — cause hypersomnia, whereas those involving more caudally the ARAS produce coma: bilateral rostral pontine or caudal midbrain infarcts (Caplan, 1996a).

Occlusion of the rostral basilar artery

The syndrome of the "top of the basilar artery" (Caplan, 1980) causes infarcts of the high midbrain and thalamus, and of the temporal and occipital lobe portions supplied by the posterior cerebral arteries (PCAs) (Caplan, 1988; Caplan, 1996b). Anatomical variations of penetrating vessels originating from a common pedicle of the basilar (mesencephalic) arteries, fully described by Percheron (Percheron 1976), explain that bilateral paramedian portions of the midbrain and thalamus are often also involved. The main signs of apex basilar artery occlusion comprise ALC associated with behavioral abnormalities (abulia, peduncular hallucinations), memory (amnesia) and neuro-ophthalmological functions. Hypersomnia is the hallmark of ALC associated with infarction in the territory of the thalamic-subthalamic (thalamoperforating) arteries and the paramedian mesencephalic arteries, which perfuse the rostral ARAS, surrounding the periaqueductal and third ventricle area. Hypersomnia following butterfly-shaped bilateral rostral paramedian thalamo-mesencephalic infarcts was reported by French neurologists in the 1950s and 60s (Castaigne et al., 1962; Facon et al., 1958). One patient reported by Facon and co-workers slept for 3 years. Segarra named this clinical syndrome due to high medial brainstem infarction "somnolent mutism," as opposed to the "coma vigil" associated with bilateral cerebral lesions (Segarra, 1970). There have been various associated oculomotor findings:

1. Vertical gaze paresis has been noted, due to lesion of the rostral interstitial nucleus of the MLF, which involves the posterior commissure, the interstitial nucleus of Cajal, and the periaqueductal gray. Upgaze and vertical gaze palsies are more common than downgaze palsy, which may be dysconjugated — i.e. contraversive skew deviation and ocular tilt reaction, vertical diplopia (asymetric posterior thalamic, midbrain tegmentum lesions), and altered or preserved when elicited by OCR.

2. Monocular elevation paresis has been noted, so-called "double monocular elevator palsy."

3. Vertical one-and-a-half syndrome was described by Hommel and Bogousslavsky (1991) and Mehler (1988).

4. Bilateral/controlateral ptosis (levator nucleus) or retraction of the upper eyelids (PC), so-called "Collier's sign," was first described by Collier (1927).

5. Disorders of convergence, including hyperconvergence or convergence spasm, and convergence retraction nystagmus, and the so-called "pseudosixth" phenomenon, was described by Miller Fischer (1961). This involves failure of full abduction without dysfunction of bilateral sixth nerves, hyperconvergence, and adducting jerks. For details, see Figure 1 in Caplan (1980).

6. Various pupils sizes have been noted, depending on whether lesions affect sympathetic fibers (myosis), Edinger—Westphal nucleus and its efferents (mydriasis), or a combination of both (midposition). Eccentric, oval-shaped, and pear-shaped (corectopia; see Figure 23.6) pupils also occur (Caplan, 1988; 1996b).

7. Bilateral ptosis due to third nucleus infarctions has been noted, which may be more prominent opposite to the side of unilateral levator subnucleus involvement.

8. There have been abnormalities of accommodation, convergence, and pupillary constriction, including the light-near dissociation simulating Argyll Robertson pupil.

Paramedian thalamic and midbrain infarcts

The syndrome of "somnolent" coma or mutism, as opposed to "vigilant coma" (akinetic mutism, see Chapter 22), was first delineated by Segarra — the so-called "syndrome of the mesencephalic artery" (Segarra, 1970). He reported two cases pooled with previously similar published observations, giving the first clinico-pathological study of ALC-associated bilateral paramedian thalamo-mesencephalic strokes. The first patient developed pseudo-clonic seizures with initial coma, with complete ophthalmoplegia, whereas the second comatose case showed vertical gaze paresis, unilateral ptosis, bilateral adductor paresis, and both had areactive pupils on examination. In both cases, ALC lasted two months and was fluctuating with episodes of coma and stupor (with generalized delta slowing on EEG) alternating with apparent awareness. Pathological findings confirmed butterfly-shaped "dimesencephalic junction" ischemic infarctions involving the periaqueductal gray, the tegmental reticular formation, the posterior commissure, the mamillothalamic tract (field H1 of Forel), and the intralaminar nuclei (and different other thalamic nuclei in each) on both sides. The vascular supply of this region originates from the so-called mesencephalic artery located between the top of the basilar artery and the PCoA, a long circumferential artery that irrigates the colliculi and gives off perforating branches (Percheron, 1976; Foix and Hillemand, 1925).

According to Segarra, bifurcation of the aforementioned perforating arteries at the midline explained that they supplied the thalamo-mesencephalic junction on both sides (Segarra, 1970). Further larger series of paramedian thalamic and midbrain ischemic infarcts with clinico-pathological studies (Bogousslavsky *et al.*, 1988a; Castaigne *et al.*, 1981) and anatomic studies (Percheron, 1976) clarified the paramedian arterial territory supply. The paramedian territory comprises two distinct groups of arteries (paramedian thalamic and superior paramedian mesencephalic, because of their common origin and analogy – common or single pedicle), which explains why paramedian infarctions of the thalamus and midbrain are frequently associated if not bilateral. The review of *unilateral paramedian thalamic infarcts* emphasized that ALC was not restricted to pure paramedian thalamic infarcts (Castaigne *et al.*, 1981). As regards cases with *bilateral thalamic infarcts*, most had ALC, characterized by coma followed by recovery of consciousness frequently followed by hypersomnia. Disturbances of behavior and ALC were frequent in bilateral paramedian thalamic infarcts (Castaigne *et al.*, 1981). The *paramedian thalamopeduncular infarcts* (Castaigne *et al.*, 1981) were more extensive and rarely isolated to the paramedian territory (the extension into the hypothalamus occurred in nearly half of the cases). Initial coma of variable depth and/or hypersomnia was associated frequently with abnormalities of the ocular motility (unilateral or bilateral more or less complete third nerve palsy). Delayed abnormal movements (tremor, myoclonus, athetosis) appeared in some cases. Overall, most patients developed hypersomnia, attributed to paramedian tegmental lesions, which may explain somnolence by interruption of ascending noradrenergic pathways from the locus ceruleus, mesencephalic reticular formation, and raphe nuclei to the core of thalamic nuclei; i.e. dorsomedial (magno-cellular part) and intralaminar (Bassetti *et al.*, 1996; Bassetti, 2001; Castaigne *et al.*, 1981). Biller *et al.* (1985) described the neuro-ophthalmological findings in two patients with *isolated bilateral paramedian and midbrain ischemic strokes* confirmed by MRI. Both cases showed sudden ALC with initial pseudo-coma or stupor, followed by hypersomnia, associated with bilateral ophthalmoplegia. The first showed complete bilateral ophthalmoplegia with areactive mydriasis (5 mm). The other had initial full left external ophthalmoplegia associated with right lid retraction (Collier's sign), downward deviation with downbeating jerks with preserved adduction, whereas later VOR produced bilateral abduction ("pseudosixth palsy"), and signs of bilateral oculosympathetic dysfunction (areactive 3.5-mm pupils to light or accommodation which dilated after hydroxyamphetamine but not after cocaine local instillation). The first large series of pure and isolated thalamic infarcts has been published by Bogousslavsky *et al.* (1988a). Overall, fluctuating ALCs were found in all patients with unilateral and bilateral paramedian territory infarctions, lasting from 15 minutes to one day and which could persist for more than two weeks. Associated neuro-ophthalmological findings included mainly vertical gaze and convergence palsy, skew deviation, pseudosixth palsy and ptosis. A recent series of patients with bilateral thalamic infarction confirmed that half of them involved the so-called paramedian arterial territory, representing the most common bilateral thalamic stroke pattern (Kumral *et al.*, 2001).

A recent review summarized the current knowledge and simplification of the stroke syndromes involving the so-called paramedian artery territory (Schmahmann, 2003), including the brain arterial cartography defined by Tatu and colleagues (Tatu *et al.*, 1998; 2001). The *interpeduncular arteries*, arising from the proximal part of the PCA (P1) between the basilar arteries bifurcation and the PCoA – i.e. mesencephalic or basilar communicating artery – include three main rami (inferior, middle, superior; see Figure 23.7), with the inferior and middle rami, corresponding together to the paramedian mesencephalic pedicle of Percheron, irrigating the pons and midbrain (Percheron, 1976; Schmahmann, 2003; Tatu *et al.*, 1998; 2001). The superior rami, by giving rise to the paramedian thalamic (thalamoperforating) arteries, supplies the following parts of thalamic nuclei: dorsomedial, internal medullary lamina, and intralaminar (central lateral, centromedian, parafascicular), and may also irrigate the paraventricular and the posteromedial part of the ventrolateral nuclei, as well as the ventromedial aspect of the pulvinar, the lateral dorsal, lateral posterior, and ventral anterior. As mentioned earlier, individual anatomical variations in the origin of the paramedian artery and middle rami might explain bilateral infarcts involving the thalamo-mesencephalic junction. *Unilateral paramedian thalamic infarcts* produce only transient ALCs lasting for hours or days with decreased arousal and wakefulness which consist of lethargy and hypersomnia, abnormalities in vertical gaze (upgaze or up-/down-gaze palsy, skew deviation), associated with memory disturbances, confusion, behavior abnormalities, aphasia (left-sided) or spatial deficits (right-sided), and rarely contralateral slight transient hemiparesis, hemisensory abnormalities, asterixis, tremor, and dystonic movements (Caplan, 1996c; Schmahmann, 2003). Conversely, patients with *bilateral infarction in the paramedian artery territory* show more persistent and deeper ALCs, ranging from hypersomnia to stupor or pseudo-coma ("somnolent coma" of Segarra), associated with: (1) constant vertical gaze paresis including downgaze palsy and convergence abnormalities, pseudosixth nerve palsies, bilateral INO, myosis, intolerance to bright light; (2) severe memory impairment in a Korsakoff-like syndrome with confabulation, sometimes with prominent time disorientation described as "chronotaraxis" (Spiegel and Wycis, 1956); and (3) severe behavioral disorders (apathy, disinterest, flattened emotions, poor insight, lack of psychic

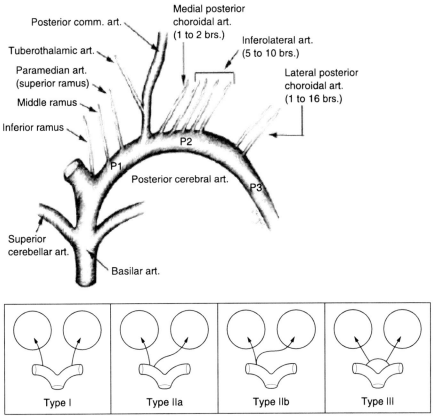

Figure 23.7 Artist's rendition of the origin of the arteries to thalamus arising from the vertebrobasilar system. Note that the inferolateral arteries may arise individually or from a common pedicle. With permission of Schmahmann (Schmahmann, 2003).

self-activation) (Bogousslavsky *et al.*, 1991; Caplan, 1996c; Schmahmann, 2003). Hypersomnia following isolated MRI-proven paramedian thalamic stroke was studied by polysomnograms in a series of twelve patients, including four with bilateral infarctions (Bassetti *et al.*, 1996). The main findings were consistent with deficient arousal during the day (stage 1 sleep), related to increased stage 1, reduced stage 2 and slow-wave (stage 3–4) non-REM sleep with reduced sleep spindles, particularly in patients with severe hypersomnia, but REM sleep was in the normal ranges (Bassetti *et al.*, 1996). These findings emphasized the functional duality of paramedian thalamic structures as a common pathway in wakefulness and generation of non-REM sleep (Bassetti *et al.*, 1996).

Some improvement of sleepiness and apathy has been observed in a single case study following the administration of bromocriptine in large doses (up to 120 mg/ day) (Catsman-Berrevoets and von Harskamp, 1988).

We report an example of a patient with bilateral thalamo-mesencephalic junction infarction due to infarction of the superior and middle rami (see case 2, Figure 23.8).

The syndrome of combined polar and paramedian thalamic infarction

In about one-third of cases the tuberothalamic (polar) artery does not exit and its vascular territory is taken over by the paramedian artery (Bogousslavsky

A.

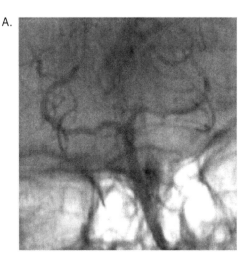

B.

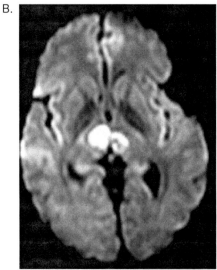

Figure 23.8 Right VA angiogram shows patent basilar artery and PCA (A) MR imaging with DWI (B) and T2-WI (C) confirms bilateral "butterfly-shaped" paramedian thalamic acute ischemic stroke, and rostral midbrain infarction (D).

C.

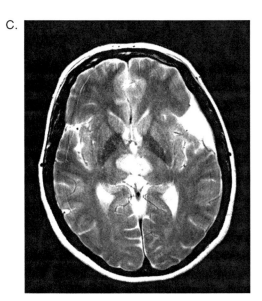

D.

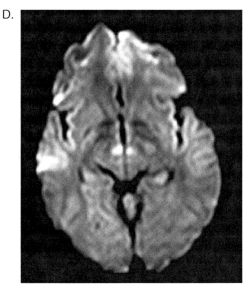

Figure 23.8 (cont.)

Clinical Case 2. A 49-year-old female developed a transient vertical diplopia, dysarthria, and right-sided hemisensory loss. One hour after admission in the ERD (regional hospital), she was found stuporous, whereas examination showed bilateral ptosis and miosis, complete vertical gaze palsy, and bilateral corticospinal signs with bilateral Babinski signs. Plain CT-scan was normal, and immediate intubation and sedation were performed for fast heliportation to our ERD. A conventional right VA angiogram at 3-hours after stroke onset revealed a patent basilar artery and PCA. After extubation, she was mildly disorientated, showed a downward gaze palsy, memory disturbances, and mild executive dysfunction. MR imaging confirmed an acute and bilateral ischemic infarct in the paramedian and middle ramus of the interpeduncular arteries territory. The etiology was a patent foramen ovale.

et al., 1986; Perren *et al.*, 2005; Schmahmann, 2003). In a recent series of such combined polar and paramedian infarctions, ALC was observed in bilateral infarct at the acute stage, including initial coma followed by persistent (>1 month) disturbances of consciousness and vertical gaze palsy, whereas hypersomnia was observed in unilateral infarction (Perren *et al.*, 2005). The clinical hallmarks of this combined paramedian and polar stroke pattern consisted of ALC followed by severe amnesia and abnormal vertical gaze, due to lesions of the anterior and dorsomedial thalamic nuclei (Perren *et al.*, 2005).

The syndrome of rostral mesencephalic–hypothalamic–thalamic infarct

We have reported nine patients with a syndrome of central Horner's syndrome (HS) and contralateral hemiparesis (Rossetti *et al.*, 2003). This diencephalic alternate syndrome consisted of central HS – i.e. classical HS (ptosis, myosis, and pseudo-enophthalmos) – and hypohydrosis of the hemibody on the same side, due to sympathicoexcitatory tract lesion at the first neuron level, alternating with ataxic hemiparesis, and asterixis, hypoesthesia, or dystonia on the opposite side (Rossetti *et al.*, 2003). Associated vertical gaze palsy was observed in a few patients, and transient somnolence in half of them (Rossetti *et al.*, 2003). MRI showed unilateral infarcts of the rostral paramedian midbrain and thalamus together with the posterior hypothalamus and polar thalamic infarction in a few cases, whereas the remaining had isolated tuberothalamic ischemic stroke. Our findings confirmed that the posterior hypothalamus is supplied by some of the 7–10 perforating branches arising from the PCoA (Tatu *et al.*, 1998; Tatu *et al.*, 2001), and that this diencephalic alternate syndrome occurs in cases with a common supply of the rostral mesencephalic–hypothalamic–thalamic junction by the superior and middle rami of the interpeduncular arteries (Bogousslavsky *et al.*, 1988a; Percheron, 1976; Rossetti *et al.*, 2003; Schmahmann, 2003; Tatu *et al.*, 1998; 2001).

The syndrome of anteromedian, central and posterolateral thalamic infarctions

In a recent series from the Lausanne Stroke Registry (Bogousslavsky *et al.*, 1988b), Carrera *et al.* (2004) studied MRI-proven isolated thalamic infarcts and delineated three deviant stroke patterns in one-third of them, involving other than the following four major arterial territories: polar or tuberothalamic or anterior; paramedian or thalamic-subthalamic; inferolateral or thalamogeniculate or ventrolateral; posterior choroidal (Bogousslavsky *et al.*, 1988a; Caplan, 1996c; Carrera *et al.*, 2004; Percheron, 1976; Schmahmann, 2003; Tatu *et al.*, 1998; 2001). The deviant thalamic territories were the following:

1. *anteromedian* – combining the polar and paramedian infarcts, found in 13% of all patients (decreased vigilance in 16% and 67% of patients with unilateral and

bilateral lesions, respectively; vertical gaze paresis (67%); memory impairment and executive dysfunction in 89% of them);

2. *central* — involving the central thalamus and adjacent parts of the four classical territories, found in 6% (ALC present in one-third of them, with vigilance impairment in unilateral lesion and vertical gaze palsy in bilateral infarct);

3. *posterolateral* (11%) — with infarction in the inferolateral and posterior choroidal arteries territory with sparing of consciousness (Carrera *et al.*, 2004).

The authors studied also the frequencies, etiologies, and clinical features of the remaining 50 patients with the four classical aforementioned thalamic artery territory ischemic strokes (detailed in Table 23.4, with permission of Carrera *et al.*, 2004). It is noteworthy that ALCs, characterized by decreased vigilance and impaired consciousness, were present in 25% and 63% of patients

Table 23.4. Stroke frequency, mechanisms, and clinical features of the remaining 50 patients with the four classical thalamic arteries territory

	Anterior ($n=8$)	Paramedian ($n=19$)	Inferolateral ($n=19$)	Posterior choroidal ($n=4$)
Frequency	11%	27%	27%	6%
Etiology	Cardiac 50%, art-to-art 13%, other 37%	Cardiac 68%, art-to-art 16%, microangiopathy 4%, other 11%	Microangiopathy 58%, cardiac 11%, art-to-art 1%, other 20%	Microangio-pathy 50%, other 50%
Clinical features				
ALC	Decreased vigilance 25%	Impaired consciousness 63%	None	None
Cognitive impairment	Executive dysfunction and memory impairment 100%	Executive dysfunction 63% memory impairment 37%	Executive dysfunction 42%	None
Vertical gaze paresis	None	63%	None	None
Hemihypesthesia	None	None	84%	75%
Hemiataxia	None	None	74%	None
Hemiparesia	None	None	26%	None
Sectoranopsia	None	None	None	25%

Source: art-to-art = arterioarterial

Adapted with permission from Carrera *et al.*, 2004.

with polar and paramedian thalamic infarctions, which represented 11% and 27% of all 71 thalamic infarcts, respectively.

The syndrome of rostral pontine and caudal midbrain infarction

Patients with acute bilateral tegmental pontine and mesencephalic large infarcts present usually with the most severe and deep ALC form: coma (Caplan, 1988; 1996a; 1996b; Chase et al., 1968; Hayem, 1868; La bauge et al., 1981). Although Kingston first reported a similar case (Kingston, 1842), the stroke syndrome of fatal basilar artery occlusion associated with coma was first recognized by Hayem (1868), and completed later by Leyden (1882). Kubik and Adams published the first clinico-pathologic series (Kubik and Adams, 1949). Subsequent series confirmed that stroke-induced coma correlated with bilateral medial pontine base and tegmentum and lower midbrain infarctions (Chase et al., 1968); although resting EEG recording in the acute stage were almost diffusely abnormal, no specific pattern could be related to the clinical state or lesion size/location. In the remaining stuporous patients with incomplete/unilateral pontine tegmental lesions, EEG was non-reactive to external stimuli (Chase et al., 1968). Later in the clinical course of these rostral pontine and caudal midbrain infarct patterns, consciousness might be recovered while subjects remained tetraplegic, deaf, with only vertical eye blinking and movements, corresponding to the definition of the locked-in syndrome. Recent modern multimodal electrophysiological studies — EEG, somatosensory, brainstem auditory, and motor evoked potentials (SEPs/BAEPs/MEPs) — showed preserved EEG alpha activity, confirming the integrity of consciousness in locked-in syndrome (Cummings and Greenberg, 1977; Bassetti et al., 1994). Pontine lesions responsible for the locked-in syndrome are located near the experimentally proven generator for sleep in animals (Jouvet, 1969; Zeman, 2001), where REM sleep was suppressed by lesions of the caudal raphe, loci ceruleus, or reticular caudal pontine nuclei (Jouvet, 1969). A recent topographic/spectral EEG performed in two patients with basilar occlusion suggests that alpha reactivity depends on the preservation of thalamo-cortical connections (Kamondi and Szirmai, 1993). Indeed, maintenance of consciousness is related to the integrity of the ARAS located in the paramedian tegmentum of the pons and midbrain (Caplan, 1996b).

Ponto-mesencephalic ischemia that induces coma is caused by occlusion of the proximal and middle portion of the basilar artery, secondary to atherothrombosis (including dolichoectasia), dissection, or embolism (cardiac or arterio-arterial) (Caplan, 1988; 1996b), or sympathetic-mediated vasospasm (cocaine, Ecstasy, amphetamine) (Vallée et al., 2003). In the first series of Kubik and Adams in 1949, who first recognized the pre-mortem clinical diagnosis of the syndrome of basilar artery occlusion, half of the patients presented with coma at stroke onset

Table 23.5. Main signs of rostral pontine and caudal midbrain stroke associated with coma

	Bilateral infarcts	Incomplete infarction
Neuro-ophthalmological signs	Bilateral horizontal gaze palsies	Ipsilesional conjugate horizontal gaze palsy
	Bilateral pinpoint pupils	
	Bilateral pontine ptosis without myosis	Unilateral or bilateral (wall-eyed bilateral) internuclear ophthalmoplegia
	Bilateral ocular bobbing	One and a half syndrome
Motor signs	Quadri-or hemiplegia	hemiplegia
	alternating hemiplegia	monoplegia
	Paraplegia, diplegia, monoplegia	
	pseudo-clonic seizures, myoclonic jerking	

(Kubik and Adams, 1949). In a review of patients with basilar artery occlusion, coma was observed in 78%, associated with motor signs and neuro-ophthalmologic abnormalities including pupils abnormalities (La bauge *et al.*, 1981).

Early recognition of warning signs of basilar artery occlusion, which is a medical emergency, is mandatory for immediate neuroimaging study (angiogram, CT-angiography, or MR imaging) (du Mesnil de *et al.*, 2002; Nighoghossian *et al.*, 1999), and further recanalization therapy (Smith and Delargy, 2005; Adams *et al.*, 2003; Brandt *et al.*, 1996). Thus, it is important to recognize signs of rostral pontine and caudal midbrain stroke (Table 23.5). The most frequent warning signs are vertigo (61−73%), headache (41−49%), dysarthria (23−30%), ALC (17−23%) (La bauge *et al.*, 1981; von campe *et al.*, 2003), and alternating hemiplegia or the appearance of contralateral deficit within 24 hours (Fisher, 1988).

We report two examples of patients with basilar artery occlusion, the first (case 1, Figure 23.2) with ventro-pontine ischemic and initial coma, evolving into classical locked-in syndrome despite IA TT. The second is a case with dramatic incomplete bilateral ponto-mesencephalic infarctions with the most catastrophic locked-in syndrome pattern (case 3, Figure 23.9).

Anterior circulation strokes
Middle cerebral artery (MCA) stroke syndrome

Hemispheric dominance for ALC associated with unilateral MCA stroke hypothesized by Plum and Posner (1980b; 1980c), has not been supported by recent studies. Indeed, in a large series of 564 MCA-associated infarcts,

73% showed drowsiness without differences between left and right hemispheric insult (Cucchiara *et al.*, 2003). In addition, somnolence has been observed in 27% of patients with M2-branch infarct ($n = 610$) versus 88% of those with large hemispheric strokes; i.e. near one-third each for complete, large superficial, and large superficial/deep MCA territory infarcts. On the other hand, stupor was a negative outcome predictor, present in 10% of patients with complete MCA territory infarct. These patients with complete MCA strokes, presenting with hemiplegia, homonymous hemianopia, and hemineglect/aphasia, are at risk for brain swelling and edema, and further uncal herniation, and may be

A.

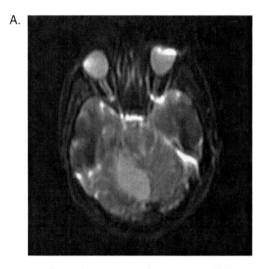

B.

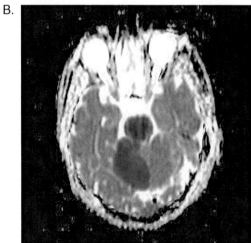

Figure 23.9

C.
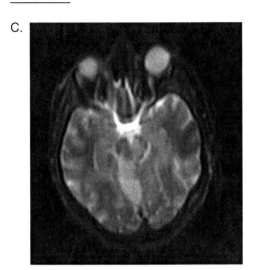

D.
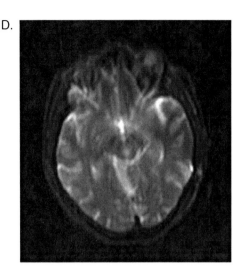

E.
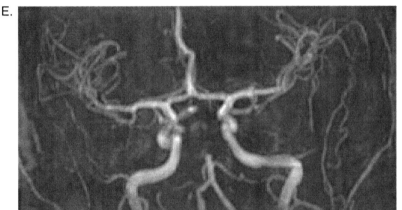

Figure 23.9   MR imaging DWI (A) and corresponding ADC (B) sequences showing prominent pontine acute infarct together with a right PICA territory infarction. MR imaging DWI sequences showing acute infarcts of the left midbrain tegmentum and cerebral peduncle (C) and periaqueductal gray (D), together with a right superior cerebellar artery territory infarction. Time-of-Flight (TOF) MRA showing acute occlusion of the middle and upper segment of the basilar artery (E).

Clinical Case 3. A 39-year-old female was found comatose (CGS 3), anarthric, with complete ophthalmoplegia, bi-facial plegia and lower cranial nerve palsies, and quadriplegia with four-limbs extension on noxious stimuli, with bilateral extensor plantar responses. Under intubation, a diagnostic procedure was performed. Thrombolysis was not performed because of evidence of poor outcome and a too long delay of 12 hours after stroke onset. EEG showed delta slow waves over the left hemisphere, and absent SEPs responses (N20). According to the family, and the wishes of the patient before stroke onset, she was extubated. Necropsy showed a PFO with a left VA and complete basilar artery occlusion.

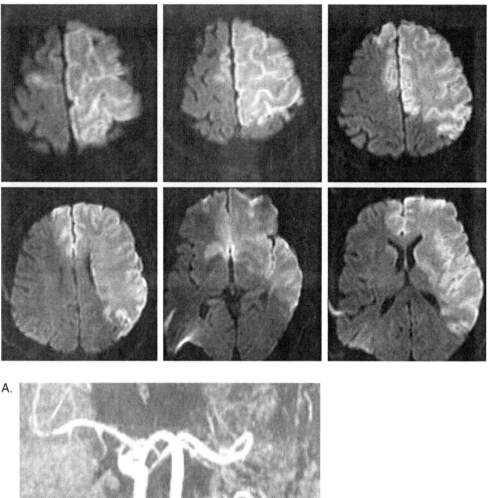

A.

Figure 23.10 MR imaging studies with DWI sequences, from the top (upper left) to the bottom (lower right) demonstrate left complete MCA-territory and bilateral ACA infarctions. (A) TOF-MRA shows occlusion of the left ICA and absent flow in the two ACA.

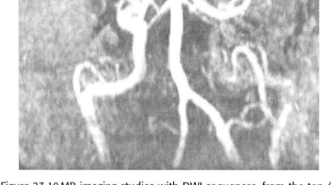

Clinical Case 4. A 52-year-old man, smoker, was transferred to our ICU, intubated, for suspected ABO with sudden coma and initial normal plain CT. Because of bilateral corticospinal tract signs with left hemiplegia and right lower limb monoplegia with extension of upper limb on noxious stimuli, MR imaging was performed.

candidates for surgical hemicraniectomy or moderate hypothermia (Maramattom *et al.*, 2004; Wijdicks, 2000a; 2000b).

Bilateral anterior circulation strokes due to bilateral internal carotid artery occlusion mimic basilar artery occlusion with sudden coma and quadriplegia, which was first described by Fisher (1954). A recent series of six patients of such a catastrophic stroke syndrome has been recently published (Kwon *et al.*, 2002); all of them died within 72 hours.

Bilateral anterior cerebral artery (ACA) stroke syndrome

In the acute stage, bilateral ACA territory infarcts may present with ALC characterized by lethargy, before evolving into akinetic mutism, as published in a case report by Minagar and David (1999). The explanation is an anatomical variant with an azygous or unilateral arterial supply of both ACAs from one ICA (Critchley, 1930; Bogousslavsky and Regli, 1990). Such an unusual situation is illustrated by a patient presenting with coma and right hemiplegia with contralateral hemiparesis, due to bilateral ACA and left-MCA territory infarctions (case 4, Figure 23.10).

Acknowledgement

I thank Dr. Stefano Binaghi, Radiology Department, for providing the CI/MRI illustrations.

REFERENCES

Adams, H. P., Jr., Adams, R. J., Brott, T., *et al.* (2003). Guidelines for the early management of patients with ischemic stroke: A scientific statement from the Stroke Council of the American Stroke Association. *Stroke*, **34**, 1056–83.

Adams, R. D. (1997). Approach to the patient with neurologic disease. In R. D. Adams, M. Victor and A. Ropper, eds., *Principles of Neurology*, Part 1, 6th edn. New York: McGraw-Hill, pp. 3–11.

Alajouanine, T. (1957). Les altérations des états de conscience causés par les désordres neurologiques. *Acta Med. Belgium*, **2**, 19–41.

Albright, T. D., Jessel, T. M., Kandel, E. R. and Posner, M. I. (2001). Progress in the neural sciences in the century after Cajal (and the mysteries that remain). *Ann. N. Y. Acad. Sci*, **929**, 11–40.

Bassetti, C. (2001). Disturbances of consciousness and sleep–wake functions. In J. Bogousslavsky and L. R. Caplan, eds., *Stroke Syndromes*, Chapter 14, Second Edition. New York: Cambridge University Press, pp. 192–210.

Bassetti, C., Mathis, J., Gugger, M., Lovblad, K. O. and Hess, C. W. (1996). Hypersomnia following paramedian thalamic stroke: A report of 12 patients. *Ann. Neurol.*, **39**, 471–80.

Bassetti, C., Mathis, J. and Hess, C. W. (1994). Multimodal electrophysiological studies including motor evoked potentials in patients with locked-in syndrome: Report of six patients. *J. Neurol. Neurosurg. Psychiatry*, **57**, 1403–6.

Bauby, J. -D. (1997). *The Diving Bell and the Butterfly*. In A. A. Knopf, ed., Alfred A Knopf, New York. English translation by J Leggatt.

Biller, J., Sand, J. J., Corbett, J. J., Adams, H. P., Jr. and Dunn, V. (1985). Syndrome of the paramedian thalamic arteries: Clinical and neuroimaging correlation. *J. Clin. Neuroophthalmol.*, **5**, 217–23.

Bogousslavsky, J. (1990). Respiratory failure and unilateral caudal brainstem infarction. *Ann. Neurol.*, **28**, 668–73.

Bogousslavsky, J. and Regli, F. (1990). Anterior cerebral artery territory infarction in the Lausanne Stroke Registry. Clinical and etiologic patterns. *Arch. Neurol.*, **47**, 144–50.

Bogousslavsky, J., Regli, F. and Assal, G. (1986). The syndrome of unilateral tuberothalamic artery territory infarction. *Stroke*, **17**, 434–41.

Bogousslavsky, J., Regli, F., Delaloye, B., *et al.* (1991). Loss of psychic self-activation with bithalamic infarction. Neurobehavioural, CT, MRI and SPECT correlates. *Acta Neurol. Scand.*, **83**, 309–16.

Bogousslavsky, J., Regli, F. and Uske, A. (1988a). Thalamic infarcts: Clinical syndromes, etiology, and prognosis. *Neurology*, **38**, 837–48.

Bogousslavsky, J., Van, M. G. and Regli, F. (1988b). The Lausanne Stroke Registry: Analysis of 1,000 consecutive patients with first stroke. *Stroke*, **19**, 1083–92.

Brandt, T., von, K. R., Muller-Kuppers, M. and Hacke, W. (1996). Thrombolytic therapy of acute basilar artery occlusion. Variables affecting recanalization and outcome. *Stroke*, **27**, 875–81.

Brazis, P. W., Masdeu, J. C., Biller, J. (1996). The localization of lesions causing coma. In P. W. Brazis, J. C. Masdeu and J. Biller, eds., *Localization in Clinical Neurology*, Chapter 21, Third Edition. Boston: Little, Brown and Company, pp. 565–95.

Bushnell, C. D., Phillips-Bute, B. G., Laskowitz, D. T., *et al.* (1999). Survival and outcome after endotracheal intubation for acute stroke. *Neurology*, **52**, 1374–81.

Caplan, L. R. (1980). "Top of basilar" syndrome. *Neurology*, **30**, 72–9.

Caplan, L. R. (1988). Vertebrobasilar system syndromes. In: P. J. Vinken, G. W. Bruyn, H. L. Klawans, eds., *Handbook of Clinical Neurology*, Chapter 14, 9th Edition. Elsevier Science Publishing Co., New York, pp. 371–407.

Caplan, L. R. (1996a). Signs and symptoms and their clinical localization. In L. R. Caplan, ed., *Posterior Circulation Diseases. Clinical Findings, Diagnosis, and Management*, Chapter 4. Cambridge, Massachussetts: Blackwell Science, Inc., pp. 73–130.

Caplan, L. R. (1996b). Basilar artery occlusive disease. In L. R. Caplan, ed., *Posterior Circulation Diseases. Clinical Findings, Diagnosis, and Management*, Chapter 11. Cambridge, Massachussetts: Blackwell Science, Inc., pp. 324–80.

Caplan, L. R. (1996c). Penetrating branch artery and lacunar disease. In L. R. Caplan, ed., *Posterior Circulation Diseases. Clinical Findings, Diagnosis, and Management*, Chapter 12, First Edition. Cambridge, Massachussetts: Blackwell Science, Inc., pp. 381–443.

Carrera, E., Michel, P. and Bogousslavsky, J. (2004). Anteromedian, central, and posterolateral infarcts of the thalamus: Three variant types. *Stroke*, **35**, 2826–31.

Castaigne, P., Buge, A. and Escourolle, R. (1962). Ramolissement pédonculaire médian, tegmento-thalamique avec ophtalmoplégie et hypersomnie. *Rev. Neurol. (Paris)*, **106**, 357–67.

Castaigne, P., Lhermitte, F., Buge, A., *et al.* (1981). Paramedian thalamic and midbrain infarct: Clinical and neuropathological study. *Ann. Neurol.*, **10**, 127–48.

Catsman-Berrevoets, C. E. and von Harskamp, F. (1988). Compulsive pre-sleep behavior and apathy due to bilateral thalamic stroke: Response to bromocriptine. *Neurology*, **38**, 647–9.

Chase, T. N., Moretti, L. and Frensky, A. L. (1968). Clinical and electroencephalographic manifestations of vascular lesions of the pons. *Neurology*, **18**, 357–68.

Collier, J. (1927). Nuclear ophthalmoplegia with special references to retraction of the lids and ptosis and to lesions of of the posterior commissure. *Brain*, **50**, 488–98.

Crick, F., Koch, C., Kreiman, G. and Fried, I. (2004). Consciousness and neurosurgery. *Neurosurgery*, **55**, 273–81.

Critchley, M. (1930). The anterior cerebral artery, and its syndromes. *Brain*, **53**, 120–65.

Cucchiara, B., Kasner, S. E., Wolk, D. A., *et al.* (2003). Lack of hemispheric dominance for consciousness in acute ischaemic stroke. *J. Neurol. Neurosurg. Psychiatry*, **74**, 889–92.

Cummings, J. L. and Greenberg, R. (1977). Sleep patterns in the "locked-in" syndrome. *Electroencephalogr. Clin. Neurophysiol.*, **43**, 270–1.

Devereaux, M. W., Keane, J. R. and Davis, R. L. (1973). Automatic respiration failure associated with infarction of the medulla. *Arch. Neurol.*, **29**, 46–52.

du Mesnil de, R. R., Neumann-Haefelin, T., Berkefeld, J., Sitzer, M. and Lanfermann, H. (2002). Magnetic resonance imaging in basilar artery occlusion. *Arch. Neurol.*, **59**, 398–402.

Dudzinski, D. (2001). The diving bell meets the butterfly: Identity lost and re-membered. *Theor. Med. Bioeth.*, **22**, 33–46.

Facon, E., Steriade, M. and Werthein, N. (1958). Hypersomnie prolongée engendrée par des lesions bilatérales du système activateur médial: Le syndrome thrombotique de la bifurcation du tronc basilaire. *Rev. Neurol. (Paris)*, **98**, 117–33.

Fisher, C. M. (1954). Occlusion of the carotid arteries: Further experiences. *Arch. Neurol. Psychiatry*, **72**, 187–204.

(1961). Clinical syndromes in cerebral hemorrhages. In W. S. Fields, ed., *Pathogenesis and Treatment of Cerebrovascular Disease*. Springfield, IL: Charles C. Thomas Publishers, pp. 316–38.

(1988). The 'herald hemiparesis' of basilar artery occlusion. *Arch. Neurol.*, **45**, 1301–3.

Foix, C. and Hillemand, P. (1925). Les artères de l'axe encéphalique jusqu'au diencéphale inclusivement. *Rev. Neurol. (Paris)*, **2**, 705–39.

Giacino, J. T., Ashwal, S., Childs, N., *et al.* (2002). The minimally conscious state: Definition and diagnostic criteria. *Neurology*, **58**, 349–53.

Ginsberg, A. (2005). Poem: Locked-in syndrome. *Neurology*, **64**, 2161.

Hayem, M. G. (1868). Sur la thrombose par artérite du tronc basilaire. Comme cause de mort rapide. *Arch. Physiol. Norm. Pathol.*, **1**, 270–89.

Hommel, M. and Bogousslavsky, J. (1991). The spectrum of vertical gaze palsy following unilateral brainstem stroke. *Neurology*, **41**, 1229−34.

Howard, R. S. and Hirsch, N. P. (1999). Coma, vegetative state, and locked-in syndrome. In D. H. Miller and E. C. R aps, eds., *Critical Care Neurology, Blue Book of Practical Neurology*, Butterworth Heinnemann, Boston, pp. 91−120.

Ingvar, D. H., Brun, A. and Johansson, L. (1978). Survival after severe cerebral anoxia with destruction of the cerebral cortex; the apallic syndrome. In S. Korein, ed., *Brain Death: Interelated Medical and Social Issues. Ann. N. Y. Acad. Sci.* 315, pp. 184−214.

Jenett, B. and Plum, F. (1972). Persistent vegetative state after brain damage: A syndrome in search of a name. *Lancet*, **1**: 734−7.

John, E. R. (2002). The neurophysics of consciousness. *Brain Res. Brain Res. Rev.*, **39**, 1−28.

Jouvet, M. (1969). Biogenic amines and the states of sleep. *Science*, **163**, 32−41.

Kamondi, A. and Szirmai, I. (1993). Topographic EEG analysis in two patients with basilar thrombosis. *Clin. Electroencephalogr.*, **24**, 138−45.

Kingston, P. (1842). Case of fatal encephalitis with hemiplegia, immediately excited by Cantharides, in consequences of intense predisposition from basilar and internal carotid aneurism. *Edinburgh Med. J.*, **57**, 69−77.

Kretschmer, E. (1940). Das apallische syndrom. *Z. Ges. Neurol. Psychiat.*, **169**, 576−9.

Kubik, C. S. and Adams, R. D. (1949). Occlusion of the basilar artery: A clinical and pathological study. *Brain*, **69**, 73−121.

Kumral, E., Evyapan, D., Balkir, K. and Kutluhan, S. (2001). Bilateral thalamic infarction. Clinical, etiological and MRI correlates. *Acta Neurol. Scand.*, **103**, 35−42.

Kwon, S. U., Lee, S. H. and Kim, J. S. (2002). Sudden coma from acute bilateral internal carotid artery territory infarction. *Neurology*, **58**, 1846−9.

La bauge, R., Pages, M., Marty-Double, J. M., Blard, M. B. M and Salvaing, P. (1981). Occlusion du tronc basilaire. *Rev. Neurol. (Paris)*, **137**, 545−71.

Levin, B. E. and Margolis, G. (1977). Acute failure of automatic respirations secondary to unilateral brainstem infarct. *Ann. Neurol.*, **1**, 583−6.

Leyden, E. (1882). Ueber di thrombose der basilar arterie. *Zeitschrift Klin. Med.*, **5**, 165−85.

Lipowsi, Z. J. (1973). Organic brain syndromes: A reformulation. *Compr. Psychiatry*, **19**, 309−22.

Llinas, R. and Ribary, U. (2001). Consciousness and the brain. The thalamocortical dialogue in health and disease. *Ann. N. Y. Acad. Sci.*, **929**, 166−75.

Maia, T. V. and Cleeremans, A. (2005). Consciousness: Converging insights from connectionist modeling and neuroscience. *Trends Cogn. Sci.*, **9**, 397−404.

Maramattom, B. V., Bahn, M. M. and Wijdicks, E. F. (2004). Which patient fares worse after early deterioration due to swelling from hemispheric stroke? *Neurology*, **63**, 2142−5.

Mehler, M. F. (1988). The neuro-ophthalmogic spectrum of the rostral basilar artery syndrome. *Arch. Neurol.*, **45**, 966.

Melo, T. P., de Mendoça, A., Crespo, M., Carvahlo, M. and Ferro, J. M. (1992). An emergency room-based study of stroke coma. *Cerebrovasc. Dis.*, **2**, 93−101.

Minagar, A. and David, N. J. (1999). Bilateral infarction in the territory of the anterior cerebral arteries. *Neurology*, **52**, 886−8.

Morison, R. Y. and Dempsey, E. W. (1942). A study of thalamo-cortical relations. *Am. J. Physiol.*, **135**, 281–92.

Moruzzi, G. and Magoun, H. W. (1949). Brainstem reticular formation and activation of the EEG. *Electroencephalogr. Clin. Neurophysiology*, **1**, 455–73.

Multi-Society Task Force on PVS (1994). Medical aspects of the persistent vegetative state. *N. Engl. J. Med.*, **330**, 1499–508,1572–1579.

Nighoghossian, N., Derex, L., Turjman, F., *et al.* (1999). Hyperacute diffusion-weighted MRI in basilar occlusion treated with intra-arterial t-PA. *Cerebrovasc. Dis.*, **9**, 351–4.

Pappas, C. T. E. and Carrion, C. (1989). Altered levels of consciousness and the reticular activating system. *BNI Quarterly*, **5**, 2–8.

Parvizi, J. and Damasio, A. (2001). Consciousness and the brainstem. *Cognition*, **79**, 135–60.

(2003). Neuroanatomical correlates of brainstem coma. *Brain*, **126**, 1524–36.

Percheron, G. (1976). Les artères du thalamus humain II. Artères et territoires thalamiques paramédians de l'artère basilare communicante. *Rev. Neurol. (Paris)*, **132**, 309–24.

Perren, F., Clarke, S. and Bogousslavsky, J. (2005). The syndrome of combined polar and paramedian thalamic infarction. *Arch. Neurol.*, **62**, 1212–6.

Pinault, D. (2004). The thalamic reticular nucleus: Structure, function and concept. *Brain Res. Brain Res. Rev.*, **46**, 1–31.

Plum, F. (1991). Coma and related global disturbances of the human conscious state. In A. Peters and E. G. Jones, eds., *Cerebral Cortex*, New York: Plenum Press, pp. 359–425.

Plum, F., Posner, J. B. (1980a). Subtentorial lesions causing coma. In F. Plum and J. B. Posner, eds., *The Diagnosis of Stupor and Coma, 3*, Third Edition. Philadelphia: F. A. Davis Company, pp. 153–75.

(1980b). Supratentorial lesions causing coma. In F. Plum, J. B. Posner, eds., *The Diagnosis of Stupor and Coma, 2*, Third Edition. Philadelphia: F. A. Davis Company, pp. 87–151.

(1980c). The pathologic physiology of signs and symptoms of coma. In F. Plum and J. B. Posner, eds., *The Diagnosis of Stupor and Coma, 1*, Third Edition. Philadelphia: F. A. Davis Company, pp. 1–86.

Ropper, A. H., Gress, D. R., Diringer, M. N., *et al.* (2004). Critical care of acute stroke. In A. H. Ropper, ed., *Neurological and Neurosurgical Intensive Care*, Fourth Edition. Philadelphia: Lippincott Williams & Wilking, pp. 208–16.

Rossetti, A. O., Reichhart, M. D. and Bogousslavsky, J. (2003). Central Horner's syndrome with contralateral ataxic hemiparesis: A diencephalic alternate syndrome. *Neurology*, **61**, 334–8.

Schmahmann, J. D. (2003). Vascular syndromes of the thalamus. *Stroke*, **34**, 2264–78.

Searle, J. R. (2000). Consciousness. *Annu. Rev. Neurosci.*, **23**, 557–78.

Segarra, J. M. (1970). Cerebral vascular disease and behavior. I. The syndrome of the mesensephalic artery (basilar artery bifurcation). *Arch. Neurol.*, **22**, 408–18.

Sieb, R. A. (2004). The emergence of consciousness. *Med. Hypotheses*, **63**, 900–4.

Smith, E. and Delargy, M. (2005). Locked-in syndrome. *BMJ*, **330**, 406–9.

Smith, W. S., Sung, G., Starkman, S., *et al.* (2005). Safety and efficacy of mechanical embolectomy in acute ischemic stroke: Results of the MERCI trial. *Stroke*, **36**, 1432–8.

Spiegel, E. A. and Wycis, H. T. O. C. F. H. (1956). Thalamic chronotaraxis. *Am. J. Psychiatry*, **113**, 97–105.

Tatu, L., Moulin, T., Bogousslavsky, J. and Duvernoy, H. (1998). Arterial territories of the human brain: Cerebral hemispheres. *Neurology*, **50**, 1699–708.

(2001). Arterial territories of human brain. In J. Bogousslavsky and L. R. Caplan, eds., *Stroke Syndromes*, Chapter 29, Second Edition. New York: Cambridge University Press, pp. 375–404.

Teasdale, G. and Jenett, B. (1974). Assessment of coma and impaired consciousness. A practical scale. *Lancet*, **2**, 81.

Toates, F. (2006). A model of the hierarchy of behaviour, cognition, and consciousness. *Conscious. Cogn.*, **15**, 75–118.

Vallee, J. N., Crozier, S., Guillevin, R., *et al.* (2003). Acute basilar artery occlusion treated by thromboaspiration in a cocaine and ecstasy abuser. *Neurology*, **61**, 839–41.

von Campe, G., Regli, F. and Bogousslavsky, J. (2003). Heralding manifestations of basilar artery occlusion with lethal or severe stroke. *J. Neurol. Neurosurg. Psychiatry*, **74**, 1621–6.

Weir, C. J., Bradford, A. P. and Lees, K. R. (2003). The prognostic value of the components of the Glasgow Coma Scale following acute stroke. *QJM*, **96**, 67–74.

Wijdicks, E. F. (2000a). Management of massive hemispheric cerebral infarct: Is there a ray of hope? *Mayo Clin. Proc.*, **75**, 945–52.

(2000b). Altered Arousal and Coma. In E. F.M. Wijdicks, ed., *Neurologic Catastrophes in the Emergency Department*, Part I. Chapter 1, First Edition. Boston: Butterworth-Heinemann, pp. 3–42.

(2001). The diagnosis of brain death. *N. Engl. J. Med.*, **344**, 1215–21.

Wijdicks, E. F. and Cranford, R. E. (2005). Clinical diagnosis of prolonged states of impaired consciousness in adults. *Mayo Clin. Proc.*, **80**, 1037–46.

Wijdicks, E. F., Kokmen, E. and O'Brien, P. C. (1998). Measurement of impaired consciousness in the neurological intensive care unit: A new test. *J. Neurol. Neurosurg. Psychiatry*, **64**, 117–9.

Wijdicks, E. F. M., Ramlet, W. R., Marattom, B. V., Manno, E. M. and McClelland, R. L. (2005). Validation of a new coma scale: The FOUR Score. *Ann. Neurol.*, **58**, 585–93.

Young, G. B. and Pigott, S. E. (1999). Neurobiological basis of consciousness. *Arch. Neurol.*, **56**, 153–7.

Zeman, A. (1997). Persistent vegetative state. *Lancet*, **350**, 795–9.

(2001). Consciousness. *Brain*, **124**, 1263–89.

24

Delirium and confusional state in stroke patients

Hilde Henon and Didier Leys

University Hospital of Lille, France

Main characteristics of delirium and confusional state

Delirium or acute confusional state (ACS) is a mental disorder characterized by acute onset, altered level of consciousness, fluctuating course, and disturbances in orientation, memory, thought, and behavior (Lipowski, 1990). This condition is frequent in stroke patients, although stroke is a rare cause of ACS. Many predisposing factors have been identified. Stroke per se may, however, induce ACS. The occurrence of this behavioral disturbance adversely influences outcome in stroke patients. However, no specific treatment is available.

ACS is an acute, transient disorder of consciousness and cognition with fluctuating intensity. The symptoms of delirium are wide ranging, and although they are non-specific, their abrupt or rapid onset and their fluctuating nature is highly characteristic and is a valuable diagnostic tool. The main feature of delirium is disordered attention with difficulties in focusing and sustaining attention on one stimulus and difficulties in shifting attention to new external stimuli: attention wanders, perseverations may be observed. Attention disturbances are not isolated and examination will reveal abnormalities of thinking, perception, and memory. The change in cognition includes impaired memory, language (anomia, incoherent speech, aphasia, agraphia), disorientation to time and place and visuospatial dysfunction. Perception disturbances may also be present with illusions, hallucinations, or delusions. Sleep−wake abnormalities are frequent with daytime sleepiness and reduced and fragmented sleep during the night with nocturnal agitation, shouting, and aggressivity. Many individuals are restless and hyperactive while others are lethargic. Two subtypes of delirium have been described according to the level of activity: the hyperactive type with agitated, disoriented, and delusional patients, and the hypoactive type with a subdued, disoriented, and apathetic patient. However, quick shifting from hyperactivity to reduced activity is frequently observed. Delirious patients may display a wide range of emotions, including fear, anxiety, apathy, depression,

Table 24.1. Diagnostic criteria for delirium (DSM-IV criteria)

A. Disturbance of consciousness (i.e., reduced clarity of awareness about the environment) with reduced ability to focus, sustain, or shift attention

B. A change in cognition (e.g., memory deficit, disorientation, language disturbance) or development of a perceptual disturbance that is not better accounted for by a pre-existing, established, or evolving dementia

C. The disturbance develops over a short period of time (usually hours to days), and tends to fluctuate during the course of the day

D. Evidence from the history, physical examination, or laboratory findings indicate that the disturbance is caused by direct consequences of a general medical condition

euphoria, with sometimes rapidly changing emotions. The diagnostic criteria for delirium from the American Psychiatric Association (2000) are given in Table 24.1.

The terms delirium, confusion, agitation, and confusional state are used variously by different neurologists and psychiatrists (Lipowski, 1990; Adams *et al.*, 1997). Several authors restrict the term *delirium* to hyperactive ACS with increased verbal, motor, and autonomic activity, hallucinations or illusions, suggesting that ACS and delirium may have pathogenic mechanisms of different types and involve different parts of the brain (Adams *et al.*, 1997). However, delirium is not a stable condition and fluctuation of symptoms is an important part of the diagnosis of ACS: many patients will present both hyperactive and hypoactive subtypes of delirium (O'Keeffe, 1999; Camus *et al.*, 2000). It is also important to notice that some authors consider as delirium only hyperactive states with accompanying confusion associated with focal stroke and exclude ACS secondary to metabolic or toxic encephalopathy. In this chapter, the terms ACS and delirium will be used interchangeably and, beside location of stroke, risk factors for confusion in stroke patients will be considered.

The main differential diagnosis of delirium is dementia (Erkinjuntti *et al.*, 1986). However, it may also be difficult to differentiate delirium from psychotic disorders such as schizophrenia or psychiatric disorders such as depression or mania. The acute onset and the fluctuating nature of confusional state are, however, key features for the differential diagnosis. The main elements for the differential diagnosis of delirium are given in Table 24.2.

ACS occurs in up to half of older patients who have been admitted to a hospital (Levkoff *et al.*, 1991; Jitapunkul *et al.*, 1992). ACS is associated with several adverse outcomes including increased functional decline during hospitalization, risk of hospital-acquired complications, increased duration of hospital

Table 24.2. Differential diagnosis of acute confusional states (ACS)

	ACS	Dementia	Depression	Psychotic disorders
Onset and course	Acute onset, fluctuating course	Progressive onset and course	Variable, single or recurrent episodes, may be chronic	Variable, usually slow onset, then chronic with exacerbations
Consciousness and orientation	Fluctuating levels of consciousness with and disorientation	Clear until late stages	Normal	Normal, perplexity may occur in acute stage
Attention	Impaired	Impaired	May be impaired	May be impaired
Memory	Impaired	Impaired	Normal	Normal
Psychotic symptoms (hallucinations, illusions)	Frequent: visual hallucinations, delusions, usually simple in content	Uncommon in the absence of associated ACS	Infrequent, complex and in keeping with prevailing mood	Frequent, complex, often paranoid
Electroencephalogram	Usually abnormal: generalized diffuse slowing in most cases	Usually abnormal: generalized diffuse slowing in most cases	Usually normal	Usually normal

stay, need for institutional care, poor long-term functional and cognitive outcome, and death (Francis *et al.*, 1990; George *et al.*, 1997; O'Keeffe and Lavan, 1997; Rockwood *et al.*, 1999; Curyto *et al.*, 2001; McCusker *et al.*, 2001; Rahkonen *et al.*, 2001; Lundstrom *et al.*, 2003). Several predisposing factors for ACS in hospitalized patients have been identified irrespective of the cause of admission: age (Lipowski, 1989; Schor *et al.*, 1992), male gender (Schor *et al.*, 1992), drugs and in particular drugs with anticholinergic effect (Lipowski, 1989; Sumner and Simons, 1994; Han *et al.*, 2001; Tune *et al.*, 1992; Caeiro *et al.*, 2004a), somatic or metabolic disorders (Lipowski, 1989; Koponen *et al.*, 1989; 1993; George *et al.*, 1997), dementia (Lipowski, 1989; Schor *et al.*, 1992; Koponen *et al.*, 1993; Pompei *et al.*, 1994; Rahkonen *et al.*, 2000), vision and hearing impairment (George *et al.*, 1997), and focal brain lesions of any origin (Lipowski, 1989; Sumner *et al.*, 1994; Koponen *et al.*, 1989; 1993), especially stroke (Lipowski, 1989). Stroke remains, however, a rare cause of delirium in patients without focal neurological signs. Among patients with ACS who underwent a computed tomography (CT) scan, 15% had a cerebral lesion (stroke, subdural hematoma, tumor), and most of them had focal neurological signs (Naughton *et al.*, 1997). Infections and stroke were, however, the most important etiological factors for ACS in elderly healthy individuals (Rahkonen *et al.*, 2000). In stroke patients, ACS has been reported in single case reports, small groups of patients, or retrospective studies. There have been only a few systematic investigations of ACS specifically prospectively performed in stroke patients (Gustafson *et al.*, 1991; Hénon *et al.*, 1999; Sandberg *et al.*, 2001; Caiero *et al.*, 2004a,b): ACS was found to occur in 13—48% of stroke patients.

The pathogenesis of ACS remains largely unknown (Lipowski, 1989; 1990; Flacker and Lipsitz, 1999; Ferro, 2001). Advances in neuropsychiatry have revealed differences between brain regions, including the hemispheres, which may underlie the constellation of symptoms among different psychiatric disorders. It has also been suggested that delirium could involve particular neural pathways and that lateralization to the right may be relevant. Prefrontal cortices, anterior and right thalamus, and right basilar mesial temporoparietal cortex may play a significant role in subserving delirium symptoms and may be the "final common pathway" for delirium from a variety of etiologies. The final common pathway may be responsible for certain "core symptoms" (disorientation, cognitive deficits, sleep—wake cycle disturbance, disorganized thinking, and language abnormalities), while other symptoms (delusions, hallucinations, illusions, and affective lability) may occur depending on the etiology causing delirium (Trzepacz, 1999a).

The stress—hypercortisolemia hypothesis postulates that delirium is a manifestation of acute stress mediated by abnormally elevated levels of cortisol. Glucocorticoid hormones are important for coping with stress but may have deleterious effects on mood and memory during prolonged excessive secretion. A key abnormality related to cortisol excess in delirium seems to be abnormal "shut-off" of the hypothalamic—pituitary—adrenal (HPA) axis tested by the dexamethasone suppression test (Olsson, 1999). Indeed, higher post-dexamethasone cortisol levels (Gustafson *et al.*, 1993) and increased levels of ACTH in the first hours after onset (Fassbender *et al.*, 1994) were observed in stroke patients with ACS. Type II receptors for glucocorticoid, which are occupied during high stress levels of hormones, are densely expressed in the hippocampus and an intact hippocampal formation seems to be necessary for adequate negative feedback responsiveness. Stroke, pain, and infections are highly stressful conditions, leading to an increase of the glucocorticoid formation, which could in some cases not be adequately suppressed.

Alternatively, delirium could be associated with a reduced oxidative metabolism leading to a decrease synthesis of acetylcholine and epinephrine. The main neurochemical correlate of delirium is a decrease of the cholinergic activity. Indeed, anticholinergic drugs frequently induce confusional state (Karlsson, 1999; Tune and Egeli, 1999; Francis, 1996; Caeiro et al., 2004a). Intake of medications with anticholinergic activity was found to increase the symptoms of delirium in patients with diagnosed ACS (Han et al., 2001). Cholinergic drugs can improve delirium induced by lithium and anticholinergic drugs (Wengel et al., 1998). In a series of surgical patients and of elderly medical patients, delirious patients were found to have higher levels of serum acetylcholinesterase activity (Fisher, 2001; Mach et al., 1995; Mussi et al., 1999). One reason why ACS is more frequent in older and in demented patients could be the age-related loss of cholinergic reserve and the focal loss of acetylcholine in the nucleus basal of Meynert (McDonald and Treolar, 1996; Reyes-Ortiz, 1997). One reason why ACS could be more frequent in stroke patients is that the production of endogenous anti-cholinergic substances is increased during acute illness (Flacker and Wei, 2001).

Other neuromediators might, however, play a role as ACS was a common side-effect of drugs that decreased release of glutamate and dopamine (Trzepacz, 1999b; Muir et al., 2000). An imbalance in the cholinergic and dopaminergic neurotransmitter systems could account for delirium symptoms (Trzepacz, 1999b).

Stroke subtypes leading to delirium and confusional state

ACS and delirium can be produced by strategic lesions involving structures subserving attention, memory, and emotional behavior. It is, however, important to notice that in the majority of the descriptions of the focal form of ACS, patients were not assessed with instruments specific for delirium, and in most cases, patients do not strictly meet DSM-IV criteria of delirium. This is well illustrated in recent negative reports. Four cases of patients with lesion involving the genu of the internal capsule were reported (Madureira et al., 1999): although patients had cognitive and behavioral disturbances, they did not fulfill criteria for ACS. In the same way, none of the 12 patients with thalamic infarcts reported by Ghika-Schmid and Bogousslavsky (2000) were delirious. Moreover, in case reports with first generations of CT scans, another vascular lesion of the brain cannot be excluded and may interfere with the neuropsychological profile (Godefroy et al., 1994). Finally, in elderly patients without follow-up after stroke, the contribution of an underlying dementia to the occurrence of ACS cannot be excluded. The frequency of ACS is influenced by numerous factors related to stroke including (1) stroke type with a higher frequency in cerebral hemorrhage (Gustafson et al., 1991; Caiero et al., 2004b) and (2) stroke location.

Key points Main types of stroke associated with acute confusional state

Stroke type	Territory/characteristics
Arterial infarct	Thalamus: paramedian and thalamopolar arteries, posterior cerebral artery (especially bilateral infarcts), anterior cerebral artery (especially bilateral infarcts), middle cerebral artery: deep (caudate nucleus, genu of the internal capsule) and superficial (especially right) territories
Ruptured aneurysm	Anterior communicating artery, intraventricular bleeding, acute hydrocephalus
Hemorrhage	Frontal and thalamus
Complication and comorbidities	Metabolic disorders, infections and fever, pain, cardiopulmonary disorders Ethanol and drugs intoxication or withdrawal Epilepsy, subdural hematoma and brain injury Pre-existing dementia

Thalamic strokes

Although acute cognitive disturbances may occur after thalamic vascular lesions, criteria for the diagnosis of delirium are usually not fulfilled and agitation and ACS are rarely observed after thalamic stroke. Among 100 patients with thalamic hemorrhages (Kumral *et al.*, 1995), only 3 patients exhibited acute hallucinosis and agitation. However, ACS has been reported in stroke involving dorsomesial and anterior thalamic locations (Graff-Radford *et al.*, 1984) as in medial thalamic lesion (Castaigne *et al.*, 1981; Mori *et al.*, 1981). The suspected mechanism is that the thalamus acts as a filter, allowing only the relevant information to travel to the cortex, but stroke could compromise the thalamic gating function, leading to sensory overload and hyperarousal (Gaudreau and Gagnon, 2005).

Uni- and bilateral posterior cerebral artery territory infarcts

Unilateral and bilateral medial temporo-occipital lesions may cause agitated delirium (Medina *et al.*, 1974; Devinsky *et al.*, 1988; Verslegers *et al.*, 1991;

Milandre *et al.*, 1994; Nicolai and Lazzarino, 1994; Garcia-Albea, 1989; Vatsavayi *et al.*, 2003). Reviewing 9 of their own patients and 49 patients from other reports, Symonds and MacKenzie (1957) noted confusion at onset in half of patients with visual loss and acute bilateral infarct in the territory of the posterior cerebral arteries. Caplan (1980; 1996; 2000) reviewed reports of patients who developed an agitated delirious state after embolism to the rostral basilar artery and its PCA branches: all the patients had bilateral infarcts involving occipital and temporal lobe cortex below the calcarine sulcus, including the lingual and fusiform gyri. The dysfunction of the fusiform-parahippocampal and hippocampal regions is thought to be responsible for delirium. Destruction of the neocortical association area or its disconnection from limbic structures, resulting in impairment of focal attention, loss of memory, and disruption of temporal sequencing, may be responsible for ACS.

Other authors report cases with unilateral posterior cerebral artery territory infarct. The influence of the left hemisphere has sometimes been underlined (Devinsky *et al.*, 1988; Fisher, 1983). Devinsky *et al.* (1988) reported 4 patients with left-sided posterior cerebral artery infarction who developed ACS. Fifteen additional patients with ACS following unilateral posterior cerebral artery infarction were identified from a review of the literature; in 14 the lesion was left-sided. For Devinsky *et al.* (1988), destruction of dominant hemisphere neocortex or its disconnection from limbic structures, resulting in impairment of focal attention, loss of linguistically organized memory, and/or disruption of temporal sequencing may be responsible for this syndrome. However, the predominance of the influence of the left hemisphere was not consistently found (Milandre *et al.*, 1994).

Anterior cerebral artery territory infarcts

Lesion of the medial frontal lobe in anterior cerebral artery territory infarction may cause ACS (Bogousslavsky and Regli, 1990; Amyes and Nielsen, 1955; Kumral *et al.*, 2002). Lesions are usually bilateral or right unilateral. ACS may, however, occur in left unilateral anterior cerebral artery stroke. ACS is supposed to result from a lesion affecting the prefrontal cortex and anterior cingulate gyrus.

Stroke lesions located in the head of the caudate nucleus

The most prominent clinical features of caudate vascular lesions are behavioral and cognitive abnormalities (Damasio *et al.*, 1982; Richfield *et al.*, 1987; Mendez *et al.*, 1989; Caplan *et al.*, 1990; Stein *et al.*, 1984; Pedrazzi *et al.*, 1990; Kumral *et al.*, 1999). ACS may be present in lesions involving the caudate nucleus (Mendez *et al.*, 1989; Caplan *et al.*, 1990; Kumral *et al.*, 1999), in right as in left lesions, probably more frequently in bilateral lesions (Kumral *et al.*, 1999) and in lesions involving the head of the caudate nucleus (Kumral *et al.*, 1999). The caudate nucleus connects associative cortex, including frontal, parietal, and temporal lobes, with deeper anatomic structures by cortico-pallido-nigra-thalamo-cortical loops (Alexander *et al.*, 1985; 1986). Frontal lobe dysfunction due to dynamic interruption of the complex striato-pallido-thalamo-frontal circuit is likely to be involved in the development of delirium. However, the role of associated multiple lesions has also been questioned (Godefroy *et al.*, 1994).

Stroke lesions located in the inferior part of the genu of the internal capsule

A few case reports suggest that ACS can result from an infarction of the inferior genu of the internal capsule (Tatemichi *et al.*, 1992). The acute syndrome featured fluctuating alertness, inattention, memory loss, apathy, abulia, and psychomotor retardation, suggesting frontal lobe dysfunction. This could result from a functional deactivation of the ipsilateral frontal cortex secondary to an interruption of the inferior and anterior thalamic peduncles by the capsular genu infarct.

Right middle cerebral artery territory infarcts

Right middle cerebral artery territory infarction is the most common stroke responsible for ACS (Mesulam *et al.*, 1976; Mullally *et al.*, 1982; Schmidley and Messing, 1984; Mori and Yamadori, 1987; Caplan *et al.*, 1986). In a prospective study, ACS was observed in up to 61% of patients with an acute middle cerebral artery territory infarct (Mori and Yamadori, 1987), sometimes leading to chronic confusional state (Mullaly *et al.*, 1989). Disturbance of global attentional tone could be the consequence of frontostriatal lesions (Mesulam *et al.*, 1976; Mori and Yamadori, 1987), while agitated delirium would be related to damage to the right temporal lobe (Caplan *et al.*, 1986; Mori and Yamadori, 1987), in particular in the middle temporal gyrus. The sensory–limbic interaction would be disrupted following damage to the right temporal lobe, where massive neural inputs from limbic regions as well as wide cortical regions merge (Caplan *et al.*, 1986; Mori and Yamadori, 1987).

Subarachnoid hemorrhage

ACS can be a presenting syndrome of subarachnoid hemorrhage (Fisher, 1975; Mobbs *et al.*, 2001). In a retrospective study, Reijneveld *et al.* (2000) found that ACS was rare at the acute stage of subarachnoid hemorrhage, observed in 1.4% of patients, and that no preferential site of hemorrhage was associated with confusion, suggesting that ACS could be related to the global cerebral dysfunction that initially occurs during aneurismal rupture. The only prospective study of ACS in patients with subarachnoid hemorrhage found ACS in 16%

of patients, ACS being more frequent in patients with intraventricular bleeding, hydrocephalus and basofrontal hemorrhage (Caeiro *et al.*, 2004c). The cingulum, frontal projections from the thalamus, the septal area and the Meynert nucleus are likely to be damaged by hematomas in such a location, probably disrupting cholinergic projections to the cerebral cortex and the hippocampus. Structures close to the lateral and the third ventricles such as anterior and medial thalamic nuclei, fornix, mammillary bodies, caudate and hippocampal formation are important in attention, working and declarative memory, and in executive functions. Their dysfunction due to intraventricular bleeding or hydrocephalus may play a role in the development of ACS (Caiero *et al.*, 2004c).

Risk factors for delirium in stroke patients

Thirteen to 48% of stroke patients experience delirium at the acute stage of stroke (Caeiro *et al.*, 2004b; Hénon *et al.*, 1999; Gustafson *et al.*, 1991). ACS can be the direct consequence of stroke and is rarely the sole manifestation of stroke. ACS can be secondary to stroke complications (such as metabolic disturbances, hypoxia, seizures, and infection) and can also be the consequence of an associated dementia. When ACS occurs in a patient with a vascular lesion involving an area not classically responsible for delirium, other causes of ACS must be looked for. ACS seems to be more frequent in patients with cerebral hemorrhage (Gustafson *et al.*, 1991; Caiero *et al.*, 2004b) compared to patients with ischemic stroke. The main risk factors for ACS in stroke patients reported in the literature are: aging (Caeiro *et al.*, 2004b; Gustafson *et al.*, 1991), pre-existing cognitive disturbances (Hénon *et al.*, 1999), the presence of medical complications such as infections and electrolyte imbalance (Caeiro *et al.*, 2004b; Hénon *et al.*, 1999), the presence of neglect (Caeiro *et al.*, 2004b), and severity of stroke (Gustafson *et al.*, 1991). The influence of stroke location is not clear as ACS has been described to occur more frequently in left-sided hemispheric lesions (Gustafson *et al.*, 1991) than in right-sided hemispheric lesions (Hénon *et al.*, 1999).

When ACS occurs in a stroke patient, a comprehensive search for precipitating factors must be performed (Ferro *et al.*, 2002), including search for: metabolic disorders (hypo- or hyperglycemia, hypoxemia, electrolyte imbalance, renal or hepatic failure, thyroid disorders), infections, fever, cardiopulmonary disorders (pulmonary embolus, cardiac or respiratory failure, myocardial infarction), epilepsy, ethanol, sedatives or illicit drugs, intoxication at stroke onset, or withdrawal during the next days, iatrogenic complication (use of psychotropic, dopaminergic, or anticholinergic drugs, cimetidine, digoxin, steroids), pain (headache, abdominal pain from fecal impaction or aerocolia, vesical distension, bed sores), subdural hematoma or cerebral contusion (especially in the case of a fall secondary to stroke onset) and pre-existing dementia.

Assessment

Delirium is under-identified in clinical practice: non-detection rates of 33–66% are typically reported (Inouye, 1994). Detection can be improved by the use of screening instruments. A number of delirium-evaluating instruments have been developed (Robertsson, 1999), mostly on the basis of the DSM criteria. The Confusion Assessment Method (CAM) is widely used because it is reliable, brief and applicable to a variety of settings (Inouye *et al.*, 1990) based on DSM-III-R criteria. The diagnostic algorithm of the CAM depends on the presence of four criteria: acute onset and fluctuating course, inattention, disorganized thinking, or altered level of consciousness (Monette *et al.*, 2001) (Table 24.3). It has two versions, with nine and four items, respectively. The Organic Brain Syndrome Scale (Jensen *et al.*, 1993) has 39 items and has been developed for use by a research assistant. The Delirium Symptom Interview (DSI) has 62 items to be used by laymen (Albert *et al.*, 1992).These scales are diagnostic instruments determining the presence or absence of symptoms. Other scales generate scores which allow quantifying the severity of the delirium. The Delirium Rating Scale (DRS) (Trzepacz *et al.*, 1988; 2001; Trzepacz, 1999a) (Table 24.3) is the most widely used scale for evaluation of the severity of the ACS; it is also useful for positive diagnosis and for differential diagnosis with dementia or depression (Trzepacz *et al.*, 2001). Delirium should, however, be rated over a 24-hour period to detect fluctuations and sleep–wake cycle abnormalities (Trzepacz *et al.*, 1999a). The DRS quantifies multiple parameters affected by delirium such as temporal onset of symptoms, perceptual disturbances, hallucinations, delusions, psychomotor behavioral disturbances, cognitive status deficits, sleep–wake cycle disturbances, lability of mood, and variability of symptoms. This scale fulfils four essential criteria for usefulness in diagnosis of delirium (Inouye *et al.*, 1994): specific validation for use in delirium; capability to distinguish delirium from dementia and depression; assessment of multiple features of delirium, and feasibility in delirious patients (Trzepacz *et al.*, 1988). Other instruments have been developed specifically for measuring the severity of the delirium syndrome. The Memorial Delirium Assessment Scale (MDAS) (Breitbart *et al.*, 1997), designed for use by experienced psychiatrists, contains 10 items concerning level of consciousness, orientation, short-term memory, digit span, attention, thinking,

Table 24.3. Delirium scales

The Confusional Assessment Method (CAM)

(1) Acute onset and fluctuating course

+

(2) Inattention

+

(3) Disorganized thinking or (4) altered level of consciousness

↓ the presence of both the first and second and of either the third or the fourth are required
   for the diagnosis of delirium

Delirium

↓ when the diagnosis is established, the assessment of other delirium symptoms is possible

Assessment of other delirium symptoms

Disorientation

Memory impairment

Perceptual disturbances

Psychomotor agitation

Psychomotor retardation

Altered sleep−wake cycle

The Delirium Rating Scale

1. Temporal onset of symptoms	quoted 0, 1, or 2
2. Perceptual disturbances	quoted 0, 1, or 2
3. hallucination type	quoted 0, 1, or 2
4. delusions	quoted 0, 1, or 2
5. Psychomotor behavior	quoted 0, 1, or 2
6. Cognitive status during formal testing	quoted 0, 1, 2, 3, or 4
7. Physical disorder	quoted 0, 1, or 2
8. Sleep−wake cycle disturbances	quoted 0, 1, 2, 3, or 4
9. Lability of mood	quoted 0, 1, or 2
10. Variability of symptoms	quoted 0, 1, 2, 3, or 4

---

perceptual disturbance, delusions, psychomotor activity, and sleep−wake cycle.
The Delirium Assessment Scale (DAS) (O'Keefe, 1994), designed for use by
physicians, is derived from the DSM-III-R criteria except for items on the onset
of symptoms and the presumed etiology of the disorder. It contains 11 items
covering orientation, memory, attention, perceptual disturbances, psychomotor
activity/alertness, coherence, global accessibility, reported psychomotor activity,
fluctuation of symptoms, and sleep−wake cycle. The items measuring impairment
of orientation, memory, and attention include sub-items from MMSE and digit
span. The other items deal with behavior observed during the interview and

behavior reported by the patient and the staff. The Confusional State Evaluation (CSE) (Robertsson et al., 1997) has been elaborated to assess delirium particularly in elderly patients and to measure changes of symptoms over time to evaluate effects of intervention: it contains 22 items, 12 of which measure key symptoms leading to a confusion score, 7 items deal with symptoms frequently observed in patients with ACS, and 3 items relate to the duration and intensity of the episode of delirium. This scale has been designed to be used by trained nurses, doctors, and psychologists. The Delirium Index has also been elaborated to assess the severity of delirium: it appears to be a reliable, valid and responsive measure of the severity of delirium, in patients with delirium, with or without dementia (McCusker et al., 1998; 2004).

The selection of a specific scale depends on the purpose, on time constraints, and on the examiner. Rating scales designed to be used by experts usually contain few items, while scales designed to be used by non-trained people are usually more detailed with many items. The CAM-A scale, despite its simplicity, has a high sensitivity and specificity. The DRS is perhaps the most widespread scale and is in use in many countries (Robertsson et al., 1999; Ferro et al., 2002).

Outcome in stroke patients with delirium

Only few data are available concerning the influence of ACS on the outcome of stroke. They all suggest that stroke patients with ACS have a worse outcome compared to patients without. Delirious stroke patients have a higher risk of in-hospital and 6-month death, a longer duration of hospital stay, and a higher risk of post-stroke dementia (Gustafson et al., 1991; Hénon et al., 1999).

Management and treatment

Despite the frequency of ACS in stroke, no therapeutic trial has been conducted in this pathology to our knowledge. Moreover, only few data are available for the treatment of ACS: they are mainly issued from studies which included post-surgical patients.

Cole (1999) made a review to evaluate the effectiveness of systematic interventions in preventing or detecting and treating delirium. The literature search identified ten studies on prevention and seven studies on detection and treatment. A broad spectrum of systematic interventions appeared to be modestly effective in preventing delirium in young and old surgical patients but not elderly medical patients. Systematic detection and treatment programs and special nursing care appeared to add large benefits to traditional medical care in young and old surgical patients and modest benefits in elderly medical patients; however, it seemed that the more precise the target of the detection and treatment program, the greater the benefit.

Treatment should be aimed at alleviating the specific symptoms of delirium and efforts should be made to identify and treat the underlying causes. Some supportive and environmental measures are recommended: simple but firm communication, reality orientation, a visible clock, and the presence of a relative contribute to a heightened sense of control during delirium (Schofield, 1997). Providing support and orientation, and an unambiguous environment, are useful. Preliminary evidence suggests that nurses trained in managing confused patients improve outcome by limiting risk factors, enhancing diagnosis of delirium, and encouraging standardized treatment (Simon *et al.*, 1997). An effective prevention of delirium was achieved through the application of practical interventions targeted towards six risk factors: cognitive impairment, immobility, sleep deprivation, vision impairment, hearing impairment, and dehydration (Inouye *et al.*, 1999).

Drug treatment of ACS requires careful consideration of the benefit/risk balance as sedative drugs may improve behavioral disturbances but worsen cognitive impairment (Meagher, 2001). Neuroleptics are effective on a wide range of symptoms of ACS (American Psychiatric Association, 1999; Breitbart *et al.*, 1996; Platt *et al.*, 1994), with a rapid onset of action (Nakamura *et al.*, 1997) which allows improvement of the patient's condition before the treatment of the underlying cause is effective. Neuroleptics seem more effective than benzodiazepines to treat ACS caused by factors other than alcohol withdrawal (American Psychiatric Association, 1999). Haloperidol is usually preferred because it has limited anticholinergic effects, and less severe sedative and hypotensive effects (American Psychiatric Association 1999, Hassan *et al.*, 1998). The use of low-dose oral haloperidol (1–10 mg/day) improves symptoms in most patients (Breitbart *et al.*, 1996; Platt *et al.*, 1994; Nakamura *et al.*, 1997).

Key points Management and treatment of acute confusional state

---

Detection of the cause (complications, comorbidities) and treatment

Supportive and environmental measures may be useful: simple but firm communication, reality orientation, a visible clock, and the presence of a relative

Systematic detection and treatment programs, trained nurses: may be useful

Pharmacotherapy:

in selected patients

careful considerations on the benefit/risk balance

benzodiazepines or low-dose oral of haloperidol or atypical antipsychotic drugs

in the future: cholinesterase inhibitors?

Olanzapine (5–10 mg) and risperidone (1.5–4 mg) have been used successfully in uncontrolled case series (Sipahimalani and Masand, 1997; 1998): these atypical compounds cause less extrapyramidal effects and sedation, and they could also have other interests in old patients with cognitive disturbances (Beuzen et al., 1999). Recent concerns have been expressed regarding a higher risk of stroke in patients using atypical antipsychotics (Brodaty et al., 2003; Wooltorton, 2004), not confirmed in a recent case–control study (Gill et al., 2005). Benzodiazepines can in some cases be useful, in particular in patients who do not tolerate antipsychotic drugs. Lorazepam seems to be of special interest because of its sedative properties, rapid onset of action, and short duration with a low risk of accumulation. Cholinesterase inhibitors may also in the future be used in the treatment of delirium in stroke patients. In cases of dementia with cholinergic deficiency (Alzheimer's, Lewy body dementia, mixed dementia), cholinesterase inhibitors have demonstrated their efficacy on the hallucinations (Kaufer et al., 1998; Wengel et al., 1998; 1999). Burke et al. (1999) also reported on the use of cholinesterase inhibitors for delirium in a patient without dementia. Kobayashi et al. (2004) recently reported a case of severe intractable delirium caused by a basal forebrain vascular lesion and its dramatic recovery after donepezil administration. Further studies are necessary to evaluate the efficacy and safety of cholinesterase inhibitors in stroke patients with ACS.

REFERENCES

Adams, R. D., Viktor, M. and Ropper, A. H. (1997). *Principles of Neurology*, 6th edn. New York: McGraw-Hill, pp. 405–16.

Albert, M. S., Levkoff, S. E., Reilly, C., et al. (1992). The delirium symptom interview: An interview for the detection of delirium symptoms in hospitalized patients. *J. Geriatr. Psychiatry Neurol.*, 5, 14–21.

Alexander, G. E. and DeLong, M. R. (1985). Microstimulation of the primate neo-striatum, I: Physiological properties of striatal microexcitable zones. *J. Neurophysiol.*, 53, 1417–32.

Alexander, G. E., DeLong, M. R. and Strick, P. L. (1986). Parallel organization of functionally segregated circuits linking basal ganglia and cortex. *Ann. Rev. Neurosci.*, 9, 357–81.

American Psychiatric Association (1999). Practice guidelines for the treatment of delirium. *Am. J. Psychiatry.*, 156, 1–20.

(2000). *Diagnostic and Statistical Manual of Mental Disorders*. 4th edn. Text Revision. DSM-IV-Washington, D.C., American Psychiatric Association, 143. Copyright 2000, American Psychiatric Association.

Amyes, E. W. and Nielsen, J. M. (1955). Clinicopathological study of vascular lesions of the anterior cingulated region. *Bull. Los Angeles Neurol. Soc.*, 20, 112–30.

Beuzen, J.N., Taylor, N., Wesnes, K. and Wood, A. (1999). A comparison of the effects of olanzapine, haloperidol and placebo on cognitive and psychomotor functions in healthy elderly volunteers. *J. Psychopharmacol.*, **13**, 152–8.

Bogousslavsky, J. and Regli, F. (1990). Anterior cerebral artery territory infarction in the Lausanne Stroke Registry: Clinical and etiologic patterns. *Arch. Neurol.*, **47**, 144–50.

Breitbart, W., Marotta, R., Platt, M.M., *et al.* (1996). A double-blind trial of haloperidol, chlorpromazine, and lorazepam in the treatment of delirium in hospitalized AIDS patients. *Am. J. Psychiatry*, **153**, 231–7.

Breitbart, W., Rosenfeld, B., Roth, A., *et al.* (1997). The Memorial Delirium Assessment Scale. *Pain Symptom Manage.*, **13**, 128–37.

Brodaty, H., Ames, D., Snowden, J., *et al.* (2003). A randomized placebo controlled trial of risperidone for the treatment of aggression, agitation, and psychosis in dementia. *J. Clin. Psychiatry*, **64**, 134–43.

Burke, W.J., Roccaforte, W.H. and Wengel, S.P. (1999). Treating visual hallucinations with donepezil. *Am. J. Psychiatry*, **156**, 1117–18.

Caeiro, L., Ferro, J.M., Claro, M.I., *et al.* (2004a). Delirium in acute stroke: A preliminary study of the role of anticholinergic medications. *Eur. J. Neurol.*, **11**, 699–704.

Caeiro, L., Ferro, J.M., Albuquerque, R. and Figueira, M.L. (2004b). Delirium in the first days of acute stroke. *J. Neurol.*, **251**, 171–8.

Caeiro, L., Menger, C., Ferro, J.M., Albuquerque, R. and Figueira, M.L. (2004c). Delirium in Acute Subarachnoid Haemorrhage. *Cerebrovasc. Dis.*, **3**; (19), 31–8.

Camus, V., Gonthier, R., Dubos, G., Schwed, P. and Simeone, I. (2000). Etiologic and outcome profiles in hypoactive and hyperactive subtypes of delirium. *J. Geriatr. Psychiatry Neurol.*, **13**, 38–42.

Caplan, L.R. (1980). Top of the basilar syndrome: Selected clinical aspects. *Neurology*, **30**, 72–9.

Caplan, L.R. (1996). *Posterior Circulation Disease: Clinical findings, Diagnosis and Management*, Boston: Butterworth-Heinemann.

Caplan, L.R. (2000). Acute confusional states and delirium. In *Behavior and Mood Disorders in Focal Brain Lesions*, ed. J. Bogousslavsky and J. L. Cummings. Cambridge: Cambridge University Press.

Caplan, L.R., Kelly, M., Kase, C.S., *et al.* (1986). Infarcts of the inferior division of the right middle cerebral artery: Mirror image of Wernicke's aphasia. *Neurology*, **36**, 1015–20.

Caplan, L.R., Schmahmann, J.D., Kase, C.S., *et al.* (1990). Caudate infarcts. *Arch. Neurol.*, **47**, 133–43.

Castaigne, P., Lhermitte, F., Buge, A., *et al.* (1981). Paramedian thalamic and midbrain infarct: Clinical and neuropathological study. *Ann. Neurol.*, **10**, 127–48.

Curyto, K.J., Johnson, J., TenHave, T., *et al.* (2001). Survival of hospitalized elderly patients with delirium: A prospective study. *Am. J. Geriatr. Psychiatry*, **9**, 141–7.

Cole, M.G. (1999). Delirium: Effectiveness of systematic interventions. *Dement. Geriatr. Cogn. Disord.*, **10**, 406–11.

Damasio, A.R., Damasio, H., Rizzo, M., Varney, N. and Gersh, F. (1982). Aphasia with nonhemorrhagic lesions in the basal ganglia and internal capsule. *Arch. Neurol.*, **39**, 2–14.

Devinsky, O., Bear, D. and Volpe, B. T. (1988). Confusional states following posterior cerebral artery infarction. *Arch. Neurol.*, **45**, 160−3.

Erkinjuntti, T., Wikstrom, J., Palo, J. and Autio, L. (1986). Dementia among medical inpatients. Evaluation of 2000 consecutive admissions. *Arch. Intern. Med.*, **146**, 1923−6.

Fassbender, K., Schmidt, R., Mossner, R., Daffertshofer, M. and Hennerici, M. (1994). Pattern of activation of the hypothalamic−pituitary−adrenal axis in acute stroke. Relation to acute confusional state, extent of brain damage, and clinical outcome. *Stroke*, **25**, 1105−8.

Ferro, M. (2001). Hyperacute cognitive stroke syndromes. *J. Neurol.*, **248**, 841−9.

Ferro, J. M., Caeiro, L. and Verdelho, A. (2002). Delirium in acute stroke. *Curr. Opin. Neurol.*, **15**, 51−5.

Fisher, C. M. (1975). Clinical syndromes in cerebral thrombosis, hypertensive haemorrhage and ruptures saccular aneurysm. *Clin. Neurosurg.*, **22**, 117−47.

(1983). Honored guest presentation: Abulia minor vs agitated behavior. *Clinical Neurosurgery*, Baltimore: Williams & Wilkins, pp. 9−31.

Fisher, P. (2001). Successful treatment of nonanticholinergic delirium with a cholinesterase inhibitor. *J. Clin. Pharmacol.*, **21**, 118.

Flacker, J. M., Lipsitz, L. A. (1999). Neural mechanisms of delirium: Current hypotheses and evolving concepts. *J. Gerontol. A. Biol. Sci. Med. Sci.*, **5**, B239−46.

Flacker, J. M. and Wei, J. Y. (2001). Endogenous anticholinergic substances may exist during acute illness in elderly medical patients. *J. Gerontol. A. Biol. Sci. Med. Sci.*, **56**, M353−5.

Francis, J. (1996). Drug-induced delirium: Diagnosis and treatment. *CNS Drugs*, **5**, 102−14.

Francis, J., Martin, D. and Kapoor, W. N. (1990). A prospective study of delirium in hospitalized elderly. *JAMA*, **263**, 1097−101.

Garcia-Albea, E. (1989). Confusional state and cerebral infarcts. *Postgrad. Med. J.*, **65**, 286−90.

Gaudreau, J. D. and Gagnon, P. (2005). Psychotogenic drugs and delirium pathogenesis: The central role of the thalamus. *Med. Hypotheses*, **64**, 471−5.

George, J., Bleasdale, S. and Singleton, S. J. (1997). Causes and prognosis of delirium in elderly patients admitted to a district general hospital. *Age Ageing*, **26**, 423−7.

Ghika-Schmid, F. and Bogousslavsky, J. (2000). The acute behavioral syndrome of anterior thalamic infarction: A prospective study of 12 cases. *Ann. Neurol.*, **48**, 220−7.

Gill, S. S., Rochon, P. A., Herrmann, N., *et al.* (2005). Atypical antipsychotic drugs and risk of ischaemic stroke: Population based retrospective cohort study. *BMJ*, **330**, 445.

Godefroy, O., Rousseaux, M., Pruvo, J. P., Cabaret, M. and Leys, D. (1994). Neuropsychological changes related to unilateral laterostriatal infarcts. *J. Neurol. Neurosurg. Psychiatry*, **57**, 480−5.

Graff-Radford, N. R., Eslinger, P. J., Damasio, A. R. and Yamada, T. (1984). Nonhemorrhagic infarction of the thalamus: Behavioral, anatomic, and physiologic correlates. *Neurology*, **34**, 14−23.

Gustafson, Y., Olsson, T., Asplund, K. and Hägg, E. (1993). Acute confusional state (delirium) soon after stroke is associated with hypercortisolism. *Cerebrovasc. Dis.*, **3**, 33−8.

Gustafson, Y., Olsson, T., Eriksson, S., Asplund, K. and Bucht, G. (1991). Acute confusional states (Delirium) in stroke patients. *Cerebrovasc. Dis.*, **1**, 257−64.

Han, L., McCusker, J., Cole, M., *et al.* (2001). Use of medications with anticholinergic effect predicts clinical severity of delirium symptoms in older medical inpatients. *Arch. Intern. Med.*, **161**, 1099−105.

Hassan, E., Fontaine, D. K. and Nearman, H. S. (1998). Therapeutic considerations in the management of agitated or delirious critically ill patients. *Pharmacotherapy*, **18**, 113−29.

Hénon, H., Lebert, F., Durieu, I., *et al.* (1999). Confusional state in stroke: Relation to preexisting dementia, patient characteristics, and outcome. *Stroke*, **30**, 773−9.

Inouye, S. K. (1994). The dilemma of delirium: Clinical and research controversies regarding diagnosis and evaluation of delirium in hospitalized elderly medical patients. *Am. J. Med.*, **97**, 278−88.

Inouye, S. K., Bogardus S. T., Jr, Charpentier, P. A., *et al.* (1999). A multicomponent intervention to prevent delirium in hospitalized older patients. *N. Engl. J. Med.*, **340**, 669−76.

Inouye, S. K., van Dyck, C. H., Alessi, C. A., *et al.* (1990). Clarifying confusion: The confusion assessment method. A new method for detection of delirium. *Ann. Intern. Med.*, **113**, 941−8.

Jensen, E., Dehlin, O. and Gustafson, L. (1993). A comparison between three psychogeriatric rating scales. *Int. J. Geriatr. Psychiatry*, **8**, 215−29.

Jitapunkul, S., Pillay, I. and Ebrahim, S. (1992). Delirium in newly admitted elderly patients: A prospective study. *Q. J. Med.*, **83**, 307−14.

Karlsson, I. (1999). Drugs that induce delirium. *Dement. Geriatr. Cogn. Disord.*, **10**, 412−15.

Kaufer, D. I., Catt, K. E., Lopez, O. L. and DeKosky S. T. (1998). Dementia with Lewy bodies: Response of delirium-like features to donepezil. *Neurology*, **51**, 1512.

Kobayashi, K., Higashima, M., Mutou, K., *et al.* (2004). Severe delirium due to basal forebrain vascular lesion and efficacy of donepezil. *Prog. Neuropsychopharmacol. Biol. Psychiatry*, **28**, 1189−94.

Koponen, H. J. and Riekkinen, P. J. (1993). A prospective study of delirium in elderly patients admitted to a psychiatric hospital. *Psychol. Med.*, **23**, 103−9.

Koponen, H. J., Stenbäck, U., Mattila, E., *et al.* (1989). Delirium among elderly persons admitted to a psychiatric hospital: Clinical course during the acute stage and one-year follow-up. *Acta Psychiatr. Scand.*, **79**, 579−85.

Kumral, E., Bayulkem, G., Evyapan, D. and Yunten, N. (2002). Spectrum of anterior cerebral artery territory infarction: Clinical and MRI findings. *Eur. J. Neurol.*, **9**, 615−24.

Kumral, E., Evyapan, D. and Balkir, K. (1999). Acute caudate vascular lesions. *Stroke*, **30**, 100−8.

Kumral, E., Kocaer, T., Ertubey, N. O. and Kumral, K. (1995). Thalamic hemorrhage. A prospective study of 100 patients. *Stroke*, **26**, 964−70.

Levkoff, S., Cleary, P., Litzin, B. and Evans, D. (1991). Epidemiology of delirium: An overview of research issues and findings. *Int. Psychogeriatr.*, **3**, 149−67.

Lipowski, Z. J. (1989). Delirium in the elderly patient. *N. Engl. J. Med.*, **320**, 578−82.

(1990). Delirium in geriatric patients. In *Delirium: Acute Confusional States*. New York: Oxford University Press, pp. 413−41.

Lundstrom, M., Edlund, A., Bucht, G., Karlsson, S. and Gustafson, Y. (2003). Dementia after delirium in patients with femoral neck fractures. *J. Am. Geriatr. Soc.*, **51**, 1002–6.

Mach, J. R., Jr, Dysken, M. W., Kuskowski, M., *et al.* (1995). Serum anticholinergic activity in hospitalized older persons with delirium: A preliminary study. *J. Am. Geriatr. Soc.*, **43**, 491–5.

Madureira, S., Guerreiro, M. and Ferro, J. M. (1999). A follow-up study of cognitive impairment due to inferior capsular genu infarction. *J. Neurol.*, **246**, 764–9.

McCusker, J., Cole, M., Bellavance, F. and Primeau, F. (1998). Reliability and validity of a new measure of severity of delirium. *Int. Psychogeriatr.*, **10**, 421–33.

McCusker, J., Cole, M. G., Dendukuri, N. and Belzile, E. (2004). The delirium index, a measure of the severity of delirium: New findings on reliability, validity, and responsiveness. *J. Am. Geriatr. Soc.*, **52**, 1744–9.

McCusker, J., Cole, M., Dendukuri, N., Belzile, E. and Primeau, F. (2001). Delirium in older medical inpatients and subsequent cognitive and functional status: A prospective study. *CMAJ*, **165**, 575–83.

McDonald, A. J. and Treloar, A. (1996). Delirium and dementia: Are they distinct? *J. Am. Geriatr. Soc.*, **44**, 1001–2.

Meagher, D. J. (2001). Delirium: Optimising management. *BMJ*, **322**, 144–9.

Medina, J. L., Rubino, F. A. and Ross, E. (1974). Agitated delirium caused by infarctions of the hippocampal formation and fusiform and lingual gyri: A case report. *Neurology*, **24**, 1181–3.

Mendez, M. F., Adams, N. L. and Lewandowsky, K. (1989). Neurobehavioral changes associated with caudate lesions. *Neurology*, **39**, 349–54.

Mesulam, M. M., Waxman, S. G., Geschwind, N. and Sabin, T. D. (1976). Acute confusional states with right middle cerebral artery infarctions. *J. Neurol. Neurosurg. Psychiatry*, **39**, 84–9.

Milandre, L., Brosset, C., Botti, G. and Khalil, R. (1994). A study of 82 cerebral infarctions in the area of posterior cerebral arteries. *Rev. Neurol. (Paris)*, **150**, 133–41.

Mobbs, R. J., Chandran, K. N. and Newcombe, R. L. (2001). Psychiatric presentation of aneurysmal subarachnoid haemorrhage. *ANZ. J. Surg.*, **71**, 69–70.

Monette, J., Galbaud du Fort, G., Fung, S. H., *et al.* (2001). Evaluation of the Confusion Assessment Method (CAM) as a screening tool for delirium in the emergency room. *Gen. Hosp. Psychiatry*, **23**, 20–5.

Mori, E., Matsunaga, K., Yokoyama, K. and Yamadori, A. (1981). The effect of bilateral thalamic infarction to human behaviour. *Clin. Neurol.*, **21**, 110–16.

Mori, E. and Yamadori, A. (1987). Acute confusional state and acute agitated delirium. Occurrence after infarction in the right middle cerebral artery territory. *Arch. Neurol.*, **44**, 1139–43.

Muir, K. W., Holzapfel, L. and Lees, K. R. (2000). Phase II clinical trial of sipatrigine (619C89) by continuous infusion in acute stroke. *Cerebrovasc. Dis.*, **10**, 431–6.

Mullaly, W., Huff, K., Ronthal, M. and Geschwind, N. (1982). Frequency of acute confusional states with lesions of the right hemisphere. *Ann. Neurol.*, **12**, 113.

Mullaly, W., Ronthal, M., Huff, K. and Geschwind, N. (1989). Chronic confusional state. *N. J. Med.*, **86**, 541–4.

Mussi, C., Ferrari, R., Ascari, S. and Salvioli, G. (1999). Importance of serum anticholinergic activity in the assessment of elderly patients with delirium. *J. Geriatr. Psychiatry Neurol.*, **12**, 82–6.

Nakamura, J., Uchimura, N., Yamada, S. and Nakazawa, Y. (1997). Does plasma free-3-methoxy-4-hydroxyphenyl (ethylene) glycol increase in the delirious state? A comparison of the effects of mianserin and haloperidol on delirium. *Int. Clin. Psychopharmacol.*, **12**, 147–52.

Naughton, B. J., Moran, M., Ghaly, Y. and Michalakes, C. (1997). Computed tomography scanning and delirium in elder patients. *Acad. Emerg. Med.*, **4**, 1107–10.

Nicolai, A. and Lazzarino, L. G. (1994). Acute confusional states secondary to infarctions in the territory of the posterior cerebral artery in elderly patients. *Ital. J. Neurol. Sci.*, **15**, 91–6.

O'Keeffe, S. T. (1994). Rating the severity of delirium: The delirium Assessment Scale. *Int. J. Geriatr. Psychiatry*, **9**, 551–6.

O'Keeffe, S. T. (1999). Clinical subtypes of delirium in the elderly. *Dement. Geriatr. Cogn. Disord.*, **5**, 380–5.

O'Keeffe, S. and Lavan, J. (1997). The prognostic significance of delirium in older hospital patients. *J. Am. Geriatr. Soc.*, **45**, 174–8.

Olsson, T. (1999). Activity in the hypothalamic–pituitary–adrenal axis and delirium. *Dement. Geriatr. Cogn. Disord.*, **10**, 345–9.

Pedrazzi, P., Bogousslavsky, J. and Regli, F. (1990). Hématomes limités á la tête du noyau caudé. *Rev. Neurol. (Paris)*, **146**, 726–38.

Platt, M. M., Breitbart, W., Smith, M., *et al.* (1994). Efficacy of neuroleptics for hypoactive delirium. *J. Neuropsychiatry Clin. Neurosci.*, **6**, 66–7.

Pompei, P., Foreman, M., Rudberg, M. A., *et al.* (1994). Delirium in hospitalized older persons: Outcomes and predictors. *J. Am. Geriatr. Soc.*, **42**, 809–15.

Rahkonen, T., Eloniemi-Sulkava, U., Halonen, P., *et al.* (2001). Delirium in the non-demented oldest old in the general population: Risk factors and prognosis. *J. Geriatr. Psychiatry*, **16**, 415–21.

Rahkonen, T., Luukkainen-Markkula, R., Paanila, S., Sivenius, J. and Sulkava, R. (2000). Delirium episode as a sign of undetected dementia among community dwelling elderly subjects: A 2 year follow up study. *J. Neurol. Neurosurg. Psychiatry*, **69**, 519–21.

Reijneveld, J. C., Wermer, M., Boonman, Z., van Gijn, J. and Rinkel, G. J. (2000). Acute confusional state as presenting feature in aneurysmal subarachnoid hemorrhage: Frequency and characteristics. *J. Neurol.*, **247**, 112–16.

Reyes-Ortiz, C. A. (1997). Delirium, dementia and brain reserve. *J. Am. Geriatr. Soc.*, **45**, 778–9.

Richfield, E. K., Twyman, R. and Berent, S. (1987). Neurological syndrome following bilateral damage to the head of the caudate nuclei. *Ann. Neurol.*, **22**, 768–71.

Robertsson, B. (1999). Assessment scales in delirium. *Dement. Geriatr. Cogn. Disord.*, **10**, 368–79.

Robertsson, B., Karlsson, I., Styrud, E. and Gottfries, C. G. (1997). Confusional State Evaluation (CSE): An instrument for measuring severity of delirium in the elderly. *Br. J. Psychiatry*, **170**, 565–70.

Rockwood, K., Cosway, S., Carver, D., *et al.* (1999). The risk of dementia and death after delirium. *Age Ageing*, **28**, 551–6.

Sandberg, O., Franklin, K. A., Bucht, G. and Gustafson, Y. (2001). Sleep apnea, delirium, depressed mood, cognition, and ADL ability after stroke. *J. Am. Geriatr. Soc.*, **49**, 391–7.

Schmidley, J. W. and Messing, R. O. (1984). Agitated confusional states in patients with right hemisphere infarctions. *Stroke*, **15**, 883–5.

Schofield, I. (1997). A small exploratory study of the reaction of older people to an episode of delirium. *J. Adv. Nurs.*, **25**, 942–52.

Schor, J. D., Levkoff, S. E., Lipstitz, L. A., *et al.* (1992). Risk factors for delirium in hospitalised elderly. *JAMA*, **267**, 827–31.

Simon, L., Jewell, N. and Brokel, J. (1997). Management of acute delirium in hospitalized elderly: A process improvement project. *Geriatr. Nurs.*, **18**, 150–4.

Sipahimalani, A. and Masand, P. S. (1997). Use of risperidone in delirium: Case reports. *Ann. Clin. Psychiatry.*, **9**, 105–7.

(1998). Olanzapine in the treatment of delirium. *Psychosomatics*, **39**, 422–30.

Stein, R. W., Kase, C. S., Hier, D. B., *et al.* (1984). Caudate hemorrhage. *Neurology*, **34**, 1549–54.

Sumner, A. D. and Simons, R. J. (1994). Delirium in the hospitalized elderly. *Cleve. Clin. J. Med.*, **61**, 258–62.

Symonds, C. and MacKenzie, I. (1957). Bilateral loss of vision from cerebral infarction. *Brain*, **80**, 415–55.

Tatemichi, T. K., Desmond, D. W., Prohovnik, I., *et al.* (1992). Confusion and memory loss from capsular genu infarction: A thalamocortical disconnection syndrome? *Neurology*, **42**, 1966–79.

Trzepacz, P. T. (1999a). The Delirium Rating Scale. Its use in consultation-liaison research. *Psychosomatics*, **40**, 193–204.

Trzepacz, P. T. (1999b). Update on the neuropathogenesis of delirium. *Dement. Geriatr. Cogn. Disord.*, **10**, 330–4.

Trzepacz, P. T., Baker, R. W. and Greenhouse, J. (1988). A symptom rating scale for delirium. *Psychiatry Res.*, **23**, 89–97.

Trzepacz, P. T., Mittal, D., Torres, R., *et al.* (2001). Validation of the Delirium Rating Scale-revised-98, comparison with the delirium rating scale and the cognitive test for delirium. *J. Neuropsychiatry Clin. Neurosci.*, **13**, 229–42.

Tune, L., Carr, S., Hoag, E. and Cooper, T. (1992). Anticholinergic effects of drugs commonly prescribed for the elderly: Potential means for assessing risk of delirium. *Am. J. Psychiatry*, **149**, 1393–4.

Tune, L. R. and Egeli, S. (1999). Acetylcholine and delirium. *Dement. Geriatr. Cogn. Disord.*, **10**, 342–4.

Vatsavayi, V., Malhotra, S. and Franco, K. (2003). Agitated delirium with posterior cerebral artery infarction. *J. Emerg. Med.*, **24**, 263–6.

Verslegers, W., De Deyn, P. P., Saerens, J., *et al.* (1991). Slow progressive bilateral posterior artery infarction presenting as agitated delirium, complicated with Anton's syndrome. *Eur. Neurol.*, **31**, 216–19.

Wengel, S. P., Burke, W. J. and Roccaforte, W. H. (1999). Donepezil for postoperative delirium associated with Alzheimer's disease. *J. Am. Geriatr. Soc.*, **47**, 379–80.

Wengel, S. P., Roccaforte, W. H. and Burke, W. J. (1998). Donezepil improves symptoms of delirium in dementia: Implications for future research. *J. Geriatr. Psychiatry Neurol.*, **11**, 159–61.

Wooltorton, E. (2004). Olanzapine (Zyprexa): Increased incidence of cerebrovascular events in dementia trials. *CMAJ*, **170**, 1395.

25

Post-stroke delusion

Pierre Thomas

University Hospital, Lille, France

Introduction

Delusion is defined as strongly held and often bizarre beliefs whose acceptance and subsequent behavior can constitute the grounds for insanity. The patient with delusion is considered to have lost touch with reality. Delusional ideation may concern one or more of the following themes: grandiosity, jealousy, persecutory thoughts, erotomania. Delusional states that are fully experienced by the subject are accompanied by various affective and behavioral symptoms such as emotionalism, negativism, dysphoria, aggressiveness, hostility, agitation, or anxiety reaction.

There are several monothematic delusions like somatic delusion (hypochondria), delusional parasitosis, belief that the skin is infested with worms, insects, or organisms, Cotard's syndrome, belief in the loss of a body organ, or the belief of being dead – Fregoli's or Capgras' delusion. Detailed investigations of such monodelusional conditions can help to generate testable theories of delusion, face recognition and normal belief formation in cognitive neuropsychiatry (Ellis and Lewis, 2001).

Acute and chronic delusions are a core symptom of several psychiatric disorders (schizophrenia, paranoia, paraphrenia, schizoaffective disorders) and they may sometimes appear during the acute phase of non-psychotic disorder. Since the nineteenth century, it has been acknowledged that psychotic mental disorders characterized by delusions or hallucinations may develop as the physiological result of various brain diseases or general medical illnesses. The DSM-IV RT defines the criteria of "Psychotic disorder due to a general medical condition" (Table 25.1). Two subtypes are proposed according to the prominence of delusion or hallucination.

According to ICD-10 and DSM-IV classifications, *delusional misidentification* syndromes are a subgroup of unspecified persistent delusional disorders. They are characterized by systematic incorrect identification with the subjective conviction that a place, person or event is duplicated. Pick has described a syndrome that he named "reduplicative paramnesia" in which a person repeatedly and consistently

Table 25.1. DSM-IV RT diagnostic criteria for psychotic disorder due to a general medical condition

A. Prominent hallucinations or delusions.
B. There is evidence from the history, physical examination, or laboratory findings that the disturbance is the direct physiological consequence of a general medical condition.
C. The disturbance is not better accounted for by another mental disorder.
D. The disturbance does not occur exclusively during the course of a delirium.
Subtype according to predominant symptom:
with delusions: if delusions are the predominant symptom
with hallucinations: if hallucinations are the predominant symptom

misidentifies a familiar place, sometimes including occupants, as a replica (Young *et al.*, 1993). Pick suggested that this reflects a memory disorder, specifically disturbing a sense of familiarity that plays an important role in recognition. Twenty years later Capgras' syndrome (also called "illusion des sosies") was described in which a family member is viewed as a stranger with an identical appearance (Capgras and Reboul-Lachaux, 1923; Samson and Picard, 1986). Other variants of delusional misidentifications have been reported such as Fregoli delusion (see later), the delusion of subjective doubles and intermetamorphosis delusions. A common denominator of these unspecific psychopathological symptoms is the patient's denial of identity with the conviction that his/her own identity or the identity of relatives has been altered. Fregoli's syndrome is characterized by the delusional identification of an emotionally close person in different persons of different shape, different age, and different sex. Intermetamorphosis delusion is a rare variant of Capgras' syndrome involving a patient's perceiving that an individual has been transformed both psychologically and physically into another person.

The Capgras delusion is characterized by the firm conviction that some emotionally close person has been replaced by an impostor, double, robots, or aliens with a strong physical resemblance. This false belief in doubles and duplicates may sometimes trigger the decision to kill the impostor. The paradox is that patients with Capgras delusion recognize the close relation but deny the authenticity of his/her identity (Debruille and Stip, 1996). These patients are mentally not confused and the disorder is not attributed to a gross impairment of visual perception and memory. Thus, Capgras delusion is attributed to an impaired sense of face familiarity contrasting with prosopagnosia which is characterized by the inability to identify faces (Barton, 2003). The patient often uses subtle differences in behavior, personality, or physical appearance to characterize the impostor (Todd *et al.*, 1981). The delusion often includes more than one subject of misidentification. The Capgras delusion has been reported across a wide range of ages with a higher prevalence within women and among various ethnic groups (Christodoulou, 1977). Capgras' syndrome is estimated to be observed in 4% of psychosis, including schizophrenia, schizoaffective disorder, and affective disorders (Kirov *et al.*, 1994; Silva and Leong, 1992). Ramachandran (1998) has suggested that Cotard's syndrome that is always associated with a severe depressive state is an extreme form of Capgras' syndrome where the kinesthetic recognition to all stimuli is absent.

Key points Main characteristics of the delusions

Delusion is often defined as strongly held and often bizarre beliefs whose acceptance and subsequent behavior can constitute the grounds for insanity. A patient with delusion is considered to have lost touch with reality.

Stroke and delusion

Frequency of delusion in stroke patients

Williams *et al.* (2004) have conducted a study examining the impact of any mental health conditions on stroke outcome. Among 51,119 patients, 9.1% received a mental disorder diagnosis, according to the ICD-9, within 3 years of their stroke (4.7% depression and 5.4% other mental health diagnosis including comorbidity with depression; 2.7% substance abuse, 1.5% anxiety disorders, 0.5% schizophrenia, 0.4% personality disorders and 0.3% other affective disorders). The presence of any mental disorder increased the mortality risk by more than 10% with a similar magnitude whatever the type of mental disorder. These results support those obtained in studies of post-stroke depression showing that it is associated with a poor outcome (e.g. Ramasubbu *et al.*, 1998). Mechanisms accounting for increased mortality are presumably multidetermined, including functional disability, unemployment, lack of exercise, poor nutrition, life stress, low level of social support and coping resources, delayed access to carers, and immune functioning (Scott *et al.*, 1997; Kiecolt-Glaser *et al.*, 2002). Thus the treatment of post-stroke mental disorders may improve not only symptoms but also the global outcome (Williams *et al.*, 2004).

Delusional ideation has been investigated in a few series of stroke patients. Post-stroke psychosis is a rare complication of cerebral infarction, occurring at a rate of 0.5–2% of all strokes (Rabin *et al.*, 1991). Some retrospective studies report a higher incidence of delusional ideation ranging from 1% to 5.3% (Price and Mesulam, 1985). In a prospective study, Kumral and Oztürk (2004) found delusional ideation defined according to DSM-IV criteria in 4% of 360 patients. Delusional state started within the first 3 days post-stroke in all cases. Delusional themes were persecutory, jealousy and suspicion of abandonment, and mixed themes which were the most frequent. Psychosis of the schizophreniform type has been reported in patients with epilepsy and right temporo-parietal lesion due to traumatic brain injury but not to stroke to our knowledge (Rabin *et al.*, 1991; Levine and Flinkelstein, 1982).

Delusion and stroke characteristics

Most studies have supported the prominence of delusion in patients with right posterior stroke. In a retrospective study, Levine and Grek (1984) observed that patients with right hemisphere infarcts show a variety of delusional ideations including reduplication of person or place, sexual, somatic, and temporal themes. There was no clear relation between lesion sites and the themes of delusion (Levine and Grek, 1984). Price and Mesulam (1985) reported five right-handed patients with inattention and paranoid delusional ideation with parieto-temporal infarction. Grandiose delusional ideation was described in eight patients with manic-like behavior who suffered from lesions of the right caudate nucleus and medio- and baso-temporal regions (Starkstein *et al.*, 1990). In the prospective study of Kumral and Oztürk (2004), all patients with delusional ideation had a right hemisphere infarct, mainly in the territory of the inferior–posterior division of the middle cerebral artery. Cotard's syndrome is reported in patients with posterior occipito-parietal lesions and delusional parasitosis, in occipito-temporal infarction (Nagaratnam and O'Neile, 2000).

Key points Strokes responsible for the delusion

Higher frequency of right hemisphere stroke
Possible correlation between delusional content and lesion location with:
– right temporoparietal stroke: disturbances in the "sense of familiarity" of places
– right inferior temporal stroke: disturbances in the "sense of familiarity" of persons (Capgras syndrome)
– parietal stroke: dysmorphic distortions

Stroke and misidentification delusion

Perceptual distortions in the internal or external environment are central in both derealization and depersonalization, which are common syndromes observed in several psychiatric conditions. Both syndromes are not sufficient to produce delusion, which is a persistent and resistant reconstruction of reality. Therefore, other mechanisms are necessary to determine delusional ideation. Fronto-limbic region, ventral striatum, and parietal cortex would be involved in the correction of misperceptions (Ramachandran, 1998). Premorbid personality, previous mental disorders, drugs or pre-existing cerebral atrophy may also contribute to facilitate the delusion production in individuals with psychogenic or organic derealization or depersonalization. Although frequently seen in psychotic states, more than a third of the reported cases of Capgras' syndrome occurred in conjunction with a brain lesion (Collins and Hawthorne, 1990). Capgras' syndrome has been observed in dementia with Lewy bodies, Alzheimer's disease, epilepsy, tumor, severe closed head injury, stroke, Parkinson's disease, acquired immunodeficiency syndrome (AIDS), alcoholism, lithium toxicity, and migraine. Delusional misidentification syndromes concerning either places, persons, or the body have been associated with different lesions which usually involve the right hemisphere (Ellis, 1994). A few studies support the idea that lesions of the right temporo-parietal region impair the "sense of familiarity" of places, lesions of the right inferior temporal region the "sense of familiarity" of persons (Cutting, 1991; Silva et al., 1993; Forstl et al., 1994) and that lesions of the parietal lobe may produce dysmorphic distortions (Alexander et al., 1979).

According to Ramachandran (1998), the "gateway" to the limbic system is the amygdala. The amygdala determines the emotional significance of the incoming visual input from visual areas of the temporal lobes and this emotional valence is transmitted to other limbic structures. Ramachandran suggested the existence in Capgras' syndrome of a disconnection within the temporal lobe between the face recognition area and the region involved in the experience of emotion. Such a disconnection accounts for the spared ability to recognize others' faces and the impaired ability to experience the appropriate emotional feeling associated with a specific person. The absence of emotional feeling for a person emotionally close results in the belief that he/she is another person. Such a disconnection suppresses the generation of affective responses accompanying face recognition (Ellis et al., 1997; Hirstein and Ramachandran, 1997). According to Young et al. (1993), lesions responsible for Capgras' syndrome disrupt neuroanatomical pathways involved in appropriate emotional responses to faces of familiar people and to their voices as showed in blind Capgras patients (Rojo et al., 1991; Reid et al., 1993). These lesions disrupt information flow between the inferior temporal lobes and the medial limbic circuit (Signer, 1994). This disconnection has also been associated with visual hypoemotionality, a visual modality-specific inability to become emotionally aroused by visual cues (Bauer, 1982). To support this view, a PET study of Capgras' syndrome in Alzheimer's disease shows abnormalities suggesting an impairment of connections between frontal, paralimbic, and association areas (Paillère-Martinot et al., 1994).

Electrodermal skin conductance response (SCR) is a valuable tool for the measure of autonomic responses and is used to examine unconscious or covert identification of stimuli. Recently, increased SCR has been found to correlate not only with activity in the amygdala but also in neuroanatomical structures, including the right fusiform gyrus, involved in affect recognition of face processing (Ellis *et al.*, 1997). Prosopagnosia results from the disorder of conscious face recognition and is frequently associated with the preservation of unconscious or covert identification, as showed by normal SCR. Conversely, patients with Capgras delusion do not demonstrate the normal enhanced SCR in response to presentation of a familiar face (Ellis *et al.*, 1997; Hirstein and Ramachandran, 1997). Such a pattern is consistent with the hypothesis that prosopagnosia represents an interruption of the overt route to recognition, whereas Capgras delusion represents an interruption of the covert route (Ellis and Young, 1990). However, some patients with Capgras' syndrome may show covert face recognition, as assessed by priming tasks (Ellis *et al.*, 2000). Further studies are necessary to elucidate how identity processes and affective response processes are integrated and the mechanisms involved in producing delusions following abnormal perceptual experiences.

Anosognosia for hemiplegia, hemiasomatognosia and somatoparaphrenia

Some patients report a feeling of strangeness concerning the contralesional limbs and attribute them to another person. This delusional variant of hemiasomatognosia usually associated with anosognosia for hemiplegia, observed in right brain damage, is labeled "somatoparaphrenia." The pathogenesis of this delusional disorder refers to a denial of the illness, a reduced sensory feedback resulting in a failure of awareness and misidentification (Paulig *et al.*, 2000).

Anosognosia after an acute lesion usually resolves within a few months. Some approaches suggest that anosognosic symptoms are related to major sensory deficits and sensory inattention leading to lack of central feedback and therefore the inability to experience the paretic limbs (Heilman *et al.*, 1998). Other psychotic symptoms co-occur with this condition: confabulations, persecutory delusional beliefs, or place misidentification (Venneri and Shanks, 2004). On the basis of Alzheimer's disease studies, such psychiatric symptoms are considered to be related to disturbances of reality monitoring (Feinberg and Shapiro, 1989; Shanks and Venneri, 2002) and they are associated with a hypometabolism of the right frontal lobe (Starkstein *et al.*, 1995; Migliorelli *et al.*, 1995).

In a few stroke patients with persistent anosognosia and bizarre beliefs on their paralyzed limbs, extensive right fronto-parietal and subcortical lesions and hypometabolism have been reported (Berti *et al.*, 1998; Venneri and Shanks, 2004).

Outcome and treatment

Patients with delusion need a detailed assessment of the consequences of the delusional syndrome: suicide or violence risk, emotional behavior, sleep disorders, and distress requiring immediate psychiatric admission or adjuvant treatments. Personal and family past history of psychosis or bipolar disorder, present anosognosia, and dysexecutive syndrome have to be identified. Those factors may increase the risk of post-stroke delusion and require specific long-term care plans. Iatrogenic factors have also to be considered, especially with glutamate antagonists acting on N-methyl-D-aspartate (NMDA) receptors with dose-dependant side-effects such as hallucinations, psychosis or catatonia (Lees, 1998).

Antipsychotic treatment should ideally produce a regression of the delusional ideation within 30 days. The usual treatment of such symptoms relies on antipsychotic drugs. New-generation antipsychotics like olanzapine, risperidone or amisulpride have been preferred to first-generation antipsychotics since they produce fewer extrapyramidal symptoms. However, recent concerns have been expressed regarding a higher risk of stroke in older patients with behavioral and psychological symptoms of dementia using atypical antipsychotics (Brodaty *et al.*, 2003; Wooltorton, 2004), not confirmed in a recent case–control study (Gill *et al.*, 2005).

Key point Assessment

> – Assessment of the consequences of the delusional syndrome: i.e. suicide or violence risk, emotional behavior, sleep disorders, and distress requiring psychiatric admission or adjuvant treatments.

Key points Management and treatment

> Antipsychotic treatment: new generation antipsychotics produce less extrapyramidal symptoms than the first generation antipsychotics
> Warning of increased vascular risk with second generation antipsychotic in older patients with behavioral and psychological symptoms of dementia: to be confirmed
> Refractory delusions: clozapine
> Recognizing and treating poststroke mental health condition not only improve patient symptoms and functioning but may also reduce subsequent mortality risk

The Capgras' syndrome (psychiatric or neurological) has been reported to respond well to antipsychotic agents, including olanzapine (Lykouras *et al.*, 2002), sulpiride, trifluoperazine (Pauw and Szulecka, 1988), as well as to drugs with antipsychotic properties, in particular pimozide (Passer and Warnock, 1991). However, some delusional states may be refractory to treatment despite various antipsychotic therapies of sufficient duration. To our knowledge, there is no report of cases with delusions of misidentification treated with clozapine. A recent study reported the remission of Capgras' syndrome by treatment with the antidepressant mirtazapine (Khouzam, 2002).

Further studies of post-stroke delusion are necessary to determine the optimal treatment strategies including pharmacological agents and rehabilitation psychotherapies.

REFERENCES

Alexander, M., Stuss, D. T. and Benson, D. F. (1979). Capgras Syndrome; a reduplicative phenomenon. *Neurology*, **29**, 334–9.

Barton, J. J. (2003). Disorders of face perception and recognition. *Neurol. Clin.*, **21**, 521–48.

Bauer, R. M. (1982). Visual hypoemotionality as a symptom of visual–limbic disconnection in man. *Arch. Neurol.*, **39**, 702–8.

Berti, A., Ladavas, E., Stracciari, A., Giannarelli, C. and Ossola, A. (1998). Anosognosia for motor impairment and dissociation with patient's evaluation of the disorder: Theoretical consideration *Cogn. Neuropsychiatry*, **3**, 21–44.

Brodaty, H., Ames, D., Snowden, J., *et al.* (2003). A randomized placebo controlled trial of risperidone for the treatment of aggression, agitation, and psychosis in dementia. *J. Clin. Psychiatry*, **64**, 134–43.

Capgras, J. and Reboul-Lachaux, J. (1923). Illusion de sosies; un delire systematisé chronique. *Bull. Soc. Med. Ment.*, **2**, 6–16.

Christodoulou, G. N. (1977). The syndrome of Capgras. *Br. J. Psychiatry*, **130**, 556–64.

Collins, M. N. and Hawthorne, M. (1990). Capgras' syndrome with organic disorders. *Postgrad. Med. J.*, **66**, 1064–7.

Cutting, J. (1991). Delusional misidentification and the role of right hemisphere in the appreciation of identity. *Br. J. Psychiatry*, **159**, 70–5.

Debruille, J. and Stip, E. (1996). Capgras syndrome: Evolution of the hypotheses. *Can. J. Psychiatry*, **41**, 181–7.

Ellis, H. D. and Lewis, M. B. (2001). Capgras delusion: A window on face recognition. *Trends Cogn. Sci.*, **5**, 149–56.

Ellis, H. D., Lewis, M. B., Moselhy, H. F. and Young, A. W. (2000). Automatic without autonomic responses to familiar faces: Differential components of covert recognition in a case of Capgras delusion. *Cogn. Neuropsychiatry*, **5**, 255–69.

Ellis, H. (1994). The role of right hemisphere in the Capgras delusion. *Psychopathology*, **27**, 177–85.

Ellis, H. D. and Young, A. W. (1990). Accounting for delusional misidentifications. *Br. J. Psychiatry*, **157**, 239–48.

Ellis, A., Young, A. W., Quayle, A. H. and de Pauw, K. W. (1997). Reduced anatomic responses to faces in Capgras delusion. *Proc. R. Soc. Lond. [Biol.]*, **264**, 1085–92.

Feinberg, T. E. and Shapiro, R. M. (1989). Misidentification reduplication and the right hemisphere. *Neuropsychiatry Neuropsychol. Behav. Neurol.*, **2**, 39–48.

Forstl, H., Besthorn, C., Burns, A., *et al.* (1994). Delusional misidentification in Alzheimer's disease: A summary of clinical and biological aspects. *Psychopathology*, **27**, 194–9.

Gill, S. S., Rochon, P. A., Herrmann, N., *et al.* (2005). Atypical antipsychotic drugs and risk of ischemic stroke: Population based retrospective cohort study. *BMJ*, **26**, 445.

Heilman, K. M., Barret, A. M. and Adair, J. C. (1998). Possible mechanism of agnosognosia: A defect in self awareness. *Philos. Trans. R. Soc. London. [Biol.]*, **353**, 1903–9.

Hirstein, W. and Ramachandran, V. S. (1997). Capgras syndrome: A novel probe for understanding the neural representation of the identity and familiarity of persons. *Proc. R. Soc. Lond. [Biol.]*, **264**, 437–44.

Khouzam, H. R. (2002). Capgras syndrome responding to the antidepressant mirtazapine. *Compr. Ther.*, **28**, 238–40.

Kiecolt-Glaser, J. K., McGuire, L., Robles, T. F. and Glaser, R. (2002). Emotion, morbidity and mortality: New perspectives from psychoneuroendocrinology. *Annu. Rev. Psychol.*, **53**, 83–107.

Kirov, G., Jones, P. and Lewis, S. W. (1994). Prevalence of delusional misidentification syndromes. *Psychopathology*, **27**,148–9.

Kumral, E. and Oztürk, O. (2004). Delusional state following acute stroke. *Neurology*, **62**, 110–13.

Lees, K. R. (1998). Does neuroprotection improve stroke outcome? *Lancet*, **351**, 1447–8.

Levine, D. N. and Finkelstein, S. (1982). Delayed psychosis after temporo-parietal stroke or trauma, relation to epilepsy. *Neurology*, **32**, 267–72.

Levine, D. N. and Grek, A. (1984). The anatomic basis for delusion after right cerebral infarction. *Neurology*, **34**, 577–82.

Lykouras, L., Typaldou, M., Gournellis, R., Vaslamatzis, G. and Christodoulou, G. N. (2002). Coexistence of Capgras and Frégoli syndromes in a single patient. Clinical, neuroimaging and neuropsychological findings. *Eur. Psychiatry*, **17**, 234–5.

Migliorelli, R., Teson, A., Sabe, L., *et al.* (1995). Anosognosia in Alzheimer's disease. A study of associated factors. *J. Neuropsychiatry Clin. Neurosci.*, **7**, 338–44.

Nagaratnam, N. and O'Neile, L. O. (2000). Delusional parasitosis following occipito-temporal cerebral infarction. *Gen. Hosp. Psychiatry*, **22**, 129–32.

Paillère-Martinot, M. L., Dao-Castellana, M. H., Masure, M. C., Pillon, B. and Martinot, J. L. (1994). Delusional misidentification: A clinical, neuropsychological and brain imaging case study. *Psychopathology*, **27**, 200–10.

Passer, K. M. and Warnock, J. K. (1991). Pimozide in the treatment of Capgras' syndrome. *Psychosomatics*, **32**, 446–8.

Paulig, M., Weber, M. and Garbelotto, S. (2000). Somatophrenia. A positive variant of anosognosia for hemiplegia. *Nervenartz*, **71**, 123–9.

Pauw, K. W. and Szulecka, T. K. (1988). Dangerous delusions. Violence and the misidentification syndromes. *Br. J. Psychiatry*, **152**, 91–6.

Price, B. H. and Mesulam, M. (1985). Psychiatric manifestations of right hemisphere infarctions. *J. Nerv. Ment. Dis.*, **173**, 610–14.

Rabin, P. V., Starkstein, S. E. and Robinson, R. G. (1991). Risk factors for developing atypical schizophreniform psychosis following stroke. *J. Neuropsychiatry Clin. Neurosci.*, **3**, 6–9.

Ramachandran, V. S. (1998). Consciousness and body image. *Philos. Trans. R. Soc. London. [Biol.]*, **353**, 1851–9.

Ramasubbu, R., Robinson, R. G., Flint, A. J., Kosier, T. and Price, T. R. (1998). Functional impairment associated with acute poststroke depression. The stroke data bank study. *J. Neuropsychiatry Clin. Neurosci.*, **10**, 26–33.

Reid, I., Young, A.W. and Hellawell, D. J. (1993). Voice recognition impairment in a blind Capgras patient. *Behav. Neurol.*, **6**, 225–8.

Rojo, V. J., Caballero, L., Iruela, L. M. and Baca, E. (1991). Capgras' syndrome in a blind patient. *Am. J. Psychiatry*, **148**, 1271–2.

Samson, E. and Picard, S. (1986). The Capgras syndrome. *Can. J. Psychiatry*, **31**, 142–5.

Scott, W. K., Macera, C. A., Cornman, C. B. and Sharpe, P. A. (1997). Functional Health status as a predictor of mortality in men and women over 65. *J. Clin. Epidemiol.*, **50**, 291–6.

Shanks, M. F. and Venneri, A. (2002). The emergence of delusional companions in Alzheimer disease an unusual misidentification syndrome. *Cogn. Neuropsychiatry*, **7**, 317–28.

Signer, S. F. (1994). Localization and lateralization in the delusion of substitution. *Psychopathology*, **27**, 168–76.

Silva, J. A. and Leong, G. B. (1992). The Capgras' syndrome in paranoid schizophrenia. *Psychopathology*, **25**, 147–53.

Silva, A. J., Leong, G. B. and Wine, D. B. (1993). Misidentification delusions, facial misrecognition and right brain injury. *Can. J. Psychiatry*, **38**, 239–41.

Starkstein, S. E., Mayberg, H. S. and Berthier, M. L. (1990). Mania after brain injury. Neuroradiological and metabolic findings. *Ann. Neurol.*, **27**, 652–9.

Starkstein, S. E., Vazquez, S., Migliorelli, R., *et al.* (1995). A single photon emission computed tomographic study of anosognosia in Alzheimer's disease. *Arch. Neurol.*, **52**, 415–20.

Todd, J., Dewhurst, K. and Wallis, G. (1981). The syndrome of Capgras. *Br. J. Psychiatry*, **139**, 319–27.

Venneri, A. and Shanks, M. (2004). Belief and awareness; reflections on a case of persistent anosognosia. *Neuropsychologia*, **42**, 230–8.

Williams, L. S., Ghose, S. S. and Swindle, R. W. (2004). Depression and other Mental Health diagnoses increase mortality risk after ischemic stroke. *Am. J. Psychiatry*, **161**, 1090–5.

Wooltorton, E. (2004). Olanzapine (Zyprexa): Increased incidence of cerebrovascular events in dementia trials. *CMAJ*, **170**, 1395.

Young, A. W., Ellis, H. D., Quayle, A. H. and De Pauw, K. W. (1993). Face processing impairments and the Capgras delusion. *Br. J. Psychiatry*, **162**, 695–8.

26

Acute behavioral and mood changes

Selma Aybek and Julien Bogousslavsky

Swiss Medical Network, Montreux, Switzerland

Introduction

Motor, sensory, and cognitive deficits are classically recognized as clinical signs of stroke. It was only during the twentieth century that modifications of affective and emotional behavior were recognized in cerebrovascular diseases, with Kraepelin (1921) first describing an association between depression and atherosclerotic diseases. Later, Goldstein (1948) described the catastrophic reaction observed in brain-injured patients, but it was only in the 1970s that Gainotti (1972) conducted the first systematic study of emotional symptoms associated with brain lesions. When talking about *mood changes* it is not always clear in the literature whether it refers to affective disorders included in psychiatric disturbances or to emotional disorders. Since other chapters in this book are dedicated to mania, depression, and delusion, we will focus on *emotional* and *behavioral* modifications related to stroke.

Emotional modifications

The study of emotion in stroke patients is particularly difficult because the variables involved are multiple and complex. One problem is the definition of emotion itself, since it can be expressed in three main ways (Eysenck, 1975, p. 439): a *subjective feeling* or state experienced by the patient (e.g. sadness, anger, happiness, fear, disgust, surprise), *physiological reactions* characterized by somatic visceral—autonomic responses (e.g. increased heart rate, blood pressure, salivation, perspiration) and a *behavioral component* that can be observed (e.g. running away when afraid or smiling when happy). As far as stroke patients are concerned, the study of subjective feelings is extremely difficult since it excludes aphasic patients. Although possible, the study of vegetative changes is not easily applicable to incapacitated patients in an acute stroke unit. Therefore, currently the only approach to emotions is through observation of the displayed behavior.

Sadness

Sadness is a displayed behavior of sad mimic accompanied by crying, complaining, groaning, or even screaming. It is rarely seen in stroke patients as a pure isolated symptom since it is often accompanied by other features of abnormal behavior such as emotionalism or apathy, which will be discussed later. In our acute stroke study (Aybek et al., 2005) we found that 40% of patients demonstrated signs of sadness and women were more prone then men at showing this behavior, when observed in the first days after stroke. This did not correlate to precise specific stroke localization, but it did correlate to a personal history of alcohol abuse, which could be interpreted as signs of premorbid affective disorder. Indeed, alcohol abuse can be interpreted as an antidepressant self-medication.

Aggressiveness and anger

Aggressiveness is a very common consequence of traumatic brain injury but has been recently described in stroke patients as well. A systematic study (Kim et al., 2002) reports a prevalence of 32% of aggressive behavior in post-stroke patients examined in the chronic phase (3–12 months post-stroke). A precise localization of the stroke was not established. It is still a matter of controversy whether anger and aggressiveness are the direct consequences of the brain damage or whether they represent a natural reaction in a handicapped person. However, in this study, there was no significant correlation with the Barthel index and Rankin score, the emotional behavior of aggression being independent of the degree of functional impairment. Our prospective study (Aybek et al., 2005) in acute stroke showed that 17% of patients presented aggressiveness in the first 4 days after the stroke and a positive correlation was found with the hemorrhagic nature of the stroke but no precise localization was found.

Joy and "fou-rire prodromique"

An acute burst of laughter has been described in the onset of ischemic strokes, in the anterior choroidal artery territory (Sibon et al., 2003) as well as in carotid dissection (Osseby et al., 1999) and brainstem infarction (Wali, 1993). This burst of laughter is usually not accompanied by a feeling a joy; on the contrary, some patients described anxiety. Different locations have been described but in all cases the lesion was subcortical and there seems to be a predominance of left hemisphere lesions.

Happiness and pleasure

In a systematic prospective study (Ghika-Schmid et al., 1999) of emotion in the first days after stroke, 24% patients reported a feeling of happiness, even though no anatomical correlate could be identified. A case report (Danziger et al., 1997) mentions that a patient presenting with a stroke in the postero-inferior cerebellar artery experienced visual hallucinations along with an intense sensation of pleasure and satisfaction five days post-stroke; this sensation, judged to be out of proportion to the stimulus, took place for the first time when he was receiving his morning body care, and the second time during lunch, which was a regular hospital meal.

Fear

Few data are available concerning fear and brain lesion, and it is worth mentioning that lack of fear feeling has been described (Sprengelmeyer *et al.*, 1999) after a stroke in a patient with a left thalamo-capsular lesion and bilateral gliosis of the amygdala. Careful testing revealed an impaired recognition of emotional faces showing fear but the patient also described himself as almost never feeling fear on a self-rating scale. The study of the subjective feeling of fear in acute stroke patients (Ghika-Schmid *et al.*, 1999) revealed that 11 out of 53 patients experienced fear during the acute hospitalization. This feeling had an inverse correlation with denial of illness, so that decreased fear relates to the manifestation of denial, which could be interpreted as a defense mechanism. This is of high clinical significance since this same study showed that this group of patients failed to seek medical attention.

Behavioral modifications

Emotionalism

Emotionalism or emotional lability is an increased frequency of crying and laughing with little warning. This symptom is very frequent in acute stroke (Carota *et al.*, 2002) with prevalence up to 40%. Various localizations have been found, frontal and temporal being the most frequently involved (House *et al.*, 1989). The prevalence then declines to 15–21% six months after stroke. The exact mechanism is not known but an implication of serotoninergic pathways is likely since some patients respond to serotonin reuptake inhibitors (Brown *et al.*, 1998).

Catastrophic reaction

Catastrophic reaction manifests as a disruptive emotional behavior when the patient is confronted with an unsolvable task. The dissociation between the degree of physical impairment and the occurrence of this behavior supports the hypothesis of a specific lesion-induced neural dysfunction. Only patients with left hemisphere lesions show catastrophic reaction, especially those with lesions in regions projecting to the amygdala (insula, temporal, frontal opercular, and parietal cortex). It is also important to recognize such a behavior since it seems to be a predictor of post-stroke depression with 66% of patients developing depression at 3 months (Carota *et al.*, 2001).

Athymormia

Athymormia is characterized by apathetic, aspontaneous, and indifferent behavior with motor and affective drive loss, without anxiety or suffering but adequate activity can be obtained on hetero-stimulation. The patient is unable to undertake any activity on auto-stimulation. This term is also referred to as "loss of self psychic activation." Only bilateral lesions can induce it and it has been described in bilateral pallidal and putamen (Milandré *et al.*, 1995), caudate (Rodier *et al.*, 1994), and thalamus (Kumral *et al.*, 2001) infarcts.

Apathy

Apathy is a state of little spontaneous actions or speech, with flat affect. In contrast to athymormia, apathy is frequently associated with hypophonia and some frontal signs (grasp reflex, perseveration, utilization behavior). It has, indeed, been associated with frontal dysfunction as demonstrated by SPECT studies (Okada *et al.*, 1997).

Modification of sexual behavior

Some cases of *hypersexual behavior* have been described in an acute setting, as in the Klüver–Bucy syndrome (see later). An interesting report (Ong Hai and Odderson, 2000) has also described a behavior of excessive masturbation in a patient presenting an alien-limb syndrome in relation to a right frontal and anterior corpus callosum stroke. Those are rare. The more common modification of sexual behavior after stroke consists of *decreased libido* and diminished coital frequency. The mechanism is multiple since post-stroke depression, sensory and motor sequelae, and functional handicap play a role. Some studies reported a prevalence of right hemisphere lesions (Coslett and Heilman, 1986), while others reported opposite results (Monga *et al.*, 1981). In acute stroke, this symptom, however, is never mentioned.

The temporal lobe seems to be involved in *sexual preference* (Gautier Smith, 1980). The case of a patient presenting temporal lobe epilepsy was reported (Mitchell and Falconer, 1954), since he showed fetishism and cross-dressing, which disappeared after temporal lobectomy. As far as stroke is concerned, few data are available but a case report was able to define a link between a temporal lobe ischemic stroke and a change of sexual preference (namely homosexuality) developing in a 70-year-old happily married man (Cheasty *et al.*, 2002).

Klüver–Bucy syndrome

This syndrome is rarely encountered in stroke patients since it is associated with bitemporal lesions. It is still worth describing, as incomplete forms can be seen (Ghika-Schmid *et al.*, 1995; Muller *et al.*, 1999). The full syndrome requires at least three of the following: loss of fear or anxiety, bulimia or loss of alimentary selectivity, aberrant sexual behavior (increased activity and/or inappropriate sexual object choice), hypermetamorphosis (excessive visual exploration of environment), hyperorality (tendency to examine all objects by mouth) and "psychic blindness" (failure in recognizing emotional visual stimuli).

Modifications of eating behavior

As discussed with Klüver–Bucy syndrome, hyperorality and hyperphagia are encountered in bitemporal lesions. The ventromesial hypothalamus, the amygdala and the fiber bundle from the substantia nigra to the basal ganglia are involved in the regulation of appetite and satiety. An interesting report described a patient presenting with acute memory loss and hyperphagia in relation to a thalamic infarct (Cerrato *et al.*, 2004). The first day of the stroke the wife described her husband as obsessed with food with compulsive eating all day long of everything he found in the refrigerator or kitchen.

Kleptomania

Although not of major clinical significance in acute stroke, it is worth mentioning that kleptomania, another compulsive behavior, has been linked with cerebral vasculitis associated with lupus erythematosus (Ampelas *et al.*, 2001). It has been better documented in association with frontal lobe lesions, such as subarachnoid hemorrhage (Gossling and Rosin, 1994) or craniopharyngioma (Nyffeler and Regard, 2001).

Assessment in stroke patients

Emotional modifications

As already stated, the study of emotions is extremely difficult in the stroke patient and the observational method is still the best, although not very precise. The development of scales is thus crucial in order to have reliable measures and to perform more research in this very interesting field. We have developed an index, the Emotional Behavior Index (Aybek *et al.*, 2005; Table 26.1), which can be completed by nurses in stroke units, who can help evaluate the behavior of patients in the very acute phase. Its aim is to assess the basic emotions of sadness and aggressiveness and the complex behaviors of denial, apathy, passivity, adaptation and disinhibition. The assessment of anger

Table 26.1. Emotional Behaviour Index Form

Sadness	Indifference	Adaptation
Cries	Indifferent	Smiles
Looks sad	Neglected	Sociable
Complains	Apathetic	Quiet
Screams	Disinhibition	Patient
Groans	Jokes	Capable of founded request
Passivity	Disinhibited	Decent
Gives up	Laughs	Interested, curious
Isolated	Impatient	Looks serious
Aggressiveness	Denial	Interactive
Tense	Minimizes	Accommodating
Agitated	Total denial	Helpful
Angry	Partial denial	Expressive
Rebellious		Tidy
Opposed		Docile
Aggressive		
Revolted		

Table 26.2. The 10-item Spielberger Trait Anger Scale

1. I am quick-tempered
2. I have a fiery temper
3. I am a hotheaded person
4. I get angry when I am slowed down by others' mistakes
5. I feel annoyed when I am not given recognition for doing good work
6. I fly off the handle
7. When I get angry I say nasty things
8. It makes me furious when I am criticized in front of others
9. When I get frustrated, I feel like hitting someone
10. I feel infuriated when I do a good job and get a poor evaluation

can be made with the Spielberger Trait Anger Scale (Spielberger *et al.*, 1983; Table 26.2).

Behavioral modifications

The interpretation of apathy, athymormia, catastrophic reaction, and emotionalism still relies on a careful bedside examination by a skilled neurologist. The well-known Neuropsychiatric Inventory used mostly for demented patients has been used in stroke patients (Angelelli *et al.*, 2004).

For other complex behaviors, such as eating behavior, sexual behavior, and social behavior, only case reports exist and no systematic review permits us to define the best way to test them. It must, then, be emphasized that clinicians should be aware of those behavior modifications and should systematically ask the family members, since the patient might not themselves report the behavior. Special attention should also be given to the nurses' descriptions of the patient's behavior since they spend most of their time at the bedside.

Prognosis and management

Emotional and behavioral modifications in acute stroke are very interesting but are still underestimated and under-reported. Clinicians have a tendency to interpret unusual acute behaviors as part of a normal reaction in hospitalized patients suddenly put in an unusual life condition. For example, catastrophic reaction might be interpreted as a normal emotional reaction to a major life event like a stroke. Careful review of this disorder, however, showed a clear left hemisphere association and some evidence that catastrophic reaction might be a predictor of post-stroke depression.

Only careful clinical examination and reports will help us to understand abnormal behaviors and their neural substrate. Now that the major concern in acute stroke is tissue salvaging, we developed practical scales like the National Institute of Health Stroke Scale to evaluate the patient quickly; but one should not neglect a detailed examination along with this evaluation. Indeed, for the time being we have not identified clear behavioral predictors of outcome, but prospective studies are needed.

REFERENCES

Ampelas, J. F., Wattiaux, M. J. and Van Amerongen, A. P. (2001). Psychiatric manifestations of lupus erythematosus systemic and Sjogren's syndrome. *Encephale*, **27**(6), 588–99.

Angelelli, P., Paolucci, S., Bivona, U., et al. (2004). Development of neuropsychiatric symptoms in poststroke patients: A cross-sectional study. *Acta Psychiatr. Scand.*, **110**(1), 55–63.

Aybek, S., Carota, A., Ghika-Schmid, F., et al. (2005). Emotional behavior in acute stroke: The Lausanne Emotion in Stroke Study. *Cogn. Behav. Neurol.*, **18**(1), 37–44.

Brown, K. W., Sloan, R. L. and Pentland, B. (1998). Fluoxetine as a treatment for post-stroke emotionalism. *Acta Psychiatr. Scand.*, **98**, 455–8.

Carota, A., Rossetti, A. O., Karapanayiotides, T. and Bogousslavsky, J. (2001). Catastrophic reaction in acute stroke: A reflex behavior in aphasic patients. *Neurology*, **57**, 1902–5.

Carota, A., Staub, F. and Bogousslavsky, J. (2002). Emotions, behaviours and mood changes in stroke. *Curr. Opin. Neurol.*, **15**, 57–69.

Cerrato, P., Grasso, M., Azzaro, C., *et al.* (2004). Transient compulsive hyperphagia in a patient with a thalamic infarct. *J. Neurol. Neurosurg. Psychiatry*, 1364–5.

Cheasty, M., Condren, R. and Cooney, C. (2002). Altered sexual preference and behavior in a man with vascular ischaemic lesions in the temporal lobe. *In. J. Geriatr. Psychiatry*, **17**, 87–90.

Coslett, H. B. and Heilman, K. M. (1986). Male sexual function. Impairment after right hemisphere stroke. *Arch. Neurol.*, **43**, 1036–39.

Danziger, N., Meary, E., Mercier, B., Samson, Y. and Rancurel, G. (1997). Visual hallucinosis and hyperhedonism in pontine and thalamic infarction. *Rev. Neurol.*, **153**, 679–83.

Eysenck, H. J. (1975). The measurement of emotion: Psychological parameters and methods. In *Emotions: Their Parameters and Measurements*, ed. L. Levi, NY: Raven Press.

Gainotti, G. (1972). Emotional behavior and hemispheric side of the lesion. *Cortex*, **8**, 41–55.

Gautier Smith, P. C. (1980). Cerebral dysfunction and disorders of sexual behavior. *Rev. Neurol.*, **136**(4), 311–19.

Ghika-Schmid, F., Assal, De Tribolet N. and Regli, F. (1995). Klüver-Bucy syndrome after left anterior temporal resection. *Neuropsychologia*, **33**, 101–13.

Ghika-Schmid, F., Van Melle, G., Guex, P. and Bogousslavsky, J. (1999). Subjective experience and behavior in acute stroke. *Neurology*, **52**, 22.

Goldstein, K. (1948). *Language and Language Disturbances*, New York: Grune and Stratton.

Gossling, H. W. and Rosin, J. (1994). Kleptomania before and after spontaneous subarachnoid hemorrhage – a neuropsychodynamic case report. *Fortschr. Neurol. Psychiatr.*, May; **62**(5), 164–8.

House, A., Dennis, M. and Molyneux, A. (1989). Emotionalism after stroke. *BMJ*, **298**, 991–4.

Kim, J. S., Choi, S., Kwon, S. U. and Seo, Y. S. (2002). Inability to control anger or aggression after stroke. *Neurology*, **58**, 1106–8.

Kraepelin, E. (1921). *Manic Depressive Insanity and Paranoia*, Livingstone: Edinburgh.

Kumral, E., Evyapan, D., Balkir, K. and Kutluhan, S. (2001). Bilateral thalamic infarction. Clinical, etiological and MRI correlates. *Acta Neurol. Scand.*, **103**, 35.

Milandré, L., Habib, M. and Royere, M. L. (1995). Athymormic syndrome caused by bilateral striato-capsular infarction. Moyamoya disease in adults. *Rev. Neurol.*, **151**, 383–7.

Mitchell, W. and Falconer, M. A. (1954). Epilepsy with fetishism relieved by temporal lobectomy. *Lancet*, **2**, 626–30.

Monga, T. N., Lawson, J. S. and Inglis, J. (1981). Sexual dysfunction in stroke patients. *Arch. Phys. Med. Rehabil.*, **62**, 286–8.

Muller, A., Baumgartner, R. W., Rohrenbach, C. and Regard, M. (1999). Persistant Klüver-Bucy syndrome after bilateral thalamic infarction. *Neuropsychiatry Neuropsychol. Behav. Neurol.*, **12**, 136–9.

Nyffeler, T. and Regard, M. (2001). Kleptomania in a patient with a right frontolimbic lesion. *Neuropsychiatry Neuropsychol. Behav. Neurol.*, **14**(1), 73–6.

Okada, K., Kobayashi, S. and Yamagata, S. (1997). Poststroke apathy and regional blood flow. *Stroke*, **28**, 2437–41.

Ong Hai, B. G. and Odderson, I. R. (2000). Involuntary masturbation as a manifestation of stroke-related alien hand syndrome. *Am. J. Phys. Med. Rehabil.*, **79**(4), 395–8.

Osseby, G., Manceau, E., Huet, F., *et al.* (1999). Fou rire prodromique as the heralding symptom of lenticular infarction caused by dissection of the internal carotid artery in a 12-year-old boy. *Eur. J. Paediatr. Neurol.*, **3**(3), 133–6.

Rodier, R., Tranchant, C. G., Mohr, M. and Warter, J. M. (1994). Neurobehavioral changes following bilateral infarct in the caudate nuclei: A case report with pathological analysis. *J. Neurol. Sci.*, **126**, 213–18.

Sibon, I., Barreau, X. and Orgogozo, J. M. (2003). Fou rire prodromique and choroidal anterior artery stroke. *Cerebrovasc. Dis.*, **15**(1–2), 149–50.

Spielberger, C. D., Jacobs Russell S. and Crane, R. S. (1983). Assessment of anger: The State-Trait Anger Scale. In J. N. Butcher and C. D. Spielberger, eds., *Advances in Personality Assessment*, Vol. 2. Hillsdale, NJ: Lawrence Erlbaum Associates, pp. 161–89.

Sprengelmeyer, R., Young, A. W., Schroeder, U., *et al.* (1999). Knowing no fear. *Proc. R. Soc. Lond.*, **266**, 2451–6.

Wali, G. M. (1993). Fou rire prodromique heralding brainstem stroke. *JNNP*, **56**(2), 209–10.

27

Stroke and personality change

Pierre Thomas

University Hospital, Lille, France

Introduction

Personality is defined as a distinctive constellation of relatively stable behaviors, thoughts, motives, and emotions that characterize a unique individual. Personality organization derives from the interaction between the individual and social learning as well as an internal set of motivated predispositions to respond. Cloninger *et al.* (1993) have developed a biosocial model of personality describing four dimensions of temperament genetically dependent and stable and three dimensions of character that are influenced by social learning. The four dimensions of temperaments include:

1. *novelty seeking*, describing genetic dispositions towards being excitable, impulsive, exploratory, and quick-tempered
2. *harm avoidance*, related to behavioral inhibition, implying a heritable bias towards being cautious, apprehensive, and pessimistic
3. *reward dependence*, involving the maintenance of behaviors previously associated with reinforcement
4. *persistence*, describing the ability to persevere despite fatigue or lack of reward. The three dimensions of character are:
1. *self-directedness*, implying an autonomous self-concept and feelings of hope and self-confidence
2. *cooperativeness*, involving identification with and acceptance of others, and compassion
3. *self-transcendence*, related to spirituality, patience, and self-forgetfulness.

Cloninger *et al.* (1993) hypothesized that each temperament dimension is regulated neurochemically by a complex distributed network of brain connections. Novelty seeking has been associated with dopaminergic activity, harm avoidance with serotonergic activity, and reward dependence with noradrenergic activity. Youn *et al.* (2002) observed that each temperament dimension is correlated with regional cerebral glucose metabolism in specific areas of paralimbic regions and temporal lobes. These findings provide further evidence that temperament dimension is associated with specific brain areas and neurotransmitters.

A personality disorder is suspected when an individual uses maladaptive, enduring, and inflexible patterns of thinking and behavior to fulfill his or her own needs and attain self-satisfaction resulting in the individual's own detriment or occurring at the expense of others and society. Personality disorders result in significant functional impairment and subjective distress, and subjects are at risk of psychiatric diseases. The DSM-IV TR (APA, 2000) has defined the criteria of a group of personality disorders characterized by pathological trends.

Personality disorders associated with structural brain damage have been defined in DSM III, IIIR and IV as *organic personality syndrome*. This diagnosis has been revisited in the DSM IV TR (APA, 2000) and is relabeled as "Personality change due to a general medical condition." The DSM IV TR criteria describe longstanding types of personality changes according to dominant behaviors (Table 27.1). The personality change might be suspected in an individual without any history of prior psychiatric disorder in a context of brain damage or other general condition.

Key points Main characteristics of the personality disorders

Use of maladaptive, enduring, and inflexible patterns of thinking and behavior to fulfill his/her own needs and attain self-satisfaction
Results in individual's own detriment
Occurs at the expense of others and society

Personality changes associated with brain damage

The case of Phineas Gage (Harlow, 1848) shed light on the presence of behavioral disorders and personality changes following traumatic lesion of the frontal lobes. A meter-long tamping iron weighing 6 kg went into and out of the front part of the skull of Gage. Notably, Gage not only survived the accident, but also had no subsequent difficulties with walking, general movement, or speech. However, his personality permanently changed ("... Gage is no longer Gage..."). The description of Gage's behavioral changes is considered as the prototype of personality change associated with frontal lobe lesion. In frontal lobe lesions, personality changes predominate over other neurological symptoms. Further descriptions of personality changes secondary to frontal lesions have led to the suggestion that mental illness might be due to abnormal frontal lobe functioning, and this formed the basis of the leucotomy procedure.

Table 27.1. DSM-IV TR diagnostic criteria for personality change due to a general medical condition

---

A. A persistent personality disturbance that represents a change from the individual's previous characteristic personality pattern. (In children, the disturbance involves a marked deviation from normal development or a significant change in the child's usual behavior patterns lasting at least 1 year.)

B. There is evidence from the history, physical examination, or laboratory findings that the disturbance is the direct physiological consequence of a general medical condition.

C. The disturbance is not better accounted for by another mental disorder (including other mental disorders due to a general medical condition).

D. The disturbance does not occur exclusively during the course of a delirium.

E. The disturbance causes clinically significant distress or impairment in social, occupational, or other important areas of functioning.

Type specification:

labile type: if the predominant feature is affective lability

disinhibited type: if the predominant feature is poor impulse control as evidenced by sexual indiscretions, etc.

aggressive type: if the predominant feature is aggressive behavior

apathetic type: if the predominant feature is marked apathy and indifference

paranoid type: if the predominant feature is suspiciousness or paranoid ideation

other type: if the predominant feature is not one of the above, e.g., personality change associated with a seizure disorder

combined type: if more than one feature predominates in the clinical picture

unspecified type

To date, numerous descriptions of personality change are available and their high frequency in closed head injuries is well documented. Blumer and Benson (1975) described two types of personality changes after frontal lobe lesion: (1) towards apathy and indifference (pseudo-depressed), and (2) towards puerility and euphoria (pseudo-psychopathic). They added that the mixture of the two types is more common than the pure types. However, the architecture of the neurobiological networks involved in the assembly of human traits and reactions known as personality remains unclear.

Personality change and stroke

As personality is a complex and dynamic integration of emotional and cognitive functions, any stroke will have an impact on personality organization by interfering with these processes. Conversely the post-stroke reorganization of personality will have an impact on an individual's functioning. A study demonstrated that the occurrence of mental disorders complicating a vascular disease is a strong determinant of disability (Kattainen *et al.*, 2004).

As a part of personality, the emotional and behavioral consequences of stroke are illustrated through some changes observed in stroke patients, especially dysprosody, apathy, emotional incontinence, and aggressive behavior. Most of these behavioral changes are components of the dysexecutive syndrome (see Chapter 19). In addition these symptoms have some resemblance to those of mood disorders (see Chapters 28 and 29).

Receptive aprosodia

Receptive aprosodia, often associated with right parietal lesions, refers to a patient's inability to recognize the affective tonality of a sentence (Starkstein *et al.*, 1993b). This results in misunderstanding or indifference to others. On the other hand, expressive or motor aprosodia, often associated with right frontal lesions, results in a lack of emotional inflection, the patient appearing inexpressive or sad. Anosognosia refers to the patient's indifference to the disease and lack of concern with stroke care, especially a rehabilitation program. The presence of aphasia makes the differential diagnosis with depression more difficult because of the patient's difficulty in expressing the content of his/her affects. Contrary to depression where mood change persists, these changes are more responsive to environmental changes.

Apathy

Apathy is defined as a lack of feeling, emotion, interest, or concern. Starkstein *et al.* (1993a) found the presence of apathy without depression in 11% of stroke patients examined at the acute phase, and it often coexisted with important cognitive disturbances. Frontal damage associated with anterior cerebral artery lesions is a classical, albeit rare, cause of apathy. In its major form, it results in akinetic mutism, usually associated with lesions of the cingulate gyrus and mesial premotor area. Marin (1990), in reviewing lesions associated with apathy, has defined four groups of pathology:

1. lesions in the unilateral cingulate gyrus, supplementary motor area, and mesial motor areas
2. right hemisphere stroke
3. bilateral lesion of the amygdala and anterior temporal lobes
4. frontal lobe damage.

A cerebral functional imaging study of stroke patients revealed that apathy scores are correlated with decreased regional cerebral blood flows in the supplementary motor area, dorsolateral and frontotemporal regions supporting the involvement of these regions in apathy (Okada *et al.*, 1997). The outcome of apathy and treatment options has not been reported. Further studies are necessary to address this issue.

Poststroke emotional incontinence

Poststroke emotional incontinence includes catastrophic reaction and the pseudobulbar syndrome. The *catastrophic reaction* first described by Goldstein (1939) is an emotional disorder appearing following stroke, characterized by excessive anger, despair, frustration, denial, and tearfulness. It is often associated with post-stroke depression and personal or family history of psychiatric disorders (Starkstein *et al.*, 1993b; Carota *et al.*, 2001). Catastrophic reaction is usually observed in patients with left hemisphere damage (Gainotti, 1972), and the lesion is often located in the anterior subcortical regions (Starkstein *et al.*, 1993b). Some authors suggested that catastrophic reaction is a behavioral symptom of depression in patients with anterior subcortical damage (Starkstein *et al.*, 1993b) while others attributed catastrophic reaction to a communication impairment related to damage to left hemispheric areas involved in emotional regulation and social communication (Carota *et al.*, 2001).

Pseudobulbar syndrome

The pseudobulbar syndrome (or *pseudobulbar palsy*) is common following stroke, observed in nearly 15% of patients (Andersen, 1999). The patient shows frequent and easily provoked spells of laughing or crying. The symptoms are usually appropriate to the context but in severe cases their occurrence is inappropriate. The symptoms often decline over time without any treatment. The pseudobulbar syndrome can be a cause of frustration and stigma for the patient and family.

Current theories on mental functions do not provide satisfactory explanations for emotional syndromes. Recently a novel interpretative framework has been proposed, based on neuropsychological experimental data on the "mirror system" which is thought to be relevant for the emotional part of human personality and behavior through imitative processes (Bodini *et al.*, 2004; Carmichael, 2004). Further studies may support this hypothesis.

Violent and aggressive behavior

Violent and aggressive behavior following stroke refers to antisocial personality traits following frontal lobe lesions. These observations report changes such as "poor impulse control, explosive aggressive outbursts, inappropriate verbal lewdness, jocularity, and lack of interpersonal sensitivity." Such dysregulation of affect and behavior may occur without major cognitive, motor, and sensory impairment. Blumer and Benson (1975) named this syndrome "pseudopsychopathy" owing to its similarities to the psychopathic personality, and Damasio (1994) called it "acquired sociopathy." This syndrome includes reactive or affective aggression, as opposed to instrumental aggression. In reactive aggression, a frustrating or threatening event without any potential goal triggers the aggressive act. In contrast, instrumental aggression or proactive aggression is a means to achieve a desired goal. Kim *et al.* (2002) found that 32% of a sample of 149 patients had an inability to control anger or aggression, suggesting that this dysregulation is one of the main post-stroke behavioral syndromes with depression and emotional incontinence.

Acquired damage to medial frontal and orbital frontal cortex is associated with increased risk of reactive aggression in humans (Grafman *et al.*, 1996). Interestingly, studies of primary personality disorders with dominant aggressive and impulsive behavior (mostly sociopathic or borderline personality disorders) have suggested the presence of brain dysfunctions consistent with those observed in post-stroke personality disorders (Herpertz *et al.*, 2001). Structural and functional neuroimaging studies of patients with personality disorders have revealed a dysfunction of a frontolimbic network involving the anterior cingulate cortex, the orbitofrontal and dorsolateral prefrontal cortex, the hippocampus, and the amygdala (Herpertz *et al.*, 2001). Such a network seems to mediate important aspects of personality disorder through a dysfunctional serotonin neurotransmission. Abnormal serotonin neurotransmission has been associated with disinhibited impulsive aggression and affect dysregulation in patients with a personality disorder. In addition, studies with emotional and stressful stimulation in personality disordered patients demonstrated a failure to activate the anterior cingulate cortex which is involved in affective control (Blair, 2004). Simultaneous limbic and prefrontal impairment has been suggested such that a weakening of prefrontal inhibitory control could contribute to amygdala hyperactivity (Blair, 2004).

Personality changes and the risk of poststroke depression

In addition to neurobiological and neuropsychological factors, psychological distress may increase the vulnerability to post-stroke depression. Experiencing post-stroke life through some personality trait like neuroticism may facilitate the onset of post-stroke depression and worsen the outcome. The way personality change after stroke is fully dependent of the location and size of the lesion, the psychosocial support, the quality of care as well as the subject's pre-stroke personality. Pre-existing personality disorders are at risk of post-stroke psychiatric disorders, mostly depression (Andersen *et al.*, 1995).

The importance of some personality characteristics on prognosis and improvement after a stroke is now established. A one-year prospective study has shown that patients with high neuroticism scores on the NEO five-factor inventory had a 4.6 times higher risk of developing post-stroke depression than did patients with low scores regardless of lesion location (Aben *et al.*, 2003). Neuroticism was the unique dimension of the five-factor model of personality to show a significant effect on the development of post-stroke depression. Neuroticism is defined as a stable disposition to experience psychological distress across time and situations consisting of negative emotions such as fear, anger, and frustration. However, it is not entirely clear whether the personality traits assessed one month after stroke reflect premorbid personality or personality change after stroke. The authors argue that their measures do not reflect a change in personality after stroke otherwise they would have observed a lesion location effect. These findings suggest that personality assessment may help to detect patients at risk of post-stroke depression early after stroke.

Assessment and outcome

Psychometric tools may help to complete the diagnosis and to reveal dominant traits of personality. Some of them have been documented in various brain pathologies: the Eysenck Personality Inventory (Harvey and Bryant, 1998), the Cloninger Temperament and Character Inventory (Flegr *et al.*, 2003), and the NEO five-factor inventory (Lannoo *et al.*, 1997). The NEO five-factor inventory is based on the five-factor model of personality defining five independent personality dimensions: neuroticism, extraversion, openness to new experiences, agreeableness, and conscientiousness. A study in a geriatric stroke population showed that the long-term functional outcome (activities of daily life) is predicted by extrovert personality (assessed using the Eysenck Personality Inventory) and active coping strategy (assessed from interviews on how the patients handle difficult events) (Elmstahl *et al.*, 1996). These results support the view that better knowledge of personality characteristics improves the possibility of setting up more individual rehabilitation programs.

Clinical diagnosis of a personality change imperatively requires a diachronic evaluation of the patients thinking, behavior, interaction, and functioning. It is important to exclude any axis-I diagnosis such as depression, mixed or hypomanic state, anxiety disorder, or psychotic disorder that would require specific treatments.

Key points Assessment of personality disorders

Diachronic evaluation of the patients thinking, behavior, interaction, and functioning
Exclusion of depression mixed or hypomanic states, anxiety disorders, or psychotic disorder
Scales: Eysenck personality inventory, Cloninger's temperament and character inventory,
   NEO-five factor inventory

Key points Management and treatment of personality disorders

Pharmacological agents: long-term efficiency remains to be established

When the pseudobulbar syndrome interferes with everyday life activities or complicates relationships with the family, pharmacotherapy must be considered. Some treatment studies have shown that the pseudobulbar syndrome improves with antidepressant treatment (nortryptilline and citalopram), raising the question of its relation with depression in a brain-damaged patient (Andersen *et al.*, 1993; Robinson *et al.*, 1993). Antidepressants, mood stabilisers, or antipsychotic treatments may improve pathological aggressiveness, impulsive behavior, and labile emotion. Conversely, the long-term efficiency of pharmacological agents on personality changes has not been established.

REFERENCES

Aben, I., Denollet, J., Lousberg, R., *et al.* (2003). Personality and vulnerability to depression in stroke patients. *Stroke*, **3**, 2391–5.

American Psychiatric Association DSM-IV TR: (2000). *Diagnostic and Statistical Manual of Mental Disorders*, 4th edn. Text Revision. American Psychiatric Association.

Andersen, G. (1999). Treatment of uncontrolled crying after stroke. *Drug Therapy*, **6**, 105–11.

Andersen, G., Vestergaard, K., Ingemann-Nielsen, M. and Lauritzen, L. (1995). Risk factors for post-stroke depression. *Acta Psychiatr. Scand.*, **92**, 193–8.

Andersen, G., Vestergaard, K. and Riis, J. (1993). Citalopram for poststroke pathological crying. *Lancet*, **342**, 837–9.

Blair, R. J. R. (2004). The roles of orbital frontal cortex in the modulation of antisocial behavior. *Brain, Cogn.*, **55**, 198–208.

Blumer, D. and Benson, D. F. (1975). Personality changes with frontal and temporal lobe lesions. In *Psychiatric Aspects of Neurological Disease*, ed. D. F. Benson and D. Blumer. New York: Grune & Stratton, pp. 151–170.

Bodini, B., Iacoboni, M. and Lenzi, G.L. (2004). Acute stroke effects on emotions: An interpretation through the mirror system. *Curr. Opin. Neurol.*, **17**, 55–60.

Carmichael, G. (2004). Left temporoparietal junction performs social reasoning. *Lancet Neurology*, **3**, 328.

Carota, A., Rosseti, A.O., Karapaianotides, T. and Bougousslavsky, J. (2001). Catastrophic reaction in acute stroke. A reflex behavior in aphasic patients. *Neurology*, **57**, 1902–5.

Cloninger, C.R., Svrakic, D.M. and Przybeck, T.R. (1993). A psychobiological model of temperament and character. *Arch. Gen. Psychiatry*, **50**, 975–90.

Damasio, A.R. (1994). *Descartes' Error: Emotion, Rationality and the Human Brain*. New York: Putnam Grosset Books.

Elmstahl, S., Sommer, M., Hagberg, B. (1996). A 3-year follow-up of stroke patients: Relationships between activities of daily living and personality characteristics. *Arch. Gerontol. Geriat.*, **22**, 233–44.

Flegr, J., Preiss, M., Klose, J., *et al.* (2003). Decreased level of psychobiological factor novelty seeking and lower intelligence in men latently infected with the protozoan parasite Toxoplasma gondii. Dopamine, a missing link between schizophrenia and toxoplasmosis? *Biol. Psychol.*, **63**, 253–68.

Gainotti, G. (1972). Emotional behavior and hemispheric side of the brain. *Cortex*, **8**, 41–55.

Goldstein, K. (1939). *The Organism*. New York: American Book.

Grafman, J., Schwab, K., Warden, D., Pridgen, B.S. and Brown, H.R. (1996). Frontal lobe injuries, violence, and aggression: A report of the Vietnam head injury study. *Neurology*, **46**, 1231–8.

Harlow, J.M. (1848). Passage of an iron rod through the head. *Boston Med. Surg. J.*, **39**, 389–93.

Harvey, A.G. and Bryant, R.A. (1998). Predictors of acute stress following mild traumatic brain injury. *Brain Inj.*, **12**, 147–54.

Herpertz, S.C., Dietrich, T.M., Wenning, B., *et al.* (2001). Evidence of abnormal amygdala functioning in borderline personality disorder: A functional MRI study. *Biol. Psychiatry*, **50**, 292–8.

Kattainen, A., Koskinen, S., Reunanen, A., *et al.* (2004). Impact of cardiovascular diseases on activity limitations and need for help among older persons. *J. Clin. Epidemiol.*, **57**, 82–8.

Kim, J.S., Choi, S., Kwon, S.U. and Seo, Y.S. (2002). Inability to control anger or aggression after stroke. *Neurology*, **58**, 1106–8.

Lannoo, E., de Deyne, C., Colardyn, F., de Soete, G. and Jannes, C. (1997). Personality change following head injury: Assessment with the NEO Five-Factor Inventory. *J. Psychosom. Res.*, **43**, 505–11.

Marin, R.S. (1990). Differential diagnosis and classification of apathy. *Am. J. Psychiatry*, **147**, 22–30.

Okada, K., Kobaiashi, S., Yamagata, S., Takahashi, K. and Yamaguchi, S. (1997). Poststroke apathy and regional cerebral blood flow. *Stroke*, **28**, 2437–41.

Robinson, R. G., Parikh, R. M., Lipsley, J. R. Starkstein, S. E. and Price, T. R. (1993). Pathological laughing and crying following stroke: Validation of a measurement scale and a double blind study. *Am. J. Psychiatry*, **150**, 286–93.

Starkstein, S. E., Fedoroff, J. P., Price, T. R., Leiguarda, R. and Robinson, R. G. (1993a). Apathy following cerebrovascular lesions. *Stroke*, **24**, 1625–30.

(1993b). Catastrophic reaction after cerebrovascular lesions. Frequency correlates and validation of a scale. *J. Neurol. Neurosurg. Psychiatry*, **5**, 189–94.

Youn, T., Lyoo, I. K., Kim, J. K., *et al.* (2002). Relationship between personality trait and regional cerebral glucose metabolism assessed with positron emission tomography. *Biol. Psychol.*, **60**, 109–20.

28

Post-stroke mania

Pierre Thomas

University Hospital, Lille, France

Introduction

Bipolar disorder is one of the two main types of mood disorder and has a strong pattern of inheritability. It concerns 1−5% of the general population (Baldessarini, 2002) and causes significant functional impairment and disability that affects the lives of patients and relatives. Suicide accounts for 18.9% of deaths in manic patients, contributing to the major mortality rate in untreated patients, higher than for many types of heart disorder and cancer (Goodwin and Jamison, 1990). The depressive phase represents one of the highest risk periods for suicide in bipolar disorder.

Mania is the unique hallmark of bipolar disorder, in contrast to unipolar (depressive) disorder. Thus the occurrence of a single episode of mania is sufficient to fit the criteria of bipolar disorder. According to the DSMIV-TR criteria (APA, 2000), a manic episode is defined as a distinct period during which patients experience abnormally and persistently raised expansive or irritable mood. Manic and hypomanic episodes have similar symptoms, but hypomanic episodes are not sufficiently severe to cause pronounced impairment in social or occupational functioning. A mixed episode is characterized by a period of at least 1 week in which the diagnosis criteria are fitted for both manic and major

Key points Main characteristic of mania

Mania: unique hallmark of bipolar disorder
    characterized by elevated, expansive, or irritable mood
    causes pronounced impairment in social or occupational functioning
Secondary mania:
    associated with general conditions and neurological lesions
    later age of onset
    outcome (including suicide risk) similar to that of primary mania

Table 28.1. DSM-IV-TR criteria for mood disorder due to a general medical condition

---

A. A prominent and persistent disturbance in mood predominates in the clinical picture and is characterized by either (or both) of the following:
    (1) depressed mood or markedly diminished interest or pleasure in all, or almost all, activities
    (2) elevated, expansive, or irritable mood
B. There is evidence from the history, physical examination, or laboratory findings that the disturbance is the direct physiological consequence of a general medical condition.
C. The disturbance is not better accounted for by another mental disorder (e.g., adjustment disorder in response to the stress of having a general medical condition).
D. The disturbance does not occur exclusively during the course of a delirium.
E. The symptoms cause clinically significant distress or impairment in social, occupational, or other important areas of functioning.
Specify type: according to the predominant mood
With depressive features
With major depressive-like episode
With manic features: if the predominant mood is elevated, euphoric, or irritable
With mixed features: if the symptoms of both mania and depression are present but neither predominates

---

depressive episodes. Mixed states are one of the most difficult forms to treat and carry an elevated risk of suicide. Bipolar mood swings may also take a more moderate form known as cyclothymia, comprising short and irregular cycles of activity and lethargy, pessimism and optimism, insomnia and oversleeping, involvement and indifference.

Comorbidities and the frequent association with substance abuse may complicate the diagnosis with confounding symptoms. An accurate diagnosis requires considering the patient and family history within the context of the number, severity, and duration of mood symptoms. Management of bipolar disorder relies on an accurate diagnosis and a long-term maintenance medication regimen (Daly, 1997).

Primary versus secondary mania

A large variety of general conditions, neurological lesions, or other states affecting brain functioning may induce secondary mania. An organic causation should be especially considered in the absence of a past or a family history of affective disorder. The DSM-IV TR has proposed the category of "Mood disorder due to a general medical condition," with manic, mixed, and depressive subtypes (Table 28.1).

Attempts to validate the primary—secondary distinction by clinical feature, biological factor, or treatment response have not been successful, with the exception of a later age of onset in secondary mania (Goodwin and Jamison, 1990). Thus primary and secondary first episodes of mania share similar outcomes in terms of mood morbidity, functioning, and suicide risk. An interesting approach is the spectrum model reflecting varying levels of vulnerability to the disorder (Akiskal *et al.*, 2000). The highest level of vulnerability favors the occurrence of primary mania with little or no external stress, and, according to a continuum, low level of vulnerability requires a major stressful event to trigger a manic episode (i.e. secondary mania).

Bipolar disorder and the brain

Recent studies have shown that individuals with bipolar disorder have some abnormalities. Neuroimaging studies using both computed tomography (CT) and magnetic resonance imaging (MRI) have revealed multiple unspecific structural abnormalities. Several studies have reported larger ventricles, smaller prefrontal lobe volumes, and larger volume of basal ganglia in patients with bipolar disorder (Strakowski *et al.*, 2002). MRI studies have revealed the high number of hyperintensities localized in the deep white matter (from 5—50%, compared with about 3% in age-matched controls (McDonald *et al.*, 1999). Studies in children and adolescents with mania continue to reveal an abundance of these white matter hyperintensities (Lyoo *et al.*, 2002; Pillai *et al.*, 2002). Their locations suggest they may disrupt communicating fibers between frontal and temporal regions, consistent with the observation of mania secondary to fronto-temporal lesions. The MRI changes in bipolar disorder are close, albeit more limited, to those of "Cerebral autosomal dominant arteriopathy with subcortical infarcts and leukoencephalopathy" (CADASIL). Interestingly, bipolar disorders are observed in CADASIL patients (Ahearn *et al.*, 2002).

Functional imaging studies showed that bipolar-depressed patients have significantly lower cortical metabolism than either controls or patients with unipolar depression (Baxter *et al.*, 1985; Buchsbaum *et al.*, 1986). Drevets *et al.*, (1997) have reported in depressed bipolar patients a decreased metabolism of the subgenual prefrontal cortex that did not alter with the remission of the episode. Convergently, studies with magnetic resonance imaging (MRI) provide indications of bilateral amygdala enlargement (Altshuler *et al.*, 1998; Strakowski *et al.*, 2002). Moreover, a functional MRI study has also reported dysfunction of the amygdala using an affect-recognition paradigm (Yurgelun-Todd *et al.*, 2000). These results provide convergent evidence of a dysfunction in prefrontal-limbic-subcortical circuitry underlying bipolar disorder (Berns *et al.*, 2003).

Post-stroke mania

Suspicion of a relationship between bipolar disorder and alteration in brain structure arose from the clinical observation that some brain lesions resulted in manic-like behavior. Kraepelin noted in 1921 an association between cerebrovascular disease and manic depressive illness. Many case reports have described manic states following stroke (Cumming and Mendez, 1984). However, mania remains a rare complication of stroke, observed in approximately 1% of patients (Huffman and Stern, 2003). This low frequency contrasts with the high prevalence of post-stroke depression. Thus only a few studies examining clinical and treatment specificity have been reported.

Symptoms of post-stroke mania are usually similar to those of primary mania, featuring a combination of major symptoms: thought acceleration, pressured speech and motor agitation, sleep disturbance, and social or sexual disinhibition. Cook et al. (1987) observed that manic patients with brain lesions were more assaultive and irritable and presented more mixed states rather than pure mania when compared with primary manic patients. In contrast to primary mania, some patients may suffer from lacunar amnesia of the manic episode, especially when the lesion includes the thalamus (Cummings and Mendez, 1984). In addition, the symptom duration is longer (2–4 months) in the majority of reported cases as compared to primary mania where the treatment related improvement usually occurs within one month.

Post-stroke mania should be differentiated from the agitation of acute delirium, and from the hyperkinetic state due to movement disorders, which may be associated with mania. The frequent association with movement disorders, such as hyperkinetic movement disorders or parkinsonism, is accounted for by the prominence of basal ganglia lesions responsible for mania. The severity of movement disorders sometimes varies as a function of mood polarity with the improvement of parkinsonism during manic switches (Bertier et al., 1996). Other symptoms require specific cares, like comorbid anxiety, catatonia of the agitated type, or psychotic symptoms (Robinson and Starkstein, 1997). Alcohol and other substance abuse are important comorbid conditions, and they worsen mania and its outcome.

A first episode of mania due to structural brain damage may show less association with prior vulnerability. Patients with personal or familial past history of bipolar disorders including cyclothymic temperaments could be at risk for post-stroke mania, since higher rates of affective disorders have been found in patients or family members (Robinson et al., 1988). However, it remains unclear whether post-stroke mania is a manifestation of bipolar spectrum vulnerability or is a secondary consequence of the lesion.

Stroke associated with mania

Lesions associated with mania involve more commonly the frontal and temporal lobes, the head of the caudate nucleus, and the thalamus (Cummings and Mendez, 1984; Starkstein *et al.*, 1991). It has been suggested that lesions of the left frontal lobe result in depression, whereas right fronto-temporal lesions produce mania. However, these generalizations about laterality are far too simplistic, and many exceptions have been observed.

Robinson (1998) observed that 8 of 9 patients (89%) with post-stroke mania had a right hemisphere lesion whereas only 7 of 31 (23%) patients with post-stroke depression had a right hemisphere lesion. When post-stroke patients with mania were compared to patients matched for lesion size and location, the manic patients had significantly greater subcortical atrophy as indicated by increased ventricular to brain ratios (Starkstein *et al.*, 1987). These findings suggest that post-stroke mania depends on the presence of two factors: (1) a predisposing factor being either genetic loading or subcortical atrophy, and (2) a lesion of specific cortico-limbic pathway involving the right hemisphere (Starkstein and Robinson, 1989). This combination is rare and this may explain the low prevalence of post-stroke mania.

Most patients suffer from lesions of the non-dominant hemisphere (Fenn and George, 1999), although cases with left brain damage have been reported (Liu *et al.*, 1996). Manic disorders in stroke patients without any personal or familial history of affective disorders result mainly from right orbito-frontal, basotemporal, basal ganglia, or thalamus lesions (Robinson *et al.*, 1988; Cumming and Mendez, 1984; Starkstein *et al.*, 1990). Manic-like behavior with grandiose delusional theme was described in eight patients who had lesions involving the right caudate nucleus and the medio- and baso-temporal regions (Starkstein *et al.*, 1990). Vuilleumier *et al.* (1998) discussed the relationship between right hemisphere lesions and deficit in processing emotions and manic disorders. Since ventral brain regions are connected to dorsal regions through visuospatial and somatosensory functions, any deficit of heteromodal ventral brain areas (basotemporal or orbitofrontal cortices) may result in a deregulation of motor, instinctive affective, and intellectual behavior (Starkstein and Robinson, 1997).

Key points Strokes responsible for mania

Post-stroke mania depends on the presence of two factors:
– a predisposing factor (genetic loading or subcortical atrophy)
– a lesion of specific corticolimbic pathway involving the right hemisphere
Lesion involving the right caudate nucleus, thalamic and fronto-temporal regions

Treatment and outcome

Mania interferes with the rehabilitation program, through inappropriate appraisal, unadjusted coping, and poor compliance. Manic states following stroke are often difficult to treat. Brain damage as well as comorbidities may enhance adverse effects and inefficiency of some antimanic agents. Rates of non-compliance up to 64% have been reported for any form of bipolar disorder (Colom *et al.*, 2000; Lingam and Scott, 2002). Non-compliance is the most frequent cause of recurrence during treatment (Colom *et al.*, 2000) and is associated with high morbidity and mortality rates (Schou, 1997). The mortality rate for late-onset bipolar disorder exceeds that of the community (Evans *et al.*, 1995).

Before prescribing any treatment, iatrogenic causes have to be excluded. Psycho-stimulants or antidepressants previously prescribed for a depressive disorder may have destabilized patients' mood by switching them into manic or mixed states. Decreased sleep duration and insomnia should systematically be assessed and treated.

Open studies of post-stroke mania have found lithium, valproate, carbamazepine, antipsychotics, clonazepam, and clonidine to be effective in some case reports (Huffman and Stern, 2003; Starkstein *et al.*, 1991; Bakchine *et al.*, 1989). Most of these treatments have sedative effects. Lithium should not be the first-intention treatment because it has a narrow therapeutic index and a high frequency of adverse effects. In addition, stroke may increase the sensitivity to

Key points Assessment

> Major symptoms: thought acceleration, pressured speech, and motor agitation associated with social or sexual drive disturbance
> Assessment also includes:
> decreased sleep duration and insomnia
> comorbid anxiety, catatonia of the agitated type, or psychotic symptoms
> alcohol and other substance abuse

Key points Management and treatment

> Avoid or stop antidepressant previously prescribed
> Treatment of insomnia and comorbidities
> Anticonvulsant mood stabilizers (valproate or carbamazepine): preferred to lithium
> Full recovery to be achieved (long duration frequent)

lithium neurotoxicity (Evans *et al.*, 1995). Anticonvulsant mood stabilizers (valproate or carbamazepine) are preferred to lithium in mania due to general medical conditions (Evans *et al.*, 1995). Full recovery from mania has to be achieved because the persistence of residual symptoms is a leading cause of recurrence and disability. The treatment has to be prolonged in most cases, because of the longer duration (2–4 months) of post-stroke mania.

REFERENCES

Ahearn, E. P., Speer, M. C., Chen, Y. T., *et al.* (2002). Investigation of Notch3 as a candidate gene for bipolar disorder using brain hyperintensities as an endophenotype. *Am. J. Med. Genet.*, **114**, 652–8.

Akiskal, H. S., Bourgeois, M. L., Angst, J., *et al.* (2000). Re-evaluating the prevalence of and diagnostic composition within the broad clinical spectrum of bipolar disorders. *J. Affect. Disord.*, **59**, 5–30.

Altshuler, L. L., Bartzokis, G., Grieder, T., Curran, J. and Mintz, J. (1998). Amygdala enlargement in bipolar disorder and hippocampal reduction in schizophrenia: An MRI study demonstrating neuroanatomic specificity. *Arch. Gen. Psychiatry*, **55**, 663–4.

American Psychiatric Association DSMIV TR (2000). *Diagnostic and Statistical Manual of Mental Disorders*, 4th edn. Text Revision. American Psychiatric Association.

Bakchine, S., Lacomblez, L., Benoit, N., *et al.* (1989). Manic-like state after bilateral orbito-frontal and right temporoparietal injury: Efficacy of clonidine. *Neurology*, **39**, 777–81.

Baldessarini, R. J. (2002) Treatment research in bipolar disorder: Issues and recommendations. *CNS Drugs*, **16**, 721–9.

Baxter, L. R., Jr., Phelps, M. E., Mazziotta, J. C., *et al.* (1985). Cerebral metabolic rates for glucose in mood disorders. Studies with positron emission tomography and fluorodeoxyglucose F 18. *Arch. Gen. Psychiatry*, **42**, 441–7.

Berns, G. S., Charles, B. and Nemeroff, C. B. (2003). The neurobiology of bipolar disorder. *Am. J. Med. Genet.*, **123**, 76–84.

Bertier, M. L., Kulisewski, J., Gironell, A. and Fernandez-Benitez, J. A. (1996). Postroke bipolar affective disorders: Clinical subtypes, concurrent movement disorders and anatomical correlates. *J. Neuropsychiatry Clin. Neurosci.*, **8**, 160–7.

Buchsbaum, M. S., Wu, J., DeLisi, L. E., *et al.* (1986). Frontal cortex and basal ganglia metabolic rates assessed by positron emission tomography with 18F 2-deoxyglucose in affective illness. *J. Affect. Disord.*, **10**, 137–52.

Colom, F., Vieta, E., Martinez-Aran, A., *et al.* (2000). Clinical factors associated with treatment noncompliance in euthymic bipolar patients. *J. Clin. Psychiatry*, **61**, 549–55.

Cook, B. L., Shukla, S., Hoff, A. L. and Aronson, T. A. (1987). Mania with associated organic factors. *Acta Psychiatr. Scand.*, **76**, 674–7.

Cummings, J. L. and Mendez, M. F. (1984). Secondary mania with focal cerebral lesions. *Am. J. Psychiatry*, **141**, 1084–7.

Daly, I. (1997). Mania. *Lancet*, **349**, 1157–60.

Drevets, W. C., Price, J. L., Simpson, J. R., Jr., *et al.* (1997). Subgenual prefrontal cortex abnormalities in mood disorders. *Nature*, **24**, 824–7.

Evans, D. L., Byerly, M. G. and Greer, R. A. (1995) Secondary mania. Diagnosis and treatment. *J. Clin. Psychiatry*, **56**, 31–7.

Fenn, D. and George, K. (1999). Poststroke mania late in life involving the left hemisphere. *J. Psychiatry*, **33**, 598–600.

Goodwin, F. K. and Jamison, K. R. (1990). *Manic-Depressive Illness*. Oxford: Oxford University Press.

Huffman, J. and Stern, T. A. (2003). Acute psychiatric manifestation of stroke; a clinical case conference. *Psychosomatics*, **44**, 65–75.

Lingam, R. and Scott, J. (2002). Treatment non-adherence in affective disorders. *Acta Psychiatr. Scand.*, **105**, 164–172.

Liu, C. Y., Wang, S. J., Fuh, J. L., Yang, Y. Y. and Liu, H. C. (1996). Bipolar disorder following stroke involving the left hemisphere. *J. Psychiatry*, **30**, 688–91.

Lyoo, I. K., Lee, H. K., Jung, J. H., Noam, G. G. and Renshaw, P. F. (2002). White matter hyperintensities on magnetic resonance imaging of the brain in children with psychiatric disorders. *Compre. Psychiatry*, **43**, 361–8.

McDonald, W. M., Tupler, L. A., Marsteller, F. A., *et al.* (1999). Hyperintense lesions on magnetic resonance images in bipolar disorder. *Biol. Psychiatry*, **45**, 965–71.

Pillai, J. J., Friedman, L., Stuve, T. A., *et al.* (2002). Increased presence of white matter hyperintensities in adolescent patients with bipolar disorder. *Psychiatry Res.*, **114**, 51–6.

Robinson, R. G. (1998). *The Clinical Neuropsychiatry of Stroke*. Cambridge, UK: Cambridge University Press.

Robinson, R. G., Boston, J. D., Starkstein, S. E. and Price, T. R. (1988). Comparison of mania and depression after brain injury: Causal factors. *Am. J. Psychiatry*, **145**, 172–8.

Robinson, R. G. and Starkstein, S. E. (1997). Neuropsychiatric aspects of cerebrovascular disorders. In *The American Psychiatric Press Textbook of Neuropsychiatry*, ed. Hales, R. E. and Yudofsky, S. C. Washington DC: American Psychiatric Press, pp. 607–633.

Schou, M. (1997). Forty years of lithium treatment. *Arch. Gen. Psychiatry*, **54**, 9–15.

Starkstein, S. E. and Robinson, R. G. (1989). Affective disorders and cerebrovascular disease. *Br. J. Psychiatry*, **154**, 170–82.

Starkstein, S. E., Pearlson, G. D. and Robinson, R. G. (1987). Mania after brain injury. A controlled study of etiological factors. *Arch. Neurol.*, **44**, 1069–73.

Starkstein, S. E., Fedoroff, P., Berthier, M. L. and Robinson, R. G. (1991). Manic depressive and pure manic states after brain lesion. *Biol. Psychiatry*, **29**, 149–58.

Starkstein, S. E., Mayberg, H. S. and Berthier, M. L. (1990). Mania after brain injury. Neuroradiological and metabolic findings. *Ann. Neurol.*, **27**, 652–9.

Starkstein, S. E. and Robinson, R. G. (1997). Mechanism of disinhibition after brain lesions. *J. Nerv. Men. Dis.*, **185**, 108–14.

Strakowski, S. M., DelBello, M. P., Zimmerman, M. E., *et al.* (2002). Ventricular and periventricular structural volumes in first- versus multiple-episode bipolar disorder. *Am. J. Psychiatry*, **159**, 1841 –7.

Vuilleumier, P., Ghika-Schmid, F., Bogousslavski, J., Assal, G. and Regli, F. (1998). Persistant recurrence of hypomania and prosopoaffective agnosia in a patient with right thalamic infarct. *Neuropsychiatry Neuropsychol. Behav. Neurol.*, **11**, 40–4.

Yurgelun-Todd, D. A., Gruber, S. A., Kanayama, G., *et al.* (2000). fMRI during affect discrimination in bipolar affective disorder. *Bipolar Disord.*, **2**, 237–48.

29

Depression after stroke

Antonio Carota[1] and Stefano Paolucci[2]

[1]CHUV, Lausanne, Switzerland
[2]IRCCS Fondazione Santa Lucia, Rome, Italy

Diagnosis of depression after stroke

Depression occurring after stroke (post-stroke depression, PSD) has been the object of many clinical studies (about 300 during the last 30 years). We will review the available data and discuss the clinical implications of the research conducted to date.

Key points Main characteristics of PSD

DSM-IV criteria are adopted for diagnosis of PSD, even if they are subject to some criticism.
Whether PSD is a different disease from ED, and whether major and minor depressions differ in neurobiological causes, remain unresolved issues.
To reduce disability, caregiver burden, and costs, diagnosis and treatment of PSD should be considered, when possible, in the early phases of stroke.
The prevalence of a depressive episode occurring within 6—12 months after stroke onset is high (globally estimated to be about 30%), albeit with marked variability among studies.
The severity of the neurological deficit is the risk factor that has most clinical relevance. On the other hand, all individuals with stroke should be evaluated for PSD even when several years have elapsed since onset.
Pathogenesis of PSD, diagnosed according to DSM-IV criteria, is multifactorial.
The link between lesion location and PSD pathogenesis remains unproven.
The role of psychodynamic factors should be carefully evaluated in the individual patient and in clinical studies.
Even if suicide is infrequent, patients with PSD should be assessed for suicidal ideas.
PSD has a very negative impact on functional autonomy of stroke patients.
Treatment of PSD should be started promptly in an attempt to reduce the unfavorable effect of PSD on rehabilitation.
Recovery is considered significant when it corresponds to a reduction of HDRS or BDI scores by 50% or more.
Pharmacological treatment may improve the degree of functional outcome but not equalize it for PSD+ and PSD− subgroups.
Treatment of PSD may improve cognitive functioning.
Treatment of PSD may reduce the risk of mortality in stroke victims.

Patients should be evaluated for PSD in the acute phase (Berg *et al.*, 2001) in the first few months after stroke onset (Pohjasvaara *et al.*, 1998), and before transfer in rehabilitation grounds (Paolucci *et al.*, 1999; Gillen *et al.*, 2001), to reduce disability, caregiver burden, and costs.

Diagnostic criteria

Key points Assessment of depression in stroke

PSD diagnosis of a depressive episode using the DSM-IV criteria requires at least two weeks of persistence of symptoms.

Cognitive (aphasia, attention, memory, and executive disorders), behavioral (apathy, emotionalism), psychiatric (anxiety), and other physical changes (immobilization, dysphagia, fatigue) can make the assessment of PSD difficult.

For diagnosing PSD scales and questionnaires have proved valuable instruments. The use of scales and questionnaires is specifically required to monitor therapeutic interventions.

In patients with aphasia PSD should be assessed with non-verbal measurements and with interviews of significant others.

PSD is a clinical diagnosis and should be reached by a multidimensional approach (interview with the patient, family, caregivers, and medical staff; analysis of the pre-morbid history, daily life, and social activities; observation of patient's behaviors in different contexts; detailed cognitive examination, validated mood questionnaires).

The DSM-IV-TR (American Psychiatric Association, 2001) defines universally adopted diagnostic criteria (Table 29.1). These criteria correspond to depression occurring with chronic medical conditions (e.g. chronic heart failure, hyperthyroidism, and others), including stroke. The only feature distinguishing PSD from endogenous depression (ED) is a persistent depressed mood that is judged to be due to the direct physiological effects of a general medical condition. The ICD-10 diagnostic criteria for an organic depressive disorder are comparable to DSM-IV criteria.

DSM-IV diagnostic criteria for a major depressive episode require the persistence of symptoms for at least two weeks. Thus, in many cases PSD cannot be formally diagnosed in an acute care setting. Common criteria notwithstanding, PSD can be overdiagnosed if too much emphasis is given to depressive equivalents (vegetative signs and cognitive slowing) that are related to the stroke itself. On the other hand, PSD diagnosis may be underestimated by non-psychiatric medical professionals. In a clinical study performed in the rehabilitation ward on a sample of 15 stroke victims, a questionnaire filled out by patients showed 50% to be suffering from PSD (Schubert *et al.*, 1992). Psychiatrists diagnosed 68% of the patients with PSD. But much more striking,

Table 29.1. DSM-IV diagnostic criteria

With depressive features – the predominant mood is depressed, but not all criteria for a
  major depressive episode are met
With major depressive-like episodes
A. At least five of the following symptoms are present over at least a 2-week period; at least
    one of the symptoms is either a depressed mood or loss of interest or pleasure
    1. Depressed mood most of the day
    2. Markedly decreased interest or pleasure
    3. Significant weight loss or weight gain
    4. Insomnia or hypersomnia
    5. Psychomotor agitation or retardation
    6. Fatigue or loss of energy
    7. Feelings of worthlessness or excessive or inappropriate guilt
    8. Diminished ability to think or concentrate
    9. Recurrent thoughts of death
B. Distress or impairment of social, occupational, or other functioning
C. No bereavement
With manic features – the predominant mood is elevated, euphoric, or irritable
With mixed features – symptoms of both mania and depression are present, but neither
  predominates

when psychiatrists were excluded from the medical team, the remaining medical
professionals diagnosed none of the patients as suffering from PSD.

Specificity of PSD

The DSM-IV criteria are based on the assumption that a unique postulate exists
for all the depressive syndromes. The DSM-IV defines a unique depressive
dimension where all the qualitative attributes of depression (dysthymia,
melancholia, anhedonia, reactive and non-reactive depression) are represented
in a continuum with different degrees of severity. Within this unidimensional
perspective, similarities and differences of symptoms between PSD and endogenous depression (ED) and baseline personality traits (depressive temperament,
neuroticism, and emotional dyscontrol) are irrelevant to diagnosis. As a consequence it is unclear why a presupposed etiological factor for PSD (e.g. stroke)
should exclude the diagnosis of a depressive disorder related to ED.

Furthermore, DSM-IV symptom criteria for PSD involve somatic conditions
(fatigue, sleep disturbances) and cognitive complaints that are also frequent in
non-depressed stroke patients. For instance, both depression and subcortical
dysfunction have apathy or loss of interest as behavioral correlates. Slowness of
speech and/or thinking may be depressive equivalents or represent a deficit in
cognitive processing.

Gainotti *et al.* (1999) considered that "non-reactive" or "unmotivated" aspects of the depressed mood (e.g. feelings of worthlessness, guilt, and suicidal ideation) together with morning aggravation of symptoms are specific for ED, whereas "reactive" or "motivated" aspects (low mood, reduced appetite, anergia), anxiety, and vegetative signs characterize PSD. According to these authors, the "unmotivated" aspects are related to neurobiological factors whereas the "motivated" symptoms are the result of a psychological reaction to disability (Gainotti *et al.*, 1999). Comparing 20 PSD with 41 ED patients, Beblo and Driessen (2002) found more physical signs in patients with PSD but not anhedonia, cyclic, or ideational disturbances. On the other hand, other studies showed that when somatic or autonomic symptoms were excluded from analysis, the prevalence of PSD was not significantly reduced (Fedoroff *et al.*, 1991; Paradiso *et al.*, 1997). Another strong argument for PSD and ED as overlapping diseases is that both conditions respond to the same classes of antidepressant drugs (serotonine-reuptake inhibitors and tricyclic antidepressants).

The DSM-IV distinction between "major" and "minor" forms of PSD is a further subject of debate. The DSM-IV diagnosis of a "major depressive-like episode" is based on the existence of five or more of these depressive symptoms, two of which must be depressed mood and a loss of interest and pleasure in almost all activities. "Minor depression" is defined as a less severe form of depression with the presence of at least two, but fewer than five, of the symptoms of major depression, including either depressed mood or loss of interest. The DSM-IV distinction between major and minor depression seems reasonable and clinically adequate for both PSD and ED (Paradiso and Robinson, 1999), but it is uncertain if the two forms correspond to different etiologies and outcomes. The distinction between major and minor forms of PSD has been configured in terms of the "continuum" versus the "categorical" hypothesis. The "continuum hypothesis" posits that major and minor forms of PSD are two expressions of the same disease, only differing in the severity of symptoms on a continuous gradient (Gainotti *et al.*, 1997a). This continuity may correspond, for both forms, to a psychological reaction that parallels the degree of disability. The "continuum hypothesis" has therefore a psychodynamic foundation. The "categorical" hypothesis considers that major and minor forms of PSD have different etiologies (related to stroke location for major PSD), and that the etiological difference is important in treating the disorder (Morris *et al.*, 1994).

Scales and questionnaires

Scales and questionnaires, based on the DSM-IV criteria, are important clinical tools because they allow monitoring of the effects of therapeutic interventions and they engender reproducible diagnoses allowing meaningful comparisons among the different studies.

The Hamilton Depression Rating Scale (HDRS) (Hamilton, 1960) is the most widely used. It is a semi-structured interview consisting of 21 items, variably rated (0−2 or 0−4). In patients with ED, a score 7−17 corresponds to mild depression, 18−24 to moderate depression and >24 to severe depression (Endicott *et al.*, 1981).

The Beck Depression Inventory (BDI) (Beck *et al.*, 1961) is a self-rating scale including 21 items, which are rated 0−3. This scale has excellent validity compared with HDRS but poorly evaluates somatic symptoms. Significant scores are: 0−13, minimal or no depression; 14−19, mild depression; 20−29, moderate depression; and 29−63, severe depression. A short version of this scale, consisting of 13 items, is also available.

The Hospital Anxiety and Depression Scale (HADS) (Zigmond and Snaith, 1983) has several advantages. It is a self-rating short scale (14 items), assesses both depression and anxiety, and is very easy to complete for elderly persons or patients with chronic medical conditions. Scores are similar for both anxiety and depression: 8−10, doubtful cases; >11, presence of the disease.

The Zung Self-Rating Depression Scale (ZSDS) (20 items; Zung, 1965) is a self-rating scale with characteristics very similar to the HADS.

The Montgomery−Asberg Depression Rating Scale (MADRS) (Montgomery and Asberg, 1979) includes 10 items, rated 0−6. Significant scores are: 6 or less, absence of depression; 6−34, mild or moderate depression; 35 or above, severe depression. The MADRS shows a greater sensitivity to change and its capacity to differentiate between those who respond to antidepressant treatment and those who do not may be better than with HDRS and BDI.

Gainotti and colleagues created the Post-Stroke Depression Scale (Gainotti *et al.*, 1997a) to evaluate depressive symptoms (especially somatic symptoms) or other conditions (e.g. the catastrophic reaction or emotionalism) considered specific to patients with stroke in comparison to patients with ED without brain damage. The scale, filled in by the examiner, evaluates ten different symptoms, each scored between 0 (absence) and 5 (maximal severity). In the last section, the depressed mood is scored between minus 2 (non-motivated depression prevailing in the morning) and plus 2 (depression related to severe disability). For the depressed mood, feelings of guilt, and suicidal ideas, the patient must indicate if these symptoms are related or not to the consequences of stroke. The scale does not supply cutoffs for the presence of a depressive disorder but provides a clinical profile of depression.

The Stroke Aphasic Depression Questionnaire (Sutcliffe and Lincoln, 1998) and the modified Analogue Dysphoria Scale (Stern and Bachman, 1991) could be useful tools for assessment of depression in patients with aphasia. They evaluate depressive symptoms (including eating and sleep disturbances) with verbal and non-verbal items together with the caregivers' reports.

The Visual Analog Mood Scale (VAMS) (Arruda et al., 1999) requires the patient to show which of the two stylized faces (sad or happy) on a vertical line (to avoid neglect inferences) better represents their mood or feelings. Clinical utility of VAMS is controversial because even these non-verbal measurements require verbal cues and instructions to some extent, and because the responses remain unreliable even for a significant number of patients without aphasia (Price et al., 1999).

Even if standardized questionnaires of depression have been shown to have concurrent validity for ED and PSD (Agrell and Dehlin, 1989; Aben et al., 2002a), there is evidence that lower cutoff scores may be more adequate for PSD in comparison to ED (Naarding et al., 2002) but these data are not universally agreed (Lincoln et al., 2003).

Stroke confounders

Evaluating depression in stroke patients may be particularly difficult because of the clinical features due to the stroke itself. The main problem is that neurobehavioral changes due to stroke may compromise the validity of patients' answers during a psychiatric interview. Even when language and attention are not impaired, patients may still fail to respond in a reliable fashion (Toedter et al., 1995; Price et al., 1999). Therefore the validity of replies of patients in psychiatric interviews should be accurately evaluated and documented.

Thus it is essential that healthcare professionals evaluating a patient for PSD carefully consider whether a "depressed response" might instead be a neurological symptom (Table 29.2).

The assessment of mood in patients with memory and/or executive dysfunction requires a detailed cognitive examination. Psychiatric interviews of patients with anosognosia for hemiparesis may be particularly difficult because they could express behavioral correlates of depression while verbally denying mood changes (Biran and Chatterjee, 2003). The degree of anosognosia for hemiparesis can be quantified by clinical criteria (Bisiach et al., 1986) and by structured clinical interviews (Marcel et al., 2004). Other questionnaires (Cummings et al., 1994; Sherer et al., 1998) also including reports of relatives, spouses, and significant others can be useful to assess and quantify an impairment of self-awareness that has a more general significance than anosognosic for hemiparesis.

Patients with affective dysprosodia, while talking, give the false impression of a lack of affection and are often considered depressed, even when they are not. Informally recorded interviews of patients or standardized tests such as the Florida

Table 29.2. Diagnostic confounders of depression in stroke

INDIRECT

Common to many severely ill hospitalized patients

Controlled appetite (e.g. NPO and tube feeding)

Frequently awakened

Confined to bed

Delirium (acute confusional states)

Of special concern in stroke patients

Immobility (potential confusion with apathy)

Dysphagia (interferes with eating habits)

Slurred speech (and resultant miscommunication)

Fatigue

DIRECT

Aphasia

Amnesia and cognitive impairment

Anosognosia

Aprosody

Neurological apathy syndromes

    Isolated abulia/apathia

    Loss of psychic auto-activation

Frontal lobe syndrome

    Klüver-Bucy syndrome

    Korsakoff's syndrome

Poststroke fatigue

Disorders of emotional expression

Pseudobulbar syndrome

Emotional lability or emotionalism

Catastrophic reaction

Dementia

Affect Battery (Blonder *et al.*, 1991) help in evaluating dysprosodia and recognition of facial and vocal expressions.

Apathy and depression are highly correlated in patients with ED but apathy may be present without depression in patients with stroke, Alzheimer's (Levy *et al.*, 1998) and vascular dementia. Structured interviews, such as the Apathy Scale (Starkstein *et al.*, 1993a) and the Apathy Evaluation Scale (Marin *et al.*, 1991) can be useful in distinguishing apathy from depression.

Fatigue is reported by up to 70% of stroke patients, even at a considerable time after stroke, and is often independent from depressive feelings, neurological deficits, and lesion location. The Fatigue Impact Scale helps in characterizing this symptom and its causes (Ingles *et al.*, 1999). The recognition of fatigue and its differentiation from PSD may be critical for therapeutical interventions.

Athymhormia or "loss of self psychic activation" refers to lack of motivation, to apathetic, unspontaneous, and indifferent behavior, reversible under repeated stimulation, and to motor and affective drive loss without anxiety or suffering. Athymhormia can be assessed by special interviews (Habib, 1995) and is generally consequent to ischemic focal lesions, involving (often bilaterally) the rostral part of the caudate nucleus, the pallidum, the putamen, the thalamus, and the gyrus cinguli.

Pathological crying, emotionalism, and catastrophic reactions in stroke patients should be differentiated from PSD because they are disorders of emotional expression rather than primary disturbances of feelings.

Pathological crying indicates reflex crying or laughing occurring even after neutral stimuli (not sad) and without congruence of internal affects (no sadness). This condition is usually associated with other pseudobulbar signs and is the consequence of bilateral lesions along the corticobulbar tracts.

Emotionalism or "emotional incontinence" refers to crying or laughing, starting with little or no warning, generally after congruent stimuli (sad) and inducing subjective feelings (sadness). After stroke, patients with emotionalism are less able to control crying or weeping, which often causes embarrassment in social contexts. A specific link between lesion location and the emergence of emotionalism has not yet been demonstrated. The underlying abnormality may be serotoninergic, and, as well for PSD, symptoms might notably improve with selective serotonine reuptake inhibitors (SSRIs) (Jeret, 1997; Nahas *et al.*, 1998). The Pathological Crying and Laughing Scale is a questionnaire constructed for screening and quantifying emotionalism and pathological crying/laughing (Robinson *et al.*, 1993b).

Catastrophic reaction presents as a disruptive emotional behavior (crying, aggressiveness, escaping) when the patient is confronted with an unsolvable task (e.g. writing for an aphasic, moving the arm for a hemiplegic patient). In the early and late phases of stroke, this reaction is generally associated with left hemisphere stroke and aphasia (Gainotti, 1972; Starkstein *et al.*, 1993b; Kim and Choi-Kwon, 2000; Carota *et al.*, 2001).

Even if emotionalism and catastrophic reactions are distinct from depression, patients with these disorders should be considered at risk for developing PSD (Kim and Choi-Kwon, 2000).

In stroke victims, other neuropsychiatric symptoms, such as anxiety, personality changes, obsessive–compulsive disorder, mania, eating and sleep disorders, can manifest themselves in isolation or in association with PSD (Angelelli *et al.*, 2004). As their repercussion on morbidity could be relevant, they should be specifically searched for when patients are assessed for PSD. The Neuropsychiatric Inventory (NPI; Cummings *et al.*, 1994), an informant-based questionnaire, provides a careful profile of both neuropsychiatric changes in stroke patients together with the impact of these changes on activities of daily living (Angelelli *et al.*, 2004).

Epidemiology and risk factors

Because of methodological differences among clinical studies (e.g. timing and contexts of investigation, exclusion of patients with aphasia or other cognitive deficits, structured interviews used for PSD diagnosis), available data are heterogeneous. PSD prevalence varies between 6–22% in the first 2 weeks, 22–53% at 3–4 months, 16–47% at 1 year, 19% at 2 years, 9–41% at 3 years, 35% at 4.9 years, and 19% at 7 years. Prevalence is higher (30–55%) in rehabilitation centers (Provinciali and Coccia, 2002; Turner-Stokes and Hassan, 2002). Major depression accounts for up to 56% of stroke patients, whereas minor depression has a prevalence of about 15%. The following are considered risk factors for developing PSD: patient aged below 65 years (Eriksson *et al.*, 2004); female (Herrmann *et al.*, 1998; Paolucci *et al.*, 1999; Eriksson *et al.*, 2004); history of prior depression (Andersen *et al.*, 1995; Ng *et al.*, 1995); history of previous stroke (Andersen *et al.*, 1995; Kim *et al.*, 2002; Eriksson *et al.*, 2004); psychosocial problems (Andersen *et al.*, 1995; Eriksson *et al.*, 2004); high level of education (Paolucci *et al.*, 1999); disability (Singh *et al.*, 2000); living in an institution (Eriksson *et al.*, 2004).

In women, major depression seems to correlate with a high level of education, the degree of cognitive impairment, and the presence of psychiatric antecedents. In men, major depression seems to be more related to the severity of physical impairment (Paradiso and Robinson, 1998). Indeed, minor PSD could be more frequent in men and be correlated with inadequate spousal or social support (Morris *et al.*, 1992a).

Pathophysiology

In the last 30 years, many clinical studies have been carried out to improve knowledge of PSD pathophysiology. These studies mostly attempted to verify the role of lesion location, using neuroradiological images (MRI and CT scans) to compare a group of stroke patients with PSD with a group without PSD. Unfortunately, the great number of variables involved, selection bias, and methodological problems compromised the validity of both positive and negative findings. The only conclusion from the available data is that the pathophysiology of PSD is still poorly understood. Even if PSD is certainly a multifactorial disorder, major insight into the role of biological and psychological mechanisms remains an important field of research in neurosciences, as it could lead to finding more appropriate therapeutic interventions.

Attempts to correlate PSD with lesion localization

One of the most intriguing working hypotheses is that brain areas involved in PSD are equally implicated in ED. These regions could be part of, and connected to, the limbic system and other brain areas processing mood and emotions for enhancing or inhibiting behaviors.

Mesial temporal lobe hypoperfusion was found with brain SPECT imaging in a group of depressed patients with subcortical lesions, but not in a non-depressed group with similar lesion location, suggesting that the involvement of the temporal lobe may be critical for the occurrence of PSD (Grasso *et al.*, 1994). The basal ganglia are also part of the neural pathways underlying motor or behavioral responses to emotional stimuli or affects. Several studies suggested the role of the basal ganglia in the development of PSD (Herrmann *et al.*, 1995; Lauterbach *et al.*, 1997) but not all (Sato *et al.*, 1999). The low incidence of depression with brainstem and cerebellar lesions supports the etiological role of anterior brain regions (anterior and middle cerebral artery vascular territories).

Localization theories

A large number of clinical studies by Robinson and colleagues (reviewed in Robinson, 1998) have suggested that frontal, subcortical, and basal ganglia lesions may play a causal role in PSD.

The main hypothesis was that a lesion in the left hemisphere and its proximity to the frontal pole are the most important variables related to the occurrence of a major depressive episode after stroke. Damage of the biogenic amine-containing pathways, which have a more anterior cortical distribution, was considered the neuroanatomical substrate. However, this localization model has been the subject of several criticisms. For instance, diffuse lesions in the middle cerebral artery territory are often proximal to both poles. Furthermore, only a small sample of patients was analyzed (30–45 subjects) and the statistical foundation of the model appeared weak. The exclusion of patients with severe aphasia or cognitive impairment was a selection bias. The confounding roles of amnesia, executive dysfunction, anosognosia, neglect, apathy, fatigue, and loss of psychic auto-activation were not evaluated, even if most of these conditions are neurobehavioral correlates of basal ganglia and anterior lesions. Finally, the possibility that the ischemic lesion had a remote effect on distant areas was not evaluated.

In fact, several other clinical studies failed to find any lateralization or any anteroposterior gradient (House *et al.*, 1990a; Andersen *et al.*, 1995; Ng *et al.*, 1995; Gainotti *et al.*, 1997b; Herrmann *et al.*, 1998; Paolucci *et al.*, 1999), while others found that right lesions were significantly associated with PSD (MacHale *et al.*, 1998). Actually, depression may be associated with an asymmetric mode of hemisphere functioning only if co-occurring with a generalized anxiety disorder (Heller *et al.*, 1995).

In successive studies, Robinson and colleagues (Shimoda and Robinson, 1999) suggested that PSD was related to left anterior and basal ganglia lesions in the acute phase (i.e. shortly after the stroke itself), to an anterior location for both hemispheres when PSD was present several months after the stroke, and to right posterior lesions when PSD was present 1–2 years after the stroke.

Localization theories were considered valid only in patients with typical asymmetry of occipital lobes (right occipital lobe greater than left); and, in case of left lesions, women were found to have a greater risk of depression than men. The authors concluded that post-stroke delay, occipital asymmetry, and gender were the principal factors explaining the inter-study differences in anatomical correlates of PSD.

A recent meta-analysis (Carson *et al.*, 2000), which evaluated 48 of 143 selected studies but included only 35 in the analysis, concluded that lesion location might contribute to PSD only to a small extent. Methodological differences might explain the conflicting results of the various studies (Singh *et al.*, 1998; Bhogal *et al.*, 2004).

Psychodynamic factors

While evaluating patients for PSD it is important to have some understanding of the patient's emotional life prior to the stroke, in order to ensure that the current disorder represents a meaningful change from the pre-morbid level of functioning. Personality traits, such as neuroticism, have been shown to be a risk factor for developing PSD (Aben *et al.*, 2002b). Furthermore, a genetic predisposition could play a role in PSD, as an increased incidence of family history of psychiatric disorders was reported in patients with PSD (Morris *et al.*, 1990).

Many psychosocial factors strictly related to the consequences of disability have been considered as major causes of PSD. Diminished physical or cognitive functioning inevitably produces conflicts with significant others with whom the patient interacts; there may be isolation, loss of a professional role, and the need for medical and rehabilitative programs; environmental changes and financial problems may ensue. Any and all of these factors are certainly a source of anxiety for the stroke survivor and they must all be considered in evaluating and caring for the victims of stroke (Ouimet *et al.*, 2001). In this regard, PSD could be considered a "reactive" depressive syndrome triggered by the process of coping with disability, as the patients themselves frequently report.

Similar prevalence of depressive disorders after stroke and other medical conditions (Fruhwald *et al.*, 2001; Aben *et al.*, 2003) supports the causative role of a non-specific psychological reaction to illness.

The "reactive" aspects of depression could correspond to two possible models.

1. In the first model, depression is a pathological disease of more general importance. The stroke may be considered as a precipitating event, acting on a preexisting vulnerability or on latent or unconscious conflicts.

2. In the second model, namely the "interactivity" model, the trigger event is considered a trauma, whereas the reaction, among a possible defined variety of responses, gives a specific configuration to the occurrence of depression. The interactivity model posits depression as an adaptive disorder next to the cognitive models of stress. The importance of life events is known for ED. Depressive episodes are often temporally linked to precipitant events, especially events that imply a loss of personal expectations.

In the "reactive" form of depression, as in PSD, a specific profile of symptoms can be frequently observed: patients complain about their difficulties and the environment, show self-pity, feel others' guilt, often report somatic symptoms that frequently are the source of obsessions, and intrusive thoughts.

The main symptom of "non-reactive" depression is considered to be anhedonia (a decreased experience of pleasure or interest in previously enjoyed activities). The DSM-IV criteria do not consider the existence of different qualitative forms of depression. Bias in selecting patients (i.e. discriminating between patients with reactive or non-reactive PSD) could be another reason for the inconclusive findings of localization studies.

Cognitive impairment

A significant association between PSD and cognitive deficits has been reported in several studies, even though stroke itself may be followed by a significant decline in cognitive performance when pre-stroke and post-stroke measurements are compared (Henon *et al.*, 2001). The main question is whether it is depression that negatively influences the outcome of cognitive impairment (*dementia of depression*) or whether cognitive impairment leads to depression (*depression of dementia*). The answer is probably that the link runs both ways.

In a group of 53 patients with single stroke lesions, Bolla-Wilson *et al.* (1989) found that, among patients with left hemisphere lesions, those with major depression were more impaired in terms of orientation, language (naming), verbal learning, visuoperceptual and visuoconstructional tasks, and executive functions (attention, concentration, non-verbal problem-solving, and psychomotor speed) than those without depression. The same neuropsychological profile applies to elderly patients with ED. The presence of dysphasia also increases the risk of major depression (Kauhanen *et al.*, 1999).

Improvement of cognitive impairment after antidepressant therapy (Kimura *et al.*, 2000) stresses the importance of recognizing and treating PSD. Nevertheless in other community studies, using MMSE (House *et al.*, 1990b; Aben *et al.*, 2002) or other measurements (Kase *et al.*, 1998), no evidence was found to support a correlation between cognitive impairment and major depression one year after a first stroke, or in a 13-year period. The issue remains open to further research.

Outcome and disability

It is an unresolved issue whether functional impairment leads to depression or whether depression itself compromises the recovery of neurological deficits. Although many studies indicated that PSD has a negative role on functional recovery (Flick, 1999), available data should be interpreted cautiously because the majority of these studies did not discriminate between groups of patients receiving treatment for PSD and those not receiving treatment. Furthermore the real impact of physical and cognitive impairment on daily life and social activities should be assessed according to the values and lifestyle of the patient. For example, the consequences of naming difficulties might be much more significant for a lawyer or secretary than for an artist or farmer.

Nevertheless some data are noteworthy. The development and intensity of depressive symptoms correlate strongly with the grade of functional impairment (Neau *et al.*, 1998; Kauhanen *et al.*, 1999) during the acute phase and the first 6 months after stroke. PSD has been shown to influence the outcome of stroke patients even at a considerable delay from stroke onset; this has been demonstrated to be true at 1 year (Herrmann *et al.*, 1998; Singh *et al.*, 2000; Aben *et al.*, 2003), at 14 months (Morris *et al.*, 1992b), at 15 months (Pohjasvaara *et al.*, 2001), and at 2 years (Parikh *et al.*, 1990). Iterative scores of questionnaires assessing the functional autonomy correlate with the progression of PSD and are better longitudinal predictors of depressive symptoms than lesion location (Singh *et al.*, 2000).

Patients with PSD are more severely compromised in activities of daily living (ADLs) than patients without PSD, in a manner that is independent of other variables (Ramasubbu *et al.*, 1998). In a study by Pohjasvaara *et al.* (1998), the presence of PSD was shown to increase 2- to 3-fold the risk of dependence in ADLs. However, in that study, only 39% of patients were treated for depression. Patients with PSD, if compared to stroke patients without PSD, show major disability both before and after specific rehabilitation programs, but the degree of functional improvement may be similar (Paolucci *et al.*, 2001). In a previous study by Paolucci and colleagues (Paolucci *et al.*, 1999), depression was shown to be a highly significant independent predictor of low response on ADLs, as indicated by previous studies (Sinyor *et al.*, 1986; van de Weg *et al.*, 1999).

Pharmacological treatment of PSD seems to influence positively the functional outcome (Robinson *et al.*, 2000; Chemerinski *et al.*, 2001; Gainotti *et al.*, 2001), although the outcome of PSD and non-PSD patients remains different and more favorable for non-PSD patients (Gonzalez-Torrecillas *et al.*, 1995). Therefore available data fail to prove that an improvement of PSD also leads to a significant improvement of functional status (Gainotti and Marra, 2002).

Suicide

Suicides among stroke patients are low compared with other depressive states. In an epidemiological survey of 37,000 stroke patients, the overall suicide prevalence was 0.37% (Stenager *et al.*, 1998). Risk factors include younger age, depression, severe insomnia, chronic illness, an organic brain syndrome, severe physical impairment, a history of alcohol abuse, poor social support, brooding, and self-blame (Kishi *et al.*, 1996; 2001). The prevalence of suicidal ideas is similar (25%) between patients with stroke and patients with other chronic medical conditions (Kishi *et al.*, 2001).

Mortality

Patients with PSD (or those with depressive feelings) before or in the first phases after a stroke have a 3-fold greater risk of mortality over the following 10 years, in comparison with patients without depression (Everson *et al.*, 1998; House *et al.*, 2001). This risk seems independent of other cardiovascular risk factors, such as age, sex, social class, type of stroke, or lesion location, and it is associated with social isolation (Morris *et al.*, 1993). Patients who are depressed may return to detrimental habits (smoking, alcohol), and might not comply with treatment recommendations (Gillen *et al.*, 2001) or health-promoting behaviors. PSD patients are also at increased risk of falling (Ugur *et al.*, 2000), which is an important factor in mortality. Increased mortality for patients with PSD may also be due to modifications of the cardiovascular system. For instance it is known that patients with ED experience a higher grade of arterial hypertension (especially of the systolic value) and myocardial infarction (Hippisley-Cox *et al.*, 1998), probably mediated by enhanced platelet aggregation. Early treatment of PSD may reduce the risk of mortality (Jorge *et al.*, 2003).

Treatment

Depression related to a medical illness responds to pharmacological treatments (Gill and Hatcher, 2000). The recovery is considered significant when it corresponds to a reduction of HDRS or BDI scores of at least 50%. However, it should be stressed that such a reduction might not correspond to disease remission.

Tricyclic antidepressants are no longer the treatment of choice, because of the severity and elevated frequency of adverse effects (orthostatic hypotension, atrioventricular block, delirium or confusion, drowsiness, agitation, life-threatening cardiac arrhythmias, heart block, urinary outlet obstruction, narrow-angle glaucoma). SSRIs have a better safety profile and have been shown to be more effective than both placebo and tricyclic antidepressants (Andersen *et al.*, 1994; Wiart *et al.*, 2000; Bak *et al.*, 2002; Fruehwald *et al.*, 2003). Side effects are rare and similar in frequency and expression in patients with PSD and ED. They consist of gastrointestinal symptoms (particularly nausea), headache, and "stimulant" effects such as agitation, anxiety, insomnia, and rarely mania. Male sexual dysfunction is very rare but must be taken into account when proposing a treatment. Only a few studies have compared the effects of SSRIs with tricyclic antidepressants and these have generally involved small numbers of patients (Robinson *et al.*, 2000). Fluoxetine may not be the first-choice SSRI if a rapid onset is required, as steady-state concentrations are not reached until after 4–5 weeks, whereas sertraline and citalopram require less than a week. The longer half-lifed fluoxetine allows less frequent administration in non-compliant patients and results in less severe discontinuation effects. Fluoxetine is helpful when depression is associated with bulimia or diabetes because it increases basal metabolism, enhances weight loss, and reduces glycemic values. For this reason the interaction with antidiabetic drugs should be closely monitored. Fluoxetine inhibits P450 isoenzymes and should not be used in stroke patients receiving anticoagulant therapy. Sertraline and citalopram seem to be more efficacious in the treatment of stroke-associated lability of mood and, compared to fluoxetine, are better tolerated, have lower risk of agitation, weight loss, dermatological adverse effects, and fewer interactions with drugs influencing cytochrome P450 enzymes. SSRIs have been associated with increased risk of bleeding complications, possibly as a result of inhibition of platelet aggregation, but this risk has been shown to be not significant (Bak *et al.*, 2002).

There are no specific guidelines for the choice of drugs in the SSRI category, and this choice should be evaluated on a clinical basis for every single patient.

Some studies have demonstrated that improvement of PSD induced by SSRIs enhances recovery of neurological and cognitive deficits (Gainotti *et al.*, 2001) and performance in activities of daily living (Gonzalez-Torrecillas *et al.*, 1995;

Chemerinski *et al.*, 2001). This effect can be quite large (30% of functional recovery) (van de Weg *et al.*, 1999), but a close relationship between appropriate early PSD treatment and functional recovery has not emerged in all studies (Robinson *et al.*, 2000; Wiart *et al.*, 2000; Paolucci *et al.*, 2001). As generally accepted, a placebo effect may also account for 35% of the therapeutic response in trials of antidepressants. Moreover, spontaneous remissions might also be frequent. Major PSD has been suggested to have a natural course of less than a year, while minor depression is often more persistent (Robinson, 1998). It is important to indicate that SSRIs probably improve cognitive functions impaired by depression, but not deficits directly due to cerebral damage. Preventive antidepressant treatment in all patients with first-ever stroke does not affect the functional outcome (Palomaki *et al.*, 1999; Anderson *et al.*, 2004). Most significant here, antidepressant treatment reduces the overall mortality in PSD patients (Jorge *et al.*, 2003). Some reports suggest that fluoxetine may improve functional recovery, independently of its antidepressant action (Dam *et al.*, 1996; Pariente *et al.*, 2001).

Trazodone, which has a high tolerability profile, may be a possible safe and efficacious alternative to SSRIs when the latter are contraindicated (Reding *et al.*, 1986).

Cognitive and behavioral therapies could be appropriate treatments (Lincoln and Flannaghan, 2003), especially if all factors contributing to depression are clearly defined, but conclusive data are not available because of methodological differences among studies (Kneebone and Dunmore, 2000; Lincoln and Flannaghan, 2003). Patients reporting only verbal distress might respond better to cognitive therapy alone, while patients with vegetative symptoms might best be treated with an antidepressant agent. Duration of pharmacological treatment is not clearly defined. Although most studies evaluated the effect of a 6-week treatment phase, longer periods (4–6 months) are probably indicated (Turner-Stokes and Hassan, 2002).

Key points Management and treatment of PSD

Pharmacotherapy

There is evidence of the efficaciousness of nortriptilyne, citalopram and fluoxetine

If PSD is diagnosed, pharmacological treatment should be started as early as possible

SSRIs are first choice drugs because of their better safety profile

Pharmacological treatment should be continued for at least 4–6 months

Other approaches

Cognitive and behavioral therapies could be appropriate treatments, especially if all factors
   contributing to depression are clearly defined, but conclusive data are not available.

Conclusions

A depressive episode occurring within 6–12 months after stroke has high prevalence (about 30%).

DSM-IV criteria are currently used for PSD diagnosis. However, the different subtypes of PSD (major and minor, standard/non-standard, reactive or non-reactive) increases the difficulty of carrying out clinical investigations on large population samples. Obtaining a complete evaluation of the impact of other cognitive, behavioral, physiological, and psychological changes due to the stroke itself (e.g. aphasia, anosognosia, apathy, fatigue) is essential for proper diagnosis of PSD. Extensive neurobehavioral and psychiatric testing, use of non-verbal measurements in aphasic patients, and interviews of families or caregivers are necessary to evaluate depressive symptoms in stroke survivors. This multidimensional approach then allows the choice of more specific therapies that may not exclusively be pharmacological. SSRIs are currently the drugs of choice because of their better tolerability profile. Early pharmacological therapy, when the diagnosis of PSD is clear, may greatly improve not only the quality of life but also recovery from neurological and cognitive deficits, and can reduce mortality.

Planning clinical studies for investigating PSD is a very difficult task, because of the many variables involved. The link between PSD and brain dysfunction is, therefore, still impossible to describe. Advances in our knowledge of the neurobiological factors of PSD may lead to new therapies and improve stroke outcome.

All psychosocial factors possibly interfering with mood changes should be evaluated. The stroke patient is coping with a serious physical illness that reduces his or her self-integrity in terms of personal vulnerability and low self-esteem and generates possible conflicts with significant others. Strategies to increase social activity and support financial security, job satisfaction, adequacy of living arrangements, and psychiatric care are strongly encouraged.

Acknowledgements

This work was supported by a grant to Antonio Carota from the Biaggi foundation. We thank Susan P. Koniak, Dr. Francesca Fusco, and Dr. Theodoros Karapanayiotides for valuable comments on the manuscript.

REFERENCES

Aben, I., Denollet, J., et al. (2002b). Personality and vulnerability to depression in stroke patients: A 1-year prospective follow-up study. Stroke, 33(10), 2391–5.

Aben, I., Verhey, F., *et al.* (2002a). Validity of the Beck depression inventory, hospital anxiety and depression scale, SCL-90, and Hamilton depression rating scale as screening instruments for depression in stroke patients. *Psychosomatics*, **43**(5), 386–93.

Aben, I., Verhey, F., *et al.* (2003). A comparative study into the one year cumulative incidence of depression after stroke and myocardial infarction. *J. Neurol. Neurosurg. Psychiatry*, **74**(5), 581–5.

Agrell, B. and Dehlin, O. (1989). Comparison of six depression rating scales in geriatric stroke patients. *Stroke*, **20**(9), 1190–4.

Andersen, G., Vestergaard, K., *et al.* (1995). Risk factors for post-stroke depression. *Acta Psychiatr. Scand.*, **92**(3), 193–8.

Andersen, G., Vestergaard, K., *et al.* (1994). Effective treatment of poststroke depression with the selective serotonin reuptake inhibitor citalopram. *Stroke*, **25**(6), 1099–104.

Anderson, C., Hackett, M., *et al.* (2004). Interventions for preventing depression after stroke. *Cochrane Database Syst. Rev.*, **2**, CD003689.

Angelelli, P., Paolucci, S., *et al.* (2004). Development of neuropsychiatric symptoms in poststroke patients: A cross-sectional study. *Acta Psychiatr. Scand.*, **110**(1), 55–63.

Arruda, J. E., Stern, R. A., *et al.* (1999). Measurement of mood states in stroke patients: Validation of the visual analog mood scales. *Arch. Phys. Med. Rehabil.*, **80**(6), 676–80.

American Psychiatric Association. (2001). DSM-IV-TR. *Diagnostic and Statistical Manual of Mental Disorders*.

Bak, S., Tsiropoulos, I., *et al.* (2002). Selective serotonin reuptake inhibitors and the risk of stroke: A population-based case-control study. *Stroke*, **33**(6), 1465–73.

Beblo, T. and Driessen, M. (2002). No melancholia in poststroke depression? A phenomenologic comparison of primary and poststroke depression. *J. Geriatr. Psychiatry Neurol.*, **15**(1), 44–9.

Beck, A. T., Ward, C. H., *et al.* (1961). An inventory for measuring depression. *Arch. Gen. Psychiatry*, **4**, 561–71.

Berg, A., Palomaki, H., *et al.* (2001). Poststroke depression in acute phase after stroke. *Cerebrovasc. Dis.*, **12**(1), 14–20.

Bhogal, S. K., Teasell, R., *et al.* (2004). Lesion location and poststroke depression: Systematic review of the methodological limitations in the literature. *Stroke*, **35**(3), 794–802.

Biran, I. and Chatterjee, A. (2003). Depression with anosognosia following a left subcortical stroke. *Clin. Neurol. Neurosurg.*, **105**(2), 99–101.

Bisiach, E., Vallar, G., *et al.* (1986). Unawareness of disease following lesions of the right hemisphere: Anosognosia for hemiplegia and anosognosia for hemianopia. *Neuropsychologia*, **24**(4), 471–82.

Blonder, L. X., Bowers, D., *et al.* (1991). The role of the right hemisphere in emotional communication. *Brain*, **114**(Pt 3), 1115–27.

Bolla-Wilson, K., Robinson, R. G., *et al.* (1989). Lateralization of dementia of depression in stroke patients. *Am. J. Psychiatry*, **146**(5), 627–34.

Carota, A., Rossetti, A. O., *et al.* (2001). Catastrophic reaction in acute stroke: A reflex behavior in aphasic patients. *Neurology*, **57**(10), 1902–5.

Carson, A. J., MacHale, S., *et al.* (2000). Depression after stroke and lesion location: A systematic review. *Lancet*, **356**(9224), 122–6.

Chemerinski, E., Robinson, R. G., et al. (2001). Improved recovery in activities of daily living associated with remission of poststroke depression. *Stroke*, **32**(1), 113–7.

Cummings, J. L., Mega, M., et al. (1994). The Neuropsychiatric Inventory: Comprehensive assessment of psychopathology in dementia. *Neurology*, **44**(12), 2308–14.

Dam, M., Tonin, P., et al. (1996). Effects of fluoxetine and maprotiline on functional recovery in poststroke hemiplegic patients undergoing rehabilitation therapy. *Stroke*, **27**(7), 1211–4.

Endicott, J., Cohen, J., et al. (1981). Hamilton Depression Rating Scale. Extracted from regular and change versions of the Schedule for Affective Disorders and Schizophrenia. *Arch. Gen. Psychiatry*, **38**(1), 98–103.

Eriksson, M., Asplund, K., et al. (2004). Self-reported depression and use of antidepressants after stroke: A national survey. *Stroke*, **35**(4), 936–41.

Everson, S. A., Roberts, R. E., et al. (1998). Depressive symptoms and increased risk of stroke mortality over a 29-year period. *Arch. Intern. Med.*, **158**(10), 1133–8.

Fedoroff, J. P., Starkstein, S. E., et al. (1991). Are depressive symptoms nonspecific in patients with acute stroke? *Am. J. Psychiatry*, **148**(9), 1172–6.

Flick, C. L. (1999). Stroke rehabilitation. 4. Stroke outcome and psychosocial consequences. *Arch. Phys. Med. Rehabil.*, **80**(5 Suppl. 1), S21–6.

Fruehwald, S., Gatterbauer, E., et al. (2003). Early fluoxetine treatment of post-stroke depression—a three-month double-blind placebo-controlled study with an open-label long-term follow up. *J. Neurol.*, **250**(3), 347–51.

Fruhwald, S., Loffler, H., et al. (2001). Relationship between depression, anxiety and quality of life: A study of stroke patients compared to chronic low back pain and myocardial ischemia patients. *Psychopathology*, **34**(1), 50–6.

Gainotti, G. (1972). Emotional behavior and hemispheric side of the lesion. *Cortex*, **8**(1), 41–55.

Gainotti, G., Antonucci, G., et al. (2001). Relation between depression after stroke, antidepressant therapy, and functional recovery. *J. Neurol. Neurosurg. Psychiatry*, **71**(2), 258–61.

Gainotti, G., Azzoni, A., et al. (1997b). Relation of lesion location to verbal and nonverbal mood measures in stroke patients. *Stroke*, **28**(11), 2145–9.

Gainotti, G., Azzoni, A., et al. (1997a). The Post-Stroke Depression Rating Scale: A test specifically devised to investigate affective disorders of stroke patients. *J. Clin. Exp. Neuropsychol.*, **19**(3), 340–56.

Gainotti, G., Azzoni, A., et al. (1999). Frequency, phenomenology and anatomical-clinical correlates of major post-stroke depression. *Br. J. Psychiatry*, **175**, 163–7.

Gainotti, G. and Marra, C. (2002). Determinants and consequences of post-stroke depression. *Curr. Opin. Neurol.*, **15**(1), 85–9.

Gill, D. and Hatcher, S. (2000). Antidepressants for depression in medical illness. *Cochrane Database Syst. Rev.*, **4**.

Gillen, R., Tennen, H., et al. (2001). Depressive symptoms and history of depression predict rehabilitation efficiency in stroke patients. *Arch. Phys. Med. Rehabil.*, **82**(12), 1645–9.

Gonzalez-Torrecillas, J. L., Mendlewicz, J., *et al.* (1995). Effects of early treatment of poststroke depression on neuropsychological rehabilitation. *Int. Psychogeriatr.*, **7**(4), 547–60.

Grasso, M. G., Pantano, P., *et al.* (1994). Mesial temporal cortex hypoperfusion is associated with depression in subcortical stroke. *Stroke*, **25**(5), 980–5.

Habib, M. (1995). Activity and motivational disorders in neurology: Proposal for an evaluation scale. *Encephale*, **21**, 563–70.

Hamilton, M. (1960). A rating scale for depression. *J. Neurol. Neurosurg. Psychiatry*, **23**, 56–62.

Heller, W., Etienne, M. A., *et al.* (1995). Patterns of perceptual asymmetry in depression and anxiety: Implications for neuropsychological models of emotion and psychopathology. *J. Abnorm. Psychol.*, **104**(2), 327–33.

Henon, H., Durieu, I., *et al.* (2001). Poststroke dementia: Incidence and relationship to prestroke cognitive decline. *Neurology*, **57**(7), 1216–22.

Herrmann, M., Bartels, C., *et al.* (1995). Poststroke depression. Is there a pathoanatomic correlate for depression in the postacute stage of stroke? *Stroke*, **26**(5), 850–6.

Herrmann, N., Black, S. E., *et al.* (1998). The Sunnybrook Stroke Study: A prospective study of depressive symptoms and functional outcome. *Stroke*, **29**(3), 618–24.

Hippisley-Cox, J., Fielding, K., *et al.* (1998). Depression as a risk factor for ischaemic heart disease in men: Population based case-control study. *BMJ*, **316**(7146), 1714–9.

House, A., Dennis, M., *et al.* (1990a). Mood disorders after stroke and their relation to lesion location. A CT scan study. *Brain*, **113**(Pt 4), 1113–29.

House, A., Dennis, M., *et al.* (1990b). The relationship between intellectual impairment and mood disorder in the first year after stroke. *Psychol. Med.*, **20**(4), 805–14.

House, A., Knapp, P., *et al.* (2001). Mortality at 12 and 24 months after stroke may be associated with depressive symptoms at 1 month. *Stroke*, **32**(3), 696–701.

Ingles, J. L., Eskes, G. A., *et al.* (1999). Fatigue after stroke. *Arch. Phys. Med. Rehabil.*, **80**(2), 173–8.

Jeret, J. S. (1997). Treatment of poststroke pathological crying. *Stroke*, **28**(11), 2321–2.

Jorge, R. E., Robinson, R. G., *et al.* (2003). Mortality and poststroke depression: A placebo-controlled trial of antidepressants. *Am. J. Psychiatry*, **160**(10), 1823–9.

Kase, C. S., Wolf, P. A., *et al.* (1998). Intellectual decline after stroke: The Framingham Study. *Stroke*, **29**(4), 805–12.

Kauhanen, M., Korpelainen, J. T., *et al.* (1999). Poststroke depression correlates with cognitive impairment and neurological deficits. *Stroke*, **30**(9), 1875–80.

Kim, J. M., Stewart, R., *et al.* (2002). Previous stroke but not vascular risk factors are associated with depression in a cognitively impaired older Korean population. *Int. J. Geriatr. Psychiatry*, **17**(5), 453–8.

Kim, J. S. and Choi-Kwon, S. (2000). Poststroke depression and emotional incontinence: Correlation with lesion location. *Neurology*, **54**(9), 1805–10.

Kimura, M., Robinson, R. G., *et al.* (2000). Treatment of cognitive impairment after poststroke depression: A double-blind treatment trial. *Stroke*, **31**(7), 1482–6.

Kishi, Y., Robinson, R. G., *et al.* (1996). Suicidal plans in patients with stroke: Comparison between acute-onset and delayed-onset suicidal plans. *Int. Psychogeriatr.*, **8**(4), 623–34.

Kishi, Y., Robinson, R. G., *et al.* (2001). Suicidal ideation among patients during the rehabilitation period after life-threatening physical illness. *J. Nerv. Ment. Dis.*, **189**(9), 623–8.

Kneebone, II and Dunmore, E. (2000). Psychological management of post-stroke depression. *Br. J. Clin. Psychol.*, **39**(Pt 1), 53–65.

Lauterbach, E. C., Jackson, J. G., *et al.* (1997). Major depression after left posterior globus pallidus lesions. *Neuropsychiatry Neuropsychol. Behav. Neurol.*, **10**(1), 9–16.

Levy, M. L., Cummings, J. L., *et al.* (1998). Apathy is not depression. *J. Neuropsychiatry Clin. Neurosci.*, **10**(3), 314–9.

Lincoln, N. B. and Flannaghan, T. (2003). Cognitive behavioral psychotherapy for depression following stroke: A randomized controlled trial. *Stroke*, **34**(1), 111–5.

Lincoln, N. B., Nicholl, C. R., *et al.* (2003). The validity of questionnaire measures for assessing depression after stroke. *Clin. Rehabil.*, **17**(8), 840–6.

MacHale, S. M., O'Rourke, S. J., *et al.* (1998). Depression and its relation to lesion location after stroke. *J. Neurol. Neurosurg. Psychiatry*, **64**(3), 371–4.

Marcel, A. J., Tegner, R., *et al.* (2004). Anosognosia for plegia: Specificity, extension, partiality and disunity of bodily unawareness. *Cortex*, **40**(1), 19–40.

Marin, R. S., Biedrzychi, R. C., *et al.* (1991). Reliability and validity of the Apathy Evaluation Scale. *Psychiatry Res.*, **38**, 143–62.

Montgomery, S. A. and Asberg, M. (1979). A new depression scale designed to be sensitive to change. *Br. J. Psychiatry*, **134**, 382–9.

Morris, P. L., Raphael, B., *et al.* (1992b). Clinical depression is associated with impaired recovery from stroke. *Med. J. Aust.*, **157**(4), 239–42.

Morris, P. L., Robinson, R. G., *et al.* (1990). Prevalence and course of depressive disorders in hospitalized stroke patients. *Int. J. Psychiatry Med.*, **20**(4), 349–64.

Morris, P. L., Robinson, R. G., *et al.* (1992a). The relationship between risk factors for affective disorder and poststroke depression in hospitalised stroke patients. *Aust. N. Z. J. Psychiatry*, **26**(2), 208–17.

Morris, P. L., Robinson, R. G., *et al.* (1993). Association of depression with 10-year poststroke mortality. *Am. J. Psychiatry*, **150**(1), 124–9.

Morris, P. L., Shields, R. B., *et al.* (1994). Are there two depressive syndromes after stroke? *J. Nerv. Ment. Dis.*, **182**(4), 230–4.

Naarding, P., Leentjens, A. F., *et al.* (2002). Disease-specific properties of the Rating Scale for Depression in patients with stroke, Alzheimer's dementia, and Parkinson's disease. *J. Neuropsychiatry Clin. Neurosci.*, **14**(3), 329–34.

Nahas, Z., Arlinghaus, K. A., *et al.* (1998). Rapid response of emotional incontinence to selective serotonin reuptake inhibitors. *J. Neuropsychiatry Clin. Neurosci.*, **10**(4), 453–5.

Neau, J. P., Ingrand, P., *et al.* (1998). Functional recovery and social outcome after cerebral infarction in young adults. *Cerebrovasc. Dis.*, **8**(5), 296–302.

Ng, K. C., Chan, K. L., *et al.* (1995). A study of post-stroke depression in a rehabilitative center. *Acta Psychiatr. Scand.*, **92**(1), 75–9.

Ouimet, M. A., Primeau, F., *et al.* (2001). Psychosocial risk factors in poststroke depression: A systematic review. *Can. J. Psychiatry*, **46**(9), 819–28.

Palomaki, H., Kaste, M., *et al.* (1999). Prevention of poststroke depression: 1 year randomised placebo controlled double blind trial of mianserin with 6 month follow up after therapy. *J. Neurol. Neurosurg. Psychiatry*, **66**(4), 490−4.

Paolucci, S., Antonucci, G., *et al.* (1999). Poststroke depression and its role in rehabilitation of inpatients. *Arch. Phys. Med. Rehabil.*, **80**(9), 985−90.

Paolucci, S., Antonucci, G., *et al.* (2001). Post-stroke depression, antidepressant treatment and rehabilitation results. A case-control study. *Cerebrovasc. Dis.*, **12**(3), 264−71.

Paradiso, S., Ohkubo, T., *et al.* (1997). Vegetative and psychological symptoms associated with depressed mood over the first two years after stroke. *Int. J. Psychiatry Med.*, **27**(2), 137−57.

Paradiso, S. and Robinson, R. G. (1998). Gender differences in poststroke depression. *J. Neuropsychiatry Clin. Neurosci.*, **10**(1), 41−7.

Paradiso, S. and Robinson, R. G. (1999). Minor depression after stroke: An initial validation of the DSM-IV construct. *Am. J. Geriatr. Psychiatry*, **7**(3), 244−51.

Pariente, J., Loubinoux, I., *et al.* (2001). Fluoxetine modulates motor performance and cerebral activation of patients recovering from stroke. *Ann. Neurol.*, **50**(6), 718−29.

Parikh, R. M., Robinson, R. G., *et al.* (1990). The impact of poststroke depression on recovery in activities of daily living over a 2-year follow-up. *Arch. Neurol.*, **47**(7), 785−9.

Pohjasvaara, T., Leppavuori, A., *et al.* (1998). Frequency and clinical determinants of poststroke depression. *Stroke*, **29**(11), 2311−7.

Pohjasvaara, T., Vataja, R., *et al.* (2001). Depression is an independent predictor of poor long-term functional outcome post-stroke. *Eur. J. Neurol.*, **8**(4), 315−9.

Price, C. I., Curless, R. H., *et al.* (1999). Can stroke patients use visual analogue scales? *Stroke*, **30**(7), 1357−61.

Provinciali, L. and Coccia, M. (2002). Post-stroke and vascular depression: A critical review. *Neurol. Sci.*, **22**(6), 417−28.

Ramasubbu, R., Robinson, R. G. *et al.* (1998). Functional impairment associated with acute poststroke depression: The Stroke Data Bank Study. *J. Neuropsychiatry Clin. Neurosci.*, **10**(1), 26−33.

Reding, M. J., Orto, L. A., *et al.* (1986). Antidepressant therapy after stroke. A double-blind trial. *Arch. Neurol.*, **43**(8), 763−5.

Robinson, R. G. (1998). *The Clinical Neuropsychiatry of Stroke*. New York: Cambridge University Press.

Robinson, R. G., Parikh, R. M., *et al.* (1993). Pathological laughing and crying following stroke: Validation of a measurement scale and a double-blind treatment study. *Am. J. Psychiatry*, **150**(2), 286−93.

Robinson, R. G., Schultz, S. K., *et al.* (2000). Nortriptyline versus fluoxetine in the treatment of depression and in short-term recovery after stroke: A placebo-controlled, double-blind study. *Am. J. Psychiatry*, **157**(3), 351−9.

Sato, R., Bryan, R. N., *et al.* (1999). Neuroanatomic and functional correlates of depressed mood: The Cardiovascular Health Study. *Am. J. Epidemiol.*, **150**(9), 919−29.

Schubert, D. S., Taylor, C., *et al.* (1992). Detection of depression in the stroke patient. *Psychosomatics*, **33**(3), 290−4.

Sherer, M., Bergloff, P., *et al.* (1998). The Awareness Questionnaire: Factor structure and internal consistency. *Brain Inj.*, **12**(1), 63–8.

Shimoda, K. and Robinson, R. G. (1999). The relationship between poststroke depression and lesion location in long-term follow-up. *Biol. Psychiatry*, **45**(2), 187–92.

Singh, A., Black, S. E., *et al.* (2000). Functional and neuroanatomic correlations in poststroke depression: The Sunnybrook Stroke Study. *Stroke*, **31**(3), 637–44.

Singh, A., Herrmann, N., *et al.* (1998). The importance of lesion location in poststroke depression: A critical review. *Can. J. Psychiatry*, **43**(9), 921–7.

Sinyor, D., Amato, P., *et al.* (1986). Post-stroke depression: Relationships to functional impairment, coping strategies, and rehabilitation outcome. *Stroke*, **17**(6), 1102–7.

Starkstein, S. E., Fedoroff, J. P., *et al.* (1993a). Apathy following cerebrovascular lesions. *Stroke*, **24**(11), 1625–30.

Starkstein, S. E., Fedoroff, J. P., *et al.* (1993b). Catastrophic reaction after cerebrovascular lesions: Frequency, correlates, and validation of a scale. *J. Neuropsychiatry Clin. Neurosci.*, **5**(2), 189–94.

Stenager, E. N., Madsen, C., *et al.* (1998). Suicide in patients with stroke: Epidemiological study. *BMJ*, **316**(7139), 1206.

Stern, R. A. and Bachman, D. L. (1991). Depressive symptoms following stroke. *Am. J. Psychiatry*, **148**(3), 351–6.

Sutcliffe, L. M. and Lincoln, N. B. (1998). The assessment of depression in aphasic stroke patients: The development of the Stroke Aphasic Depression Questionnaire. *Clin. Rehabil.*, **12**(6), 506–13.

Toedter, L. J., Schall, R. R., *et al.* (1995). Psychological measures: Reliability in the assessment of stroke patients. *Arch. Phys. Med. Rehabil.*, **76**(8), 719–25.

Turner-Stokes, L. and Hassan, N. (2002). Depression after stroke: A review of the evidence base to inform the development of an integrated care pathway. Part 1: Diagnosis, frequency and impact. *Clin. Rehabil.*, **16**(3), 231–47.

Ugur, C., Gucuyener, D., *et al.* (2000). Characteristics of falling in patients with stroke. *J. Neurol. Neurosurg. Psychiatry*, **69**(5), 649–51.

van de Weg, F. B., Kuik, D. J., *et al.* (1999). Post-stroke depression and functional outcome: A cohort study investigating the influence of depression on functional recovery from stroke. *Clin. Rehabil.*, **13**(3), 268–72.

Wiart, L., Petit, H., *et al.* (2000). Fluoxetine in early poststroke depression: A double-blind placebo-controlled study. *Stroke*, **31**(8), 1829–32.

Zigmond, A. S. and Snaith, R. P. (1983). The hospital anxiety and depression scale. *Acta Psychiatr. Scand.*, **67**(6), 361–70.

Zung, W. W. (1965). A Self-Rating Depression Scale. *Arch. Gen. Psychiatry*, **12**, 63–70.

30

Fatigue

Fabienne Staub

CHUV, Lausanne, Switzerland

Introduction

Fatigue is a non-specific symptom associated with a wide range of states and diseases. The feeling of fatigue is a frequent complaint in various medical conditions, including psychiatric diseases (mainly depression, anxiety, and somatoform disorders), cancer, autoimmune, endocrinological, infectious, rheumatological and neurological affections, and sleep disorders. Fatigue may also develop without any antecedent condition other than a viral infection, leading to what is known as "chronic fatigue syndrome" (Holmes *et al.*, 1988). Some medical and pharmacological treatments (cytokines, interferon, radiotherapy, chemotherapy), physical or mental exertions, or particular environmental or psychological conditions (extreme temperature, stress, inactivity) can also induce fatigue.

Fatigue is an extremely widespread, and often benign, symptom in the general population, headaches being the only somatic complaint occurring at a higher frequency. In general practice, fatigue is a significant symptom in 10–30% of outpatients, presenting as an isolated symptom in only 1–3% of these (Kroenke and Price, 1993; Fuhrer and Wessely, 1995). Because the phenomenon constitutes an evil of modern society, the distinction between normal benign fatigue and abnormal fatigue is very difficult to make. Severity, chronicity, and an association with other symptoms or functional disability all point to a pathological condition.

The origin of fatigue can be attributed to general non-specific factors characterizing most diseases, such as pain, sleep disorders, depression, anxiety, inactivity, or to specific variables related to disease pathophysiology or treatment. The pathophysiological mechanisms are usually divided into central and peripheral causes, the latter being better known and better understood. Peripheral muscular fatigue, defined as a failure to sustain force of voluntary muscle contraction, is classically associated with altered motor control, including impaired muscle excitation, contraction, or metabolism. Myasthenia gravis and metabolic myopathies are typical examples of this type of fatigue. On the other hand, central fatigue, defined as the failure to initiate and/or sustain mental and physical tasks requiring self-motivation and sustained attention, involves the central nervous system. The pathophysiological processes involved in central fatigue are largely unknown. Nevertheless, current evidence suggests the involvement of a complex and multidimensional circuit including the nervous, endocrinological, and immune systems, which might explain why highly diverse "stresses" (physical, chemical, emotional, infectious, etc.), acting at various levels, are likely to disrupt a system homeostasis and induce fatigue.

The present chapter will concentrate on central fatigue.

The problem of definition

The first issue to resolve about fatigue concerns its definition. Although "fatigue" as a term and phenomenon is widely known by the general population, the vagueness which surrounds the concept makes any operational definition difficult. The first and most obvious distinction is between the objective and subjective dimensions of fatigue. *Objective fatigue* corresponds to an observable and measurable decrement in performance occurring during the repetition of a physical or mental task, while *subjective fatigue* is a feeling of early exhaustion, weariness, and aversion to effort. It is important to stress that the feeling of fatigue is, as a general rule, poorly correlated with the behavioral aspects of fatigue.

It can also be useful to distinguish between "fatigability" (fatigue developing in connection with activities requiring a sustained effort) and fatigue as a primary state, which stresses the lack of initiative due to an imbalance between motivation (preserved) and effectiveness (decreased). Finally, it is also possible to divide the concept of fatigue into various subtypes, namely "physical" fatigue occurring after muscular exertion, "somatic" fatigue related to the occurrence of a medical illness, "mental" fatigue appearing with cognitively demanding tasks or with the presence of cognitive disorders, and "psychological" fatigue associated with lack of interest, poor motivation, or depressive thoughts. These subtypes of fatigue, which are not mutually exclusive, can be revealed at a behavioral level (corresponding to objective fatigue) or at a psychological level (corresponding to subjective fatigue).

Key points Main characteristics of fatigue

Subjective fatigue: feeling of early exhaustion, weariness, and aversion to effort
Objective fatigue: measurable decrement in performance occurring during the repetition
    of a physical or mental task
Fatigability: fatigue developing in connection with activities requiring a sustained effort
Fatigue as a primary state: lack of initiative due to an imbalance between motivation
    (preserved) and effectiveness (decreased)
*Various subtypes of fatigue which can be revealed at a behavioral level (objective fatigue) or
    at a psychological level (subjective fatigue)*:
"physical" fatigue: after muscular exertion
"somatic" fatigue: related to the occurrence of a medical illness
"mental" fatigue: appearing with cognitively demanding tasks
"psychological" fatigue: lack of interest, poor motivation, or depressive thoughts
Specifically for PSF, we proposed the terms of:
"task-specific fatigue": directly caused by a specific cognitive/neurological sequela
"primary PSF": occurring in absence of depression, significant cognitive or neurological
    impairment, or any other clinical dysfunction which may cause fatigue
Have also to be considered:
fatigue linked to post-stroke sleep disturbances
fatigue resulting from coping factors (risk of disease recurrence, acceptance of deficits)

Post-stroke fatigue (PSF)

Fatigue has been extensively studied in other neurological disorders, such as Parkinson's disease, post-polio syndrome, immune-mediated polyneuropathies, systemic lupus erythematosus, Lyme disease, and amyotrophic lateral sclerosis. Conversely, there have been very few studies on fatigue occurring after stroke (Leegaard, 1983; van Zandvoort *et al.*, 1998; Ingles *et al.*, 1999; van der Werf *et al.*, 2001; Glader *et al.*, 2002, Röding *et al.*, 2003; Carlsson *et al.*, 2003; Schuitemaker *et al.*, 2004).

Incidence and time-course

In clinical practice, many neurologists have observed that stroke patients frequently complain of a disabling fatigue, which is, in some cases, the only significant sequela of the stroke. Fatigue is reported in 30–72% of patients and in 16–36% of controls (Ingles *et al.*, 1999; van der Werf *et al.*, 2001; Glader *et al.*, 2002; Carlsson *et al.*, 2003, Staub *et al.*, 2004). As with post-stroke depression (PSD; see Chapter 29), the large variation in the reported prevalence is probably explained by the use of different scales and cutoff scores, the choice of different selection criteria, and different delays of investigations.

Fatigue appears to be a persisting and longlasting symptom. In cross-sectional studies, the time elapsed since the stroke was found to have no influence on the presence and severity of fatigue (Ingles *et al.*, 1999; van der Werf *et al.*, 2001). The only longitudinal prospective study showed that rated (subjective) fatigue remained stable when evaluated at 6 and 12 months, despite a significant improvement in neurological and functional outcome and depression over this time (Staub *et al.*, 2004).

Overlap between PSF and depression and other similar phenomena

Given that the term "fatigue" covers a vast and poorly delimited semantic field, it is important that the clinician establishes a semiology of the phenomenon of fatigue and other related and similar phenomena by a rigorous use of terminology. Asthenia, lack of energy, lack of motivation, weakness, fatigability, sleepiness, weariness, lassitude, boredom, adynamia, anhedonia, and abulia are all terms used, sometimes inappropriately, as synonyms for fatigue. Conversely, the term "fatigue" is sometimes used by the patient to describe similar phenomena, such as depression or other abnormal body states (dizziness, dyspnea, etc.).

The overlap between fatigue and depression is undeniable, and the presence of fatigue constitutes one of the main diagnostic criteria for depression in most standardized scales for assessment of depression. Nevertheless, fatigue can also occur in the absence of depression, a dissociation already highlighted for patients with Parkinson's disease (Friedman and Friedman, 1993) or multiple sclerosis (Vercoulen *et al.*, 1996; van der Werf *et al.*, 1998) and which is equally valid in stroke patients (Ingles *et al.*, 1999; van der Werf *et al.*, 2001). For example, only 38% of patients with severe fatigue after stroke were found to be depressed (van der Werf *et al.*, 2001).

Apathy, severe reduction of initiative, and emotional flatness are the hallmarks of the abulic states, which must also be differentiated from PSF and PSD.

Nature of post-stroke fatigue

There are different types of PSF and the causes that may lead to a fatigue syndrome after stroke are varied. *Neuropsychological deficits* could generate mental fatigue, not only because of the increased cognitive demands, but also because they force the subject to additional mental effort to match previous performance. Even with apparent total recovery in standardized psychometric assessments, performance at the previous level may be possible only at a higher psychophysiological cost. We have proposed the use of the term "task-specific fatigue" to designate fatigue that is directly caused by a specific cognitive sequel (Staub and

Bogousslavsky, 2001). A typical example is a subject with residual aphasia who develops mental fatigue after speaking for a certain time. In this case, the feeling of fatigue probably results from the loss of automatisms, with the patient having to voluntarily control activities that are usually automatic, thus generating a feeling of effort and early exhaustion.

Stroke patients also experience physical fatigue due to the presence of *motor disability and vegetative symptoms*. The above remarks on the loss of automatisms also apply to physical tasks, such as walking, and the term "task-specific" fatigue can again be used.

In stroke patients, the necessity of accepting neurological and cognitive deficits and their attempts to mask or overcome deficits also lead to *psychological stress*, anxiety, and sadness, with subsequent "psychological" fatigue.

Post-stroke *sleep disturbances* must also be considered. Insomnia, hypersomnia, and obstructive apnea are frequently reported after stroke and are manifested clinically as diurnal fatigue (Blanco *et al.*, 1999, Mohsenin and Valor, 1995). Fatigue induced by concomitant sleep disorders is usually characterized by diurnal somnolence, rather than loss of drive, but this distinction may be particularly difficult to make clinically.

Once the relationships between fatigue and stroke sequelae, psychological factors and sleep disorders have been considered, it must be determined whether the PSF is "primary" — i.e. occurring in the absence of depression, significant cognitive or neurological impairment, or any other clinical dysfunction which may cause fatigue. "Primary" PSF may be linked to specific damage to the reticular formation and other cortex-activating systems involved in the functioning of the neural attentional network.

Key points Factors associated with fatigue

Lesion location may contribute only to a small extent to the risk of developing PSF
Most studies: No association with stroke site and side
Staub et al. (2000; 2002):
patients with cortical stroke may be at greater risk to develop "task-specific" PSF
patients with brainstem stroke may be at greater risk to develop "primary" PSF
Other association:
frequent association with depression

Impact of fatigue on stroke outcome

Patients showing good neurological recovery are the group most likely to feel themselves disabled by the presence of fatigue, which may prevent them from resuming social, familial, and professional activities, even when neurological or cognitive sequelae cannot be found (Staub and Bogousslavsky, 2001;

Carlsson *et al.*, 2003). The explanation may be that patients with severe neuro-psychological and neurological impairment see fatigue as only a "minor" symptom compared to their other symptoms. Furthermore, patients with major disability are generally partially or completely dependent and thus not confronted by the demands of an active social and professional life. It is striking to note that only a small proportion of young stroke patients return to full-time work after disease onset, even in the absence of neurological and cognitive deficits detectable during classical clinical examination. Young stroke patients often report non-specific symptoms, such as fatigue, irritability, anxiety, headache, emotional lability, forgetfulness, and concentration difficulties (Röding *et al.*, 2003; Carlsson *et al.*, 2003; Leegaard, 1983). Unfortunately, such complaints tend to be ignored by doctors and rehabilitation professionals, who generally concentrate on the patient's loss of a specific function. Thus, the first step in the management of fatigue is its acknowledgment by the clinician as a potentially disabling post-stroke condition interfering with the rehabilitation process and compromising the patient's ability to regain functions. By interviewing young patients on their subjective experience of the rehabilitation process, Röding *et al.* (2003) found that fatigue affected their entire existence, being considered as an overwhelming and uncontrollable effect of stroke. Furthermore, the presence of fatigue often leads to questions and worry about its significance and its impact on disease course and functional recovery. In the specific case of small subcortical strokes, which do not usually lead to major cognitive dysfunction, the patients' quality of life has been found to be less favorable than expected, and patients commonly complain of fatigue and of "being different from before stroke," despite good functional recovery (van Zandvoort *et al.*, 1998). These data point out the necessity of informing stroke patients (especially younger patients) about PSF and its potential repercussions on everyday life. In cases of minimal physical and cognitive impairment, fatigue may be the main factor preventing resumption of full-time work (Röding *et al.*, 2003). When confronted with such cases, clinicians should take a cautious approach and prescribe a progressive return to professional activity.

As we have already mentioned, PSF is a longlasting symptom. In a large general stroke population assessed 2 years after stroke and followed up for 3 years, PSF was found to be an independent predictor for institutionalization and for reduced autonomy in daily-living activities, and, like PSD, was shown to increase the case fatality rate (Glader *et al.*, 2002).

Fatigue and stroke location

The study of PSF would seem to be a particularly promising approach for research into the neurobiological mechanisms underling central fatigue, as it should make it possible to explore the effects of well delimited lesions on the genesis of fatigue in the absence of concomitant immune, endocrinological, viral, or infectious pathologies. However, the majority of existing studies have found no correlation between fatigue and stroke site or side (Ingles *et al.*, 1999; van der Werf *et al.*, 2001; Carlsson *et al.*, 2003). In contrast to this general tendency, our group obtained some data suggesting potential links between PSF and stroke location (Staub *et al.*, 2000; 2002). By focusing on patients with a first-ever acute "non-disabling" stroke and after excluding subjects with a standard diagnosis of depression, we found that two groups had higher fatigue severity scores, these being patients with lesions involving the cortex, in whom fatigue was often associated with specific cognitive disorders, and patients with brainstem strokes. The latter group appears particularly interesting because they *a priori* do not have relevant cognitive dysfunction and may be particularly at risk of developing the condition we have called primary PSF. We hypothesize that primary PSF is the result of subtle attentional deficits in association with specific damage to the reticular formation and other cortex-activating systems.

The incrimination of specific brain structures and areas in the genesis of fatigue is not new. Colombo *et al.* (2000) hypothesized that, in multiple sclerosis patients, fatigue might be the result of functional deafferentation of the cortex due to cortical—subcortical damage, the main structures involved being the periventricular areas, internal capsule, and trigone. In Parkinson's disease, basal ganglia lesion and striatal dopaminergic input impairment, both of which are known to diminish cortical activation and reduce voluntary attention, have been associated with fatigue (Owen *et al.*, 1993). In post-polio and other post-viral chronic fatigue syndromes, Bruno *et al.* (1998) postulated that viral damage to the reticular formation, lenticular, hypothalamic and thalamic nuclei, cortical motor areas, and especially dopaminergic neurons in the substantia nigra is responsible for the development of a feeling of fatigue, exhaustion, and aversion to effort, mediated by a decrement in cortical activation, with attentional impairment, slowing of information processing, and motor activity inhibition. Finally, Chaudhuri and Behan (2000) proposed that the central fatigue observed in central nervous system disorders may be due to dysfunction of the striato-thalamo-cortical loop connecting the neostriatum with the prefrontal cortex, a hypothesis supported by the marked association of central fatigue with basal ganglia diseases, whether structural, metabolic, or neurochemical.

Even if the neurobiological substrate of central fatigue is far from completely understood, there is now evidence that specific brain structures and circuits are involved in its genesis.

Whatever the mechanism, the link between fatigue and brain lesions appears to be very complex. Like PSD, PSF is a complex, heterogeneous, and mainly subjective phenomenon which cannot be easily explained by lesion localization. In fact, published studies (Leegaard, 1983; van Zandvoort et al., 1998; Ingles et al., 1999; van der Werf et al., 2001; Glader et al., 2002, Röding et al., 2003; Carlsson et al., 2003; Schuitemaker et al., 2004) and our unpublished data have shown that it is difficult to find very good predictors for PSF. Lesion location may contribute only to a small extent to the risk of developing PSF which may develop irrespective of the stroke site. Nevertheless, patients with lesions in the abovementioned structures may be at greater risk. In addition, the type of fatigue may vary according to lesion topography. Cortical involvement, associated with specific cognitive impairment, may play a predominant role in the development of task-specific fatigue, while damage to the reticular formation and other cortex-activating systems, linked to subtle attentional difficulties, may preferentially be associated with primary PSF.

Assessment of PSF

In a clinical setting, the practitioner is confronted not with fatigue itself, but with a patient who complaints (usually spontaneously) about fatigue. Thus, it is of utmost importance to consider not only the symptoms, etiology, and pathophysiology of the fatigue, but also the inner state (cognition and mood) of the patient and the context and circumstances associated with fatigue development.

Subjective Component

Assessment of the subjective component of fatigue is not easy, because the feeling of fatigue is a complex phenomenon with multimodal components (motor–perceptive, emotional, and cognitive) and because it is poorly correlated with objective measurements. A variety of self-reporting instruments have been developed to measure subjective fatigue. Some were created for specific disorders, such as multiple sclerosis or chronic fatigue syndrome (Schwartz et al., 1993; Fisk et al., 1994), while others have more general applications and are included in a less specific health assessment. Some questionnaires assess a general feeling of fatigue (Lee et al., 1991), others selectively assess the mental (Bentall et al., 1993) or physical (Vercoulen et al., 1994; 1996) dimensions, while others are more comprehensive (Schwartz et al., 1993; Fisk et al., 1994). Currently, there is no validated scale for the specific evaluation of PSF. Thus scales used to assess fatigue in other disorders, such as the Fatigue Impact Scale (Fisk et al., 1994), Fatigue Assessment Instrument (Schwartz et al., 1993), or the fatigue subscale of the Checklist Individual Strength (Vercoulen et al., 1994; 1996), have been used in stroke populations. Even though the choice of a multidimensional self-estimation instrument is undoubtedly more appropriate for capturing the complexity of

PSF, a single-item strategy might be a suitable alternative in the general stroke population, including patients with severe cognitive impairment. Indeed, the neurobehavioral consequences of stroke, especially aphasia, often compromise patient evaluation. An easily understandable single-item questionnaire should make it possible to assess a large percentage of stroke patients, a factor indispensable in the collection of epidemiological data.

Objective component

As far as we are aware, only one study has tried to evaluate the objective component of PSF (Van Zandvoort *et al.*, 1998). Objective mental fatigue, defined as a decreased capacity for mental effort, was evaluated by detailed psychometric assessment in patients with a single supratentorial small infarction and in controls. Although globally "normal," the patients' performance in tests involving greater concentration was impaired. Thus, subtle attentional deficits seem to be the main determinants of mental fatigue in stroke patients, reflecting a problem of performance, rather than competence.

An interesting approach would be to correlate objective changes in cognitive performance with the self-reported feeling of fatigue. Such a study was carried out in multiple sclerosis patients and healthy controls before and after a difficult continuous cognitive task requiring intense concentration (Krupp and Elkins, 2000). Interestingly, although both groups reported an increased feeling of fatigue, performance improved in controls and declined in patients. This lack of correlation between performance-based measurement of fatigue and subjective fatigue emphasizes the complexity of the phenomenon and the need to consider the patient's inner state.

Key points Assessment of fatigue

Clinical setting
Identification of fatigue as a problem: interferences with daily functioning
Nature of fatigue:
is fatigue consecutive to stroke?
is fatigue different in quality and quantity from that experienced before stroke?
type of fatigue
Screening for coexisting and aggravating factors:
mood disorders
sleep disorders
medications (antispastic agents, tricyclic antidepressants, anticonvulsants...)
medical comorbidities (anemia, hypothyroidism...)
Fatigue scales: currently, no validated scale for PSF
Neurological and neuropsychological assessment

Guidelines for the clinician

Identification of fatigue as a problem

PSF is often spontaneously reported by the patients. The following questions have to be addressed. (a) Does fatigue constitute a problem interfering with daily functioning? (b) Is the fatigue consecutive to the stroke? (c) Is the present fatigue different in nature from that experienced before stroke?

Screening for factors that can induce or worsen fatigue

1. *Mood evaluation.* Pay particular attention to depression and anxiety. The only relevant and constant factor consistently found to be associated with PSF in different studies is depression (Ingles *et al.*, 1999; van der Werf *et al.*, 2001; Glader *et al.*, 2002, Carlsson *et al.*, 2003). Anxiety, which has not been specifically considered in existing studies, may be an even more crucial variable (Staub *et al.*, 2004).

2. *Identification of sleep disorders.* Insomnia, hypersomnia, and obstructive apnea are frequently reported in stroke patients. After a detailed interview, possibly accompanied by the administration of questionnaires (i.e. the Epworth Sleepiness Scale), it may be useful to perform formal sleep studies on some patients.

3. *Listing of medications.* Fatigue can be caused by many drugs, such as antispastic agents, tricyclic antidepressants, and anticonvulsants.

4. *History of coexisting diseases and medical comorbidities.* A laboratory screen is especially useful in order to exclude conditions typically associated with fatigue, such as anemia or hypothyroidism.

Identification of PSF

PSF is frequently reported by the patients as a new phenomenon, quantitatively and qualitatively different from the fatigue experienced before stroke. Its repercussions on the patient's life are often considered overwhelming and uncontrollable.

1. *Fatigue scales.* If the patient is able to understand the questionnaires, their use provides useful and quantifiable information.

2. *Neurological and neuropsychological evaluations.* In some patients, fatigue is clearly linked to cognitive or neurological sequelae. We have already proposed the term "task-specific" fatigue to describe this kind of fatigue, which appears when the patient is asked to perform an impaired function. The rehabilitation of such impaired abilities (i.e. language and motility) should result in improvement of fatigue symptoms. The diagnosis of primary PSF should be

reserved for those cases in which fatigue occurs in the absence of significant detectable stroke sequelae, depression, or other clinical conditions that can explain fatigue. Special care should be paid to the evaluation of attentional functions, since primary PSF may be linked to specific damage to cortex-activating systems involved in the functioning of the neural attentional network.

Management and treatment

Because of the multidimensional nature of PSF, the management and treatment of fatigue must be individually tailored as much as possible.

As already mentioned, our understanding of the neurobiological basis of fatigue is poor. As a consequence, there is a lack of specific pharmacological treatments and there have been few therapeutic successes. In addition, fatigue is still often considered as a medically unexplained symptom and due to somatization or a feature of depression.

The first step in the management of fatigue is therefore its acknowledgement as a potentially invalidating post-stroke condition interfering with the patient's social, familial and professional life and compromising their ability to regain impaired functions. Because of the potential deleterious aspects of PSF, relevant information should be given to the patient at an early stage (especially younger patients). In cases of minimal physical and cognitive impairment, fatigue may be the main factor preventing resumption of full-time work (Röding et al., 2003). When confronted with such cases, clinicians should take a cautious approach and propose a progressive return to professional activity.

The presence of a persisting fatigue syndrome after stroke often requires lifestyle changes, including a reduction in work, an increase in sleep quantity, the introduction of naps, and the fragmentation of activities. Together, the patient and physician must determine the level of disability caused by the fatigue in order to establish an acceptable range of mental and physical daily activities and avoid exhaustion and burnout.

The consideration and treatment of comorbidities and coexisting aggravating factors is essential. The treatment of pain, sleep disorders, and spasticity are examples of such conditions. Special attention must be paid to mood disorders because of their very frequent association with fatigue. Sedative antidepressants should be avoided. Cognitive behavioral therapy and psychosocial framing may help the patient cope, both by minimizing negative changes in self-perception and by providing advice and help for the resolution of concrete socio-professional difficulties (i.e. loss of employment and failure to fulfill family responsibilities).

On the other hand, the physician should, as far as possible, avoid iatrogenic aggravation of existing fatigue. Sedation and fatigue are common side-effects of many drugs. Among the pharmacological substances most frequently associated with fatigue are the psychotropic drugs, antiepileptics, opiates, and analgesics. Antihypertensives and antidiabetics must also be mentioned because of their frequent use in the stroke population. When prescribing such categories of drugs, the physician should be especially attentive to their propensity to induce fatigue as a collateral effect.

Neuropsychological rehabilitation, physiotherapy, and ergotherapy are also valuable instruments, especially when fatigue is directly linked to specific cognitive or neurological sequel ("task-specific" fatigue).

Finally, there is unfortunately no antifatigue drug. Psychostimulants (pemoline, modafinil, methylphenidate = ritalin, amphetamine), antiasthenic drugs (amino acids, trace elements, ginseng), antiviral (amantadine), and "stimulant" antidepressants (fluoxetine and nortriptyline) have sometimes been used, with variable benefit, in multiple sclerosis, chronic fatigue syndrome, multiple system atrophy, and post-polio syndrome. As far as we are aware, there have been no controlled studies on the use of pharmacological treatment in a stroke population. We are currently carrying out an experimental study with Modafinil, a psychostimulant enhancing wakefulness and vigilance, which is successfully used in the treatment of narcolepsy (Becker *et al.*, 2004). Experimental trials with Modafinil have been carried out in other disorders, in particular in multiple sclerosis, closed-head brain injury, and depression (Zifko *et al.*, 2002; Elovic, 2000; DeBattista *et al.*, 2004). Our current investigation on a population of non-depressed patients who suffered a minor stroke and developed a PSF syndrome is not very encouraging. Fewer than 20% of patients reported a subjective positive effect of medication, and, even in these patients, this was considered to have little effect on daily life and had no statistically significant effect on fatigue and mood scores or neuropsychological performance. Thirty percent of patients were forced to discontinue treatment because of side-effects (excitability, anxiety, headache, nausea, sleep disorders), which appeared to be more frequent and severe in stroke patients than in narcoleptics, despite the use of smaller doses (50–100 mg/day). Significant success was seen in a few cases with thalamic and brainstem lesions. In stroke patients, Modafinil may be effective in individuals with hypersomnia and excessive daytime sleepiness (Staub *et al.*, unpublished data).

These data must be regarded with caution and larger trials are needed before any treatment efficacy can be confirmed for stroke patients.

Key points Management and treatment of fatigue

Because of its multidimensional nature, management and treatment of PSF must be
  individually tailored

Acknowledgment of fatigue as a potentially invalidating post-stroke sequelae

Progressive return to professional activity

Life-style changes: reduction in work, increase in sleep quantity, fragmentation of activities...

Treatment of comorbidities and coexisting aggravating factors

Rehabilitation of impaired neurological and cognitive abilities

Cognitive behavioral therapy and psychosocial framing

Psychostimulant drugs in selected cases

Conclusion

PSF was previously misleadingly regarded as a mere component of PSD. It is
now established that, even though they are often strongly correlated, these
two phenomena can develop independently. Like PSD, PSF is a frequent and
disabling consequence of stroke. Its study is complex because of (1) difficulties in
the choice of an operational definition, (2) the lack of objective tools for its
measurement, (3) the diversity of its manifestations, and (4) our ignorance of
the underlying neurobiological mechanisms. In patients with excellent neurological and neuropsychological recovery, PSF may be the only persisting sequel, but
can severely limit the return to previous activities. For these reasons, recognition
of PSF may be critical during recovery and rehabilitation after stroke.

Further studies are needed to understand the clinical and biological pathophysiology of PSF. This could lead to the treatment of PSF which is currently only
experimental and anecdotal.

REFERENCES

Becker, P. M., Schwartz, J. R., Feldman, N. T. and Hughes, R. J. (2004). Effect of modafinil
  on fatigue, mood, and health-related quality of life in patients with narcolepsy.
  Psychopharmacology, **171**(2), 133–9.

Bentall, R. P., Wood, G. C., Marrinan, T., Deans, C. and Edwards, R. H. (1993). A brief mental
  fatigue questionnaire. *Br. J. Clin. Psychol.*, **32**, 375–9.

Blanco, M., Espinosa, M., Arpa, J., Barreiro, P. and Rodriguez-Albarino, A. (1999).
  Hypersomnia and thalamic and brain stem stroke: A study of seven patients. *Neurologia*,
  14(6), 307–14.

Bruno, R. L., Creange, S. J. and Frick, N. M. (1998). Parallels between post-polio fatigue
  and chronic fatigue syndrome: A common pathophysiology? *Am. J. Med.*, **105**(suppl. 1),
  66–73.

Carlsson, G. E., Möller, A. and Blomstrand, C. (2003). Consequences of mild stroke in persons < 75 years—A 1-year follow-up. *Cerebrovasc. Dis.*, **16**, 383—8.

Chaudhuri, A. and Behan, P. O. (2000). Fatigue and basal ganglia. *J. Neurol. Sci.*, **179**, 34—42.

Colombo, B., Martinelli Boneschi, F., Rossi, P., *et al.* (2000). MRI and motor evoked potential findings in nondisabled multiple sclerosis patients with and without symptoms of fatigue. *J. Neurol.*, **247**(7), 506—9.

DeBattista, C., Lembke, A., Solvason, H. B., Ghebremichael, R. and Poirier, J. (2004). A prospective trial of modafinil as an adjunctive treatment of major depression. *J. Clin. Psychopharmacol.*, **24**(1), 87—90.

Elovic, E. (2000). Use of provigil for underarousal following TBI. *J. Head Trauma Rehabil.*, **15**(4), 1068—71.

Fisk, J. D., Ritvo, P. G., Ross, L., *et al.* (1994). Measuring the functional impact of fatigue: Initial validation of the fatigue impact scale. *Clin. Infect. Dis.*, **21**, 9—14.

Friedman, J. and Friedman, H. (1993). Fatigue in Parkinson's disease. *Neurology*, **43**, 2016—19.

Fuhrer, R. and Wessely, S. (1995). Fatigue in French primary care. *Psychol. Med.*, **25**, 895—905.

Glader, E. L., Stegmayr, B. and Asplund, K. (2002). Poststroke fatigue: A 2-year follow-up study of stroke patients in Sweden. *Stroke*, **33**, 1327—33.

Holmes, G. P., Kaplan, J. E., Ganz, N. M., *et al.* (1988). Chronic fatigue syndrome: A working case definition. *Ann. Intern. Med.*, **108**, 387—9.

Ingles, J. L., Eskes, G. A. and Phillips, S. J. (1999). Fatigue after stroke. *Arch. Phys. Med. Rehabil.*, **80**, 173—8.

Kroenke, K. and Price, R. (1993). Symptoms in the community: Prevalence, classification and psychiatric comorbidity. *Arch. Intern. Med.*, **153**, 2474—80.

Krupp, L. B. and Elkins, L. E. (2000). Fatigue and declines in cognitive functioning in multiple sclerosis. *Neurology*, **55**(7), 934—9.

Lee, K. A., Hicks, G. and Nino-Murcia, G. (1991). Validity and reliability of a scale to assess fatigue. *Psychiatry Res.*, **36**, 291—8.

Leegaard, O. F. (1983). Diffuse cerebral symptoms in convalescents from cerebral infarction and myocardial infarction. *Acta Neurol. Scan.*, **67**, 348—55.

Mohsenin, V. and Valor, R. (1995). Sleep apnea in patients with hemispheric stroke. *Arch. Phys. Med. Rehabil.*, **76**(1), 71—6.

Owen, A. M., Roberts, A. C., Hodges, J. R., *et al.* (1993). Contrasting mechanisms of impaired attentional set-shifting in patients with frontal lobe damage or Parkinson's disease. *Brain*, **116**, 1159—75.

Röding, J., Lindström, B., Malm, J. and Öhman, A. (2003). Frustrated and invisible — younger stroke patients' experiences of the rehabilitation process. *Disabil. Rehabil.*, **25**(15), 867—74.

Schuitemaker, G. E., Dinant, G. J., van der Pol, G. A. and Appels, A. (2004). Vital exhaustion as a risk indicator for first stroke. *Psychosomatics*, **45**, 114—18.

Schwartz, J. E., Jandorf, L. and Krupp, L. B. (1993). The measurement of fatigue: A new instrument. *J. Psychosom. Res.*, **37**(7), 753—62.

Staub, F. and Bogousslavsky, J. (2001). Fatigue after stroke: A major but neglected issue. *Cerebrovasc. Dis.*, **12**, 75—81.

Staub, F., Annoni, J. M. and Bogousslavsky, J. (2000). Fatigue after stroke: A pilot study. *Cerebrovasc. Dis.*, **10**(suppl. 2), 62.

Staub, F., Annoni, J. M. and Bogousslavsky, J. (2002). Post-stroke fatigue: a major problem in "non-disabling" stroke. *Cerebrovasc. Dis.*, **13**(suppl. 3), 96.

Staub, F., Annoni, J. M., Gramigna, S. and Bogousslavsky, J. (2004). Time dynamics of post-stroke fatigue. *Cerebrovasc. Dis.*, **17**(suppl. 5), 49.

Van der Werf, S. P., van den Broek, H. L. P., Anten, H. W. M. and Bleijenberg, G. (2001). Experience of severe fatigue long after stroke and its relation to depressive symptoms and disease characteristics. *Eur. Neurol.*, **45**, 28−33.

Van der Werf, S. P., Jongen, P. J., Lycklama a Nijeholt, G. J., *et al.* (1998). Fatigue in multiple sclerosis: Interrelations between fatigue complaints, cerebral MRI abnormalities and neurological disability. *J. Neurol. Sci.*, **160**(2), 164−70.

Van Zandvoort, M. J. E., Kappelle, L. J., Algra, A. and De Haan, E. H. F. (1998). Decreased capacity for mental effort after single supratentorial lacunar infarct may affect performance in everyday life. *J. Neurol. Neurosurg. Psychiatry.*, **65**, 697−702.

Vercoulen, J., Hommes, O. R., Swanink, C., *et al.* (1996). The measurement of fatigue in patients with multiple sclerosis: A multidimensional comparison with patients with chronic fatigue syndrome and healthy subjects. *Arch. Neurol.*, **53**, 642−49.

Vercoulen, J., Swanink, C., Fennis, J., *et al.* (1994). Dimensional assessment of chronic fatigue syndrome. *J. Psychsom. Res.*, **38**, 383−92.

Zifko, U. A., Rupp, M., Schwarz, S., Zipko, H. T. and Maida, E. M. (2002). Modafinil in treatment of fatigue in multiple sclerosis. Results of an open-label study. *J. Neurol.*, **249**(8), 983−7.

31

Vascular dementia

Hugues Chabriat[1] and Olivier Godefroy[2]

[1]University Hospital Lariboisière and IFR 49, Paris, France
[2]University Hospital, Amiens, France

Introduction

Vascular dementia (VaD) is the second most common cause of dementia with a frequency ranging from 15% to 25% in autopsy and epidemiological studies (Tomlinson *et al.*, 1970; Stevens *et al.*, 2002). In addition, dementia is observed a few months post-stroke with prevalence as high as 25–33%, and about two-thirds of these patients meet the criteria of VaD (Tatemichi *et al.*, 1993; Pohjasvaara *et al.*, 1998). VaD may be a preventable type of dementia since it is due to vascular pathology and usually concerns patients with modifiable vascular risk factors. The diagnosis of VaD has several implications, including a high risk of stroke recurrence and mortality (Tatemichi *et al.*, 1994b; Moroney *et al.*, 1997b). VaD is due to several vascular pathologies, the most frequent being small vessel disease responsible for lacunes and leukoaraïosis (reported in about 40% of poststroke dementia) and multiple territorial infarcts. Because of the vascular mechanisms of underlying lesions, VaD is characterized by the frequency of stroke history, abrupt onset, stepwise deterioration, and the early presence of non-cognitive signs such as motor and perceptual deficits, gait disorders, speech and swallowing disorders, and incontinence. However a third of autopsy-confirmed VaD did not report stroke history and about a quarter presented with a progressive worsening (Moroney *et al.*, 1997a). Although the neuropsychological pattern was found to be variable in an autopsy-confirmed VaD (Reed *et al.*, 2004), most studies highlighted the prominence of executive dysfunction and response slowing.

VaD remains probably largely underdiagnosed as suggested by a survey of statistics from Stroke Unit and Memory Clinics. Failure to identify VaD may stem from several difficulties: (1) the underrecognition of dementia in stroke patients is frequently due to failure to identify cognitive deficits or to the erroneous attribution of social decline to motor-perceptual deficits (Gauthier *et al.*, 1999); (2) the underrecognition of vascular lesions in demented patients may be due to the lack of stroke history and stepwise worsening, to underrecognition of

Table 31.1. DSM-IV criteria for vascular dementia

Dementia according to DSM-IV criteria

A.1. Memory impairment

A.2. One or more of the following cognitive disturbances

    a. aphasia

    b. apraxia

    c. agnosia

    d. disturbance in executive functioning

B.   Cognitive deficits in criteria A1 and A2 each cause significant impairment in social or occupational functioning and represent a significant decline from a previous level of functioning

C.   Factors judged to be etiologically related to the disturbance

      focal neurological signs and symptoms

      laboratory evidence indicative of cerebrovascular disease (e.g., multiple

        infarctions involving cortex and underlying white matter)

D. Not occurring exclusively during the course of delirium

early non-cognitive neurological signs, or to inadequate brain imaging study. These considerations underline the importance of careful history taken, neurological examination, adequate brain imaging, and neuropsychological studies.

Definition and diagnostic criteria for vascular dementia

Both the concept and definition of VaD were debated at the beginning of this century. The term "vascular dementia" does not actually correspond to a single or specific pathophysiological entity. It characterizes a severe cognitive impairment associated with different types of cerebrovascular diseases. For this reason, the course and prognosis of VaD can widely vary according to the underlying vascular disorder.

Different criteria have been proposed for the definition of VaD. The DSM-IV criteria are sensitive but poorly specific (American Psychiatric Association, 1994). When dementia is present, focal neurological signs and symptoms with laboratory evidence indicative of cerebrovascular disease are required to satisfy the corresponding definition (Table 31.1). Based on the DSM-IV criteria, patients with Alzheimer's disease who had a recent stroke are considered to have VaD. Elsewhere, demented patients without any visible tissue lesions on CT-scan and who had transient ischemic attacks and a carotid stenosis will also fulfill the DSM-IV diagnostic criteria for VaD. Noteworthily, this broad definition will cover not only "pure" VaD but also mixed dementias (VaD associated with Alzheimer's disease). In contrast, the definition proposed by the National Institute

Table 31.2. NINDS-AIREN criteria for the diagnosis of probable VD

1. *Dementia*
   Impairment of memory
   Impairment of memory and ≥2 cognitive domains
   orientation
   attention
   language
   visuospatial functions
   executive functions, motor control, and praxis

2. *Cerebrovascular disease*
   Focal signs on neurological examination (hemiparesis, lower facial
     weakness, Babinski's sign, sensory deficit, hemianopia, and dysarthria)
   Evidence of relevant cerebrovascular disease by brain imaging (CT)
   large-vessel infarcts
   single strategically placed infarct
   multiple basal ganglia and white matter lacunes
   extensive periventricular white matter lesions
   combinations thereof

3. *A relationship between the above disorders manifested or inferred by the*
   presence of 1 of the following
   onset of dementia within 3 months after a recognized stroke
   abrupt deterioration in cognitive functions
   fluctuating, stepwise progression of cognitive deficits

4. *Clinical features consistent with the diagnosis of probable VD*
   early presence of a gait disturbance
   history of unsteadiness or frequent, unprovoked falls
   early urinary incontinence
   pseudobulbar palsy
   personality and mood changes

5. *Features that make the diagnosis of VD uncertain*
   Early onset of memory deficit and progressive worsening of memory and other cognitive
   functions in the absence of focal neurological signs and cerebrovascular lesions on CT or
   MRI

of Neurological Disorders and Stroke (NINDS) and the Association Internationale pour la Recherche et l'Enseignement en Neurosciences (AIREN) criteria (Roman *et al.*, 1993) appear more specific for VaD and are now currently used for research and clinical trials. The NINDS-AIREN criteria (Table 31.2) require both the presence of dementia, cerebral tissue lesions known to alter cognitive performances, a temporal relationship between the vascular event and the

Table 31.3. ICD-10 research criteria (DCR-10) for vascular dementia

Dementia

A. Evidence of each of the following
   1. Decline in memory (mainly short-term memory)
   2. Decline in other cognitive abilities

Deficits in criterion A cause a significant impairment of social functioning

B. Absence of clouding of consciousness

C. Decline in emotional control or motivation or a change in social behavior

D. Symptoms in criterion A have been present ≥6 months

Unequal distribution of deficits in higher cognitive functions

Evidence of focal brain damage

Evidence of cerebrovascular disease

Table 31.4. Hachinski ischemic score

Score

Abrupt onset: 2

Stepwise deterioration: 1

Fluctuating course: 2

Nocturnal confusion: 1

Relative preservation of personality: 1

Depression: 1

Somatic complaints: 1

Emotional incontinence: 1

History of hypertension: 1

History of strokes: 2

Evidence of associated atherosclerosis: 1

Focal neurological symptoms: 2

Focal neurological signs: 2

cognitive alteration, clinical features usually associated with diffuse vascular lesions, and the lack of cognitive decline suggestive of a degenerative process. Although these criteria appear useful to better circumscribe VaD, this definition will exclude mixed dementia, a frequent cause of cognitive impairment during the elderly and also progressive cognitive decline related to the accumulation of "silent" ischemic or hemorrhagic lesions in the brain. Other criteria for VaD are available, the ICD-10 (Table 31.3) are close to the DSM-IV criteria but require the evidence of focal brain damage (Wetterling *et al.*, 1996). The Hachinski ischemic score (Table 31.4) was initially developed to separate multi-infarct dementia related to the accumulation of ischemic lesions (score >7) from

Alzheimer's disease (score < 4) (Hachinski *et al.*, 1974). However, this definition is restrictive and does not take into account single stroke dementia caused by isolated vascular insults or dementia secondary to repeated cerebral hemorrhages.

In the last decade, the limitations and utility of the concept of VaD have been repeatedly disputed. Recently, the term "vascular cognitive impairment" was proposed to better account for the whole spectrum of cognitive alterations secondary to ischemic or hemorrhagic cerebral insults which expand well beyond to dementia (Roman *et al.*, 2002). This approach is probably of crucial importance for prevention of VaD detected only at the end stage of various progressive vascular disorders. However, the framework of VaD still remains useful for the development of drugs such as cholinesterase inhibitors capable of improving cognitive functions at the most severe stage of cognitive impairment after the occurrence of cerebral tissue lesions of vascular origin.

Key points Main causes of vascular dementia

Primary vascular mechanisms
    Large artery diseases
    Small vessel diseases
    Specific arteriopathies
    Venous diseases
    Hematological factors
    Cardiac embolic events
        Leading to
        Infarcts (single strategic or multiple)
        Hemorrhages (single strategic or multiple)
        Hemodynamic mechanisms
Secondary vascular factors
    Arterial hypertension
    Cardiac abnormality
    Diabetes
    Lipid abnormalities
    Genetic factors

Modified according to Erkinjuntti, 1996.

Various Categories of VaD

In clinical practice, the diagnosis of VaD is usually raised in the presence of a demented patient who presents with cerebral lesions suggestive of a vascular origin on CT-scan or MRI. MRI is actually the most sensitive technique for the diagnosis of these lesions that can be of various types: hyperintense signals on T2-weighted MR images (or hypodensities on CT-scan) in the white-matter are presumably related to demyelination and axonal loss previously called "leukoaraïosis" and associated with diffuse small vessel diseases (Hijdra and Verbeeten, 1991), "so-called" silent infarcts detected in the absence of stroke events are most often of small size (lacunar infarcts) and located in the white-matter or subcortical grey matter (Vermeer *et al.*, 2003a), large subcortical or cortical ischemic lesions are caused by the occlusion of large vessels, micro hemorrhages are easily detected on specific MRI sequences and due to the rupture of small vessels (Kato *et al.*, 2002); large hemorrhages have most often the same origin and have a different distribution according to the underlying vessel disease. Finally, the contribution of these different lesions will largely depend on their location and number and on the presence of associated degenerative lesions.

The most important categories of VaD include: single stroke dementia, multi-infarct dementia, subcortical ischemic vascular dementia, dementia related to cerebral hemorrhages, and mixed dementia.

Dementia in patients with a single vascular lesion or single stroke dementia

Dementia may be observed in patients with isolated vascular lesions (hemorrhage or infarct) in the cortical or subcortical regions (Pullicino and Benedict, 1996). However, such a diagnosis requires a detailed neuroradiological study to exclude associated small lesions and leukoaraïosis and to exclude other causes of dementia, especially Alzheimer's disease.

Cortical stroke

In the cortex, vascular lesions can cause dementia when they involve regions with heteromodal functions, particularly the limbic system or the cortical association areas (Tatemichi, 1995). Isolated cortical infarctions causing dementia have been reported in 3 main locations: the angular gyrus (middle cerebral artery lower division), the inferomesial temporal lobe (posterior cerebral artery division) or the mesial frontal lobe (anterior cerebral artery) (Benson *et al.*, 1982; Tatemichi, 1995). All are responsible for anterograde amnesia. The angular gyrus syndrome secondary to a lesion of the dominant hemisphere also includes aphasic disturbances, constructional difficulties, and the Gerstmann tetrad (left–right disorientation, finger agnosia, dyscalculia, and dysgraphia). In angular gyrus infarcts of the non-dominant-hemisphere, spatial hemineglect and visuoconstructive disorders are associated with memory impairment (Benson *et al.*, 1982; Saver and Biller, 1995). In inferomesial temporal lobe infarctions, amnesia is due to lesions of the hippocampus region and may be associated with language, visuospatial difficulties, and/or constructional apraxia according to the affected hemispheric side (Caplan and Hedley-White, 1974; Ott and Saver, 1993). Mesial frontal lobe infarcts mainly occur after a complicated rupture of an anterior communicating artery aneurysm (Alexander and Freeman, 1984; Damasio *et al.*, 1987; Sawada and Kazui, 1995).

Subcortical stroke

Isolated subcortical vascular lesions (mainly small deep infarcts) can lead to a dementia syndrome when they disrupt specific subcortical–cortical loops which are crucial for the maintenance of the cortical functional integrity and finally for the cognitive status (Baron *et al.*, 1992). The main locations for a single small deep hemorrhage or ischemic lesion causing dementia are the thalamus, genu of internal capsule, and possibly the caudate nucleus.

Thalamic infarctions leading to dementia are mainly located either in the territory of the polar artery irrigating the anterior thalamus or in that of paramedian arteries which frequently arise from a common stem and irrigate in 50% of cases both thalami and both sides of the midbrain (Bogousslavsky *et al.*, 1988). Infarcts in the territory of the polar artery may induce executive disorders, deficit of episodic memory (Graff-Radford *et al.*, 1990), associated in left brain damage with aphasia close to the transcortical motor syndrome. In some cases, a total loss of psychic self activation has been reported (Barth *et al.*, 1995). Patients with unilateral paramedian thalamic infarct usually present an acute decrease of consciousness, neuropsychological disturbances, and abnormalities of vertical gaze (Bogousslavsky *et al.*, 1988). The cognitive alterations become evident with the resolution of consciousness impairment. Amnesia is sometimes prominent leading to confabulations and may be related to the lesion of the mamillothalamic tract (Castaigne *et al.*, 1981). The cognitive impairment is more severe in the presence of bilateral paramedian thalamic–subthalamic infarcts responsible for amnesia associated with executive disorders such as abulia, aspontaneity, and inertia (Barth *et al.*, 1995). The clinical presentation of thalamic hemorrhages is similar to that of thalamic infarcts and depends mainly on the size and location of the hematoma. Thus, both anterolateral (corresponding to the territory of polar artery) and medial (corresponding to paramedian thalamic–subthalamic arteries) thalamic hemorrhages can cause a definite dementia syndrome (Walshe *et al.*, 1977). Baron *et al.* confirmed by Positron Emission Tomography that the cognitive impairment after unilateral thalamic lesion was correlated to the ipsilateral cortical hypometabolism in support of a depression of the cortical synaptic activity (Baron *et al.*, 1992). These remote cortical effects might be related to the damage of the "non-specific" thalamic nuclei involved in the neocortical activation. This contrasts with vascular lesions of specific nuclei such as the ventroposterolateral nucleus which spares the cognitive status (Baron *et al.*, 1992; Chabriat *et al.*, 1992).

Capsular genu infarction on left side is another case of "focal dementia." Tatemichi *et al.* previously reported 4 patients having such a lesion with severe memory verbal loss associated with various cognitive deficits suggesting dementia (Tatemichi *et al.*, 1992). They inferred that this lesion was responsible for cortical deactivation (mainly the frontal cortex) by interrupting the inferior and anterior thalamic peduncles (Pullicino and Benedict, 1996; Tatemichi, 1995). The persisting dementia syndrome after recovery is possibly favored by the presence of other old cerebral ischemic lesions (Pantoni *et al.*, 2001).

Isolated *caudate* vascular lesions may also be responsible for behavioral or cognitive disturbances (Bhatia and Marsden, 1994). Caplan *et al.* (1990) reported neuropsychological alterations in 14 of 18 patients (78%) with unilateral infarcts. The clinical presentation includes various neuropsychological symptoms with prominent disorders of executive functions: reduced activity and abulia or affective symptoms (depression) with psychotic features (dorsolateral caudate), restlessness, hyperactivity, and decreased attention (ventromedial caudate) (Mendez *et al.*, 1990). The cognitive testing can reveal memory disturbances sometimes with poor recall of long-term memory (Wenchiang Han and Caplan, 1995) most often associated with abnormalities in executive functions and attention and in few cases with aphasic difficulties (left caudate infarcts) or hemineglect (right caudate infarcts) (Caplan *et al.*, 1990; Mendez *et al.*, 1990). Godefroy *et al.* (1992; 1994) did not observe dementia but only mild cognitive alterations in patients with pure unilateral lenticulostriate infarcts including caudate infarcts. Dementia was only observed in patients with multiple infarcts (especially lacunes) and/or extensive leukoaraïosis which were noticeably underestimated on CT. Therefore, caudate stroke induces severe cognitive deficit matching dementia criteria in a few cases only (Trillet *et al.*, 1990).

Dementia secondary to multiple cortical and subcortical ischemic lesions ("multi-infarct dementia")

In the presence of severe vascular disorders leading to repeated cortical and subcortical infarctions, the increased risk of dementia with the accumulation of lesions is obvious. However, the exact contribution of different tissue lesions in cognitive decline was disputed for a long time since there is no specific criterion to ensure the vascular origin of dementia in a given patient and due to the high frequency of both Alzheimer's disease and vascular disorders with aging. During the last decades, some authors reported that

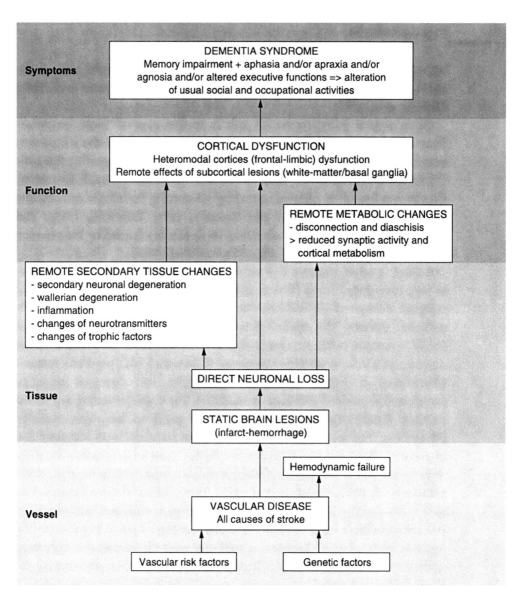

Figure 31.1 Main mechanisms of vascular dementia.

the abrupt onset of dementia, a history of stroke, the presence of focal symptoms or focal signs with the presence of isolated or multiple CT-low-density areas were the most discriminating parameters in favor of a vascular origin (Loeb and Gandolfo, 1983). However, Chui *et al.* showed that scales based on these clinical features were fairly sensitive and specific (70–80%) to differentiate pure Alzheimer's disease and multi-infarct dementia but insensitive to the presence of mixed dementia (17–30%) (Chui *et al.*, 1992). Another debated issue was the role played by the location or volume of the lesions in the dementia syndrome. This was recently settled by Zekry *et al.* who demonstrated in patients with pure VaD and mixed dementia that the location of infarctions was the main contributor of the variability of the Mini-Mental Status Examination score (at equal level with degenerative lesions in mixed dementia) in contrast with the insignificant role played by the volume of lesions (Zekry *et al.*, 2003). Therefore, it is now quite clear that the location of cerebral tissue lesions in strategic cortical or subcortical areas involved in the higher cortical functions (those entering in the definition of dementia) is finally the most important factor leading to dementia in vascular disorders.

Dementia secondary to multiple deep infarcts and leukoencephalopathy in small cerebral artery diseases

Binswanger's disease

In 1894, Otto Binswanger called "encephalitis subcorticalis chronical progressiva" a condition characterized by dementia, recurrent stroke with white-matter atrophy at pathological examination. Only in 1902, this latter was related to severe arteriolosclerosis of the long perforating arteries of deep white-matter by Alzheimer (Alzheimer, 1902). Since this date, various definitions of Binswanger's disease have been reported, particularly after the explosion of neuroimaging methods leading to the frequent identification of white-matter abnormalities in the elderly. However, Binswanger's disease should be actually considered only in cases with solid pathological data particularly focusing on the microscopic aspects of the underlying vessel disease, since both the clinical and neuroimaging features of this condition appear undoubtedly non-specific. In Japan, Tomonaga *et al.* reported a prevalence of 45 cases among 1000 autopsies (Babikian and Ropper, 1987). Its exact frequency remains however largely unknown.

Pathological examination of cases designated as having " Binswanger's disease " showed diffuse or patchy rarefaction of myelin predominating in the periventricular and occipital regions of the centrum semi-ovale associated with gliosis and spongiosis. The U fibers, internal capsules and the corpus callosum are usually spared (Babikian and Ropper, 1987). These white-matter changes are typically associated with small deep infarcts and/or dilatation of perivascular spaces or "état criblé" (Bogousslavsky, 1988) in white-matter and basal ganglia. The underlying cause is a disease of small perforating medullary arteries with thickening and hypertrophy of the media associated with lipohyalinosis and fibrosis of the adventitia. The vessel wall alterations are probably secondary to hypertension reported in nearly 100 percent of cases and considered as one cardinal feature of this condition.

Dementia is one of the main features of the disease. The typical presentation includes a progressive neurological decline marked by a few episodes of mild hemiparesis ending with mental decline, dysarthria, dysphagia, a short-step gait (described as "marche à petits pas"), imbalance, and incontinence. Patients may also exhibit spasmodic laughing or crying and sometimes a parkinsonian-like state (rigidity, bradykinesia) commonly without tremor (Caplan, 1979). Dementia usually follows the onset of gait disturbances. Deficit of executive functions are prominent with apathy, aspontaneity, attention impairment, slowing of mental processing (Babikian and Ropper, 1987; Roman *et al.*, 2002) while personality and insight are frequently preserved (Erkinjuntti *et al.*, 2000). This is in contrast with the typical presentation of Alzheimer's disease. The average duration of the disease varies from 5 to 22 years (Babikian and Ropper, 1987).

Finally, Binswanger's disease should not be considered as a pathophysiological entity but rather as the final stage of a long history of a small artery disease related to hypertension. During the two last decades, longitudinal studies showed that the extent of T2 signal abnormalities detected in the white-matter of 95% of subjects older than 65 years was strongly related to hypertension (Longstreth *et al.*, 1996), that these lesions were associated with subtle executive dysfunctions and a 2–3 fold increased risk of stroke. Noteworthily, it is now demonstrated that the occurrence of silent infarcts as detected on MRI and of ischemic stroke increases the risk of dementia (2–3 fold increase after 4 years) (Vermeer *et al.*, 2003b). Therefore, prevention strategies are crucial in patients with white-matter lesions, silent infarcts and lacunar stroke to prevent the occurrence of Binswanger's type dementia that can occur probably several decades later.

Because Binswanger's disease is usually considered in cases with solid pathological data, the term subcortical ischemic vascular dementia (SIVD) may be more appropriate in clinical practice. SIVD refers to dementia resulting from small-vessel diseases, which produces either arteriolar occlusion and lacunes or widespread incomplete infarction of white matter due to critical stenosis of medullary arterioles and hypoperfusion (Erkinjuntti *et al.*, 2000). Signs include dysarthria, mood changes, urinary symptoms, and short-stepped gait, motor and cognitive slowing, dysexecutive and episodic memory disorders. Brain imaging (computed tomography and magnetic resonance imaging) is then essential for correct diagnosis.

CADASIL

CADASIL has been identified since 1993 as a new cause of "pure vascular dementia". It is an autosomal dominant arteriopathy secondary to *Notch3 gene* mutations on chromosome 19 (Tournier-Lasserve *et al.*, 1993). In one third of symptomatic patients, the disease starts with attacks of migraine with aura at a mean age of 30 years (Chabriat *et al.*, 1995b). The most frequent clinical manifestations are subcortical transient ischemic attacks or strokes occurring between 40 and 50 years (Chabriat *et al.*, 1995b; Dichgans *et al.*, 1998). Dementia is the second commonest clinical manifestation observed in one third of symptomatic patients and it is present in 90% of patients before death (Chabriat *et al.*, 1995b). The mean age of demented patients is 60 years. The exact onset of cognitive impairment in CADASIL is difficult to ascertain. Taillia *et al.* showed that non-demented symptomatic patients, the youngest of whom was aged 35 years, had altered performances using the Wisconsin Card Sorting test, a task very sensitive to frontal dysfunction (Taillia *et al.*, 1996). A long period of mild cognitive impairment can precede the occurrence of dementia. Changes in working memory and executive function were detected before transient ischemic attack or stroke in a recent study (Amberla *et al.*, 2004). In 90% of demented cases, the cognitive impairment occurred step by step and was associated with recurrent strokes. In 10% of cases, the neuropsychological decline was isolated and progressive mimicking the course of Alzheimer's disease (Chabriat *et al.*, 1997). Most demented CADASIL patients satisfy the NINDS-AIREN and DSM-IV criteria for diagnosis of vascular dementia. The cognitive deficit is typically of subcortical type with predominating dysexecutive disorders (especially apathy) and memory impairment. Aphasia, apraxia, or agnosia are rare or observed only at the end-course of the disease (Sabbadini *et al.*, 1995). Dementia is always associated with pyramidal signs, pseudobulbar palsy, gait difficulties, and/or urinary incontinence. MRI is always abnormal in symptomatic subjects (Figure 31.2). It shows, on T2-weighted images, more or less confluent hypersignals in the white-matter and basal ganglia and, on T1-weighted images, hyposignals in the same regions corresponding to small infarcts (Chabriat *et al.*, 1996). Histologic studies show a widespread palor of white-matter and multiple small infarcts in the white-matter and basal ganglia (Baudrimont *et al.*, 1993; Gutierrez-Molina *et al.*, 1994). Electron microscopy studies show that the media of the small white-matter and leptomeningeal arteries is thickened by a granular, eosinophilic, and non-amyloïd material of undetermined origin adjacent to the smooth muscle cells. These ultrastructural wall abnormalities have been observed in other arteries, particularly in muscular and skin arteries (Ruchoux *et al.*, 1995). The severity and location of the brain ischemic lesions are probably crucial for the occurrence of dementia in CADASIL. In a positron emission tomography study of one demented patient and of his asymptomatic cousin, both with equally widespread white-matter lesions at MRI examination, Chabriat *et al.* reported a decreased cortical metabolism only in the demented subject who had the most severe basal ganglia lesions (Chabriat *et al.*,

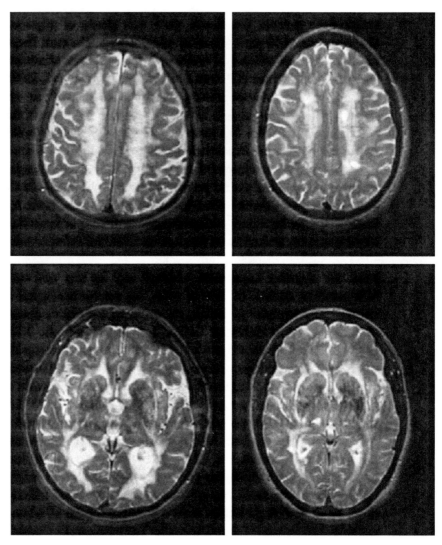

Figure 31.2 MRI from 2 CADASIL patients: note the extensive white-matter signal abnormalities and the presence of small deep infarcts in the white-matter or basal ganglia.

1995a). In the absence of cortical lesions, these findings suggest that remote metabolic effects of basal ganglia infarcts (diaschisis) at the cortical level are causing dementia in CADASIL. Other authors observed that decreased glucose consumption in the cortex of CADASIL patients was actually of various pattern and related to the location and severity of subcortical tissue lesions (Tatsch *et al.*, 2003). Recently, Mesulam *et al.* (2003) found a severe decrease of cholinergic neurons within the cortex in CADASIL. This is in favor of secondary cholinergic denervation in the cortex of CADASIL patients after the accumulation of subcortical ischemic lesions (Mesulam *et al.*, 2003). Otherwise, the presence of typical lesions of Alzheimer's disease has been reported in anecdotal cases in association with typical ischemic lesions caused by CADASIL (Gray *et al.*, 1994; Thijs *et al.*, 2003).

Other arteriolopathies leading to small deep infarcts and leukoencephalopathy

Other rare specific vascular conditions leading to multiple small brain infarcts have been recognized as possible causes of VaD. In most of them, the exact origin of the vessel disease remains to be ascertained. In a few isolated cases with extensive pathological data, the clinical and pathologic features were close to that of Binswanger's disease except for the lack of hypertension and the young age of onset (Berthier *et al.*, 1992; Loizou *et al.*, 1982) or because of distinct ultrastructural wall abnormalities involving both capillaries, arterioles, and venules (Estes *et al.*, 1991). Hereditary conditions leading to vascular dementia distinct from CADASIL have been also reported. Fukutake reviewed 17 cases affected by a familial young-adult-onset arteriosclerotic leukoencephalopathy with alopecia and lumbago without arterial hypertension in Japan (Fukutake and Hirayama 1995). The transmission was presumably autosomal recessive with a male to female ratio of 7.5. All patients except one presented with dementia which occurred in half of them after recurrent strokes. The dementia was of subcortical type and associated with pseudobulbar palsy, pyramidal signs, and incontinence. The onset was between 25 and 30. Alopecia was present in 15 patients, a prior history of acute lumbago in 13, cervical and lumbar spondylosis deformans in 12. Six of the 7 deceased patients died within 10 years after onset. Pathological data showed a diffuse demyelination associated with multiple lacunar infarcts in basal ganglia or white-matter underlaid by a small-artery disease with fibrous intimal proliferation, severe hyalinosis, and splitting of the intima and/or internal elastic membrane (Maeda *et al.*, 1976).

Progressive mental deterioration associated with visual loss was also reported in 3 of 8 members of a family with a hereditary syndrome characterized by retinal capillary obliteration and central nervous system vasculopathy called "cerebroretinal vasculopathy" (Grand *et al.*, 1988). Infarcts in basal ganglia and white-matter were underlaid by an inflammatory process with prominent fibrinoid necrosis and obliterative fibrosis involving both arteries and veins of medium and small calibers (Grand *et al.*, 1988). Other hereditary vascular conditions unlinked to *Notch3 gene* mutations and responsible for brain ischemic insults have been recently identified as potential causes of VaD (Adair *et al.*, 1997; Jen *et al.*, 1997).

Dementia related to multiple brain hemorrhages and amyloid angiopathies

The inclusion or exclusion of cerebral hemorrhages (intracerebral and subarachnoid) as classical causes of vascular dementia is a matter of debate. Some authors previously proposed to consider them separately since they usually present primarily as major strokes with neurological deficit overshadowing the cognitive impairment (Bowler and Hachinsky, 1996; Pasquier and Leys, 1997). Nevertheless in amyloid angiopathy, dementia is a prominent symptom which sometimes occurs progressively.

Amyloid angiopathy is only one aspect of cerebral diseases with amyloid deposits (Haan *et al.*, 1994). Amyloid is merely a descriptive term for proteins with particular physical characteristics (Glenner, 1980) which can be present in the neurons as neurofibrillary tangles, in the neuropil as plaques or in the vessel wall as amyloid angiopathy. Various chemical types of amyloid deposition have been recognized; ßA4 (Aß), cystatin C, transthyretin or Prion protease resistant protein (PrP). Mutations of PrP are responsible for the Creutzfeldt-Jakob disease and the Gerstmann-Straussler syndrome which are clearly distinct from vascular dementia (Haan *et al.*, 1994). Conversely mutations of ßA4 (Aß), cystatin C or transthyretin induce amyloid angiopathies that lead to dementia (Greenberg and Hyman, 1997; Greenberg *et al.*, 1993).

Most cases of amyloid angiopathy are usually sporadic and more than 40% of them are associated with Alzheimer's disease (Vinters, 1987). While the ε4 allele of apoE has been identified as a risk factor for Alzheimer's disease by promoting the aggregation and deposition of Aß within the cortex (Strittmatter *et al.*, 1993), apoE ε2 seems to play a major role in the deposition of Aß in the vascular wall leading to amyloid angiopathy and hemorrhages (Greenberg and Hyman, 1997; Nicoll *et al.*, 1997). The location of cerebral hemorrhages is probably critical in the occurrence of cognitive impairment. Elsewhere, associated lesions such as small silent infarcts in cortical watershed areas (Hashiguchi *et al.*, 2000), white-matter lesions and/or subcortical infarcts also related to amyloid angiopathy may participate in the alteration of the cognitive status.

In hereditary amyloid angiopathies, mutations in the ßA4 amyloid precursor protein (ßAPP) gene are responsible for both brain and vascular deposits. Consequently, dementia can be secondary to a combination of lesions typical of Alzheimer's disease and hemorrhages. This is observed in "hereditary cerebral hemorrhages with amyloidosis of Dutch type" and in "presenile dementia with cerebral hemorrhage" caused respectively to mutations of codon 693 and 692 of ßAPP. In contrast, mutations in the cystatin C gene can cause a familial amyloid angiopathy distinct from Alzheimer's disease responsible for cerebral hemorrhages and leading to a "pure" form of vascular dementia. Hereditary cystatin C amyloid angiopathy (HCAA) is an autosomal dominant condition described in families originating from Iceland. The clinical manifestations of HCAA are various. Onset is usually in the twenties or thirties. Some patients died after a first brain hemorrhage. Others present with recurrent focal deficits, most of them due to hemorrhagic lesions, and develop a stepwise dementia after the occurrence of several strokes (Blondal *et al.*, 1989). In some cases, long periods with neither focal manifestations nor cognitive decline were observed (Haan *et al.*, 1994). Others presented with a progressive dementia and leuko-encephalopathy with a late onset (Sveinbjfornsdfottir *et al.*, 1996). Therefore, the cognitive impairment is of various presentations; it is related to subcortical infarcts and/or most often to the subcortical and cortical sequelae of recurrent hemorrhagic lesions. The amyloid deposition is found in the proximity of blood vessels and in their walls (Blondal *et al.*, 1990). In HCAA, the amyloid deposits are not limited to the cerebral vasculature; they are also found in nodes, spleen, salivary glands, seminal vesicles, testes, and skin but remain asymptomatic. Punch skin biopsies have been proposed for the diagnosis (Benedikz *et al.*, 1990).

Oculoleptomeningeal amyloidosis results from amyloid deposits in the leptomeninges (especially the leptomeningeal vessels), the brain parenchyma, and the eye. Neurological signs are due to hydrocephalus, atrophy, and infarction of cerebral and cerebellar cortexes. Slowly progressive dementia, seizures, ataxia, hemiparesis, and decreased vision are observed in these patients. Clinical practice shows that cognitive disorders may be observed in peripheral hemosiderosis of the central nervous system but their characteristics remain to be determined.

Dementia related to hemodynamic mechanisms

Hypoperfusion secondary to carotid diseases is a very rare cause of vascular dementia. Unilateral or bilateral occlusion of carotid arteries is the most common precipitating factor (Tatemichi *et al.*, 1995). Hemodynamic failure in the frontal border-zone supplied by the distal and most pial branches of the middle and anterior cerebral arteries can lead to ischemic lesions at distance from the sylvian area. The clinical presentation often includes only aphasia, apraxia or hemineglect without prominent motor deficit (Rabinstein *et al.*, 2004). In most cases, pathological examination reveals widespread or multifocal infarction in regions including the association areas of the anterior and posterior cerebrum.

Chronic ischemia without infarction in the carotid territory is an exceptional cause of dementia. Rarely has the cognitive alteration been attributed to a "misery perfusion" with positron emission tomography investigations (Baron *et al.*, 1981). This type of dementia is reversible after correction of the hemodynamic deficit. In one documented case, extra-intracranial arterial bypass surgery was efficient to improve the cognitive status (Baron *et al.*, 1981).

The neuropsychology of vascular dementia

The development of neuropsychology has led to three major findings in the field of vascular dementia. First of all, vascular dementia is frequent and its prevalence is probably underestimated. For example, systematic assessments several months post-stroke have revealed a prevalence of dementia as high as 25% to 33%, and about two-thirds of patients meet the criteria for vascular dementia (Tatemichi *et al.*, 1993; Pohjasvaara *et al.*, 1998). This suggests that dementia is underestimated by routine assessment of stroke patients. Secondly, vascular dementia does not present a unique pattern of neuropsychological and behavioral disorders, supporting the use of a behavioral inventory and a large battery of tests. Thirdly, some neuropsychological patterns of vascular dementia are different from those observed in Alzheimer's disease and this may contribute to the diagnosis especially when other typical features of vascular dementia are lacking.

The heterogeneity of neuropsychological findings in vascular dementia is well known and can be explained by the diversity of the sites of lesions and mechanisms, which include lacunar and territorial infarcts, ischemic lesions of the white matter, and hemorrhage. The neuropsychological pattern may also be influenced by concomitant Alzheimer's disease observed in about one-third of post-stroke dementia patients (Tatemichi *et al.*, 1993; Pohjasvaara *et al.*, 1998). Finally, the pattern of cognitive deficits may differ according to the severity of dementia (Kertesz and Clydesdale, 1994), although this has not been replicated in all studies (Sachdev *et al.*, 2004).

Nevertheless, dominant features emerge from several studies. Firstly, slowing of response rate (see Chapter 19) has been reported in most studies of post-stroke cognitive disorders including vascular dementia (Tatemichi *et al.*, 1994a). Comparison with Alzheimer's disease has shown that reaction time tests and the Trail Making test may be more prolonged in vascular dementia (Starkstein *et al.*, 1997; Mendez *et al.*, 1997). Secondly, the importance of executive dysfunction is frequently underlined (Wolfe *et al.*, 1990; for review, Looi and Sachdev, 1999). Behavioral changes similar to those reported in dysexecutive syndrome (see Chapter 19) are frequently observed in vascular dementia, even at an early stage; in addition, a few studies have shown that emotional lability and anosognosia are more severe than in Alzheimer's disease or mixed dementia (i.e., dementia due to a combination of stroke and degenerative disease, especially Alzheimer's disease) (Hachinski *et al.*, 1975; Moroney *et al.*, 1997b; Starkstein *et al.*, 1997). Neuropsychological tests used in the early stage have shown more severe impairment of executive functions than in Alzheimer's disease in most studies (Looi and Sachdev, 1999; Tierney *et al.*, 2001). However, there is a marked overlap between vascular dementia and Alzheimer's dementia, limiting the value of these tests in individual patients. In addition the high variability of neuropsychological pattern has been recently showed in autopsy defined vascular dementia (Reed *et al.*, 2004). The high frequency of executive dysfunction is not specific to the stage of dementia and is also observed in non-demented stroke patients (e.g., Sachdev *et al.*, 2004) and in the early stages of CADASIL (Taillia *et al.*, 1998; Amberla *et al.*, 2004). It is especially marked in subcortical ischemic disease (Wolfe *et al.*, 1990; Kramer *et al.*, 2002; Pohjasvaara *et al.*, 2003) and is attributed to white matter abnormalities (Pohjasvaara *et al.*, 2000; Mungas *et al.*, 2001; O'Brien *et al.*, 2002; Tullberg *et al.*, 2004). Thirdly, the pattern of deficit of episodic memory has been shown to differ from that of Alzheimer's disease in some studies, a finding not replicated in others (for review, see Almkvist *et al.*, 1999; Looi and Sachdev, 1999). However, in a study focusing on subcortical ischemic dementia, recognition was relatively spared compared to Alzheimer's dementia (Tierney *et al.*, 2001). This is consistent with the hypothesis that a memory pattern suggestive of fronto-subcortical pathology (Pillon *et al.*, 1993) is more frequent in subcortical ischemic vascular dementia. A few studies have shown that a deficit of episodic memory may be initially observed for retention of visual material only (Sachdev *et al.*, 2004; Amberla *et al.*, 2004).

From a clinical point of view, two main neuropsychological patterns emerge from the literature. The first pattern consists of "subcortical" dementia with response slowing, executive disorders, impairment of retrieval processes in episodic memory, and relative sparing of spatial exploration, language, gestural, constructional, and visuognosic abilities. This pattern may be more frequent in subcortical ischemic vascular dementia (Vataja *et al.*, 2003) and may contribute to the diagnosis: it may be especially useful when other criteria of vascular dementia are missing, such as history of stroke and abrupt onset or stepwise deterioration of deficits. The second pattern, consisting of cognitive deficits "unequally" distributed or with "patchy" distribution (i.e., affecting some functions, but not others), is considered to be suggestive of vascular dementia and is used in the International Statistical Classification of Diseases criteria (WHO, 1992). It is particularly illustrated in the major hemispheric syndrome of the dominant (association with various degrees of Broca's, Wernicke's, or motor transcortical aphasia, gestural apraxia, constructional apraxia, acalculia) or nondominant (association with various degrees of hemineglect, anosognosia, hemiasomatognosia, constructional apraxia, topographical disorientation, dressing apraxia) hemisphere. Major hemispheric syndrome of the dominant hemisphere is observed in 15% to 20% of post-stroke dementia patients and its presence increases the risk of post-stroke dementia (Tatemichi *et al.*, 1993;

Pohjasvaara *et al.*, 1998). Major hemispheric syndromes are a well known consequence of hemispheric strokes and their presence should raise the possibility of a focal lesion rather than Alzheimer's disease. Other causes of major hemispheric syndrome, such as tumors, Creutzfeldt-Jakob disease, progressive primary aphasia, posterior lobar atrophy, and corticobasal degeneration, are easily excluded by the temporal course of deficits and imaging findings.

Assessment of vascular dementia

The examination of a patient with vascular dementia should include the assessment of the underlying cerebrovascular disease, the complete evaluation of the neurological and neuropsychological deficits, and estimation of the rate of functional decline.

Assessment of cerebrovascular disease

All causes of stroke can be responsible for VaD. Erkinjuntti *et al.* classified the causes of vascular dementia into primary and secondary (Erkinjuntti, 1996). Large-artery atherosclerosis is a main cause of artery-to-artery embolism and thrombosis leading to cortical and subcortical infarcts. Heart diseases, the most frequent being atrial fibrillation, are the source of small or large subcortical or cortical infarcts. Small-artery diseases change autoregulation of perforating vessels and promote small deep infarcts in basal ganglia with leukoaraiosis. Some specific vasculopathies, inflammatory or not, including giant cell arteritis, Takayasu's arteritis, isolated angiitis, Susac's syndrome, and those connected with systemic diseases such as Sjogrën's syndrome or systemic lupus erythematosus can lead to multiple and widespread small infarcts resulting in cognitive impairment. Non inflammatory arteriopathies such as fibromuscular dysplasia or moya-moya diseases can also cause VaD because of multiple ischemic or hemorrhagic lesions. Cerebral venous thrombosis is another potential cause of ischemic and/or hemorrhagic brain insults. Hematological factors such as antiphospholipid antibodies promoting the risk of thrombosis or polycythemia causing repeated ischemic lesions or a "hyperviscosity-induced dementia" should also be considered as potential causes of VaD. Obviously, this listing cannot be exhaustive. Therefore a comprehensive approach of the vascular disorder leading to the dementia syndrome is crucial to determine the mechanisms underlying the clinical status as observed in a given patient (Figure 31.3).

In the presence of VaD, the first step will consist in analyzing the cerebral tissue lesions based on imaging data. Cerebral MRI is the method of choice

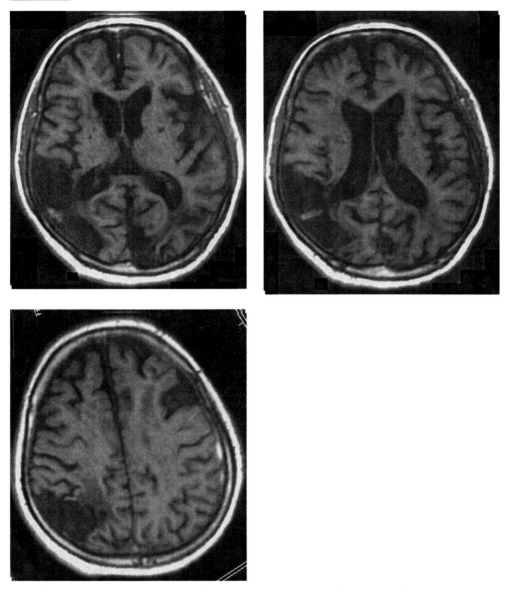

Figure 31.3 Multiple-territorial and small deep infarcts in a 77-year-old patient with dementia.

to assess the spectrum of cerebral lesions in patients with VaD. Multiple MRI sequences are necessary for this purpose and should include T1-weighted images, T2 or FLAIR images, $T2^*$ or gradient-echo images, and magnetic resonance angiography. Diffusion weighted MRI is particularly useful to detect recent ischemic insults (less than 10 days). The assessment of tissue lesions on

MRI will concern: (1) the presence of ischemic lesions (recent or old), (2) presence of absence of hemorrhagic lesions (recent or old, best evaluated on gradient-echo images), (3) size of lesions (large territorial infarction or small deep infarcts; recent large hematoma or microbleeds), (4) location of lesions in strategic areas (heteromodal cortices, mesio-temporal or frontal cortex, internal thalamus, or genu of internal capsule), (5) presence and extent of white-matter changes and location of these corresponding signal changes. According to the location, number, and type of these different lesions, the vascular mechanism can be suspected in the vast majority of cases. Thereafter, the work-up is identical to that performed in stroke patients: EKG, cardiac echography, ultrasound examination of cervical arteries, blood cell count, lipid profile, and sedimentation-rate. Other examinations such as the analysis of CSF, coagulation factors, or genetic testing will be appropriate in only a few cases and according to the context (familial disorder, cancer, other peripheral vascular events . . .).

Neuropsychological assessment

It is essential for the diagnosis of dementia and must be adapted to the severity of the deficits. The bedside assessment may reveal aphasia, gestural apraxia, hemineglect, facilitatory and oppositional paratonia (Beversdorf and Heilman, 1998), and frontal release signs (snout or glabellar) that are observed in 66% of post-stroke dementia patients (Tatemichi et al., 1993). The presence of motor and perceptual disorders that may affect interpretation of cognitive tests must be identified. Behavioral changes, such as emotional lability or apathy—abulia, may be clinically evident and the use of a behavioral inventory is useful. Some behavioral inventories have been developed for dementia testing, such as the Frontal Behavioral Inventory and the Frontotemporal Behavioral scale and they usually reveal more marked behavioral disturbances in frontotemporal dementia than in vascular dementia (Lebert et al., 1998; Kertesz et al., 2000). Screening tests, such as the Mini Mental State Examination (Folstein et al., 1975), are also part of the clinical examination. When the cognitive impairment is not too severe, cognitive assessment is based on neuropsychological tests. Given the diversity of vascular cognitive impairment, the usual neuropsychological assessment of dementia must be extended and should include accurate examination of aphasia, perceptual (hemineglect, agnosia) disorders, and executive dysfunction. The memory test must distinguish between basic associative processes and strategic retrieval processes. A visual memory test must also be performed, at least when the verbal memory test reveals normal performance.

Key points Neuropsychological assessment of vascular dementia

Neuropsychology
Clinical examination
Clinical assessment of behavior
Grasp and sucking reflexes; facilitatory and oppositional paratonia
Word generation (verbal fluency)
Behavioral changes
Behavioral inventory
Cognitive disorders
Perceptual (hemineglect, agnosia)
Language (including aphasia battery)
Gestural apraxia
Constructional abilities
Executive functions and attention
Short term and working memory
Episodic memory and strategic mnemonic processes; visual memory test
General intellectual efficiency

Treatment of VaD

The treatment of VaD includes both prevention and curative strategies.

Prevention of VaD

There are different observational studies showing that dementia (as observed in stroke) is more frequent in the presence of vascular risk factors such as carotid atherosclerosis, cardiac pathology, hypertension, and diabetes and is less frequent with moderate alcohol intake.

However, only recent interventional studies demonstrated that manipulation of vascular risk factors is actually effective in reducing the risk of dementia. In the Syst-Eur Trial and Progress trial, a significant reduction in the risk of dementia was detected with a decrease of blood pressure (from 5 to 10 mmHg). The Syst-Eur study was recently updated for the incidence of dementia in patients treated since randomization (calcium channel blocker vs. placebo) and showed a reduction of dementia from 7.4 to 3.3 cases per 1000 patient-years under the antihypertensive drug with a reduction of the incidence of both Alzheimer's disease and VaD (Forette *et al.*, 1998; Hanon and Forette, 2004). In the Progress trial determined to balance the benefit and risk of perindopril (ACE inhibitor) ± indapamide (diuretic) versus placebo in patients with a history of stroke, the active treatment was also found to decrease by 19% the risk of cognitive decline in the whole population and by 45% in subjects with recurrent stroke (Tzourio *et al.*, 2003). These results strongly support that the reduction of blood pressure is crucial to reduce the risk of dementia in general and particularly of VaD.

At the individual level, the prevention of VaD should be considered in patients with transient ischemic attack or stroke who usually have a complete work-up for their underlying vascular disease but may also involve in the near future patients with newly identified risk factors as detected now by imaging such as silent white-matter lesions and silent cerebral infarcts.

Stabilization or improvement of cognitive performances in VaD

When VaD is diagnosed, treatment to improve cognition should be considered. Drugs evaluated for cognitive impairment in Alzheimer's disease have been recently tested for VaD. The evaluation of such molecules in pure types of VaD is ongoing.

Cholinesterase inhibitors have been tested in vascular dementia during recent years. Galantamine was tested in patients with either vascular dementia (most of them had strokes) or Alzheimer's disease associated with cerebrovascular changes (most of them with only white-matter changes). The results showed that patients with VaD under the treatment improved over baseline (ADAS-Cog score) while patients with AD did not change, contrasting with the placebo group that worsened during the study period (Malouf and Birks, 2004). Two studies were performed with donepezil in VaD patients selected based on the NINDS-AIREN criteria (Black *et al.*, 2003; Wilkinson *et al.*, 2003). The results showed a significant improvement of cognitive performances with the drug in the absence of decline in the placebo group (Malouf and Birks, 2004). In the donepezil trials (Black *et al.*, 2003; Wilkinson *et al.*, 2003), 57% of patients had cortical or subcortical strokes without white-matter lesions and about 17% had white-matter lesions without strokes. Trials with Rivastigmine are on-going (Craig and Birks, 2005).

Memantine — an N-methyl-D-aspartate (NMDA) receptor antagonist — was also found to stabilize cognitive performances in VaD as measured on the Alzheimer's Disease Assessment Scale cognitive subscale (ADAS-cog) and the Mini Mental State Examination (MMSE) contrasting with the worsening detected in the placebo group (Wilcock *et al.*, 2002; Orgogozo *et al.*, 2002; Areosa *et al.*, 2004). In these trials, more than one third of patients had large cortical or subcortical lesions and more than 80% presented with lacunar infarcts or white-matter changes on MRI.

Finally, propentofylolline, a xanthin derivative that is presumably interacting on the overactivation of microglial cells by free radicals, glutamate, and calcium overload, was also found beneficial in patients who had mild to moderate AD

Key points Management and treatment of vascular dementia

Prevention
  Control and treatment of vascular risk factors: hypertension, carotid atherosclerosis, atrial fibrillation, and diabetes
    Treatment of arterial hypertension
Treatment
Promising results with recent studies using cholinesterase inhibitors and memantine

or VaD in a single double-blind trial (Marcusson *et al.*, 1997). Noteworthy, the diagnosis of VaD was not based on predefined criteria in this trial but on the judgment of the clinician (Marcusson *et al.*, 1997).

The limitations concerning the definition of VaD, the variable categories of VaD and the countless potential combinations of ischemic and hemorrhagic, small and large, subcortical and cortical lesions makes the interpretation of the results obtained in these trials extremely difficult to extrapolate at the individual level. Actually, little is known concerning the effects of these drugs according to the location and/or extent of lesions, nature of lesions (hemorrhagic versus ischemic), and presence of associated degenerative processes. This may be a challenge in the near future to develop therapeutic strategies in VaD at the individual level using both clinical and imaging data.

REFERENCES

Adair, J., Graham, G., Hart, B., *et al.* (1997). Hereditary neuropsychiatric syndrome secondary to familial vascular leukoencephlopathy. *Neurology*, **48**(3), A99.

Alexander, M. and Freeman, M. (1984). Amnesia after anterior communication artery aneurysm rupture. *Neurology*, **34**, 752–7.

Almkvist, O., Fratiglioni, L., Aguero-Torres, H., *et al.* (1999). Cognitive support at episodic encoding and retrieval: Similar patterns of utilization in community-based samples of Alzheimer's disease and vascular dementia patients. *J. Clin. Exp. Neuropsychol.*, **21**(6), 816–30.

Alzheimer, A. (1902). Die Seelenströrungen auf arteriosklerotischer Grundlage. *Allg. Z. Psychiatr.*, **59**, 695–711.

Amberla, K., Waljas, M., Tuominen, S., *et al.* (2004). Insidious cognitive decline in CADASIL. *Stroke*, **35**(7), 1598–602.

Areosa, S. A., McShane, R. and Sherriff, F. (2004). Memantine for dementia. *Cochrane Database Syst. Rev.*, CD003154.

American Psychiatric Association. (1994). *Diagnostic and Statistical Manual for Mental Disorders*.

Babikian, V. and Ropper, A. H. (1987). Binswanger's disease: A review. *Stroke*, **18**, 2–12.

Baron, J., Bousser, M., Comar, D., *et al.* (1981). Reversal of focal "misery-perfusion syndrome" by extra-intracranial arterial bypass in hemodynamic cerebral ischemia. *Stroke*, **12**, 454–9.

Baron, J., Mazoyer, B., Legault-Demare, F., *et al.* (1992). Thalamocortical diaschisis: Positron emission tomography in humans. *J. Neurol. Neurosurg. Psychiatry*, **55**, 935–42.

Barth, A., Bogousslavsky, J. and Caplan, L. (1995). Thalamic infarcts and hemorrhages. In J. Bogousslavsky and L. Caplan, eds., *Stroke Syndromes*. Cambridge University Press.

Baudrimont, M., Dubas, F., Joutel, A., *et al.* (1993). Autosomal dominant leukoencephalopathy and subcortical ischemic strokes: A clinicopathological study. *Stroke*, **24**, 122–5.

Benedikz, E., Blondal, H. and Gudmundsson, G. (1990). Skin deposits in hereditary cystatin C amyloidosis. *Virchows Arch. A. Pathol. Anat. Histopathol.*, **417**, 325–31.

Benson, D., Cummings, J. and Tsai, S. (1982). Angular gyrus syndrome simulating Alzheimer's disease. *Arch. Neurol.*, **39**, 616–20.

Berthier, E., Broussole, E., Garcia-Jacquier, M., *et al.* (1992). Leucoencephalopathie artèr-iopathique: Etude anatomoclinique d'un cas. *Rev. Neurol. (Paris)*, **148**(2), 146–9.

Beversdorf, D. Q. and Heilman, K. M. (1998). Facilitory paratonia and frontal lobe functioning. *Neurology*, **51**(4), 968–71.

Bhatia, K. and Marsden, C. (1994). The behavioural and motor consequences of focal lesions of the basal ganglia in man. *Brain*, **117**, 859–76.

Black, S., Roman, G. C., Geldmacher, D. S., *et al.* (2003). Efficacy and tolerability of donepezil in vascular dementia: Positive results of a 24-week, multicenter, international, randomized, placebo-controlled clinical trial. *Stroke*, **34**(10), 2323–30.

Blondal, H., Gudmundsson, G., Benedikz, E., *et al.* (1989). Dementia in hereditary cystatin C amyloidosis. *Prog. Clin. Biol. Re.*, **317**, 157–64.

(1990). Hereditary cerebral hemorrhage. Dementia with cystatin C amyloidosis. *Nord. Med.*, **105**(3), 76–7.

Bogousslavsky, J. (1988). Leucoencéphlopathie, leucoaraïose et infarctus cérébraux. *Rev. Neurol. (Paris)*, **144**(1), 11–17.

Bogousslavsky, J., Regli, F. and Uske, A. (1988). Thalamic infarcts: Clinical syndromes, etiology, and prognosis. *Neurology*, **38**, 837–48.

Bowler, J. and Hachinsky, V. (1996). History of the concept of vascular dementia: Two opposing views on current definitions, and criteria for vascular dementia. In I. Prohovnik, J. Wade, and T. Knezevic *et al.*, eds., *Vascular Dementia: Current Concepts*. Wiley.

Caplan, L. (1979). Chronic vascular dementia. *Primary Care*, **6**, 843–8.

Caplan, L. and Hedley-White, T. (1974). Cuing and memory dysfunction in alexia without agraphia – a case report. *Brain*, **97**, 251–62.

Caplan, L., Schmahmann, J., Kase, C., *et al.* (1990). Caudate infarcts. *Arch. Neurol.*, **47**, 133–43.

Castaigne, P., Lhermitte, F., Buge, A., *et al.* (1981). Paramedian thalamic and midbrain infarcts: Clinical and neuropathological study. *Ann. Neurol.*, **10**, 127–48.

Chabriat, H., Bousser, M. and Pappata, S. (1995a). Cerebral autosomal dominant arteriopathy with subcortical infarcts and leukoencephalopathy: A positron emission tomography study in two affected family members. *Stroke*, **26**, 1729–30.

Chabriat, H., Joutel, A., Vahedi, K., *et al.* (1997). CADASIL (Cerebral Autosomal Dominant Arteriopathy with Subcortical Infarcts and Leukoencephlopathy). *Rev. Neurol.* (Paris), **153**(6–7), 376–85.

Chabriat, H., Pappata, S., Levasseur, M., *et al.* (1992). Cortical metabolism in posterolateral thalamic stroke, PET study. *Acta Neurol. Scand.*, **86**, 285–90.

Chabriat, H., Taillia, H., Iba-Zizen, M., *et al.* (1996). MRI features of Cerebral Autosomal Dominant Arteriopathy with Subcortical Infarcts and Leukoencephalopathy. *Neurology*, **46**, A212.

Chabriat, H., Vahedi, K., IbZizen, M., *et al.* (1995b). Clinical spectrum of CADASIL: A study of 7 families. *Lancet*, **346**, 934–9.

Chui, H. C., Victoroff, J. I., Margolin, D., *et al.* (1992). Criteria for the diagnosis of ischemic vascular dementia proposed by the State of California Alzheimer's Disease Diagnostic and Treatment Centers. *Neurology*, **42**, 473–80.

Craig, D. and Birks, J. (2005). Rivastigmine for vascular cognitive impairment. *Cochrane Database Syst. Rev.*, **2**, CD 004447.

Damasio, A., Graff-Radford, N., Eslinger, P., *et al.* (1987). Amnesia following basal forebrain lesions. *Arch. Neurol.*, **42**, 263–71.

Dichgans, M., Mayer, M., Uttner, I., *et al.* (1998). The phenotypic spectrum of CADASIL: clinical findings in 102 cases. *Ann. Neurol.*, **44**(5), 731–9.

Erkinjuntti, T. (1996). Clinicopathological study of vascular dementia. In I. Prohovnik, J. Wade, T. Knezevic *et al.*, eds., *Vascular Dementia: Current Concepts*. Wiley.

Erkinjuntti, T., Inzitari, D., Pantoni, L., *et al.* (2000). Research criteria for subcortical vascular dementia in Clinical trials. *J. Neural. Transm. Suppl.*, **59**, 23–30.

Estes, M., Chimowitz, M., Awad, I., *et al.* (1991). Sclerosing vasculopathy of the central nervous system in non-elderly demented patients. *Arch. Neurol.*, **48**, 631–6.

Folstein, M. F., Folstein, S. E. and McHugh, P. R. (1975). "Mini-mental state". A practical method for grading the cognitive state of patients for the clinician. *J. Psychiatr. Res.*, **12**(3), 189–98.

Forette, F., Seux, M. L., Staessen, J. A., *et al.* (1998). Prevention of dementia in randomised double-blind placebo-controlled Systolic Hypertension in Europe (Syst-Eur) trial. *Lancet*, **352**(9137), 1347–51.

Fukutake, T. and Hirayama, K. (1995). Familial young-onset arteriosclerotic leukoencephalopathy with alopecia and lumbago without arterial hypertension. *Eur. Neurol.*, **35**, 69–79.

Gauthier, S., Rockwood, K., Gelinas, I., *et al.* (1999). Outcome measures for the study of activities of daily living in vascular dementia. *Alzheimer Dis. Assoc. Disord.*, **13**(Suppl. 3), S143–7.

Glenner, C. Amyloid deposits and myoïdosis. (1980). *N. Engl. J. Med.*, **302**, 1283–92.

Godefroy, O., Rousseaux, M., Leys, D., *et al.* (1992). Frontal lobe dysfunction in unilateral lenticulostriate infarcts. Prominent role of cortical lesions. *Arch. Neurol.*, **49**, 1285–9.

Godefroy, O., Rousseaux, M., Pruvo, J. P., Cabaret, M. and Leys, D. (1994). Neuropsychological changes related to unilateral lenticulostriate infarcts. *J. Neurol. Neurosurg. Psychiatry*, **57**, 480–5.

Graff-Radford, N., Tranel, D. Van-Hoesen, G., *et al.* (1990). Diencephalic amnesia. *Brain*, **113**, 1–25.

Grand, M., Kaine, J., Fulling, K., *et al.* (1988). Cerebroretinal vasculopathy. A new hereditary syndrome. *Ophthalmology*, **95**, 649–58.

Gray, F., Robert, F., Labrecque, R., *et al.* (1994). Autosomal dominant arteriopathic leuko-encephalopathy and Alzheimer's disease. *Neuropath. Applied Neurobiol.*, **20**, 22–30.

Greenberg, S. and Hyman, B. (1997). Cerebral amyloid angiopathy and apolipoprotein E: bad news for the good allele? *Ann. Neurol.*, **41**, 701–2.

Greenberg, S., Vonsattel, J., Stakes, J., *et al.* (1993). The clinical spectrum of cerebral amyloid angiopathy. *Neurology*, **43**, 2073–9.

Gutierrez-Molina, M., Caminero-Rodriguez, A., Martinez Garcia, C., *et al.* (1994). Small arterial granular degeneration in familial Binswanger's syndrome. *Acta Neuropath.*, **87**, 98–105.

Haan, J., Olafsson, I. and Jensson, O. (1994). Non-Alzheimer familial cerebral amyloid angiopathy. In D. Leys and P. Scheltens, eds., *Vascular Dementia*, Vol. 6. ICG Publications.

Hachinski, V., Iliff, L., Zihlka, E., *et al.* (1975). Cerebral blood flow in dementia. *Arch. Neurol.*, **32**, 632–7.

Hachinski, V. C., Lassen, N. A. and Marshall, J. (1974). Multi-infarct dementia. A cause of mental deterioration in the elderly. *Lancet*, **2**(7874), 207–10.

Hanon, O. and Forette, F. (2004). Prevention of dementia: Lessons from SYST-EUR and PROGRESS. *J. Neurol. Sci.*, **226**(1–2), 71–4.

Hashiguchi, S., Mine, H., Ide, M., *et al.* (2000). Watershed infarction associated with dementia and cerebral atrophy. *Psychiatry Clin. Neurosci.*, **54**(2), 163–8.

Hijdra, A. and Verbeeten, B. (1991). Leukoaraiosis and ventricular enlargement in patients with ischemic stroke. *Stroke*, **22**, 447–50.

Jen, J., Cohen, A., Yue, Q., *et al.* (1997). Hereditary systemic vasculopathy with stroke, retinopathy and nephropathy. *Neurology*, **48**(3), A328.

Kato, H., Izumiyama, M., Izumiyama, K., *et al.* (2002). Silent cerebral microbleeds on T2*-weighted MRI: correlation with stroke subtype, stroke recurrence, and leukoaraiosis. *Stroke*, **33**(6), 1536–40.

Kertesz, A. and Clydesdale, S. (1994). Neuropsychological deficits in vascular dementia vs Alzheimer's disease. Frontal lobe deficits prominent in vascular dementia. *Arch. Neurol.*, **51**(12), 1226–31.

Kertesz, A., Nadkarni, N., Davidson, W., *et al.* (2000). The Frontal Behavioral Inventory in the differential diagnosis of frontotemporal dementia. *J. Int. Neuropsychol. Soc.*, **6**(4), 460–8.

Kramer, J. H., Reed, B. R., Mungas, D., *et al.* (2002). Executive dysfunction in subcortical ischaemic vascular disease. *J. Neurol. Neurosurg. Psychiatry*, **72**(2), 217–20.

Lebert, F., Pasquier, F., Souliez, L., *et al.* (1998). Frontotemporal behavioral scale. *Alzheimer Dis. Assoc. Disord.*, **12**(4), 335–9.

Loeb, C. and Gandolfo, C. (1983). Diagnostic evaluation of degenerative and vascular dementia. *Stroke*, **14**, 399–401.

Loizou, L., Jefferson, J. and Smith, W. (1982). Subcortical arteriosclerotic encephalopathy (Binswanger's type) and cortical infarcts in a young normotensive patient. *J. Neurol. Neurosurg. Psychiatry*, **45**, 409–17.

Longstreth, W. T., Jr., Manolio, T. A., Arnold, A., *et al.* (1996). Clinical correlates of white matter findings on cranial magnetic resonance imaging of 3301 elderly people. The Cardiovascular Health Study. *Stroke*, **27**(8), 1274–82.

Looi, J. C. and Sachdev, P. S. (1999). Differentiation of vascular dementia from AD on neuropsychological tests. *Neurology*, **53**(4), 670–8.

Maeda, S., Nakayama, H., Isaka, K., *et al.* (1976). Familial unusual encephlopathy of Binswanger's type without hypertension. *Folia Psychiatr. Neurol. Jpn.*, **1976**(30), 165–77.

Malouf, R. and Birks, J. (2004). Donepezil for vascular cognitive impairment. *Cochrane Database Syst. Rev.*, (**1**), CD004395.

Marcusson, J., Rother, M., Kittner, B., *et al.* (1997). A 12-month, randomized, placebo-controlled trial of propentofylline (HWA 285) in patients with dementia according to DSM III-R. The European Propentofylline Study Group. *Dement. Geriatr. Cogn. Disord.*, **8**(5), 320–8.

Mendez, M., Adams, N. and Lewandowski, K. (1990). Neurobehavioural changes associated with caudate lesions. *Neurology*, **39**, 349–54.

Mendez, M. F., Cherrier, M. M. and Perryman, K. M. (1997). Differences between Alzheimer's disease and vascular dementia on information processing measures. *Brain Cogn.*, **34**(2), 301–10.

Mesulam, M., Siddique, T. and Cohen, B. (2003). Cholinergic denervation in a pure multi-infarct state: Observations on CADASIL. *Neurology*, **60**(7), 1183–5.

Moroney, J. T., Bagiella, E., Tatemichi, T. K., *et al.* (1997a). Dementia after stroke increases the risk of long-term stroke recurrence. *Neurology*, **48**, 1317–25.

Moroney, J. T., Bagiella, E., Desmond, D. W., *et al.* (1997b). Meta-analysis of the Hachinski Ischemic Score in pathologically verified dementias. *Neurology*, **49**(4), 1096–105.

Mungas, D., Jagust, W. J., Reed, B. R., *et al.* (2001). MRI predictors of cognition in subcortical ischemic vascular disease and Alzheimer's disease. *Neurology*, **57**(12), 2229–35.

Nicoll, J., Burnett, C., Love, S., *et al.* (1997). High frequency of apolipoprotein E e2 allele in hemorrhage due to cerebral amyloid angiopathy. *Ann. Neurol.*, **41**, 716–21.

O'Brien, J. T., Wiseman, R., Burton, E. J., *et al.* (2002). Cognitive associations of subcortical white matter lesions in older people. *Ann. N. Y. Acad. Sci.*, **977**, 436–44.

Orgogozo, J. M., Rigaud, A. S., Stoffler, A., Mobius, H. J. and Forette, F. (2002). Efficacy and safety of memantine in patients with mild to moderate vascular dementia: A randomized, placebo-controlled trial (MMM 300). *Stroke*, **33**, 1834–9.

Ott, B. and Saver, J. (1993). Unilateral amnesic stroke: Six new cases and a review of the literature. *Brain*, **24**, 1033–42.

Pantoni, L., Basile, A. M., Romanelli, M., *et al.* (2001). Abulia and cognitive impairment in two patients with capsular genu infarct. *Acta Neurol. Scand.*, **104**(3), 185–90.

Pasquier, F. and Leys, D. (1997). Why are stroke patients prone to develop dementia? *J. Neurol.* **244**, 135–42.

Pillon, B., Deweer, B., Agid, Y., *et al.* (1993). Explicit memory in Alzheimer's, Huntington's, and Parkinson's diseases. *Arch. Neurol.*, **50**(4), 374–9.

Pohjasvaara, T., Erkinjuntti, T., Ylikoski, R., *et al.* (1998). Clinical determinants of poststroke dementia. *Stroke*, **29**(1), 75–81.

Pohjasvaara, T., Mantyla, R., Salonen, O., *et al.* (2000). How complex interactions of ischemic brain infarcts, white matter lesions, and atrophy relate to poststroke dementia. *Arch. Neurol.*, **57**(9), 1295–300.

Pohjasvaara, T., Mantyla, R., Ylikoski, R., *et al.* (2003). Clinical features of MRI-defined subcortical vascular disease. *Alzheimer Dis. Assoc. Disord.*, **17**(4), 236–42.

Pullicino, P. and Benedict, R. (1996). Structural imaging in vascular dementia. In I. Prohovnik, J. Wade, T. Knezevic *et al.* eds., *Vascular Dementia: Current Concepts.*, Vol. 247–292. Wiley.

Rabinstein, A. A., Romano, J. G., Forteza, A. M., *et al.* (2004). Rapidly progressive dementia due to bilateral internal carotid artery occlusion with infarction of the total length of the corpus callosum. *J. Neuroimaging*, **14**(2), 176–9.

Reed, B. R., Mungas, D. M., Kramer, J. H., *et al.* (2004). Clinical and neuropsychological features in autopsy-defined vascular dementia. *Clin. Neuropsychol.*, **18**, 63–74.

Roman, G. C., Erkinjuntti, T., Wallin, A., *et al.* (2002). Subcortical ischaemic vascular dementia. *Lancet Neurol.*, **1**(7), 426–36.

Roman, G. C., Tatemichi, T. K., Erkinjuntti, T., *et al.* (1993). Vascular dementia: Diagnostic criteria for research studies. Report of the NINDS-AIREN International Workshop. *Neurology*, **43**(2), 250–60.

Ruchoux, M. M., Guerrouaou, D., Vandenhaute, B., *et al.* (1995). Systemic vascular smooth muscle cell impairment in Cerebral Autosomal Dominant Arteriopathy with Subcortical Infarcts and Leukoencephlopathy. *Acta Neuropathol.*, **89**, 500–12.

Sabbadini, G., Francia, A., Calandriello, L., *et al.* (1995). Cerebral autosomal dominant arteriopathy with subcortical infarcts and leukoencephalopathy (CADASIL). Clinical, neuroimaging, pathological and genetic study of a large Italian family. *Brain*, **118**, 207–15.

Sachdev, P. S., Brodaty, H., Valenzuela, M. J., *et al.* (2004). The neuropsychological profile of vascular cognitive impairment in stroke and TIA patients. *Neurology*, **62**(6), 912–19.

Saver, J. and Biller, J. (1995). Superficial middle cerebral artery. In J. Bogousslavsky and L. Caplan, eds., *Stroke Syndromes.* Cambridge University Press.

Sawada, T. and Kazui, S. (1995). Dementia. In J. Bogousslavsky and L. Caplan, eds., *Stroke Syndromes.* Cambridge University Press.

Starkstein, S. E., Sabe, L., Vazquez, S., *et al.* (1997). Neuropsychological, psychiatric, and cerebral perfusion correlates of leukoaraiosis in Alzheimer's disease. *J. Neurol. Neurosurg. Psychiatry*, **63**(1), 66–73.

Stevens, T., Livingston, G., Kitchen, G., *et al.* (2002). Islington study of dementia subtypes in the community. *Br. J. Psychiatry*, **180**, 270–6.

Strittmatter, W., Saunders, A., Schmechel, D., *et al.* (1993). Apolipoprotein E: high-avidity binding to B-amyloid and increased frequency of type 4 allele in late-onset familial Alzheimer disease. *PNAS*, **90**, 1977–81.

Sveinbjfornsdfottir, S., Blfondal, H., Gudmundsson, G., *et al.* (1996). Progressive dementia and leucoencephlopathy as the initial presentation of late onset hereditary cystatin-C amyloidosis. Clinicopathological presentation of two cases. *J. Neurol. Sci.*, **140**(1–2), 101–8.

Taillia, H., Chabriat, H., Kurtz, A., *et al.* (1996). Neuropsychological alterations in CADASIL (Cerebral Autosomal Dominant Arteriopathy with Subcortical Infarcts and Leukoencephalopathy): A study of 10 patients. *Cerebrovascular Dis.*, **6** (suppl. 2), 122.

Taillia, H., Chabriat, H., Kurtz, A., *et al.* (1998). Cognitive alterations in non-demented CADASIL Patients. *Cerebrovasc. Dis.*, **8**, 97–101.

Tatemichi, T. (1995). Dementia. In J. Bogousslavsky and L. Caplan, eds., *Stroke Syndromes.* Cambridge University Press.

Tatemichi, T. K., Desmond, D. W., Paik, M., *et al.* (1993). Clinical determinants of dementia related to stroke. *Ann. Neurol.*, **33**(6), 568–75.

Tatemichi, T., Desmond, D., Prohovnik, I., *et al.* (1992). Confusion and memory loss from capsular genu infarction: A thalamocortical disconnection syndrome? *Neurology*, **42**, 1966–79.

(1995). Dementia associated with bilateral carotid occlusions: Neuropsychological and haemodynamic course after extracranial to intracranial bypass surgery. *J. Neurol. Neurosurg. Psychiatry*, **58**(5), 633–6.

Tatemichi, T. K., Desmond, D. W., Stern, Y., *et al.* (1994a). Cognitive impairment after stroke: Frequency, patterns, and relationship to functional abilities. *J. Neurol. Neurosurg. Psychiatry*, **57**(2), 202–7.

Tatemichi, T. K., Paik, M., Bagiella, E., *et al.* (1994b). Risk of dementia after stroke in a hospitalized cohort. Results of a longitudinal study. *Neurology*, **44**, 1885–91.

Tatsch, K., Koch, W., Linke, R., *et al.* (2003). Cortical hypometabolism and crossed cerebellar diaschisis suggest subcortically induced disconnection in CADASIL: An 18F-FDG PET study. *J. Nucl. Med.*, **44**(6), 862–9.

Thijs, V., Robberecht, W., De Vos, R., *et al.* (2003). Coexistence of CADASIL and Alzheimer's disease. *J. Neurol. Neurosurg. Psychiatry*, **74**(6), 790–2.

Tierney, M. C., Black, S. E., Szalai, J. P., *et al.* (2001). Recognition memory and verbal fluency differentiate probable Alzheimer disease from subcortical ischemic vascular dementia. *Arch. Neurol.*, **58**(10), 1654–9.

Tomlinson, B. E., Blessed, G. and Roth, M. (1970). Observations on the brains of demented old people. *J. Neurol. Sci.*, **11**, 205–42.

Tournier-Lasserve, E., Joutel, A., Melki, J., *et al.* (1993). Cerebral autosomal dominant arteriopathy with subcortical infarcts and leukoencephalopathy maps on chromosome 19q12. *Nat. Genet.*, **3**, 256–9.

Trillet, M., Croisile, B., Tourniaire, D., *et al.* (1990). Perturbations de l'activité motrice et lésions des noyaux caudés. *Rev. Neurol.*, **146**, 338–44.

Tullberg, M., Fletcher, E., DeCarli, C., *et al.* (2004). White matter lesions impair frontal lobe function regardless of their location. *Neurology*, **63**(2), 246–53.

Tzourio, C., Anderson, C., Chapman, N., *et al.* (2003). Effects of blood pressure lowering with perindopril and indapamide therapy on dementia and cognitive decline in patients with cerebrovascular disease. *Arch. Intern. Med.*, **163**(9), 1069–75.

Vataja, R., Pohjasvaara, T., Mantyla, R., *et al.* (2003). MRI correlates of executive dysfunction in patients with ischaemic stroke. *Eur. J. Neurol.*, **10**(6), 625–31.

Vermeer, S. E., Den Heijer, T., Koudstaal, P. J., *et al.* (2003a). Incidence and risk factors of silent brain infarcts in the population-based Rotterdam Scan Study. *Stroke*, **34**(2), 392–6.

Vermeer, S. E., Prins, N. D., den Heijer, T., *et al.* (2003b). Silent brain infarcts and the risk of dementia and cognitive decline. *N. Engl. J. Med.*, **348**(13), 1215–22.

Vinters, H. V. (1987). Cerebral amyloid angiopathy. A critical review. *Stroke*, **18**(2), 311–24.

Walshe, T., Davis, K. and Fisher, C. (1977). Thalamic hemorrhage: A computed tomographic-clinical correlation. *Neurology*, **27**, 217–22.

Wenchiang Han and Caplan, L. (1995). Caudate hemorrhages and infarcts. In J. Bogousslavsky and L. Caplan, eds., *Stroke Syndromes*. Cambridge University Press.

Wetterling, T., Kanitz, R. D. and Borgis, K. J. (1996). Comparison of different diagnostic criteria for vascular dementia (ADDTC, DSM-IV, ICD-10, NINDS-AIREN). *Stroke*, **27**(1), 30–6.

Wilcock, G., Mobius, H. J. and Stoffler, A. (2002). MMM 500 group. A double-blind, placebo-controlled multicentre study of memantine in mild to moderate vascular dementia (MMM500). *Int. Clin. Psychopharmacol.*, **17**, 297–305.

Wilkinson, D., Doody, R., Helme, R., *et al.* (2003). Donepezil in vascular dementia: A randomized, placebo-controlled study. *Neurology*, **61**(4), 479–86.

Wolfe, N., Linn, R., Babikian, V. L., *et al.* (1990). Frontal systems impairment following multiple lacunar infarcts. *Arch. Neurol.*, **47**(2), 129–32.

World Health Organization. (1992). In S. W. H. O. Geneva ed., The ICD-10 Classification of Mental and Behavioural Disorders: Clinical Descriptions and Diagnostic Guidelines.

Zekry, D., Duyckaerts, C., Belmin, J., *et al.* (2003). The vascular lesions in vascular and mixed dementia: The weight of functional neuroanatomy. *Neurobiol. Aging*, **24**(2), 213–19.

32

Right versus left hemisphere syndromes

Isabel P. Martins, Lara Caeiro, and José M. Ferro

Hospital de Santa Maria, Lisboa, Portugal

Introduction

Although the brain is a symmetrical organ, its functional architecture is rather asymmetric. Beyond a certain degree of functional hierarchy, there is a lateralized distribution of cerebral functions, each hemisphere being dominant for a specific type of information processing. This functional asymmetry is evident in the association and multimodal cortices and extends to the subcortical networks.

The mechanisms of hemispheric specialization are not completely understood. Yet, there is converging evidence that the phenomenon of cerebral dominance is based on hemispheric differences in cortical cytoarchitecture and inter-area connectivity that create neural networks with specific styles of information processing (Hustler and Galuske, 2003). Innate computational differences between the two hemispheres are likely to be enhanced or modulated by experience, function acquisition (Gaillard et al., 2003; Castro-Caldas et al., 1998), timing of brain maturation, as the development of the right hemisphere precedes the development of the left (Chiron et al., 1997), and by the degree of expertise achieved in specific functions (Tatsuno and Sakai, 2005; Pascual-Leone et al., 1994). Neurochemical asymmetries may also explain some aspects of behavior (Mohr et al., 2003).

The left cerebral hemisphere is characterized by a discreet organization of functions and a rather sequential, linear, and analytic processing style. This is probably responsible for its ability to extract and process perceptual detail (Delis et al., 1988) and for its advantage in the temporal resolution of events (Zatorre & Belin, 2001), such as the rapidly changing speech sounds. The right hemisphere, on the contrary, has its functions distributed in large-scale networks, and a more "configurational" processing style, making it particularly suited to integrate across inputs and to process global percepts, such as human faces and voices, comprehension of the metaphoric and emotional components of language (Brownell et al., 1995), and monitoring context appropriate behavior (Lesak, 2004). Differences in processing styles also concern the novelty of stimuli. The right hemisphere possesses a better ability to handle new information, while the left is superior in automatized processes, like reading or writing. Different types of approach, namely lesion studies, split-brain cases, observations during the sodium amytal procedure and neurophysiological or functional activation studies, have produced evidence of these differences.

In general, it is well accepted that the left hemisphere is dominant for verbal abilities (oral and written language), in particular in what concerns the production and comprehension of phonology and syntax, motor planning, gesture communication, number processing, calculation, and verbal memory (namely semantic memory). The right hemisphere is specialized in visuospatial and other "non-verbal" (or difficult to verbalize) abilities, such as the capacity to orient, engage and shift attention, the processing and recognition of complex visual patterns, visual learning, topographic memory, music, and emotions.

Yet, the functional asymmetry between the two hemispheres is not just "material-specific" (i.e. determined by the nature of the stimuli to be processed). It is also dependent upon the type of processing required. The same stimulus can be analyzed from a linguistic or a visuospatial perspective, which in turn determines which hemisphere is recruited for the task (Stephan *et al.*, 2003). This interaction between the nature of the stimulus, planning and control of the required cognitive task, and other variables, makes the interpretation of functional specialization particularly difficult. In fact, in normal circumstances most cognitive tasks are accomplished by the integrated action of both cerebral hemispheres, which is quite evident in functional imaging studies, where sophisticated paradigms and imaging subtractions are necessary to identify localized patterns of cerebral activation.

Left and right hemispheres are also dominant for distinct emotions, affects, and behaviors. The left hemisphere is more liable for positive emotions such as happiness. Thus, after its lesion, sadness, despair, emotionalism, depression, and catastrophic reaction become apparent. As the right hemisphere is responsible for negative affects and emotions, a lesion in this hemisphere tends to produce indifference, elation, anosognosia or apathy, agitation, or abulia. Although left-side stroke patients and their partners report the same emotional changes in patients, right-side stroke patients report fewer emotional changes compared with their partners (Visser-Keizer *et al.*, 2002).

Studies of the ontogenesis of cerebral specialization suggest that hemispheric differences are established early in life. Differences in the morphology and morphometry of the planum temporale (the left hemisphere region involved in language processing) can be found in the newborn and the human fetus by the 29th week of gestation (Wada *et al.*, 1975), well before language acquisition, and functional asymmetries have been observed in 3-month-old babies in response to speech sounds, with a preferential activation of the left temporal cortex (Dehaene-Lambertz *et al.*, 2002). This early left hemisphere specialization for language has also been corroborated by the rarity of aphasias following right brain lesions in children (Marien *et al.*, 2001) and functional magnetic resonance (fMRI) studies (Ahmad *et al.*, 2003). An early pattern of right hemisphere specialization for selective attention and visuospatial processing has also been shown (Stiles-Davis *et al.*, 1988; Ferro *et al.*, 1984). In addition, asymmetries in frontal activation during childhood are markers of emotional reactivity, approach-related positive affect, or inhibition and withdrawal reactions, patterns that persist into adult life (Davidson, 1994).

Reversal of hemispheric dominance has been observed following left hemispherectomies in childhood, early focal brain lesions, and chronic epilepsy (Hertz-Pannier *et al.*, 2002; Staudt *et al.*, 2002). Besides, there are individual variations in the pattern of functional dominance among healthy subjects, particularly in left-handed individuals (Knecht *et al.*, 2000).

In this chapter we will contrast the cognitive and neuropsychiatric syndromes that occur after unilateral right or left hemisphere stroke lesions, and we will also summarize the manifestations observed in the rare cases whose lesions involve identical areas in both hemispheres (Table 32.1). A detailed localization and description of the different symptoms has been presented in previous chapters. We will organize syndromes according to the usual vascular territories, since strokes do not respect natural anatomical boundaries. It should be emphasized that the typical cognitive syndromes presented here are usually observed during the first months post-stroke, but not in the hyperacute nor in the chronic period. Anatomical correlations are blurred by diaschisis in the acute stage and become less accurate as functional recovery takes place. Neuropsychiatric syndromes will be discussed according to time after onset.

Left syndromes

Left hemisphere cognitive syndromes

Different cognitive and behavioral disorders may follow infarcts in the anterior cerebral artery (ACA) territory. These lesions usually involve the medial frontal lobe, supplementary motor area (SMA), and anterior cingulate gyrus, and may include the anterior two-thirds of the corpus callosum. Damage to the medial frontal lobe tends to reduce initiative, motivation, and spontaneous activity, leading to abulia or, in the acute stage, akinetic mutism (Nagaratnam *et al.*, 2004). Different disturbances of speech (mutism, a tendency to speak in whispers, acquired stuttering) (Hamano *et al.*, 2005; Kakishita *et al.*, 2004) and motor behavior (perseveration, forced grasp and groping, compulsive motor behavior,

Table 32.1. Syndromes of cognitive dysfunction: left versus right hemisphere stroke syndromes

Arterial territories	Localization of lesion	Left hemisphere	Right hemisphere	Bilateral damage
	Frontal lobe			
ACA	Mesial-basal PFC	Transient abulia, mutism	Motor neglect (mesial PFC)	Persistent abulia,
	Anterior cingulate gyrus SMA	Transcortical motor aphasia	Transient mutism	Akinetic mutism
	Anterior corpus callosum	Callosal disconnective syndrome	Alien hand	
			Callosal disconnection	
		Depression	Mania	
Anterior cortical division of MCA	Dorso-lateral PFC	Mutism (acute stage)	Impaired speech prosody	Dysexecutive syndrome
	Precentral gyrus	Broca's/Transc. motor aphasia	Motor neglect, anosognosia	Impaired memory (retrieval)
	Postcentral gyrus	Agraphia, dysarthria	Motor impersistence	Perseveration
		Buccolinguofacial apraxia	Perseverations	
		Executive dysfunction	Delusions	
Perforating branches MCA	Insula and opercular cortex	Speech apraxia	Dysarthria	Anarthria (bi-opercular syndrome)
		Broca's aphasia Conduction aphasia		
	Parietal lobe			
Posterior division of MCA	Superior	Visuo-motor ataxia	Visuo-spatial disorientation	Neglect syndrome
			Visuo-motor ataxia	Visuo-motor ataxia

Table 32.1(cont.)

Arterial territories	Localization of lesion	Left hemisphere	Right hemisphere	Bilateral damage
			Neglect syndrome Confusional states Constructional apraxia	
PCA branches (parieto-occipital arteries)	Inferior	Limb apraxia	Anosognosia	Apraxia
		Anomia, poor repetition	Left hemineglect	Neglect syndrome
		Agraphia, alexia, acalculia		Bálint's syndrome
Borderzone MCA–PCA infarcts	Parieto-occipital	Transcortical sensory aphasia	Neglect Reduplicative paramnesia	Bálint's syndrome
	Temporal lobe			
Posterior cortical branches of MCA	Anterior	Anomia		
	Posterior	Poor phonological processing Fluent aphasia (Wernicke's, conduction) Verbal auditory agnosia	Impaired prosodo-affective/ emotional gesture comprehension Agitated delirium	Cortical deafness Auditory agnosia
PCA temporal branches	Hippocampus and neighbor regions	Anterograde amnesia (verbal)	Poor visuo-spatial memory and learning	Dense anterograde amnesia Retrograde amnesia

Table 32.1 (cont.)

Arterial territories	Localization of lesion	Left hemisphere	Right hemisphere	Bilateral damage
			Topographic amnesia Prosopagnosia	Topographic disorientation Prosopagnosia
	Occipital lobe			
PCA calcarine arteries	Association cortex and splenium	Visual agnosia Pure alexia, color anomia	Visuo-spatial neglect	Apperceptive visual agnosia Associative visual agnosia
	Primary visual cortex	Visual hallucinations hemiachromatopsia	Visual hallucinations	Cortical blindness, achromatopsia Simple visual hallucinations

Legend: ACA (anterior cerebral artery); MCA (middle cerebral artery); PCA (posterior cerebral artery); Transc (transcortical); PFC (pre-frontal cortex); SMA (supplementary motor area)

intermanual conflicts, "alien hand" phenomenon) may occur independently of lesion side.

If the lesion is on the left ACA territory, the initial period of mutism is often followed by transcortical motor aphasia (characterized by hypospontaneity of speech with intact comprehension and normal or compulsive repetition), usually due to lesions of the SMA and underlying white matter (Bogousslavsky *et al.*, 1987). "Alien hand" phenomenon and loss of bimanual coordination, involving the right hand, have been described following left ACA infarcts (McNabb *et al.*, 1988), possibly due to impaired inhibition and programming of motor routines by a damaged left SMA and interconnected anterior cingulate cortex. If the infarct extends to the anterior corpus callosum it may produce disconnection syndromes, whereby the left hand (without access to the left hemisphere verbal information) becomes agraphic, apraxic to verbal commands and anomic to tactile stimuli, while the right hand has no such impairment. However, complete callosal disconnection syndromes are rarely observed following ACA stroke (Bogousslavsky and Regli, 1990).

Aphasia is the most typical cognitive dysfunction following left middle cerebral artery (MCA) infarcts. The type and severity of aphasia vary with the site and size of lesion in the perisylvian region and its subcortical extension, which depends upon the vascular territory involved (Kreisler *et al.*, 2000). Infarcts or hemorrhages of the anterior (frontal) language cortex impair syntactic programming and comprehension, word production (verbs more than nouns), while strokes involving the posterior temporal region (superior and middle temporal gyrus, including Wernicke's area) interfere with phonological decoding and lexical selection and retrieval (nouns more than verbs). Anosognosia can be observed in subjects with jargon aphasia; in this case, the patient is unaware of his speech disturbance (Venneri and Shanks, 2004). Damage to the periphery of the Sylvian fissure, outside the main language areas (borderzone infarcts between the middle and posterior cerebral arteries), may spare language repetition producing the syndrome of transcortical aphasia. Therefore, occlusion of the anterior MCA branches tend to elicit Broca's and transcortical motor aphasias, often associated with bucco-linguo-facial apraxia, while isolated lesions of the posterior MCA territory will produce fluent aphasia (Wernicke's, conduction or anomic aphasia) or isolated word-finding difficulties. Extensive infarcts involving all the MCA territory are associated with global aphasia.

Different aphasic syndromes have been described, in adults and children, in association with left subcortical stroke (territory of the lenticulostriate arteries) (Martins, 2000; Kirk and Kertesz, 1994; Alexander *et al.*, 1987). Although lesions in the territory of the anterior choroidal artery (AChA) do not typically cause cognitive disorders, there are rare reports describing anterograde amnesia, due to infarcts of the anterior hippocampus and amygdala, secondary to occlusion of the left AChA (Ott and Saver, 1993).

Aphasia is always associated with agraphia and, often, with other cognitive deficits that can have a localizing value. Among non-aphasic disorders of speech, dysarthria results from lesions in different sites, the posterior inferior frontal cortex, anterior subcortical white matter, and basal ganglia. Apraxia of speech (also called phonemic disarticulation or disintegration syndrome), an inability to program speech resulting in a paraphasic discourse with normal oral comprehension and writing ability (Peach, 2004), is a rare disorder produced by damage to the left frontal or prefrontal cortex (anterior branches of the MCA), subcortical structures and their connections. Damage of the premotor cortex has been occasionally associated with foreign accent syndrome, characterized by a disruption of the prosody, tone, rhythm and accent of speech, making it sound like a foreign language (Christoph *et al.*, 2004).

Infarcts or hemorrhages in the territory of the posterior divisions of the MCA, involving the left inferior parietal lobe, may produce a variable constellation of linguistic and cognitive symptoms: conduction aphasia (supramarginal gyrus), anomia, alexia with agraphia, right−left disorientation, acalculia and digito-agnosia (angular gyrus syndrome), constructional and limb apraxia, and poor comprehension of gestures. Pure acalculia (anarithmetia), with intact number processing, is typical of parietal lobe lesions. Damage to the posterior parietal cortex may disrupt visually guided hand movement (ipsilateral visuomotor ataxia). The left hemisphere is dominant for learned skilled and symbolic movements and limb apraxia can result from different lesion sites, dorsolateral frontal, parietal, and subcortical.

The left anterior temporal neocortex (temporal pole and anterior second and third temporal gyri), supplied by the temporal branches of the MCA, are involved in lexical comprehension and retrieval. Its damage may cause word-finding difficulties, sometimes involving specific lexico-semantic categories (proper names versus common names, for instance) (Damasio *et al.*, 1996).

Infarcts or hemorrhages in the territory of the left posterior cerebral artery (PCA), involving the left occipital and the medial temporal lobe, usually produce memory and learning impairments (anterograde amnesia) associated with visual field defects, aphasia or word finding difficulties, and additional symptoms, depending upon the subcortical or callosal extension of the lesion (Brandt *et al.*, 2000). Several syndromes result from disconnections between the left hemisphere language areas and the remaining visual pathways: associative visual agnosia (whereby visual stimuli can be copied but cannot be recognized or named), optic aphasia (visually presented stimuli are recognized but not named), alexia without agraphia (patients are unable to read printed words, perceived in the remaining visual field, but they can write and spell words with no difficulty), and color anomia. Pure alexia, with color anomia, is usually associated with lesions of the splenium. PCA infarcts that involve the inferior parietal lobe, including the angular gyrus, may produce the symptoms already described as more typical of the posterior MCA infarcts.

Memory impairment following unilateral PCA infarcts is much more common after left (85%) than right lesions (Ott and Saver, 1993). If the lesion is restricted to the left medial temporal lobe (inferior PCA temporal branches), including the hippocampus and surrounding structures (parahippocampus, ento- and peri-rhinal cortex) a persistent amnesia (especially for declarative episodic memory) and learning impairment are the major complaints. Amnesia due to unilateral left temporal infarcts may affect verbal and visuospatial material.

Left thalamic infarcts, due to occlusion of the proximal penetrating branches of the PCA, or of the posterior communicating artery, have been associated with a variety of cognitive and behavioral disorders including fluctuating aphasia and memory disorders, involving the encoding and retrieval of new material. Anterior thalamic lesions (tuberothalamic artery territory) may cause loss of initiative, abulia, poor expression of emotions, memory impairment, and aphasia, characterized by hypophonia, reduced speech output and normal repetition (Bogousslavsky *et al.*, 1988). Palipsychism, a superimposition of sequential mental activities, sensitivity to interference and perseveration, has also been described in left or right pure anterior thalamic infarcts (Ghika-Schmid and Bogousslavsky, 2000). Left dorsomedial infarcts (thalamo-perforating arteries) are characterized by an initial period of somnolence followed by distractibility, with an inconsistent performance in memory tasks, or anterograde amnesia. Amnesia following unilateral thalamic infarcts is much more common after left than right side lesions (Ott and Saver, 1993). Thalamic infarcts with atypical topography, involving the anteromedian region, tend to cause aphasia, amnesia and executive dysfunction (Carrera *et al.*, 2004).

Left hemisphere neuropsychiatric syndromes

Post-stroke depression (PSD) is one of the most frequent psychiatric syndromes after stroke. The association of PSD to left hemisphere lesions is widely accepted. Left anterior (cortical or subcortical) lesions are associated with PSD in the acute phase (Biran and Chatterjee, 2003; Robinson, 2000; Astrom *et al.*, 1993) and in the chronic phase (Vataja *et al.*, 2004; Lauterbach *et al.*, 1997). Still right posterior hemisphere lesions may also be associated with PSD (Verdelho *et al.*, 2004; Shimoda and Robinson, 1999; Ghika-Schmid *et al.*, 1999; Herrmann *et al.*, 1998; Singh *et al.*, 1998), particularly if there is a familial history of affective or anxiety disorder (Robinson, 2000; Morris *et al.*, 1990). In PSD following right hemispheric stroke, a personal or familial history of psychiatric disorders, social and interpersonal factors, and neuropsychological disturbances become increasingly important to determine the affective state, eventually obscuring the effects of lesion location per se. Recent systematic reviews did not support an association between PSD and left hemisphere lesions, or with the anterior-left/posterior-right hemispherical lesion location dichotomy (Bhogal *et al.*, 2004; Berg *et al.*, 2001; Carson *et al.*, 2000). The reason for these conflicting results could either be misdiagnosis of PSD with several depressive-like syndromes (catastrophic reaction, apathy, fatigue, emotional incontinence), or the result of the different diagnostic criteria used.

Catastrophic reaction occurs when a patient is confronted with a stressor. This reaction is most frequent in acute stroke patients with cerebral infarcts, affecting the left hemisphere (Caeiro *et al.*, 2002), mostly involving the superficial territory of the superior division of the MCA (Carota *et al.*, 2001; Teasell, 1993), and the basal ganglia or anterior areas (Robinson, 1998a; Teasell, 1993). In some cases, anxiety is included in the psychological profile of the patient with catastrophic reaction, in particular when the right hemisphere is involved (Starkstein *et al.*, 1993a).

Right syndromes

Right hemisphere cognitive syndromes

Unilateral spatial inattention, or neglect, for the left side of the space is the most frequent and typical cognitive dysfunction of right hemisphere lesions, occurring in 12–100% of cases with right hemisphere stroke, in different series (Bowen *et al.*, 1999). Since hemispatial attention depends upon a widely distributed (or large-scale) neuronal network (LaBerge, 2000), neglect may result from lesions at different sites (prefrontal, anterior cingulate, parietal, and subcortical). The key brain region responsible for hemispatial neglect has been localized, according to different authors, to the right temporoparietal cortex (Ringman *et al.*, 2004; Vallar and Perani, 1986), inferior parietal lobe or parahippocampal region (Mort *et al.*, 2003), and the superior temporal gyrus (Karnach *et al.*, 2001). Neglect may have different presentations (in the extrapersonal, representational, and personal space) and affect different sensory modalities, according to the part of the network involved. Extensive lesions involving the temporoparietal cortex produce more severe and lasting neglect and anosognosia (Ringman *et al.*, 2004). Left-sided neglect may affect reading, writing, and calculation, as the patient ignores most written information on their left side.

Left-sided motor neglect may follow abulia in right ACA infarcts (Bogousslavsky and Regli, 1990). Patients with motor neglect show a tendency to underutilize the left limbs despite intact motor strength and sensation. Disturbances of speech and motor behavior, already described (transient mutism, abulia, akinesia, "alien hand" phenomenon, utilization behavior), can also be present. A case of hypergraphia following a cingulate lesion of the right ACA territory has been reported (Carota *et al.*, 2003).

Infarcts or hemorrhages in the right MCA territory produce, in addition to hemispatial neglect, other symptoms that may help in localizing the lesion. Right frontal lobe lesions (anterior branches of the MCA division) may impair certain aspects of narrative discourse such as prosody and pragmatics (metaphoric comprehension, jokes, contextual and emotional adequacy of discourse). Patients may also present poor motivation, verbal memory retrieval, and working memory.

Damage to the right temporal neocortex (posterior superior temporal gyrus), due to occlusion of the temporal branches of the right MCA, may impair the comprehension of emotional aspects of speech and gestures and cause amusia (impaired musical perception or instrument amusia). Infarcts of the posterior divisions of the MCA involving the right parietal lobe produce, in addition to neglect, visuospatial dysgraphia, spatial dyscalculia, and constructional apraxia, from the lack of systematic visuospatial scanning and simultagnosia.

Dressing apraxia can also be encountered (Hier *et al.*, 1983). An unusual syndrome designated "acute hemiconcern" has been observed in a few cases, following infarcts of the right temporoparietal region (anterior parietal artery territory). It is a transient phenomenon during which patients show an excessive concern with the left side of their bodies that they manipulate and explore with the right hand (Bogousslavsky *et al.*, 1995).

Right subcortical infarcts and hemorrhages involving the internal capsule and the basal ganglia (right AChA and lenticulostriate territory) may produce cognitive dysfunction, namely visuospatial hemineglect, anosognosia, constructional apraxia, and motor impersistence. Unilateral infarcts in the territory of the right AChA may produce left-sided neglect, but memory impairment is unusual (in contrast with the left AChA).

Right PCA cortical stroke may involve the right occipital and medial temporal lobes, lingual and fusiform gyri, hippocampus, parahippocampal gyrus, and the retrosplenium region. These lesions impair visuospatial learning and memory and may cause prosopagnosia (more often when the lesion is bilateral), an inability to recognize faces, and environmental agnosia (also called topographic disorientation), whereby patients cannot recognize or orient themselves in familiar surroundings, often with poor visual imagery for places. Delusions of identification (Capgras' syndrome) and place (reduplicative paramnesia) are more common in right- than left-sided lesions, particularly in infarcts involving the temporo-parieto-occipital cortices.

Damage of right thalamus can produce difficulties with shape, face or pattern recognition, spatial localization and matching, design reconstruction, and hemispatial neglect (LaBerge, 2000). Cognitive impairment can result from right thalamic infarcts, more often involving the tuberothalamic and paramedian territory. Patients present perseveration, confabulations, sensitivity to interference, neglect, visuospatial impairment, and poor visual anterograde memory (Ghika-Schmid and Bogousslavsky, 2000; Ott and Saver, 1993; Bogousslavsky *et al.*, 1988b). Right laterothalamic infarcts may produce chronic impairment of executive abilities, namely verbal fluency (probably due to disruption of frontothalamic loops), as well as defects of learning and recall of verbal and visuospatial material (Annoni *et al.*, 2003).

Right hemisphere neuropsychiatric syndromes

Right MCA superficial lesions (Caeiro *et al.*, 2004; Hénon *et al.*, 1999; Mori and Yamadori, 1987; Caplan *et al.*, 1986b; Mesulam *et al.*, 1976) can induce delirium.

Behavioral changes can be observed in lesions of the right middle temporal gyrus including agitation, delirium, hallucinations, and autonomic hyperactivity (Mori and Yamadori, 1987), a syndrome that has been called the mirror image of Wernicke's aphasia (Caplan *et al.*, 1986a). Right MCA infarcts or right or left caudate infarcts are largely responsible for hyperactive delirium (Caplan *et al.*, 1990), while hypoactive delirium is mostly related to ACA infarcts or to lesions extending to the inferior parietal lobe (Caplan *et al.*, 1986b). However, strokes in other locations, including the left hemisphere, can cause delirium (Ferro *et al.*, 2002).

Mania is also associated with infarcts in the right hemisphere, above all if they damage limbic-connected areas such as infarcts of the right inferior temporal lobe, head of the caudate, thalamus, orbitofrontal cortex, or basotemporal cortex (Robinson, 1998b; Starkstein *et al.*, 1991; Drake *et al.*, 1990; Starkstein *et al.*, 1988; Robinson *et al.*, 1988), or the middle third of the parenchyma, in both right and left hemispheres (McDonald *et al.*, 1991). The description of cases with mania related to the left hemisphere lesion includes mainly cases of post-stroke bipolar affective disorder (Fenn and George, 1999; Liu *et al.*, 1996; Jampala and Abrams, 1983).

Apathy can be the result of a right hemisphere stroke involving the anterior cingulate circuit and the limbic system (Robinson, 1998c; Marin *et al.*, 1994; Starkstein *et al.*, 1993b). This motivational disturbance can be observed also after a lesion in the right dorsolateral frontal and anterior temporal lobe (Okada *et al.*, 1997), right or left anterior thalamus (Ghika-Schmid and Bogousslavsky, 2000), or a right or left stroke lesion of the inferior capsular genu (Madureira *et al.*, 1999).

Anosognosia is a lack of awareness of one's self-deficit. Anosodiaphoria describes the absence of emotional reaction to the presence of a deficit. In acute stroke, anosognosia is a short-lived deficit secondary to a lesion affecting the territory of the right MCA, such as the superior temporal cortex, inferior parietal cortex, basal ganglia, or thalamus (Ghika-Schmid *et al.*, 1999; Ellis and Small, 1997; Starkstein *et al.*, 1993c; Stone *et al.*, 1993; Starkstein *et al.*, 1992; Babinsky, 1914). Right thalamic lesions secondary to right thalamogeniculate and posterior choroidal artery (Karussis *et al.*, 2000) has been reported as inducing anosognosia. Patients with right-side lesions can present an anosognosia for their own memory and attention impairment and, consequently, construct a confabulation in substitution (Venneri and Shanks, 2004).

Generalized anxiety disorder is rather frequent in acute stroke and is associated with right posterior hemisphere stroke, whereas co-occurrence of anxiety and depression is more frequent after a left hemisphere lesion (Robinson, 1998d; Aström, 1996; Castillo *et al.*, 1993; Starkstein *et al.*, 1990). Furthermore, post-stroke generalized anxiety disorder is most frequent after right hemisphere lesions involving the anterior circulation (Leppävuori *et al.*, 2003). Obsessive—compulsive disorder is not very common in acute stroke, but when it is present it may become apparent after a right inferior parietal infarct (Simpson and Baldwin, 1995).

Post-stroke atypical schizophreniform psychosis has been described after right hemisphere lesions (Rabins *et al.*, 1991).

Emotional incontinence is described in patients presenting right-side cortical anterior (frontal or temporal) or lenticulocapsular or dorsal pallidum lesions or bilateral stroke lesions (Tang *et al.*, 2004; Kim, 2002; Kim and Choi-Kwon, 2000; House *et al.*, 1989). Kim (2002) also stated that crying emotional incontinence was most predominant after a right-side lesion, laughter emotional incontinence after a left-side lesion, and crying/laughing emotional incontinence after bilateral lesions.

Syndromes resulting from bilateral cortical–subcortical lesions

Occasionally, strokes produce roughly symmetrical lesions causing severe and lasting cognitive defects or dementia (Román *et al.*, 1993). This may result from a particular vascular anatomy or sequential infarcts or hemorrhages.

Persistent abulia or akinetic mutism is observed after bilateral mesial frontal infarcts in the ACA territory. Marked anterograde amnesia with confabulation has been described following rupture of anterior communicating artery aneurysms, with infarcts in the basal forebrain, areas supplied by perforating branches of the ACA (Damasio *et al.*, 1985).

Bilateral dorsolateral frontal lesions produce a dysexecutive syndrome (impaired ability to program and monitor actions, poor cognitive flexibility, and perseveration), while orbitofrontal lesions may produce a marked change in personality with dysinhibition, inappropriate laughing, and jocularity.

Bilateral anterior opercular syndrome (Foix–Chavany–Marie syndrome) is characterized by anarthria, or severe dysarthria, a condition that must be distinguished from aphasia. It is due to loss of voluntary control of the facio-lingual pharyngeal muscles.

Bilateral temporal neocortical lesions may produce different agnosic syndromes depending upon the areas involved: central or cortical deafness (bilateral lesions of the Heschl gyri), auditory agnosia (auditory association cortex), or verbal auditory agnosia (left lesion and callosal disconnection).

Bilateral and simultaneous lesions of the temporo-parieto-occipital cortex (bilateral PCA territory infarcts) can occur during thrombosis of the basilar artery or after hypotensive/hypoperfusion episodes, in which case they tend to involve the border zones between the PCA and MCA territories. The most frequent symptoms are visual (cortical blindness or bilateral visual field defects, often with hallucinations in the acute stage) and variable degrees of amnesia. Some patients deny their visual impairment, presenting confabulatory explanations for their inability to see (anosognosia for the cortical blindness or Anton syndrome).

If lesions affect predominantly the temporo-occipital regions (the "what" pathways) it will produce visual agnosia (apperceptive or associative agnosia depending upon the location of lesions), poor visual imagery, prosopagnosia, environmental agnosia, and severe anterograde amnesia, due to bilateral middle temporal lobe impairment. Achromatopsia, an inability to perceive colors, with or without impaired color imagery, can follow bilateral lesions of the lingual and fusiform gyri. When the infarcts involve predominantly the dorsal parieto-occipital cortex (involving the "where" pathways), in PCA—MCA watershed infarcts damaging both angular gyri, it may produce elements of Bálint's syndrome ("psychic palsy of gaze" or gaze apraxia, visuomotor ataxia, and sim-ultagnosia, an inability to perceive a visual scene as a whole), associated with saccadic inaccuracy, visual inattention, and spatial disorientation.

Bilateral and simultaneous thalamic infarcts (involving both intralaminar, anterior or dorsomedial nuclei) usually cause marked and lasting behavioral disorders (lack of motivation, abulia, poor attention, and amnesia), and constitute a mechanism of vascular dementia (Román *et al.*, 1993). A syndrome identical to Bálint's syndrome was described following bilateral pulvinar lesions.

REFERENCES

Ahmad, Z., Balsamo, L. M., Sachs, B. C., Xu, B. and Gaillard, W. D. (2003). Auditory comprehension of language in young children: Neural networks identified with fMRI. *Neurology*, **60**(10), 1598—605.

Alexander, M. P., Naeser, A. and Palumbo, C. L. (1987). Correlations of subcortical CT lesions sites and aphasia profiles. *Brain*, **110**, 961—91.

Annoni, J. M., Khateb, A., Gramigna, S., *et al.* (2003). Chronic cognitive impairment following laterothalamic infarcts: A study of 9 cases. *Arch. Neurol.*, **60** (10), 1439—43.

Aström, M. (1996). Generalized anxiety disorder in stroke patients. A 3-year longitudinal study. *Stroke*, **27**, 270—5.

Astrom, M., Adolfsson, R. and Asplund, K. (1993). Major depression in stroke patients. A 3-year longitudinal study. *Stroke*, **24**, 976—82.

Babinski, J. (1914). Contribution a l'étude des troubles mentaux dans l'hemiplégie organique cérébrale (anosognosie). *Rev. Neurol.*, **1**, 845—8.

Berg, A., Palomäki, H., Pehtihalmes, M., Lönnqvist, J. and Kaste, M. (2001). Post-stroke depression in acute phase after stroke. *Cerebrovasc. Dis.*, **12**, 14—20.

Bhogal, S. K., Teasell, R., Foley, N. and Speechley, M. (2004). Lesion location and post-stroke depression. Systematic review of the methodological limitations in the literature. *Stroke*, **35**, 794—802.

Biran, I. and Chatterjee, A. (2003). Depression with anosognosia following a left subcortical stroke. *Clin. Neurol. Neurosurg.*, **105**, 99—101.

Bogousslavsky, J., Assal, G. and Regli, F. (1987). Infarctus du territoire de l'artère cérébrale antérieure gauche. II. Troubles du langage. *Rev. Neurol.*, **143**, 121−7.

Bogousslavsky, J., Ferrazini, M., Regli, F., *et al.* (1988a). Manic delirium and frontal-like syndrome with paramedian infarction of the right thalamus. *J. Neurol. Neurosurg. Psychiatry*, **51**, 116−19.

Bogousslavsky, J., Kumral, E., Regli, F., Assal, G. and Ghika, J. (1995). Acute hemiconcern: A right anterior parietotemporal syndrome. *J. Neurol. Neurosurg. Psychiatry*, **58**, 428−32.

Bogousslavsky, J. and Regli, F. (1990). Anterior cerebral artery territory infarction in the Lausanne Stroke Registry. Clinical and etiologic patterns. *Arch. Neurol.*, **47**, 144−50.

Bogousslavsky, J., Regli, F. and Uske, A. (1988b). Thalamic infarts: Clinical syndromes, etiology, and prognosis. *Neurology*, **38**, 837−48.

Bowen, A., McKenna, K. and Tallis, R. C. (1999). Reasons for variability in the reported rate of occurrence of unilateral spatial neglect after stroke. *Stroke*, **30**, 1196−202.

Brandt, T., Steinke, W., Thie, A., Pessin, M. S. and Caplan, L. R. (2000). Posterior cerebral artery territory infarcts: Clinical features, infarct topography, causes and outcome. *Cerebrovasc. Dis.*, **10**, 170−82.

Brownell, H., Gardner, H., Prather, P. and Martino, G. (1995). Language, communication and the right hemisphere. In *Handbook of Neurological Speech and Language Disorders*, ed. M. Dekker. New York: Howard S. Kirshner pp. 325−49.

Caeiro, L., Ferro, J. M., Albuquerque, R. and Figueira, M. L. (2002). Catastrophic reaction in acute stroke. *Cerebrovasc. Dis.*, **13**, 52−3.

(2004). Delirium in the first days of acute stroke. *J. Neurol.*, **251**, 171−8.

Caplan, L. R., Kelly, M., Kase, C. S., *et al.* (1986a). Mirror image of Wernicke's aphasia. *Neurology*, **36**, 1015−20.

Caplan, L. R., Kelly, M., Kase, C. S., *et al.* (1986b). Infarcts of the inferior division of the right middle cerebral artery: Mirror image of Wernicke's aphasia. *Neurology*, **36**, 1015−20.

Caplan, L. R., Schmahmann, J. D., Kase, C. S., *et al.* (1990). Caudate infarcts. *Arch. Neurol.*, **47**, 133−43.

Carota, A., Annoni, J. M., Combremont, P., Clarke, S. and Bogousslavsky, J. (2003). Hypergraphia, verbal aspontaneity and post-stroke depression secondary to right cyngulate and corpus callosum infarction. *J. Neurol.*, **250** (4), 508−10.

Carota, A., Rosseti, A. O., Karapanayiotides, T. and Bogousslavsky, J. (2001). Catastrophic reaction in acute stroke: A reflex behavior in aphasic patients. *Neurology*, **57**, 1902−5.

Carrera, E., Michel, P. and Bogousslavsky, J. (2004). Anteromedian, central, and posterolateral infarcts of the thalamus: Three variant types. *Stroke*, **35** (12), 2826−31.

Carson, A. J., MacHale, S., Allen, K., *et al.* (2000). Depression after stroke and lesion location: A systematic review. *Lancet*, **356**, 122−6.

Castillo, C. S., Starkstein, S. E., Fedoroff, J. P., Price, T. R. and Robinson, R. G. (1993). Generalized anxiety disorder after stroke. *J. Nerv. Ment. Dis.*, **181**, 100−6.

Castro-Caldas, A., Petersson, K. M., Reis, A., Stone-Elander, S. and Ingvar, M. (1998). Learning in childhood determines the functional organisation of the adult brain. *Brain*, **121**, 1053−63.

Chiron, C., Jambaqué, I., Nabbout, R., *et al.* (1997). The right brain hemisphere is dominant in human infants. *Brain*, **120**, 1057−65.

Christoph, D. H., de Freitas, G. R., dos Santos, D. P., *et al.* (2004). Different perceived foreign accents in one patient after prerolandic hematoma. *Eur. Neurol.*, **52**(4), 198–201.

Damasio, H., Grabowski, T. J., Tranel, D., Hichwa, R. D. and Damasio, A. R. (1996). A neural basis for lexical retrieval. *Nature*, **380**, 499–505.

Damasio, A. R., Graff-Radford, N. R., Eslinger, P. J., Damasio, H. and Kassell, N. (1985). Amnesia following basal forebrain lesions. *Arch. Neurol.*, **42**, 263–71.

Davidson, R. J. (1994). Temperament, affective style, and frontal lobe asymmetry. In *Human Behavior and the Developing Brain*, ed. G. Dawson and K. W. Fisher. London, UK: The Guildford Press, pp. 518–36.

Dehaene-Lambertz, G., Dehaene, S. and Hertz-Pannier, S. (2002). Functional neuroimaging of speech perception in infants. *Science*, **298**, 2013–15.

Delis, D. C., Kiefner, M. G. and Fridlund, A. J. (1988). Visuospatial dysfunction following unilateral brain damage: Dissociations in hierarchical and hemispatial analysis. *J. Clin. Neuropsychol.*, **10**, 421–31.

Drake, M. E., Pakalnis, A. and Phillips, B. (1990). Secondary mania after ventral pontine infarction. *J. Neuropsychiatry Clin. Neurosci.*, **2**, 322–5.

Ellis, S. and Small, M. (1997). Localization of lesion in denial of hemiplegia after acute stroke. *Stroke*, **28**, 67–71.

Fenn, D. and George, K. (1999). Post-stroke mania late in life involving the left hemisphere. *Aust. N. Z. J. Psychiatry*, **33**, 598–600.

Ferro, J. M., Caeiro, L. and Verdelho, A. (2002). Delirium in acute stroke. *Curr. Opin. Neurol.*, **15**, 51–5.

Ferro, J. M., Martins, I. P. and Távora, L. (1984). Neglect in children. *Ann. Neurol.*, **15**, 281–4.

Gaillard, W. D., Sachs, B. C., Whitnah, J. R., *et al.* (2003). Developmental aspects of language processing: fMRI of verbal fluency in children and adults. *Hum. Brain Mapp.*, **18**(3), 176–85.

Ghika-Schmid, F. and Bogousslavsky, J. (2000). The acute behavioral syndrome of anterior thalamic infarction: A prospective study of 12 cases. *Ann. Neurol.*, **48**, 220–7.

Ghika-Schmid, F., van Melle, G., Guex, P. and Bogousslavsky, J. (1999). Subjective experience and behavior in acute stroke. The Lausanne emotion in acute stroke study. *Neurology*, **52**, 22–8.

Hamano, T., Hiraki, S., Kawamura, Y., *et al.* (2005). Acquired stuttering secondary to callosal infarction. *Neurology*, **64**, 1092–3.

Hénon, H., Lebert, F., Durieu, I., *et al.* (1999). Confusional state in stroke. Relation to preexisting dementia, patient characteristics, and outcome. *Stroke*, **30**, 773–9.

Herrmann, N., Black, S. E., Lawrence, J., Szekely, C. and Szalai, J. P. (1998). The sunnybrook stroke study. A prospective study of depressive symptoms and functional outcome. *Stroke*, **29**, 618–24.

Hertz-Pannier, L., Chiron, C., Jambaqué, I., *et al.* (2002). Late plasticity for language in a child's nondominant hemisphere. A pre- and post-surgery fMRI study. *Brain*, **125**, 361–72.

Hier, D. B., Mondlock, J. and Caplan, L. R. (1983). Behavioral abnormalities after right hemisphere stroke. *Neurology*, **33**, 337–44.

House, A., Dennis, M., Molyneau, A., Warlow, C. and Hawton, K. (1989). Emotionalism after stroke. *Br. Med. J.*, **198**, 991–4.

Hutsler, J. and Galuske, R. A. W. (2003). Hemispheric asymmetries in cerebral cortical networks. *Trends Neurosci.*, **26** (8), 429–35.

Jampala, V. C. and Abrams, R. (1983). Mania secondary to left and right hemisphere damage. *Am. J. Psychiatry*, **140**, 1197–9.

Kakishita, K., Sekiguchi, E., Maeshima, S., *et al.* (2004). Stuttering without callosal apraxia resulting from infarction in the anterior corpus callosum. A case report. *J. Neurol.*, **251**(9), 1140–1.

Karnach, H. O., Ferber, S. and Himmelbach, M. (2001). Spatial awareness is a function of the temporal not the posterior parietal lobe. *Nature*, **411**, 905–3.

Karussis, D., Leker, R. R. and Abramsky, O. (2000). Cognitive dysfunction following thalamic stroke: A study of 16 cases and review of the literature. *J. Neurol. Sci.*, **172**, 25–9.

Kim, J. S. (2002). Post-stroke emotional incontinence after small lenticulocapsular stroke: Correlation with lesion location. *J. Neurol.*, **249**, 805–10.

Kim, J. S. and Choi-Kwon, S. (2000). Post-stroke depression and emotional incontinence. Correlation with lesion location. *Neurology*, **54**, 1805–10.

Kirk, A. and Kertesz, A. (1994). Cortical and subcortical aphasias compared. *Aphasiology*, **8**, 65–82.

Knecht, S., Drager, B., Deppe, M., *et al.* (2000). Handedness and hemispheric language dominance in healthy humans. *Brain*, **123**, 2512–8.

Kreisler, A., Godefroy, O., Delmaire, C., *et al.* (2000). The anatomy of aphasia revisited. *Neurology*, **54** (5), 1117–23.

LaBerge, D. (2000). Networks of attention. In *The New Cognitive Neurosciences*, ed. M. S. Gazzaniga. 2nd edn. Cambridge, MA: MIT Press.

Lauterbach, E. C., Jackson, J. G., Wilson, A. N., Dever, G. E. and Kirsh, A. D. (1997). Major depression after left posterior globus pallidus lesions. *Neuropsychiatry Neuropsychol. Behav. Neurol.*, **10**, 9–16.

Leppävuori, A., Pohjasvaara, T., Vataja, R., Kaste, M. and Erkinjuntti, T. (2003). Generalized anxiety disorders three to four months after ischaemic stroke. *Cerebrovasc. Dis.*, **16**, 257–64.

Lesak, M. D. (2004). The behavioral geography of the brain. In *Neuropsychological Assessment*, ed. Muriel D. Lesak, Diane B. Howieson, and David W. Loring. Oxford: Oxford University Press, pp. 39–85.

Liu, C. Y., Wang, S. J., Fuh, J. L., Yang, Y. Y. and Liu, H. C. (1996). Bipolar disorder following a stroke involving the left hemisphere. *Aust. N. Z. J. Psychiatry.*, **30**, 688–91.

Madureira, S., Guerreiro, M. and Ferro, J. M. (1999). A follow-up study of cognitive impairment due to inferior capsular genu infarction. *J. Neurol.*, **246**, 764–9.

Marien, P., Paquier, P., Engelborghs, S. and Deyn, P. (2001). Acquired crossed aphasia in dextral children revisited. *Brain Lang.*, **79** (3), 426–43.

Marin, R. S., Firinciogullari, S. and Biedrzycki, R. C. (1994). Group differences in the relation between apathy and depression. *J. Nerv. Dis.*, **182**, 235–9.

Martins, I. P. (2000). Basal ganglia lesions, language and neuropsychological dysfunction. In *Localization of Brain Lesions and Development Functions*, ed. D. Riva and A. Benton. Eastleigh: John Libbey Company Ltd, pp. 57–65.

McDonald, W. M., Krishnan, K. R., Doraiswamy, P. M. and Blazer, D. G. (1991). Occurrence of subcortical hyperintensities in elderly subjects with mania. *Psychiatry Res.*, **40**, 211–20.

McNabb, A. W, Carroll, W. M, Mastaglia, F. L. (1988). "Alien hand" and loss of bimanual coordination after dominant anterior cerebral artery infarction. *J. Neurol. Neurosurg. Psychiatry*, **51**, 218–22.

Mesulam, M., Waxman, S., Geschwind, N. and Sabin, T. (1976). Acute confusional states with right middle cerebral artery infarctions. *J. Neurol. Neurosurg. Psychiatry*, **39**, 84–9.

Mohr, C., Landis, T., Bracha, H. S. and Brugger, P. (2003). Opposite turning behavior in right-handers and non-right-handers suggests a link between handedness and cerebral dopamine asymmetries. *Behav. Neurosci.*, **117**(6), 1448–52.

Mori, E. and Yamadori, A. (1987). Acute confusional state and acute agitated delirium. Occurrence after infarction in the right middle cerebral artery territory. *Arch. Neurol.*, **44**, 1139–43.

Morris, P. L., Robinson, R. G. and Raphael, B. (1990). Prevalence and course of depressive disorders in hospitalized stroke patients. *Int. J. Psychiatr. Med.*, **20**, 349–64.

Mort, D. M., Malhotra, P., Mannan, S. K., *et al.* (2003). The anatomy of visual neglect. *Brain*, **126**, 1986–97.

Nagaratnam, N., Nagaratnam, K., Ng, K. and Diu, P. (2004). Akinetic mutism following stroke. *J. Clin. Neurosci.*, **11**(1), 25–30.

Okada, K., Kobayashi, S., Yamagata, S., Takahashi, K. and Yamaguchi, S. (1997). Post-stroke apathy and regional cerebral blood flow. *Stroke*, **28**, 2437–41.

Ott, B. R. and Saver, J. L. (1993). Unilateral amnesic stroke. Six new cases and a review of the literature. *Stroke*, **24**, 1033–42.

Pascual-Leone, A., Grafman, J. and Hallet, M. (1994). Modulation of cortical neurons output maps during development of implicit and explicit knowledge. *Science*, **263**, 1287–9.

Peach, R. K. (2004). Acquired apraxia of speech: Features, accounts, and treatment. *Top Stroke Rehabil.*, **11** (1), 49–58.

Rabins, P. V., Starkstein, S. E. and Robinson, R. G. (1991). Risk factors for developing atypical (schizophreniform) psychosis following stroke. *J. Neuropsychiatry Clin. Neurosci.*, **3**, 6–9.

Ringman, J. M., Saver, J. L., Woolson, R. F., Clarke, W. R. and Adams, H. P. (2004). Frequency, risk factors, anatomy, and course of unilateral neglect in an acute stroke cohort. *Neurology*, **63**, 468–74.

Robinson, R. G. (1998a). Catastrophic reaction. In *The Clinical Neuropsychiatry of Stroke*, ed. R. G. Robinson. Cambridge: Cambridge University Press, pp. 413–420.

Robinson, R. G. (1998b). Poststroke mania. In *The Clinical Neuropsychiatry of Stroke*, ed. R. G. Robinson. Cambridge: Cambridge University Press, pp. 297–340.

Robinson, R. G. (1998c). Apathy. In *The Clinical Neuropsychiatry of Stroke*, ed. R. G. Robinson. Cambridge: Cambridge University Press, pp. 421–9.

Robinson, R. G. (1998d). Poststroke anxiety disorders. In *The Clinical Neuropsychiatry of Stroke*, ed. R. G. Robinson. Cambridge: Cambridge University Press, pp. 341–84.

Robinson, R. G. (2000). Depression and lesion location in stroke. In *Behavior and Mood Disorder in Focal Brain Lesions*, ed. J. Bogousslavsky and J. L. Cummings, Cambridge: Cambridge University Press, pp. 95–121.

Robinson, R. G., Boston, J. D., Stakstein, S. E. and Price, T. R. (1988). Comparison of mania and depression after brain injury: Causal factors. *Am. J. Psychiatry*, **145**, 172–8.

Román, G. C., Tatemichi, T. K., Erkinjuntti, T., *et al.* (1993). Vascular dementia: Diagnostic criteria for research studies. Report of the NINDS-AIREN International Workshop. *Neurology*, **43**, 250–60.

Shimoda, K. and Robinson, R. G. (1999). The relationship between post-stroke depression and lesion location in long-term follow-up. *Biol. Psychiatry*, **45**, 187–92.

Simpson, S. and Baldwin, B. (1995). Neuropsychiatry and SPECT of an acute obsessive-compulsive syndrome patient. *Br. J. Psychiatry*, **166**, 390–2.

Singh, A., Herrmann, N. and Black, S. E. (1998). The importance of lesion location in post-stroke depression: A critical review. *Can. J. Psychiatry*, **43**, 921–7.

Starkstein, S. E., Boston, J. D. and Robinson, R. G. (1988). Mechanisms of mania following brain injury: 12 case reports and review of the literature. *J. Nerv. Ment. Dis.*, **176**, 87–100.

Starkstein, S. E., Cohen, B. S., Fedoroff, P., *et al.* (1990). Relationship between anxiety disorders and depressive disorders in patients with cerebrovascular injury. *Arch. Gen. Psychiatry*, **47**, 246–51.

Starkstein, S. E., Fedoroff, P., Berthier, M. L. and Robinson, R. G. (1991). Manic-depressive and pure manic states after brain lesions. *Biol. Psychiatry*, **29**, 149–58.

Starkstein, S., Fedoroff, P., Price, T., Leiguarda, R. and Robinson, R. (1992). Anosognosia in patients with cerebrovascular lesions: A study of causative factors. *Stroke*, **10**, 1446–53.

(1993a). Catastrophic reaction after cerebrovascular lesions: Frequency, correlates and validation of a scale. *J. Neuropsychiatry Clin. Neurosci.*, **5**, 189–94.

(1993b). Apathy following cerebrovascular lesions. *Stroke*, **24**, 1625–30.

Starkstein, S. E., Fedoroff, P., Price, T. and Robinson, R. (1993c). Denial of illness scale. A reliability and validity study. *NNBN*, **6**, 93–7.

Staudt, M., Lidzba, K., Groodd, W., *et al.* (2002). Right-hemispheric organization of language following early left sided brain lesion: Functional MRI topography. *NeuroImage*, **16**, 954–67.

Stephan, K. E., Marshall, J. C., Friston, K. J., *et al.* (2003). Lateralized cognitive processes and lateralized task control in the human brain. *Science*, **301**, 384–6.

Stiles-Davis, J., Janowsky, J., Engel, M. and Nass, R. (1988). Drawing ability in four young children with congenital unilateral brain lesions. *Neuropsychologia*, **26** (3), 359–71.

Stone, S. P., Halligan, P. W. and Greenwood, R. J. (1993). The incidence of neglect phenomena and related disorders in patients with an acute right or left hemisphere stroke. *Age Ageing*, **22**, 46–52.

Tang, W. K., Chan, S. S. M., Chiu, H. F. K., *et al.* (2004). Emotional incontinence in Chinese stroke patients. Diagnosis, frequency, and clinical and radiological correlates. *J. Neurol.*, **251**, 865–9.

Tatsuno, Y. and Sakai, K. L. (2005). Language-related activations in the left prefrontal regions are differentially modulated by age, proficiency, and task demand. *J. Neurosci.*, **25** (7), 1637–44.

Teasell, R. (1993). Catastrophic reaction after stroke: A case study. *Am. J. Phys. Rehabil.*, **72**, 151–3.

Vallar, G. and Perani, D. (1986) The anatomy of unilateral neglect after right-hemisphere stroke lesions. A clinical/CT-scan correlation study in man. *Neuropsychologia*, **24**, 609–22.

Vataja, R., Leppavuori, A., Pohjasvaara, T., *et al.* (2004). Post-stroke depression and lesion location revisited. *J. Neuropsychiatry Clin. Neurosci.*, **16**, 156–62.

Venneri, A. and Shanks, M. F. (2004). Belief and awareness: Reflections on a case of persistent anosognosia. *Neuropsychologia*, **42**, 230–8.

Verdelho, A., Hénon, H., Lebert, F., Pasquier, F. and Leys, D. (2004). Depressive symptoms after stroke and relationship with dementia. *Neurology*, **62**, 905–11.

Visser-Keizer, A. C., Jong, B. M., Deelman, B. G., Berg, I. J. and Gerritsen, M. J. J. (2002). Subjective changes in emotion, cognition, and behavior after stroke: Factors affecting the perception of patients and partners. *J. Clin. Exp. Neuropsychol.*, **24**, 1032–45.

Wada, J. A., Clarck, R. and Hamm, A. (1975). Cerebral hemispheric asymmetry in Humans. Cortical speech zones in 100 adults and 100 infant brains. *Arch. Neurol.*, **32**, 239–46.

Zatorre, R. J. and Belin, P. (2001). Spectral and temporal processing in human auditory cortex. *Cereb. Cortex*, **11**, 946–53.

Index